HAHNEMANN
Revisited

HAHNEMANN
Revisited

A Textbook of Classical Homeopathy
For the Professional

Luc De Schepper
M.D., Lic. Ac.

FULL OF LIFE PUBLISHING ❦ SANTA FE

DISCLAIMER

The information in this book is presented for informational purposes only. All therapies, treatments, or energetic interventions of any nature should be undertaken only under the direct guidance and care of a properly trained and legally qualified health care professional specializing in the services rendered. Nothing described in this book should be construed by any reader or any other person to be a diagnosis or treatment for any disease or condition. Neither the author nor the publisher can accept any responsibility for any ill effects resulting from the use or misuse of the information contained herein. Any uses or misuses of the information presented here for educational purposes are the responsibility of the reader.

CONTACTING THE AUTHOR

The author welcomes feedback from readers, mailed to the publisher's address below, but regrets being unable to answer questions. Updated information about studying with Dr. Luc at the Renaissance Institute of Classical Homeopathy is available on his website, www.drluc.com.

© 2001 by Luc De Schepper. All rights reserved.
Printed in the United States of America.
    Full of Life Publications
    P.O. Box 31025
    Santa Fe, NM 87594

ISBN 0-942501-12-8

Front cover photo: Gilbert Temple, courtesy of Julian Winston
Back cover photo: Myron of Santa Fe
Cover design: Begabati Lennihan

Dedication

To Samuel Hahnemann

Non inutilis vixit

He did not live in vain

Acknowledgements

My greatest thanks go out to my editor and my most brilliant student, Begabati Lennihan. Begabati brought this book from manuscript form through all the stages of editing, typography, layout, and printing. More importantly, she challenged my ideas at every step of the way, forcing me to clarify, expand, illustrate, and document my statements. The result is a much better book, and a beautiful one, thanks to her.

I want to thank Julian Winston for contributing the cover portrait of Hahnemann, and the description of it which follows the brief biography of Hahnemann, as well as for checking the historical sections of the book for accuracy. I greatly appreciate Bob Rosa's skill in creating the illustrations. Several of my students contributed information from their areas of expertise: Margo Roman, D.V.M.; Barry Rector, R.Ph.; and Susan De Cristofaro, R.N., M.S.N., O.C.N., Clinical Nurse Specialist, and Anne Kelly, R.N., B.S.N., O.C.N., Gyn. Program Nurse, both at Dana Farber Cancer Institute. Many of my students sharpened their pencils and brought forward their best Arsenicum qualities as proofreaders, most notably Cat Weeks. I am grateful to all my students for inspiring me to write this book and to my patients for their love and support. Last but not least, my thanks to my wonderful wife, Yolanda, who gives me the joy and energy to keep going in all my projects. I am truly blessed to have such good people in my life. May we all share the passion of homeopathy.

Contents

Introduction x
A Brief Overview of Hahnemann's Life xiii

Part One: The Foundation

1 The Rapid, Gentle, and Permanent Cure 3
2 The Vital Force in Health and Healing 12
3 Laws and Principles 26
4 Pathology 48
5 Potencies 56
6 LM Potencies 88
7 Case-Taking 112
8 Constitution, Timeline, and Temperament 142

Part Two: The Healing Process

9 Prescribing 169
10 Golden Rules and Special Forms of Prescribing 199
11 Delusions 221
12 Aggravations, Accessory Symptoms, and Natural Healing Crises 240
13 Suppression 251
14 Obstacles to the Cure 266
15 Management of the Case 286
16 Palliation and Incurable Diseases 307
17 The Nosodes 316
18 The Bowel Nosodes 338

Part Three: The Chronic Miasms

19 The Roots of Chronic Disease 355
20 Psora: The Sensitizing Miasm 363
21 Sycosis: The Miasm of Excess and Overgrowth 376
22 Syphilis: The Destructive Miasm 397
23 The Tubercular and Cancer Miasms 413
24 Homeopathy and Cancer 425
25 Conclusion: Homeopathy, Medicine for the New Millennium 455

Appendices, Notes, and Resources

App. 1 Forms for the Practice 459
App. 2 The Never Well Since, or Ailments From 473
App. 3 Symptoms and their Miasms 480
App. 4 Sample Cases 504
        Solutions to Sample Cases 518
        Solutions to Cancer Cases 540
App. 5 Homeopathy and Traditional Chinese Medicine 546

        Notes 563
        Resources and Bibliography 571

List of Illustrations

2-1	The Homeopathic Paradigm of Healing	20
2-2	The Evolution of a Chronic Disease	25
3-1	Primary and Secondary Actions of a Homeopathic Remedy	30
6-1	Hahnemann's Directions for Trituration	93
6-2	How to Make LM2	96
6-3	Possible Scenarios Following the First Dose of LM1	105
6-4	Administration of 1M After LM2	106
7-1	Areas of the Tongue Associated with Each Organ in TCM	126
8-1	Layers in a Patient's Timeline	145
8-2	Changes in the Constitution of a Child Born Calcarea	148
8-3	Lifelong Effects of a Nat. mur. Event on a Sensitive Phosphorus Constitution	150
8-4	Constitutional Treatment for Hypersensitives	152
8-5	The Hippocratic Temperaments	156
9-1	Simile and Simillimum	170
9-2	Similes Leading to the Simillimum	172
9-3	Prioritizing the Levels of the Rubrics	190
9-4	Sample Scoring Chart	194
9-5	The Perfect Prescription	196
11-1	Delusions at the Deepest Level of Suppression	237
12-1	The Similar Aggravation	241
12-2	The Dissimilar Aggravation Requiring Treatment	244
12-3	Accessory Symptoms Appearing at the End of Treatment	247
12-4	Accessory Symptoms Appearing Due to Lack of Fit	248
13-1	Effects of Nat. mur. and the Miasms on the Thyroid	258
13-2	Levels of Suppression	260
15-1 *through* 15-10	Scenarios for Management of the Case	288ff.
17-1	Some Uses for a Nosode	326
18-1	Bowel Nosodes, Clinical Indications and Associated Remedies	346
19-1	The Sycotic Miasm and Suppression	386
24-1	Homeopathic and Allopathic Approaches to Treating Cancer	437
A5-1	The Six Great Meridians in Acupuncture	550
A5-2	The Generation Cycle	551
A5-3	The Ko Cycle	552
A5-4	The Anti-Ko Cycle	552
A5-5	The Organ Clock in Traditional Chinese Medicine	559

Introduction

When an allopathic physician converts to homeopathy, there is usually an interesting story behind it. Mine begins on my first day in practice—a disaster from beginning to end.

When I graduated from medical school in Belgium 27 years ago, I felt like Dr. Schweitzer and Superman combined: my black bag was filled with pills and injections, my heart full of good intentions, and my enthusiasm was at its zenith. The day I opened my office, I instructed my wife (I could not afford a receptionist) that in case a patient showed up, to tell her or him that the doctor was very busy and let the patient wait a little. It never looks good for the doctor to sit around waiting for a patient. When the doorbell finally rang, hopes were high for the first catch of the day. My wife rushed down the stairs while I tried to hide. Having been well instructed, she said to the man at the door, "My husband will be right with you. He is talking on the phone with a patient." The man looked puzzled and then replied, "That's very strange, I am from the phone company and I came to install the phone."

What an embarrassment! However, my painful journey was not finished yet. My first real patient was a young girl of 15 with a complaint of chronic headaches. Her headaches were triggered by a change of weather, which was unfortunate as the weather in Belgium changes four times a day. She had tried all the existing headache medications from her previous doctors, but she thought this new young gun fresh from medical school would have some new weapons in his arsenal. Of course I had none.

After the telephone and headache debacle, I took an aspirin for my own headache and decided there and then that there must be life beyond allopathic medicine. That was 27 years ago, and I have never stopped studying since then. I discarded all my medical textbooks and replaced them with acupuncture and homeopathy books. Since then I have learned and practiced a number of different holistic modalities, also including natural foods nutrition, vitamins, supplements, and herbs. For the last eight years I have practiced only homeopathy, because it is more powerful, goes deeper, acts more quickly, and benefits the patient more than any other modality. To this day I have not regretted this change. On the contrary, I feel that I have earned far more gratitude and appreciation from my patients and derived far more satisfaction than I ever could have dreamed of if I had remained an allopathic practitioner.

Of all the healing modalities I have studied, I have found homeopathy the most fulfilling. Homeopathy *individualizes* to the patient. The remedies are tailored not only to the patients' symptoms but also to their personality types and to the reason they became ill. If a patient feels ill even when her lab tests are normal, we take her seriously and listen carefully. As a result, we spend time really getting to know our patients, and the patients often say they feel better just from being listened to non-judgementally. Homeopathy is interested in the *why* of our patients: why did they fall sick? why do they react to particular life situations in a particular way? why do they experience certain emotions? It involves plumbing the depths of human nature, and the *mental/emotional makeup* of the patient takes high priority in our prescribing. Homeopathy works with the body's own *natural healing energy,* the Vital Force. And it *empowers the patient:* the practitioner listens to the patient for guidance in prescribing and assessing the patient's reaction to the remedy, encouraging the patient to listen to her body. The dynamic between practitioner and patient is more evenly balanced in homeopathy than in most other forms of healing, to the benefit of both.

Homeopathy has unchanging *laws and principles,* which once mastered, will unfailingly guide the prescription and the management of the case. Unfortunately the information has not been easily available, and the homeopathic tradition has largely been lost, at least in the United States. Ideally homeopathy would be learned best in a clinic, as an apprentice to a master who had learned from earlier masters, but this is not possible in this country. In this book I hope to make available to a wider audience the information I have gleaned from an extensive study of old books and journals, many of which are out of print.

In particular I have been fortunate enough to study Hahnemann's casebooks from his last years in Paris.[1] The more I read of Hahnemann's writings, the more I am convinced of his genius. On every page of his casebooks are brilliant observations and cures. I call this book Hahnemann Revisited because I believe he has answers and guidance highly relevant for us today, although sometimes inaccessible because they are couched in his old-fashioned language. I have also been greatly inspired by the master homeopaths of the past, like von Boenninghausen, Hering, Lippe, Kent, Dunham, Grimmer, Tyler, Wright-Hubbard, and Schmidt; their wisdom fills these pages. I have attempted to elucidate their teachings with examples from my own practice as well as theirs.

Certain aspects of this book may seem to depart from the mainstream of modern homeopathy—in particular the emphasis on miasmatic prescribing and LM potencies—but these were an integral part of Hahnemann's great teaching and I believe they deserve to hold a central position in homeopathy today. I like to believe that they are not widely used simply for lack of sufficient training. It would give me great joy and fulfillment if this book could serve to spread the knowledge of these powerful healing tools of homeopathy.

This book is meant for the serious student of homeopathy, for the practicing professional homeopath, and for the health care practitioner interested in learning more about it. For the student, I hope that it fulfills a need for a thorough introduction to homeopathic therapeutics and methodology. I hope that my fellow homeopaths will find something of value in it, and that allopathic practitioners will gain a window on a different way of viewing health and healing. This book is not intended for laypeople, for whom there are a number of excellent books on family and first aid health care with homeopathy. Many medical terms and abbreviations appear in the text without explanation, since professional homeopaths need a solid knowledge base in anatomy, physiology, and pathology comparable to that of our colleagues in medicine, chiropractic, acupuncture, and the other healing professions.

I would like to share a few words, if I may, with the students who read this book. Healing is a gift, and your presence as a healer can be a gift in itself, if you give your patients your attention, your respect and your love. As Mother Theresa said, "From the abundance of the heart, the mouth speaks. If your heart is full of love, you will speak of love." And you will help your patient heal even before you give a remedy. Don't be discouraged if you make a mistake. I have made many mistakes along the way, and I have always learned from them. I have been practicing alternative medicine for nearly 30 years and I have never stopped learning. I wish for all those who read this book the same enthusiasm for life-long learning. I have never placed any priority on financial rewards; instead, I have been more than rewarded by the love and gratitude of my patients. I would hope that all my readers would share the same values. Just as in tennis (my favorite game), it is better to serve than to receive.

A Brief Overview of Hahnemann's Life

Samuel Hahnemann, the founder of homeopathy, was a Renaissance genius who was gifted in many fields: he was a master pharmacist who developed procedures still used in pharmacy today, a skilled linguist and translator who was fluent in seven languages, and the forerunner of today's natural healers who promote a natural diet and healthy life-style. He could also be called the first psychiatrist, because he was the first person in modern times to promote the humane treatment of the mentally ill in addition to curing them with his remedies. Decades before Koch and Pasteur, he understood the principles of contagious illnesses and successfully treated the deadly epidemics which ravaged Europe in the first half of the nineteenth century. Hahnemann could even be considered a pioneer of modern public health and sanitation measures.

Hahnemann would merit a prominent place in the history of medicine for any of his contributions. His greatest contribution, of course, is the founding of the system of homeopathy, an unparalleled achievement. So far as we know, Hahnemann is the only person in history to have envisioned an entire system of medicine and then fully developed it into a powerful and practical tool within the span of a single lifetime. He was a true visionary whose understanding of the energetic basis of health and healing anticipated by a century the paradigm of matter as energy in modern physics. And allopathic medicine has barely begun to incorporate an understanding of the mind-body connection which Hahnemann delineated nearly two centuries ago.

I would like to begin this exposition of Hahnemann's system with a brief overview of his life, and I would encourage interested readers to explore the topic further. Rima Handley's *A Homeopathic Love Story* provides an enjoyable introduction, with her *In Search of the Later Hahnemann* helpful for understanding how Hahnemann practiced at the culmination of his career. Of the several biographies of Hahnemann available, my favorites are Haehl's *Life and Works of Hahnemann* and Bradford's *Life and Letters of Hahnemann*. These worthwhile books will provide a deep insight into Hahnemann's struggles and the obstacles he had to overcome.

Hahnemann was born on April 10, 1755, in Meissen, Saxony, Germany where his father was employed as a porcelain painter. Money was scarce, and in his early years the young Samuel was frequently taken out of school for lack of money. From the age of 12 he helped pay for his own education by tutoring his fellow students in Latin and Greek. Hahnemann's father cultivated original thinking in Samuel from the time he was young. He would often shut Samuel up in a room, giving him a knotty question to ponder. "Prove all things, hold fast to what is good, dare to be wise" was the substance of his advice to his son. He petitioned the Prince's school, St. Afra, in Meissen where Hahnemann was admitted in 1770. Hahnemann was such a brilliant student that one of his professors arranged for him to have free tuition. He left this school in 1775 after presenting a dissertation in Latin on "The wonderful construction of the human hand."

With very little money, Hahnemann left for Leipzig in the spring of 1775 to study medicine. He supported himself by giving private lessons in French and German as well as translating treatises on medicine, botany, and chemistry, a work he would continue for the next 20 years. One of his professors, Dr. Bergrath, was so impressed with the young student that he obtained for Hahnemann the privilege of attending lectures for free. Not satisfied with the dull book-knowledge that this university had to offer (they had no hospital of their own), he soon moved to Vienna.

Wandering from one location to another was to become a major theme in Hahenmann's life. From Vienna he went to Hermanstadt (now Sibu, Romania), where another benefactor, Dr. Quarin, helped him find a job. He finally completed medical school in Erlangen, and his detractors later criticized him for having received his degree from a relatively obscure school. After receiving his degree in 1779, Hahnemann settled down to practice medicine in various small villages in Germany. Within five years he had given up his practice, candidly admitting that his patients would do better without his help. In the mean time he had married Johanna Leopoldine Henriette Küchler, an apothecary's daughter, in 1782. He supported his growing family (the couple eventually had 11 children) exclusively with writing and chemistry in Dresden from 1785 until 1789. For a while he tried private practice again but found he could not count on it as a source of income: "I can only look upon my practice as good for the heart."[1]

Hahnemann published many works on chemistry, the most celebrated being a treatise on arsenic poisoning. Some of his critics would later say that Hahnemann would have been a great chemist had he not turned into a great "quack." In 1789 the family moved to Leipzig and Hahnemann published a treatise on syphilis, remarkable for its description of a new preparation of mercury which he had developed and which is still known to chemists as Hahnemaniann soluble mercury. Hahnemann's writing and chemistry provided only a meager income for his family, however, and they often lacked the bare necessities for survival. In one touching vignette, Hahnemann recounts scrubbing the family's laundry with raw potatoes because they could not afford soap.

Hahnemann began attacking the medical practices of his time as early as 1784, attracting notoriety, ridicule and rejection by his colleagues. Emperor Leopold of Austria died unexpectedly in 1792 after having been bled four times in 24 hours for a high fever and abdominal distension. Hahnemann publicly criticized the emperor's physicians and continued to speak out strongly against bloodletting, although he himself was denounced as a murderer because he denied his patients the "benefits" of bleeding. (Hahnemann had begun practicing medicine again, but soon gave it up out of frustration with the ineffective methods available and with his difficulty in collecting adequate reimbursement from his patients.) He and his family, including five children at that point, were living in one room in the direst circumstances. Hahnemann stayed up every other night doing translation work, the family's main source of income, so that he could pursue his passion, researching more effective methods of healing, during the day. During this period he also picked up his "useless" habit of pipe smoking, as he called it. However, Hahnemann was already concerned with hygienics and diet at this point, advocating the consumption of as little meat as possible and encouraging the use of goat's and sheep's milk rather than cow's milk.

The year 1791, when Hahnemann was 46, marked a turning point in the development of his thought. Up to that point he could see the limitations, even the dangers, of the medicine he had been trained in, but he had no good alternative to offer. In 1791 Hahnemann had a remarkable insight while translating Cullen's *Materia Medica*. Cullen attributed the antimalarial properties of Cinchona bark (from which quinine is made) to its bitter and astringent properties, but Hahnemann knew that other bitter herbs are not active against malaria. He began a practice which he would continue throughout his life and which demonstrated his great integrity and love of knowledge: he experimented on himself. He found that Cinchona bark (from which the homeopathic remedy China is made) could induce in him, a healthy person, the same symptoms it would cure in the sick person. This discovery led to the first law of homeopathy: the Law of Similars, or "Like Cures Like."

It was also around this time that Hahnemann made his mark as a psychiatrist. Asylums were usually run in connection with prisons; the mentally ill were crowded in close quarters with insufficient food. Worse, they were abandoned by physicians, who believed that insanity was contagious. Instead, the mentally ill were chained, flogged, and teased for the amusement of visitors. The first real asylum for mental patients was opened by Hahnemann in Georgenthal, where Duke Ernst of Gotha put one of the wings of his castle at Hahnemann's disposal. It was designed for the wealthy insane and melancholic. He had only one patient, the well-known author Klockenbring of Hannover, who was suffering from a full-blown mania which modern psychiatrists would have great difficulty treating. Yet Hahnemann cured him completely in seven months. In order to get a sense of this magnificent cure, I urge the reader to read the case in Dudgeon's *Lesser Writings of Samuel Hahnemann*.[2] It was the first time in the modern era that insane people were treated with gentleness, humaneness and compassion instead of coercion.

After this, mainly out of financial need he moved again from one village to another, violently attacked by doctors and pharmacists. His practice of making his own medicines aroused their jealousy, and the pharmacists brought action against him for interfering with their privileges. Unfortunately his enemies won and Hahnemann was prohibited from dispensing his own medicines. It was during one of those moves in 1794 that he lost a newborn son in a carriage accident in which his son Friedrich (the only one of the family who would become a homeopathic physician) was also injured.

In 1800 a scarlet fever epidemic gave Hahnemann the opportunity to demonstrate the effectiveness of the new type of medicine he was researching, based not only on the Law of Similars but also on the concept of highly diluted, potentized doses. Hahnemann created a sensation when he successfully used Belladonna in homeopathic doses as a cure and preventive for the epidemic. Hahnemann was attacked again because he asked a small remuneration for his discovery (which was understandable, considering his poverty-stricken circumstances), although he made his Belladonna available free of charge to poor patients.

In 1810 Hahnemann published the first edition of the *Organon of the Healing Art,* his most important work. This book laid out the foundations of his new approach to healing, including the Law of Similars, the principle of using a single medicine which had been potentized, administering it in the smallest possible dose, and only giving remedies which had been proven on healthy people. (These principles are all explained in detail in Chapter Three.) In the next few years Hahnemann proved many remedies on himself and his family members, and from 1814 on, he expanded the group to include his closest friends and associates (called the "Prover's Union"). These provers included some of his earliest disciples, like Gross, Stapf, Hartmann, and Rückert.

Success was achieved again in 1813 when Hahnemann used homeopathy to treat an epidemic of typhus, which affected Napoleon's soldiers after their invasion of Russia. Even Napoleon himself was treated successfully with a homeopathic remedy for a case of pthiriasis. Soon the epidemic spread to Germany, where Hahnemann cured the first stage with Bryonia and Rhus tox. Again he was attacked by the pharmacists for encroaching on their privileges by dispensing his own medicines. The Leipzig city council ordered Hahnemann to cease such activity in 1820. This persecution reached its climax in 1821, forcing Hahnemann to move to Köthen. There he was protected by Duke Ferdinand of Anhalt-Köthen, who was one of his patients and who allowed him to practice as a doctor and dispense his own medications. (Germany at that time was a loose association of duchies and city-states, each with its own laws.)

For a dozen years Hahnemann was able to practice and further develop his ideas in peace and quiet, settled in Köthen under the Duke's protection. Patients traveled from all over

Europe to see him. His wife Johanna, who had borne her husband eleven children, died in 1830 from severe lung catarrh, but Hahnemann was well taken care of by his surviving daughters, especially Charlotte and Luise. He was joined by Dr. Theodore Mossdorf, one of his students, who became his assistant and son-in-law.

During this time Hahnemann developed the next stage of his understanding of chronic diseases, the concept of miasms. He published his discovery in 1828 in the first edition of *Chronic Diseases*. Although the concept was well received by Hahnemann's staunchest supporters (Stapf, Gross, Hering, and von Boenninghausen), most homeopaths felt it was too farfetched and disavowed it. A Dr. Trinks had schemed behind Hahnemann's back with Hahnemann's publisher to delay its publication, another of the many obstacles Hahnemann faced in developing and publicizing his new system.

In 1831 homeopathy triumphed again, this time over the cholera epidemic which spread westward from Russia, while allopathic medicine was helpless against the virulent disease. The remedies Hahnemann used—Camphor, Cuprum and Veratrum—would still be among the top remedies used in a cholera epidemic today.

Hahnemann was joined in Köthen by his next energetic assistant, Dr. Gottfried Lehmann, who turned out to be the most faithful of Hahnemann's helpers. But Hahnemann was dissatisfied with the "pseudo-homeopaths" of nearby Leipzig, and he distanced himself from them more and more. In 1833 the first homeopathic hospital was opened in Leipzig under the direction of Dr. Moritz Müller; its founders hoped it would benefit from its proximity to the internationally-famous Hahnemann. At first Hahnemann was very enthusiastic, providing financial support and traveling to inspect it in 1834. But the clinic ran into financial problems after Hahnemann left for Paris in 1835 and closed for good in 1842.

This brings us to the last chapter of Hahnemann's life, which reads like a romance novel. In 1834, a beautiful and vivacious Parisienne, Marie Mélanie d'Herville-Gohier, undertook the lengthy journey to consult Hahnemann in Germany, ostensibly for the treatment of her neuralgic pains. (Later Mélanie stated that her real reason was her interest in Hahnemann's new system of medicine and a curiosity about its famous founder. Based on the turn of events, we can speculate as to whether Mélanie had ulterior motives in mind.) Mélanie gave her age as 32, although others said she was 35 (she must have been a Phosphorus!). She swept the 80-year-old widower off his feet, and they were married only three months after their first meeting.

Mélanie's role in Hahnemann's life is controversial. After eight decades of struggles, poverty, and adversity, he was able to enjoy the evening of his life with his young, beautiful, well-to-do and well-connected wife, who brought many members of the French nobility and high society to see him. On the other hand, Mélanie successfully isolated him from his children for the rest of his life. Mélanie convinced Hahnemann to come back to Paris with her, holding out the promise of his enjoying rest and the adulation of French society, many of whose members had adopted homeopathy. But after a long and strenuous trip to Paris, she convinced Hahnemann to practice again. The practice was probably tiring for the elderly Hahnemann, but we can be grateful to Mélanie because it gave him the opportunity to experiment and perfect his LM method. Mélanie learned homeopathy from her husband and worked as his assistant in the afternoon, running her own clinic for poor people in the morning. She even printed her business cards as Dr. Mélanie Hahnemann, the first female "physician" in France.

Hahnemann had great fame and success in France and completed his "most complete and best method," described in the sixth edition of the *Organon*. The manuscript was in the hands of his publisher when Hahnemann died in 1843, at the ripe old age of 88. Mélanie has been blamed for her role in withholding publication of this all-important edition, as well as for burying her husband in a private ceremony in an unmarked grave in her family's mausoleum. However, she was apparently too overcome with grief to publicize the funeral for his followers, and she buried him with the two other important men in her life, her painting teacher and her namesake, M. Gohier. Hahnemann's body was later moved to an individual grave, marked by a monument with the epitaph he had chosen: *Non inutilis vixi,* "I have not lived in vain."

To conclude this little prologue about Hahnemann, it is fitting to mention Hahnemann's great qualities of character which we homeopaths, his intellectual heirs, could all aspire to. First, Hahnemann had tremendous *perseverance* in pursuing what he believed to be true. At every step in developing his system he met with great discouragement and abuse. Hahnemann suffered from the attacks of the orthodox medical establishment of his time, which used all the legal and political weapons at their disposal to stop him. The journals of his time printed scathing, even libelous, critiques. The criticisms he endured only stimulated him to perfect his system. But many letters found after his death revealed how much Hahnemann suffered from this undeserved and unceasing persecution.

Next, Hahnemann's *integrity* was strikingly displayed in his abandoning his medical practice when he found it harmful to his patients, instead trying to support his large family on a meager income from translating books. He also demonstrated his integrity by doing something which physicians and pharmacists of today would never think of: he experimented on himself with the remedies he gave to his patients. This brings us to another admirable quality, his *industriousness.* In addition to developing an entire system of medicine and proving about a hundred remedies, he wrote about 70 original works on chemistry and medicine and translated two dozen works from English, French, Latin, and Italian. Finally, he was *humble.* He wrote to his friend Dr. Stapf, "Be as sparing as possible with your praises. I do not like them, I feel that I am only an honest, straightforward man who does no more than his duty."

Hahnemann had an unfortunate limitation which in some ways hindered the development of homeopathy, and which we modern homeopaths would do well to learn from. At a later stage in his life he became intolerant of contradiction, viewing with suspicion anyone who did not agree with him in every detail. He said: "He who does not walk exactly on the same line with me, who diverges, if it be but the breadth of a straw to the left or right, is a traitor and I will have nothing to do with him." Dr. Gross, one of Hahnemann's first and best disciples, wrote to Hahnemann that the loss of his child had taught him that homeopathy did not suffice in every case. Hahnemann never forgave him for this remark. Hahnemann alienated many of his followers with his rigidity and intolerance, although it is also true that he felt betrayed by many of them.

Millions of people owe the relief of their suffering to the greatest genius in medical history. This book is the exposition of his system. While it also draws from many of his greatest followers—von Boenninghausen, Hering, Kent, Lippe and others—Hahnemann provided the foundation, the laws and principles, on which everything else is built.

About the portrait of Hahnemann on the cover: This studio portrait was done by Gilbert Temple, a photographer in Clinton, Iowa, from an authentic engraving of Hahnemann and is currently in the collection of Julian Winston. On the reverse side is the following note:

This photograph of Samuel Hahnemann is believed to be the best likeness in existence. The original engraving of which this is a copy, having come into my possession in 1838 when I was fifteen years old. It was given to me because I had been a patient of Hahnemann, the circumstances being as follows:

I was born in Paisley, Scotland, December 4, 1823. When twelve years of age I contracted a severe cold which proved to be the beginning of serious pulmonary trouble. After having been confined to the bed for a year, I was finally sent to Paris in 1836 when I was thirteen years old, that I might be put under Hahnemann's treatment. There had been much question as to whether it were possible for me to make the trip, but it was accomplished by easy stages, including a rest of two weeks in London. These two weeks were spent at the house of the Queen's physician, Sir Andrew Clark, who examined me carefully. I overheard him say to his wife that he doubted if they ever got me to Paris, but if they did, they would never get me out again.

Upon my arrival in Paris, Hahnemann subjected me to a very thorough examination, lasting about an hour and a half, at the end of which he announced that I could be cured, but that it would take considerable time. This opinion was fully justified by subsequent events, for I was restored to health, but only after I had been under his care for nine months. Owing to circumstances unnecessary to detail, I was at his office frequently and spent a good deal of time there, sometimes remaining as long as half a day. This unusual and prolonged association with him and his work of necessity made me familiar with his face and his ways.

Some two years after my return to Scotland, Dr. Geddes M. Scott, a physician of wealth and high standing in Glasgow who had become a convert to Homeopathy, went to Paris to see Hahnemann. Upon his return he showed me an engraving of Hahnemann which he had brought with him, and asked me what I thought of it. I said at once that the likeness could not be better and Dr. Scott then said that was his opinion also. He gave me two copies, and this photograph is from a negative made from one of them. This negative was obtained only after repeated efforts and with the aid of an artist as well as the photographer, and is wholly successful in catching the likeness and expression both of the engraving and of Hahnemann himself as I knew him well in his later years.

It is no small pleasure to one who not only holds Hahnemann in grateful remembrance, but who reveres him both as a physician and as a man, to be able to place in the hands of his followers so authentic and lifelike a portrait.

—*John B. Young, 527 Ninth Ave., Clinton, Iowa*

Editorial Notes

Patient confidentiality: Patients' names and circumstantial details of their lives have been changed to protect their anonymity. All quotes are word-for-word from patients, and the actual details of their conditions, remedies, and case development are all accurate.

Names of remedies: Remedy names are given as they would be used in conversation, with common sense prevailing: Arsenicum is of course Arsenicum album, Aurum is Aurum metallicum, Calcarea is Calcarea carbonica, and so forth, with the most common and frequently used remedy assumed. When there might be any doubt, the second part of the name is given, usually abbreviated, e.g., Ferrum met. and Ferrum phos. Long remedy names are abbreviated as they would be in conversation, such as Nat. mur., Rhus tox., and Kali bich (as in the mnemonic about stringy mucus, "When it sticks, use Kali bich.").

Gender of pronouns: To avoid the awkward "he or she" or "s/he," the pronoun referring to a practitioner is sometimes male and sometimes female, with the opposite gender assigned to the patient to avoid confusion.

Quotations from the *Organon*: The word "Aphorism" always refers to the *Organon*. All quotations are from the 6th edition unless otherwise noted. (The 5th edition is quoted primarily in the section of Chapter 5 on the history of how Hahnemann developed LM potencies.) The highly recommended O'Reilly edition was used for quotations for the 6th edition and the Dudgeon translation for the 5th edition. Italics were so frequently added that it seemed tiresome to keep adding the note *[italics added]* at the end of each quotation. The reader should assume that any italics were added; occasionally they were in the translated version, as the reader will easily see by referring to it. Bracketed comments interpolated into quotes are by the translator if in roman type [thus], and by the author of this book if in italics *[thus]*.

References are included in the text if it can be done unobtrusively, otherwise they are placed in endnotes at the end of the book.

Page numbers in Kent's *Repertory* are abbreviated thus: K36.

Part One

The Foundation

※

Laws and Principles of Homeopathy

Who Is the Patient?

Chapter One

The Rapid, Gentle, and Permanent Cure

> The physician's highest and *only* calling is to make the sick healthy, to cure, as it is called.
>
> The highest ideal of cure is the rapid, gentle and permanent restoration of health; that is, the lifting and annihilation of the disease in its entire extent in the shortest, most reliable, and least disadvantageous way, according to clearly realizable principles.
>
> —Samuel Hahnemann, *Organon of the Medical Art,* Aphorisms 1 and 2

These wise words are the opening of the *Organon,* homeopathy's bible and the culmination of the life work of its founder, Samuel Hahnemann. Written 150 years ago, they have much to say about the state of medicine today. Modern medicine (allopathy) does not claim to cure chronic diseases such as diabetes, arthritis and auto-immune diseases, but merely to control the symptoms, using drugs which the patient must take for the rest of her life. Far from being gentle, many medications have side effects which are uncomfortable, harmful or even fatal for the patient, requiring multiple other medications to alleviate problems caused by the first set.[1] As for being "advantageous," modern medicine is enormously expensive, overly reliant on technology, and—perhaps most importantly of all—an unsatisfying experience for patient and practitioner alike, in which overly brief consultations are dominated by the cost parameters of HMOs and the perennial fear of a malpractice suit.

Not surprisingly, both patients and practitioners are looking for an alternative. It is my belief, after having studied and practiced several different major approaches to healing, that homeopathy has the best answers to the crisis facing modern medicine. And it has been my great joy to share what I know of homeopathy with my students, including many allopathic medical professionals. Through this textbook it is my hope to share this knowledge with a wider audience of students and practitioners, both homeopathic and allopathic, so that we may all offer our patients the best possible care.

What constitutes a real cure? How can we make it as rapid and gentle as possible? Is it possible to permanently cure chronic diseases? Homeopathy has profound answers to these questions, which will be explored in this chapter along with an introduction to homeopathy's approach to this ideal of a cure.

A True Cure

The definition of a cure seems simple at first: the disappearance of the patient's symptoms. Homeopathy aims much higher than this, however, and medical practitioners who learn to treat their patients with classical homeopathy see the difference right away. Far from giving side effects, homeopathic remedies improve the patient's life on all levels. How many times have I heard a patient say, "I have never felt better in my life!" In fact, often the first sign that a remedy is working, even before relief of the Chief Complaint, is a change on a much deeper level: the patient falls asleep right away and has a deep and restful sleep; she feels more energy; she no longer catches every cold and flu that comes around; she is no longer binging on chocolate.

These kinds of changes on the physical level are remarkable enough, but in homeopathy we expect changes on an even deeper level, the mental-emotional level: a patient will often report feeling better about herself, feeling more self-confidence and self-esteem, organizing piles of papers that have been gathering dust, finishing a half-done project, no longer snapping at her children, even enjoying sex with her husband again. Patients often report dreams in which they are able to finally say goodbye to departed loved ones or "get something off their chest" with someone who they can't "tell off" in real life (their boss, for example), waking with a feeling that they have put something behind them and can move on. Sometimes the energy and self-confidence they feel from a remedy inspires them to make necessary changes in their life, changes they have been putting off for years. I have seen many cases in which a woman finds the courage to end an abusive relationship of many years' duration within a month or two of starting a remedy.

The result is obvious to the patient's friends and family. They comment on how the patient looks younger, seems healthier, and is getting along with everyone better. They often ask, "What have you been doing? You look so good."

These changes may seem miraculous but to the homeopath they are all in a day's work. They are possible because homeopathy goes directly to the core of the person, to the body's own healing energy, strengthening it and balancing it, so that not only do the specific disease symptoms disappear, the entire spiritual-mental-emotional-physical being is restored to the natural state it was created in.

Treating the Whole Person

One of the fundamental tenets of homeopathy is that we do not treat a disease, we treat a patient with a disease. This may sound obvious, but it comes as a surprise to patients when they see the questions we need to ask (as in the sample patient intake in Appendix 1). Patients often say that a doctor has never listened to them so attentively, asked so many interesting questions, or noted down what they felt was important, until they came to a homeopath. In treating a chronic disease, we need to know about the patient's personality and physical constitution, different traumatic events in his life, his work and home environment, and his preferences in food and temperature. Most important of all is the question, "What was going on in your life when you became ill?"

One of my students, a nurse at a prominent Boston-based national cancer institute, repeated this question to the patients in her cancer support group. They were immediately inspired by it and went around the room; each person knew exactly what traumatic event in her life triggered the cancer, and in none of the cases had the oncologist shown the slightest interest in this information! Of course, we cannot blame the oncologists, because this information would not be useful to them in devising their protocol. But in homeopathy it is the *most* important information in matching the remedy to the whole person. The patient's disease symptoms come *last* in the priority. This is because homeopathy heals from the inside out, and the physical symptoms are what appear last, on the surface so to speak. This does not necessarily mean that they are on the skin, but that the physical body is an expression of the internal mental, emotional and energetic aspects of the being. By restoring the inner core, the homeopathic remedy heals the more external symptoms profoundly and permanently.

Homeopathy does not place the same value on lab tests, blood work or even on the disease name itself as does allopathic medicine. Of course there is a value in the information available through the advances in modern medical technology, as explained in Chapter 3, Pathology. Our focus on the patient includes how he feels and why. What we learn from our patients is that they feel their "regular" doctors are overly focused on these tests, lending more credence to a printout of lab values or looking at a monitor instead of the patient. Many times I have had patients tell me that when they feel better, even though their blood work is a little off, their doctor tells them they "must" feel worse. And doctors report being really stumped by the patient who reports feeling ill but whose lab tests are all normal. They may refer these patients out, pacify them with Prozac, or write them off as a hypochondriac. To a homeopath, a hypochondriac is a patient we can work with effectively, because we use their subjective symptoms to find a remedy which relieves the symptoms, restoring their health and peace of mind.

Patients also tell us they feel their "regular" doctors are overly focused on finding the diagnosis, as if their work stopped right there. There is a natural human tendency for the practitioner to relax once the disease is pinpointed. But this does not help the patient at all. It often means the patient can then be plugged into a standard protocol (with side effects, for the rest of the patient's life), and sometimes it means a death sentence: "You have six months to live." How many times in my practice have I seen patients' health suddenly spiral downwards when receiving such a diagnosis. I used to have a practice in the same building as an oncology center, and I would see patients both before and after their diagnosis of cancer. One day they could be asymptomatic and full of energy, and only a few days later they would have turned into a cancer patient, complete with fatigue and aches and pains never felt before. Fortunately in homeopathy we have remedies for what we call "hearing bad news." After receiving such a remedy, the patient would at least have the strength and presence of mind to cope with the news. How I wish that allopathic medicine, even if it adopted nothing else from homeopathy, would support the patient with one of these simple remedies when giving such a crushing diagnosis.

Individualizing to the Patient

A true homeopath has no need for a disease name. Hahnemann, on being asked by one of his grateful patients what saved his life, said it eloquently: "The name of the disease does not concern me, the name of the remedy is of no importance to you."[1] (Even to his students he would not divulge the name of the remedy—not out of secrecy or egotism, but to avoid having it become a standard prescription for any patient with the same disease.) Hahnemann taught us that the names of diseases such as nephritis, arthritis, or gastritis do not help us to cure the patient and should only be referred to as *"a kind of"* nephritis, arthritis, gastritis. What kind of "itis" depends on *who* is suffering. Ten different patients with gastritis are likely to receive ten different remedies from a homeopath depending on their entire mental-emotional-physical makeup, their life history, and the context of their relationships. Many times patients will ask: "Do you have a remedy for tinnitus?" (or back pain, vertigo, or arthritis). The homeopath's answer must be: "We have a remedy for *a person with* tinnitus" (back pain, vertigo, or arthritis).

Again, homeopathy does not focus on finding the "culprit" in the form of the microbe which causes a disease. Microbes are everywhere but only certain patients are susceptible, and by strengthening the body's Vital Force, we can change the susceptibility. Take Chronic Fatigue Syndrome, for example. Millions of dollars have been spent on pinpointing the elusive virus, variously named the EBV virus, the "yuppie virus," HHV-6, spuma virus, retrovirus, etc., yet finding a virus is only a small step because allopathic medicine lacks effective treatments for viral diseases. Nor is naming the disease any help in healing. I was sad to see that at a recent conference on the disease, fully half the time was spent trying to decide on the proper name.[2]

I am sad for the patients when the experts' time is spent like this and even sadder that the practitioners are not aware of the power of homeopathy in this condition. I have been able to help hundreds of patients with this problem, many of whom traveled from all over the country to see me. I was able to do this only because I used the gentle power of homeopathy, which does not care what virus caused the disease or what the diagnosis is. I followed the method outlined in this book and found that one patient might have chronic fatigue since a heartbreak, another since taking the birth control pill, and another since undergoing an operation. Even though they have the same symptoms, each patient would receive a different remedy. One might need Nat. mur. for the longterm effects of grief, another Sepia for the effects of synthetic hormones, and another Phosphorus for the sequelae of anesthesia. The results were a consistent restoration of the patient's energy and overall health, such as they had never experienced even with the best antiviral medications.

Basically we search for the leakage in their Vital Force, which can come about through a physical trauma like a car accident or overuse of antibiotics, a mental trauma like studying too hard or worrying about something too much, or (most frequently) an emotional trauma like the death of a loved one, the end of a relationship, devastating financial loss, or an abusive relationship. We look at the whole person who is suffering this leakage and at how the body is expressing it. All this information is put together into a totally individualized prescription. This work requires the knowledge of the human body which an allopathic practitioner must have, plus much more: an understanding of the human condition, the capacity to identify with our patients and sense the essence of their struggle in life. This is what makes homeopathy so satisfying and why the allopathic practitioners who study it find it so rewarding, as I have seen many times in my school. Most health care practitioners embark on their careers full of compassion for their patients and in homeopathy they find a way to help their patients better than they could before.

One more aspect of homeopathy which makes it so satisfying to the practitioner is that we address the whole person, and not just an organ or a part. We can treat patients of all ages and both genders, suffering from almost any ailment. What a joy to be a true family practitioner, treating three or four generations of a family and seeing the overall family dynamics improve. In a typical family, it is the mother who is helped first, perhaps for exhaustion and burnout. Next the ADD child is helped to be more calm and focused and to stop hitting his little sister, and the little sister is helped to have more self-esteem and to recover from years of being beaten up. Then the teenager comes in for help with his skin and leaves with a more congenial attitude towards his parents and teachers. Then the grandmother comes in for help with her failing memory or eyesight, and even the dog is given a remedy to stop him from relieving himself on the Oriental rug. Finally the husband (usually the last) comes for help with his stress ulcers caused by overseeing all this chaos.

In my own practice, I saw patients referred by gynecologists, pediatricians, dermatologists, internists, cardiologists, ophthalmologists, oncologists and other specialists—patients for whom these specialists had no more answers. It was gratifying indeed to see them heal (unless their pathology was too far advanced, in which case at least their quality of life improved) thanks to the gentle power of homeopathy. We have no need for specialists in homeopathy; a homeopath is trained to take all comers. I am grateful to Hahnemann that I am able to practice in this way and I do not have to treat only one little piece of my patients, referring them to another practitioner when another little piece is out of balance.

The Rapid and Gentle Cure

One of the misconceptions about homeopathy which I hear from my patients is that "it takes a long time for homeopathy to work." Of course what they refer to here is the cure of *chronic* diseases. Patients will often say something like, "I am giving you one month to show me that homeopathy can cure my ulcerative colitis [or longstanding depression, etc.] or else I am going back to my *real* doctor." Anyone who has used remedies for *acute* conditions such as traumas, infections, or childbirth knows firsthand the lightning speed with which remedies work. How many times have I given a remedy to a patient and as soon as it touches the tongue they are saying, "Is it possible that it already worked?" I have seen a patient who was up all night two nights in a row with a suffocating cough until he was cyanotic, who stopped coughing the moment he received the right remedy (Cuprum). In acute conditions, a remedy given in water touches the nerve endings in the mouth and works almost instantaneously, faster than any pharmaceutical I have ever worked with, even those given by IV push.

In chronic diseases, however, common sense must prevail: an illness of thirty years' duration cannot be cured in a week or a month. It is in the nature of a chronic disease to develop slowly over a long period, and it makes sense that a cure must come in the same way. "Nature never leaps in jumps; it always goes slow," as the old saying goes. This is a hard lesson for patients who have become used to the sudden, jerky action of medications: if you take a sleeping pill, you will fall asleep in half an hour (but if you keep taking them, you will need more and more to fall asleep). In a way it is actually worse to lull the patient into believing that her condition can be "cured" with a pill. True cure takes deep healing, such as that stimulated by a homeopathic remedy, plus a partnership between the patient and the practitioner. The patient needs to make a commitment to a new lifestyle and to actively cooperate with the practitioner in managing the course of the treatment. In homeopathy we empower the patient: the homeopath is the navigator, but the patient is the driver. We depend on the patient's observations of her symptoms and her energy level to adjust the remedy. How often have I heard patients say, when I explain this, "You mean I have to pay attention to how I *feel?*" Not only do we encourage the patient's self-observation, we teach him to make his own adjustments in the remedy. The patient-practitioner relationship is more balanced, less one-sided in homeopathy, which is healthier for both sides.

And let us remember that no other modality can even cure chronic disease in *any* length of time (especially if the definition of cure includes preventing recurrence, as discussed below). Given that it requires many months, perhaps several years, to cure a chronic disease, Hahnemann wanted to speed up the cure as much as possible within that time frame. He experimented throughout his long life to improve his system of medicine for the benefit of the patient. He felt that his greatest discovery was the LM potency, one of the major focuses of this book, which speeded up the cure, to half or a quarter of the time that other potencies required.

While homeopathic remedies do not cause side effects (as explained in Chapter 3, Laws and Principles), they can cause what are called "aggravations," usually a temporary intensification of the patient's symptoms on the way to a cure. Hahnemann felt that these aggravations caused unnecessary suffering to the patient and his experiments were also directed towards eliminating them. The LM potencies, which provided the fastest cure, also minimized aggravations to the point of almost entirely eliminating them. Hahnemann also recommended assessing the patient's individual level of sensitivity to the remedies, so that the dosage could be reduced to a small fraction, if necessary, for the very sensitive patients. (This is another concept of homeopathy which I wish my allopathic colleagues would be willing to learn from us. Even if they never prescribe a homeopathic remedy, they could save their sensitive patients so much suffering if they would only adjust the dosage of their prescriptions to the patient's sensitivity.) And let us not forget the big picture: the entire healing process in homeopathy takes a few years at the most. After that the patient no longer needs remedies, unlike the conventional process in which a patient needs medications for the rest of her life, suffers from their side effects, and needs ever-increasing dosages as she develops a tolerance to the medication.

The Permanent Cure

I have often heard from the mothers of my favorite patients, the little children, that they asked their pediatricians what seemed like a simple question: "What can you do to keep these ear infections from coming back so I don't have to keep giving my child antibiotics?" Or from my women patients that they asked their gynecologist, "What can you give me so that I don't keep getting one yeast infection after another?" Doctors are still searching for an answer to these seemingly simple questions. While allopathic medicine may seem effective at quelling the symptoms of a particular outbreak, the prevention of recurrence has never been resolved.

And we might even question the effectiveness of the symptomatic treatment. According to allopathic research, up to 50% of ear infections are viral,[3,4,5,6] yet antibiotics are universally prescribed despite their known ineffectiveness against viruses. The result is a disturbed intestinal flora and a weakened immune system for the child, who is then more susceptible to the next ear infection and becomes subject to a never-ending round of increasingly powerful antibiotics. These are powerful medications and not to be given lightly, not to mention the dangers of developing resistant bacteria. In recent Senate hearings on the problem of drug-resistant microbes, the head of the CDC estimated that 50 million unnecessary prescriptions are written in the US each year. With otitis media the most frequently-diagnosed condition in this country, many of those unnecessary prescriptions are for ear infections, which could be treated gently and effectively with homeopathy.*

**The abstract of a recent study reads as follows:* In a prospective observational study carried out by 1 homoeopathic and 4 conventional ENT practitioners, the 2 methods of treating acute pediatric otitis media were compared. Group A received treatment with homoeopathic single remedies (Aconitum napellus, Apis mellifica, Belladonna, Capsicum, Chamomilla, Kalium bichromicum, Lachesis, Lycopodium, Mercurius solubilis, Okoubaka, Pulsatilla, Silicea), whereas group B received nasal drops, antibiotics, secretolytics and/or antipyretics. The main outcome measures were duration of pain, duration of fever, and the number of recurrences after 1 year, whereby alpha < 0.05 was taken as significance level. The secondary measures were improvement after 3 hours, results of audiometry and tympanometry, and necessity for additional therapy. These parameters were only considered descriptively. The study involved 103 children in group A and 28 [sic] children in group B, aged between 6 months and 11 years in both groups. For duration of pain, the median was 2 days in group A and 3 days in group B. For duration of therapy, the median was 4 days in group A and 10 days in group B: this is due to the fact that antibiotics are usually administered over a period of 8-10 days, whereas homoeopathics can be discontinued at an earlier stage once healing has started. Of the children treated, 70.7% were free of recurrence within a year in group A and 29.3% were found to have a maximum of 3 recurrences. In group B, 56.5% were free of recurrence, and 43.5% had a maximum of 6 recurrences. Out of the 103 children in group A, 5 subsequently received antibiotics, though homoeopathic treatment was carried through to the healing stage in the remaining 98. No permanent sequels were observed in either group.

In homeopathy, the standard of cure includes the prevention of recurrence. I have treated many children with recurrent otitis, asthma attacks, or URIs who were on antibiotics for years. To the amazement of parents and doctors alike, simply strengthening the child's constitution with the proper remedy made antibiotics totally unnecessary for years afterwards. How is this possible? The simple answer is the that remedies strengthen the body's own healing energy, the Vital Force. The more complicated answer lies in miasmatic prescribing. This is homeopathy's analogue to genetic therapy, which is so intricate and detailed, so essential to homeopathic prescribing, that I have devoted the entire last section of this book to it.

From what I have said so far, homeopathy may seem like a miracle. It is not. It is a science. It works because it is based on the infallible natural laws of healing that are described in the next two chapters. The miracle, if any, is that Samuel Hahnemann was able to develop this entire system of healing in one lifetime. Perhaps it was a divine gift to Hahnemann, who was a deeply religious man and passionately committed to helping his patients. Homeopathy has certainly been a gift in my life. When I look back at all the twists and turns, all the apparent coincidences that led me to homeopathy, I wonder whether some guiding spirit or guardian angel led me to it, and I am grateful. This book is my attempt to share this gift of healing which I have been so fortunate to encounter. We begin with the basic principles on which homeopathy was founded, the immutable pillars of our science.

Chapter Two

The Vital Force in Health and Healing

> In the healthy human state, the spirit-like life force … that enlivens the material organism *[the body]* … governs without restriction and keeps all parts of the organism in admirable, harmonious, vital operation, as regards both feelings and functions, so that our indwelling, rational spirit can freely avail itself of this living, healthy instrument for the higher purposes of our existence.
>
> The material organism, thought of without life force, is capable of no sensibility, no activity, no self-preservation. It derives all sensibility and produces its life functions solely by means of the immaterial *wesen* (the life principle, the life force), that enlivens the material organism in health and in disease.
>
> —Aphorisms 9 and 10

The concept of health and healing in homeopathy is based on the energy force within the body, which Hahnemann refers to in terms variously translated as the life force, the life principle, the dynamis, the spiritual force, and the Vital Force. As Hahnemann explains in Aphorisms 9 and 10, the Vital Force animates the body and maintains a harmony among all its members; without the Vital Force, the body would be an inert corpse. And when a human being is attacked by a disease-causing agent (remember that this can be an emotional trauma as well as a physical blow or a microbe), it is the Vital Force which resists it, attempting to restore order and harmony. Hahnemann often talks of the Vital Force being "roused up" against the "morbific force" or disease-causing agent, as if it were a slumbering giant in the depths of the being. (When we say the Vital Force is "deep inside" we do not mean interior in the anatomical sense, "deep to" the skin, but rather existing on a subtler level because it is energetic rather than physical. Similarly, when we talk about healing from the inside to the outside, this means not only symptoms going from deeper organs to the surface, but also from the mental, emotional and energetic planes to the physical.)

The roused Vital Force repels the morbific agent if the Vital Force is healthy enough and the morbific agent is not too strong. This is the scenario in homeopathy's basic paradigm of how the body heals itself. The Vital Force may be weakened, however, if the person is elderly, malnourished, chronically ill, or suffering from a trauma such as a heartbreak. The Vital Force is strongest in young children, which is why they have such resilience and can suddenly spike a high fever. This is a sign of a powerful Vital Force at work. This is also why we can give young children (although not infants) larger doses of remedies than adults, the opposite of allopathic medication in which dosage is based on body weight rather than on energy level. Hahnemann encouraged his patients to strengthen their Vital Force through simple, healthy food; pure fresh air and water; exercise; and the nineteenth-century equivalents of meditation, Tai Chi, Chi Kung, and other energy-based practices like Polarity and Reiki.

Sometimes the disease-causing agent is strong enough to overwhelm even the strongest Vital Force. For example, in a rampant epidemic of a virulent disease such as cholera or bubonic plague, most people who are exposed will succumb. Except in epidemics, homeopathy rarely targets microbes, because they usually only affect susceptible people; instead, we simply reduce the patient's overall susceptibility by enhancing the Vital Force. And instead of searching for the microbe which causes chronic illness, we look for a mental or emotional trigger. We use the image of the Vital Force as a balloon: a trauma pokes a hole in the balloon, causing a leakage of energy. If we can find and patch up that energy leak, the Vital Force will heal the illness naturally.

When I describe this concept to my patients—looking for the leak in their energy balloon—most of them immediately understand the onset of their chronic illness. One patient might remember how she felt when she received the phone call that her teenager had been killed in a car accident, another the shock at finding that his trusted business partner had betrayed him or that his wife was having an affair with his best friend. Still another might recall her frustration at being passed over for a major promotion which she clearly deserved, and another how his world caved in when he received a "Dear John" letter. For many of my patients, the leakage began when receiving a diagnosis of an incurable disease. Interestingly enough, they may have been healthy, energetic and totally asymptomatic up to the point when a pathology was discovered in a routine screening, or had only minor symptoms which triggered the screening. The news that they had cancer, for example, hit them like a powerful blow, and their Vital Force was punched down like a boxer staggering to his knees, never to recover. Their health would suddenly begin a downward spiral, and almost overnight they would become "cancer patients."

The Healing Action of the Vital Force

If natural healing occurs when the Vital Force is roused against the disease, how does a homeopathic remedy work? To understand this, it helps to consider the graceful Japanese martial art of aikido, in which the opponent's own energy is used to defeat him. The more powerfully an opponent rushes at an aikido master, the faster he will soon be rushing away from him. The aikido master does not push against or resist the opponent, which would create a crash of opposing negative energies. Instead he works with the opponent's energy and just redirects or deflects it slightly. Allopathic medicine works more like two knights on horseback charging at each other and creating a tremendous crash: by attacking the symptoms (the Vital Force's attempts to throw a dangerous internal disorder to the surface) a drug crashes headlong into the Vital Force and undoes its attempts at healing. A great example is the body's use of fever: each degree of fever greatly increases the number of immunomodulators and white blood cells at the site of infection.[1,2] Hippocrates knew the value of a fever more than two thousand years ago: "Give me a fever," he said, "and I shall cure all disease." By suppressing a fever with antipyretics we actually prolong the course of illness. In fact a recent study showed that suppressing a fever actually prolonged the duration of childhood illnesses, yet acetaminophen continues to be the "gold-standard" recommendation for children with fever from acute illnesses.[3,4,5,6,7]

A homeopathic remedy, on the other hand, strengthens the Vital Force in its efforts to throw the disease out of the body. It does this by creating a sort of shadow of the disease, what Hahnemann called the artificial disease picture, to further stimulate the healing action of the Vital Force. This artificial disease picture does not harm the body because it does not exist on the physical level (as explained in the next chapter: the remedies are so dilute that they only exist as energy and do not contain a single molecule of the original remedy substance). Instead the energy of the remedy goes directly to the energetic level of the being, the Vital Force, and rouses it more powerfully to push out the disease. This concept will be explored in much more depth in the next chapter, as it is one of the fundamental principles of homeopathy.

For those who know Traditional Chinese Medicine (TCM), the Vital Force will be a familiar concept: it is very much like *qi* or *chi,* the healing energy in TCM. (The possibility that Hahnemann was actually inspired by TCM is explored in Appendix 5.) Most traditional societies have a concept of health and healing which includes an energetic or spiritual force as well as the physical body. In fact this concept was very much a part of the origins of modern medicine, as we trace our roots back to ancient Greece. The Greeks considered the human being as a trinity of body, mind and spirit, of which the last was perhaps the most important part. They viewed disease as disharmony, and their early attempts at treatment were aimed at restoring the natural balance. Hahnemann resurrected this concept, based on his study of the ancient Greeks. He declared, "Man is a composite being, a multidimensional entity, a synthetic unity of life, consciousness and intelligence," and "Mind is the key to man." Dr. James T. Kent, the famous turn-of-the-century American homeopath, wrote, "Man consists in what he thinks and what he loves and there is nothing else in man."

Historical Background

As a medical student, I wondered how the concept of disease as a disharmony in this trinity disappeared from modern medicine, and I studied the history of medicine voraciously. I found that Hippocrates, called the Father of Medicine, advocated many of the same sound principles of healthy diet and life-style advocated by Hahnemann in his time and by many health professionals today. Hippocrates conceived an early version of the mind-body connection, exemplified in his concept of the four temperaments explained in Chapter 8, in which the body's life-giving fluids reflected the patient's emotional state. In the fifth century BC he had already become the first to attest to the Law of Similars on which homeopathy is founded. As explained in the next chapter, Hippocrates formulated this law as follows: "Illnesses arise by similar things and by similar things can the sick be made well." Claudius Galen in the second century AD became the greatest authority in medicine for the next five hundred years and probably deserves the title "Father of Medicine" more than Hippocrates does. He introduced "treatment by the opposite," the Law of Contraries explained in the next chapter. Galen considered the brain the seat of the rational soul and of the animal spirit. The great medieval Swiss physician Paracelsus called for a return to Hippocratic principles and "like cures like" as a sound rule for prescribing. In developing the laws of homeopathy, Hahnemann in turn based his concepts (which he then demonstrated empirically) on those of Hippocrates and Paracelsus.

While modern medicine reveres Hippocrates as its founder, in fact its paradigm of healing is quite different from that of the ancient Greeks. Descartes' sixteenth-century statement, "I think, therefore I am," paradoxically heralded an era of mind-body split in which medicine focused only on the physical body because it is observable and objectifiable. Van Leeuwenhoek's seventeenth-century discovery of microbes as causative agents of disease, using the newly-invented microscope, began medicine's love affair with technology and its fascination with that which can be seen and measured. In a laudable effort to accept only what is rational, scientific, and experimentally reproducible, medicine focuses only on the *physical* aspect of the trinity: that which can be verified by lab tests and blood work. Consciousness (whether a thought, a feeling or a spiritual state) is difficult to quantify and is thus almost always eliminated as a variable. The human being is seen in terms of gross anatomy (organs, tissues, nerves and blood vessels), microbiology (cells and their functions), and biochemistry (molecules essential to life such as proteins and hormones, together with their structure and interaction). In a belated attempt to recognize the role of thoughts and emotions in immune function, modern medicine in the 1980s developed the field of psychoneuroimmunology, which reduces the effect of emotions to the interplay of neurotransmitters—in other words to chemicals whose structure can be analyzed and synthesized in the laboratory.

Two Views of Health and Healing

Disease in allopathic medicine is equated with pathology, which in homeopathy is viewed as the *last* stage of disease, a *late outer representation* of a long-standing disharmony in the Vital Force. To translate this into allopathic terms, a disturbance in the body's energy field may result in changes in electromagnetic charges which then influence molecular interactions which finally produce observable symptoms. Allopathic medicine defines healing as removing the pathology. This is understandable, since pathology is observable. The rash disappears, the wart is burned off, the tumor is removed, the symptoms disappear. Because it does not see the interconnectedness of all parts of the being as homeopathy does, allopathy does not include in its outcomes research the appearance of asthma after eczema disappears, or of seizures after the asthma is treated, or of cervical cancer after a genital wart is removed—let alone depression or anxiety attacks after an itch is relieved. The great 19th century homeopath Compton Burnett recorded many cases of organ tumors following the suppression of a local tumor, and even of death directly following the suppression of a rash.

Homeopathy acknowledges the connection of mind and emotions, body and spirit. Better yet, it puts a powerful tool in the hands of the practitioner. The right remedy stimulates the Vital Force to throw off the depression, the anxiety, the asthma, to make the skin eruption reappear, and then to throw this off in turn until all the symptoms are gone. Through two centuries of clinical research with hundreds of thousands of patients, homeopathy has demonstrated the truth of the mind-body connection.

As a result of its reliance on the objective and the observable, modern medicine has put on blinders when it comes to mind, emotions and spirit. It is true that recent medical studies have validated the effectiveness of such spiritual practices as simple prayer (in which, for example, prayer for an unknown, unrelated person significantly reduced the need for post-surgical interventions to the extent that "if a new medication achieved these outcomes it would be adopted immediately").[8] Yet these studies exist at the fringes of medicine. They have not yet challenged the paradigm. They are like the observations of planetary motions in Copernicus' time which just did not fit with the accepted world view that the earth was the center of the universe. These observations kept accumulating, swept aside by the "scientific establishment" of the time, until they just could not be ignored any longer. Suddenly the lens shifted and the foundations of the medieval universe were shaken, as scientists realized that the only way to explain this data meant a total shift in world view to a sun-centered universe.

Modern medicine is on the verge of such a paradigm shift right now. The evidence is mounting for the curative role of mind and emotions, energy and spirit. At this point the evidence is not being assimilated because the medical establishment does not know what to do with the information. But soon the world view will crack, this belief that health and healing are ultimately reducible to *Gray's Anatomy* and molecular interactions. And when it does, homeopathy will be ready: the visionary creation of Samuel Hahnemann two centuries ago will come to the rescue, because it has the tools already in hand to work with the Vital Force. The oncologist may ignore her patient's belief that his cancer was triggered by the death of his wife of 50 years, not only because it does not fit her paradigm, but also because this information is not useful for her prescription. The homeopath finds it supremely useful and in fact orients her whole prescription around this all-important leakage of the Vital Force, choosing among our many remedies for "ailments from grief."

The Microbe and the Terrain

It has become almost a cliché to observe the military terminology in modern medicine: patients are attacked by germs, we need to win the war on cancer, and so forth. When the microbes gain the upper hand in the body's ongoing battle against hostile microorganisms, then disease ensues, and the patient's body becomes the battleground between the germs and the toxic chemicals used to attack them. As in real warfare, there are no real winners: perhaps the microbes are subdued, but often at the expense of "heavy losses" on the winning side, in the form of hair loss or nausea, impotence or constipation. The focus of allopathic medicine is on "the enemy," the specific microbe which "causes" disease.

Homeopathy, like other forms of holistic medicine, sees life in terms of balance, perhaps best represented by the Yin-Yang symbol *(right)*. Trillions of microbes occur naturally within each human body, many of them essential to digest our food and synthesize certain vitamins. But there must be a balance between different species of our intestinal flora. What upsets that balance? Why do some people succumb to an epidemic while others do not? How can we restore the balance by strengthening the Vital Force, the natural upholder of order and harmony in the body?

Koch and Pasteur are commonly credited with founding the modern science of microbiology, but half a century earlier Hahnemann had demonstrated a profound understanding which actually reached beyond Koch and Pasteur to a more modern view of the interaction between microbe and host. (As a historical footnote, Hahnemann had also demonstrated the power of homeopathy to control and even prevent epidemics of fatal diseases such as cholera and typhoid fever. Hering, one of his top students, "vaccinated" against diseases like rabies with no fatal outcomes, unlike Pasteur's experiments with vaccinations which killed thousands of people before he reduced his dosages as Hering had done decades earlier.)

Hahnemann focused on the individual's susceptibility to a microbe or other disease trigger, explaining it in terms of a lack of natural defenses because of a weakened Vital Force. As long as the defense system is intact, we are resistant to most exterior aggressions. Hahnemann was perhaps the first Western scientist to declare what Traditional Chinese Medicine had asserted for thousands of years: the primordial importance of the individual "terrain" or "soil" on which the microbes would grow. Illness occurs, he said, only when the organism is susceptible to the "morbific cause." As he explains in Aphorism 31:

> We become diseased ... only when our organism is just exactly and sufficiently disposed and laid open to be assaulted by the cause of disease that is present, and to be altered in its condition, mistuned and displaced into abnormal feelings and functions. Hence these inimical potencies do not make everyone sick every time.

Pasteur, who initiated modern medicine's focus on the microbial culprit, actually came to the same realization at the end of his life. On his deathbed he said, *"Bernard a raison ... le terrain est tout! Le microbe n'est rien!"* ("Bernard is right ... the terrain is everything! The microbe is nothing!" He referred to Dr. Claude Bernard, today honored as the father of modern physiology.) And Virchow, the celebrated German anatomist and physiologist, said: "If I could live my life over again, I would devote it to proving that germs seek their natural habitat—unhealthy tissue—rather than being the cause of unhealthy tissue."

Unfortunately this realization has not seeped into modern medicine. Focusing on strengthening the Vital Force rather than on finding the culprit microbe would greatly enhance the effectiveness of medicine while minimizing its cost. Research into a single microbe such as that causing AIDS or CFIDS (chronic fatigue and immune dysfunction syndrome) can cost millions of dollars. Once the microbe is isolated, this does not in any way guarantee a cure, especially in the case of viruses which can "hide" inside the body's own cells. Even if a pharmaceutical can be developed which is effective against one microbe, it will not necessarily work as well against another; and a microbe can mutate much faster than a new drug can be developed. Microbes can even "teach" drug-resistance to other species by sharing plasmids.

Focusing on the microbe is thus an expensive and losing proposition. Testing each drug that comes to market costs an estimated $359 million,[9] yet this drug may be specific to a particular pathogen and ineffective against any other. However, if we focus on strengthening the Vital Force, we increase the body's ability to resist *all* microbes and *all other disease triggers,* in addition to enhancing the patient's overall experience of well-being. To the allopath, this talk of fighting microbes by enhancing the Vital Force probably sounds flimsy, vague and esoteric. But let us examine the facts. Few diseases known to modern medicine are considered as virulent as cholera. Hahnemann *cured* cholera 150 years ago—with the same remedies that could be used today in a cholera epidemic. He rescued Napoleon's army by curing typhoid fever in 1813 and saved the lives of thousands of people in a scarlet fever epidemic with simple preventive prescribing. In the great flu pandemic of 1918 in London, 45% of patients in allopathic hospitals died, while homeopathic hospitals had a death rate of less than 5%. All of this is a matter of historical record. (The flu statistics are from the London Homeopathic Hospital.) The remedies, in today's currency, cost a fraction of a cent per day.* Homeopathy could save millions of lives worldwide in the current resurgence of TB, malaria, cholera, STDs and other infectious diseases.

Strengthening the Vital Force

Health is the balanced state of body, mind and spirit. As Hahnemann states in Aphorism 9, "In the healthy human state, the spirit-like life force *[Vital Force]*... keeps all parts of the organism in admirable, harmonious, vital operation, as regards both feelings and function." The Vital Force creates and sustains this harmony between body and mind. This normal health and the harmonious Vital Force depend on a healthy life-style (nutrition, pure fresh air and water, good sanitation) and the absence of a miasm, the hereditary tendency to disease (explained in

---

*References to the expense of homeopathic remedies throughout this book are made based on the following calculations. If a consumer buys a remedy in a health food store or pharmacy, a typical tube might cost $5 and contain 80 pellets (6¢ per pellet). If she uses the remedy according to the instructions in this book, dissolving one pellet in water to make the daily dose, the cost is 6¢ per day. If she buys a remedy kit, a kit might contain 50 remedies, each with 1500 pellets per tube, at a cost of about $100 ($2 per tube or less than two-tenths of a cent per pellet and per day). A professional might buy a kit of 100 remedies for $275, each containing 1500 pellets, at a cost of $2.75 per tube, still less than two-tenths of a cent per pellet. Chronic illnesses are frequently resolved when a few cents' worth of the pellets have been used.

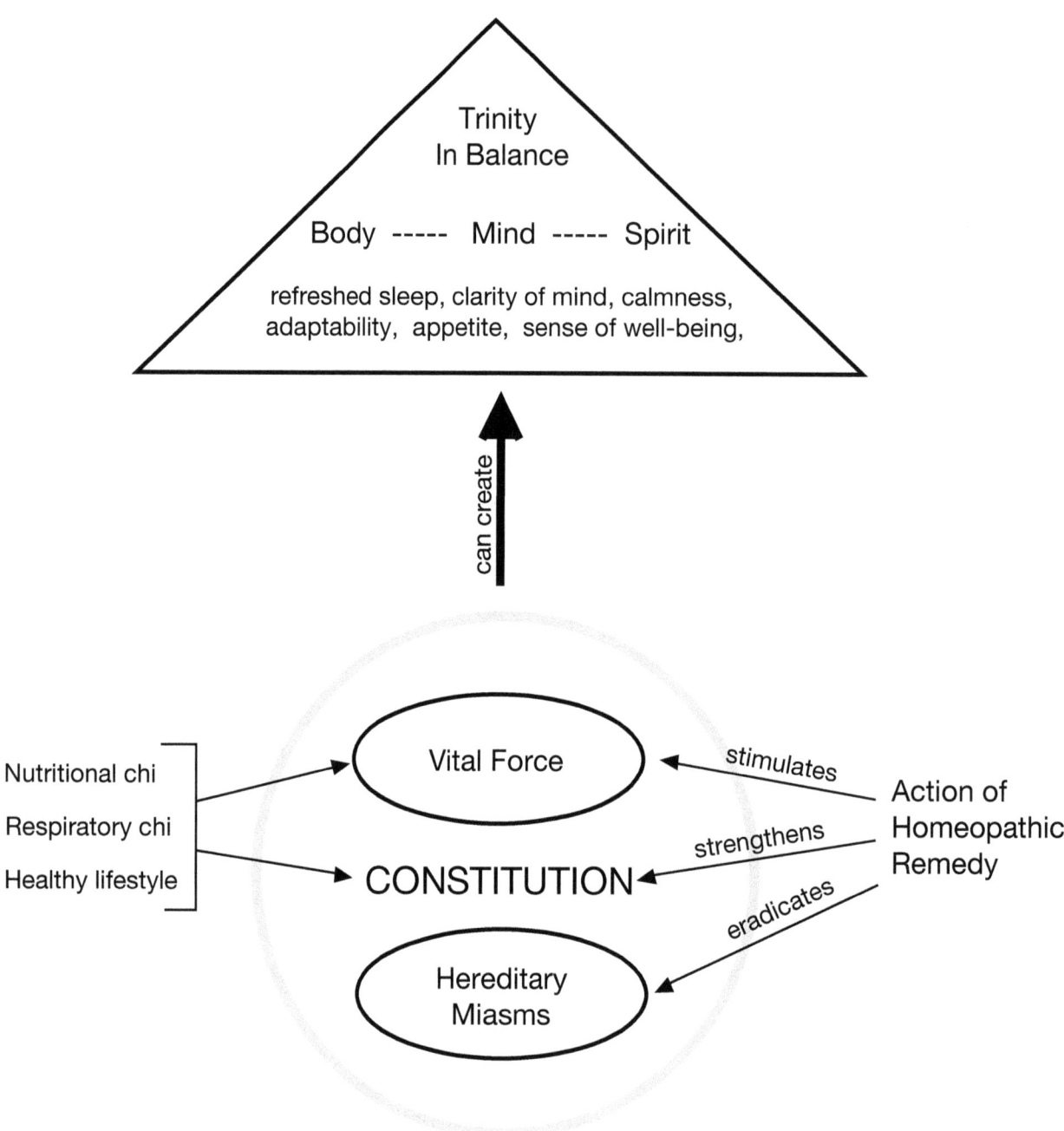

Fig. 2-1: The Homeopathic Paradigm of Healing

the last section of this book). Homeopathic remedies can successfully *prevent* the development of many chronic diseases by eradicating these miasms and by "plugging the leak in the energy balloon" caused by a mental, emotional or physical trauma (see Figure 2-1).

Homeopathic remedies cannot cure everything, however. Hahnemann was one of the first healers of his era to acknowledge the role of nutrition and life-style. He noted that many conditions which were considered chronic diseases were actually the result of deficiencies in these two areas. As he states in Aphorism 77:

Those diseases are inappropriately named chronic that are suffered by people who:
1. continually expose themselves to avoidable malignities,
2. habitually partake of harmful food or drink,
3. abandon themselves to intemperances to all kinds, which undermine health,
4. undergo prolonged deprivation of things that are necessary for life,
5. live in unhealthy places …
6. reside only in cellars, damp workplaces or other confined quarters,
7. suffer lack of exercise or open air,
8. deprive themselves of health by excessive mental or bodily deprivations,
9. live in constant vexation, etc.

These kinds of ill-health that people bring upon themselves disappear spontaneously under an improved life-style, provided no chronic miasm lies in the body. These cannot be called chronic diseases.

In modern terms, this would be like saying that if a patient is suffering from chronic indigestion *just* from eating greasy, spicy junk food all the time, we need to teach him about proper diet, not give him a palliative remedy that allows him to continue abusing his body. If his indigestion is also due to stress at work, we can give him a remedy to help his Vital Force cope with the stress, but we would be neglecting our duty to the patient if we did not *also* teach him about proper diet and stress reduction methods. Or if the patient complains of recurrent colds and rheumatic pains and you find out that she lives in a cold, damp basement, the patient may not need a homeopathic remedy, but she definitely needs a different apartment.

Hahnemann thus differentiated between what he called true chronic diseases (truly arising from within the person) and those caused by outside forces or by medical malpractice. The remainder of this book is devoted to discussing how to treat true chronic diseases with homeopathic remedies. Hahnemann also felt it was the role of the homeopath to teach patients the value of life-style changes in treating conditions which were really due to life-style factors. Most modern homeopaths do not follow Hahnemann's example in this area. Some even discourage their patients from making changes in diet. From my own experience as a holistic doctor, I have seen the value of proper diet, exercise and other life-style factors in my patients' healing. I believe that as homeopaths we can be proud that Hahnemann was a true pioneer in this, as in so many areas of healing, and I would urge my readers to consider following his good example. Hahnemann made many suggestions for a healthy life-style, most with a surprisingly modern ring to them, including the following:

- avoiding too much alcohol, salt and sugar, and overeating in general
- avoiding pornography and other "dissipations"
- avoiding unhealthy living spaces
- exercising regularly and breathing pure fresh air; avoiding a sedentary life-style and staying up too late at night
- thinking and reading too much after meals
- putting too much energy into ambition and acquisition
- protecting oneself as much as possible from emotional stresses (grief, anger, fear, etc.)
- enjoying a happy home life and a healthy sex life.*

---

*Hahnemann shows his concern with a healthy lifestyle in a letter to a young scholar:

Mental exertion and study are in themselves very unnatural occupations for young people whose bodies are not yet fully developed, especially for such as are gifted with sensitive feelings (this nearly cost me my life between the age of 15 and 20 years). Strenuous study and profound thought absorb a greater portion of life's energy than is required to thresh corn in a barn. How then can the body which has to put forth so much power in order to complete its growth endure the withdrawal not only of forces withdrawn by study, but also those which are so essential for digestion, especially as the necessary muscular exertion is absent and the requisite enjoyment of fresh air is missing. … Had I appreciated this as clearly, at your age, as I do now, I should have progressed much further in my knowledge than I have done, and I should have been able to render much greater service to the world.

The development of the body and its forces comes long before the development of the mind. The mind can only grow in a stable and strong body, and only then can it carry out important deeds. The more cheerful, firm and healthy the bodily conditions are, the keener the mental activity becomes. Not less than one hour after dinner must you touch a book. In the evening at eight o'clock all reading and writing must cease; the blood must then gradually return to its placid course throughout the body and stop rushing violently to the head. The pulse must remain quiet until you go to bed at ten o'clock. These two hours can be occupied by a friendly talk that is not too tiring. You must go out for a walk in the fresh air for an hour daily, whatever be the condition of the weather. In the evening you must eat no meat, and only a little white bread. The mid-day meal must be strengthening and nourishing, almost without spices. No tea, no coffee, no wine.[10]

In terms of dietary advice, common sense must prevail. Most Americans will benefit from simple recommendations to eat less sugary, fatty, empty-calorie foods and to stop drinking sodas. They should eat more whole grains and fresh fruits and vegetables. Personally, I do not recommend any complicated artificial system of diet. A universal diet is no more practical than a universal remedy. I have also seen patients whose Vital Force has actually been weakened by a so-called healing diet. Some of these extreme diets can induce nutritional deficiencies. It is safer to follow Hippocrates, who said, "Foods must be in the condition in which they are found in nature, or at least in a condition as close as possible to that found in nature."

Iatrogenic Diseases

We mentioned that Hahnemann differentiated between *true* chronic diseases and those arising from external influences, including medical mistreatment. As he states in Aphorism 74:

> Among chronic diseases, we must unfortunately still include those widespread diseases that are artificially induced by allopathic treatments and by prolonged use of violent, heroic medicines in large and increasing doses.

Once again Hahnemann was ahead of his time. Most of the drugs he specifies later in this aphorism have fallen into disuse, except digitalis, which is responsible for 18% of all drug-drug interactions and 26% of all drug toxicities.[11,12]

According to the National Institutes of Health, one-third of all diseases are iatrogenic. Studies suggest that adverse drug reactions may be responsible for as many as 140,000 deaths each year in the United States; the actual number is difficult to determine because many adverse reactions go unreported. A recent study of hospital care published in the *Journal of the American Medical Association* found 3.99 errors per 1,000 medication orders; researchers noted that adverse drug events, if extrapolated to the population at large, put between 770,000 and 2 million people at risk annually.[13] Another study published in JAMA in April of the previous year stated that 100,000 people die each year from bad reactions to legal prescription drugs. Another 2.2 million suffer side effects so severe that they are permanently disabled or require long hospital stays.[14] Adverse drug reactions are the fourth leading cause of death in the US, killing more people than car accidents, plane crashes, and all other accidents combined.[15]

The True Chronic Disease

Now we can appreciate Hahnemann's description of a true chronic disease in Aphorism 78:

> The true, natural, chronic diseases are those that arise from a chronic miasm. When left to themselves (without the use of remedies that are specific against them) these diseases go on increasing. Even with the best mental and bodily dietetic conduct, they mount until the end of life, tormenting the person with greater and greater sufferings. Besides those diseases that are engendered by medical malpractice, these are the most numerous and greatest torments of the human race, in that the most robust bodily *anlage [constitution]*, the best regulated life-style, and the most vigorous energy of the life force are not in a position to eradicate them.

In this aphorism Hahnemann says that these true chronic diseases are the worst kind in his era, but in a way our modern situation is worse. Instead of the clearly defined miasmatic state (which at least indicates a specific prescription), we tend to see a murky mixture of all three states, with iatrogenic and life-style-induced factors superimposed on the true chronic disease picture. By the time patients come to see us they have already been treated with medications that fight directly against the Vital Force, driving the disease deeper inward. And the average life-style in America is not conducive to health. Most people's Vital Force is weakened by a deficient diet, chemicals in the air and water, a sedentary life-style, relationship difficulties and/or unsatisfying work. Figure 2-2, Evolution of a Chronic Disease, illustrates this situation. This jungle of symptoms creates confusion for the homeopath and makes selecting the correct remedy increasingly difficult.

Fortunately Hahnemann has given us sound laws and principles to follow in finding the remedy and treating the patient. The healing action of the Vital Force is a basic concept of classical homeopathy. The laws and principles are discussed in the next chapter.

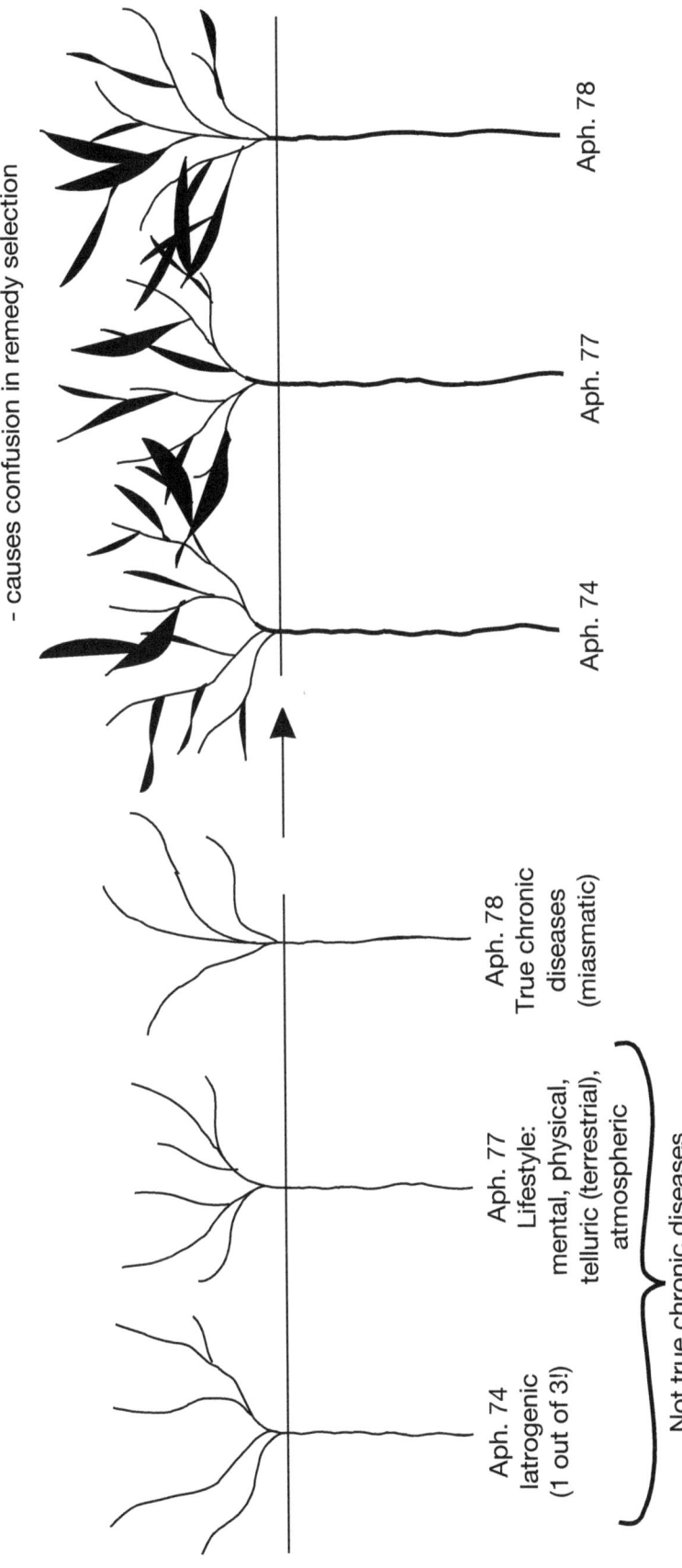

Fig. 2-2: Evolution of a Chronic Disease

CHAPTER THREE

Laws and Principles

The Importance of Laws and Principles

Every medical modality is a mixture of art and science. However, before understanding the art of homeopathy, the student must master the science—the infallible Laws of Nature upon which it is founded. The art of healing depends on the experience of the practitioner. Why did he see that case that way? What was his perception and reason for the selection of such remedy? The student, trying to imitate only the art of the teacher, will fail. It is like trying to learn chess by watching a Grand Master of chess without knowing the rules of how the pieces move. As Kent observed, homeopathy cannot be learned from the clinic: "The art of healing must not be taught first. The science must be taught first, and the art next—the law first and the experience following. The successful man is the one who has worked out the reasons for his doings." [1]

Too often I see a homeopath presenting a case at a conference and coming up with an obscure remedy, like a magician pulling a rabbit from a hat, leaving participants suitably impressed with his knowledge of Materia Medica but no wiser as to how he found the remedy. From each case presentation we should be able to garner universal methods which we can apply to any case in our practice, based on the following Laws and Principles. (We are using the word "law" and not "rule" because laws are made by infallible Nature and rules by fallible human beings.)

Like Cures Like

The foundation of homeopathy is "Like Cures Like," i.e. the principle that a substance which produces certain symptoms in healthy people can cure the same symptoms in the sick. (The substance must be administered in minute doses.) Hahnemann arrived at this conclusion from firsthand experience. At age 35, while translating Cullen's *Materia Medica,* he was struck by the described method of action of quinine, derived from Cinchona or the Peruvian bark. The description did not match what Hahnemann, already a master pharmacist, knew about the medicinal action of drugs. So he decided, as a true and inquiring physician, to try it on himself. After taking it for several days, he began to experience the episodic fever symptoms of malaria, similar to those for which quinine was prescribed. After he stopped taking the Cinchona (China), his symptoms disappeared without affecting his health at all. Soon after, he experimented with other substances and came to the same conclusion: a substance can cure the symptoms it induces, or "Like Cures Like."

We must admire Hahnemann for his courage and integrity in trying his medicines first on himself, as he did throughout his career. His example has unfortunately never been followed in allopathic medicine, whose experimental drugs are tested first on those whose systems are least able to handle them—sick patients. As Hahnemann wrote two hundred years ago in Aphorism 61:

> Had physicians been capable of reflecting on such sad results of opposed medicinal application, they would have long since found the great truth: *the true enduring curative mode must be found in the exact opposite of such an antipathic treatment of disease symptoms.*

Homeopathic remedies produce an artificial medicinal disease state that is *similar and stronger* than the natural disease but it is not the *same*. This artificial "disease" induced by the dynamic properties of the remedy is just slightly stronger than the natural disease and exists only on the dynamic or energetic plane, not on the chemical or physiological plane. It does not contain any molecules of the original substance which could cause side effects or adverse reactions. It strikes the Vital Force in almost the exact same way the disease force does, rousing the Vital Force to react against it with a stronger counterattack than against the disease itself, because the artificial disease is slightly stronger. The Vital Force has no difficulty throwing off the last removing traces of the artificial disease, because there are no molecules of the original remedy substance remaining and the Vital Force can handle a dynamic (energy-based) disease more easily than a natural one. In Hahnemann's own words, in Aphorism 68:

> In homeopathic cures ... experience shows us that, at times, initially some small amount of medicinal disease still continues on *alone* ... However, because of the extraordinary minuteness of the dose *[unlike toxic drugs]*, the transitory medicinal disease disappears so easily and so quickly by itself, that the life force has no more considerable counter-action to take up against this small artificial mistunement of its condition than the counter-action of elevating the current condition up to the healthy station ... to which end, the life force requires little effort ...

How can a homeopathic medicine, being similar to the disease but stronger, cure the patient instead of making the condition worse? The stronger remedy-induced "disease" has no toxicity because any material substance has been eliminated through the process of dilution and potentization.

The remedy thus produces a stronger disease picture, expelling the similar weaker illness, according to Nature's Law: "Two similar diseases cure each other." The Vital Force is freed now from the influence of the natural disease, while the influence of the remedy is transient because of its minuteness. Soon the Vital Force becomes free of the influence of the artificial disease too, leading ultimately to a cure (the *curative secondary action*).

All this is expressed in Aphorisms 63 and 64:

> Every agent that acts on the vitality *[Vital Force]*, every medicine or remedy, deranges more or less the vital force, and causes a certain alteration in the health of the individual for a longer or shorter period. This is called *primary action*. To its action our *vital force* endeavors to oppose its own energy. This resistant action is a property, is indeed an automatic action of our life-preserving power which goes by the name of *secondary action*.
>
> During the primary action of the medicines (remedies) on our healthy body, our vital force seems to conduct itself merely in a *passive receptive manner*. It then however appears to rouse itself again and to develop the *exact opposite condition* in the organism *(counteraction or secondary reaction)* to the effect (primary action) produced upon it.

The primary and secondary action of a remedy action is entirely different from those of allopathic drugs or substances such as coffee. Both homeopathic remedies and allopathic drugs have primary and secondary actions. But in the case of homeopathy, the primary action is similar to the effect of the disease itself, so that the secondary action of the Vital Force against the remedy parallels its action against the disease and enhances its efforts to throw off the disease state. In allopathy, the opposite happens. The drug acts *against the symptoms* of the disease (which in turn are simply expressions of the Vital Force acting *against the disease*) and thus the secondary action of the Vital Force enhances the disease itself, requiring ever-increasing doses to keep suppressing the symptoms. Figure 3-1 illustrates the action not only of a homeopathic remedy but also of many other triggers which "shock" our Vital Force. (It also demonstrates how homeopathy's concept of disease etiology is similar to that of Traditional Chinese Medicine, which sees disease as caused by internal factors or the Seven Emotions; external or climatic factors; and "not internal, not external factors" such as homeopathic remedies.)

Normally our Vital Force tries to oppose the primary action of an incoming influence by producing an opposite state, in accordance with the Law of Nature that *every action is followed by an equal and opposite reaction*. For example, if we take a laxative for constipation, the primary action of the drug causes an excessive motility of the bowels and we get diarrhea. The next day, however, the secondary action of the Vital Force will cause the bowels to do exactly the opposite, resulting in more constipation and requiring *ever-increasing* amounts of the drug to get the same result. This is an *antagonistic* reaction of the Vital Force, *not* a curative one, and leads to *iatrogenic* (physician-induced) diseases. After the administration of allopathic drugs, or another stimulus too strong for the Vital Force to handle, symptoms exactly opposite to those of the primary action will be produced.

A healing action takes place if the Vital Force is intact and has the strength to throw the symptoms to the exterior, healing from within without as shown in Figure 3-1.

We see this principle of primary and secondary action every day. For instance, if we immerse our hand in hot water, first it becomes hotter than the other one (primary effect) but shortly after it is withdrawn from the water and well dried, it becomes colder than the other one (secondary effect). Strong coffee stimulates the mind (primary effect) but it leaves behind sensations of heaviness and drowsiness (secondary effect) which continue until we drink more coffee (palliative effect). This is true in healthy people with their Vital Force intact; when the Vital Force is weak the patient may not respond at all or may overreact to environmental influences. (See Chapter 5 on treating hypersensitives.)

How then can we explain the alternation of symptoms such as constipation and diarrhea which sometimes appears in provings (discussed later in this chapter)? At first glance it seems to be a primary and *opposite* secondary action, such as we would expect to find with an allopathic drug rather than a homeopathic remedy, but in fact this is known as the *alternating action* of the remedy. The contradictory symptoms run *in cycles* if these symptoms are *true alternating primary actions* of the remedy. If one symptom were an expression of the secondary action of the remedy, it would persist until another dose was given. For instance, the diarrhea (primary action) of a laxative is followed by constipation (secondary action) and the patient remains constipated till another dose is administered. There is no spontaneous cycling of the symptoms.

The Use of a Single Remedy

As we have just seen, the homeopathic remedy works by stimulating the Vital Force. Ideally, the symptom picture of the remedy's "artificial disease" matches as closely as possible the symptom picture of the patient's illness. The totality of the patient's symptoms is matched to

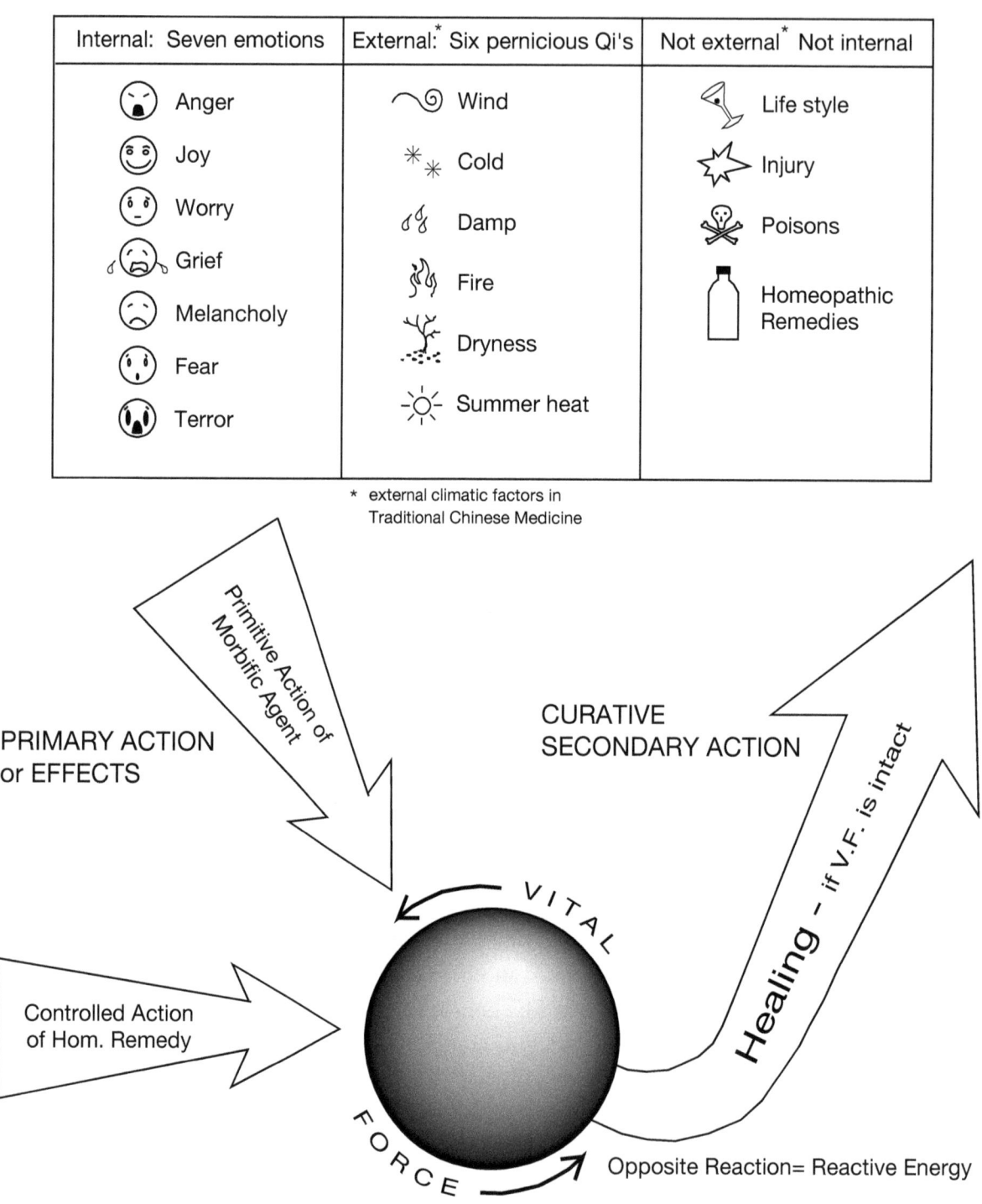

Fig. 3-1: Primary and Secondary Action of a Homeopathic Remedy and Morbific Agents

the unique "disease" picture of the remedy. It does not make sense to confuse the Vital Force by stimulating it with two or more remedies, each with its own unique picture. Each remedy has its own rhythm; two or more remedies with separate rhythms would create a disharmony.

Moreover, by administering one remedy at a time, the practitioner will be able to distinguish its actions from the interfering effects of other substances. In Aphorism 274, Hahnemann himself said: "It is still impossible to predict *how* two or more medicinal substances might hinder or alter each other's actions upon the human body." Using mixed remedies can confuse the Vital Force, neutralize the remedial effects, disorder the state of sickness, and obscure the disease picture.

Thus the next principle of homeopathy: administer only one remedy at a time. Patients should not take "mixed" preparations of homeopathic remedies, so common on the market today. Practitioners using these mixtures do a disservice to their patients and the profession. Hahnemann would have nothing but contempt for such practitioners who have the audacity to call themselves "classical" homeopaths.

As you can see, the mixing of homeopathic medicines is not only contrary to the fundamental idea of homeopathy, but it does not allow us *a posteriori* to obtain knowledge about the actions of our medicines. If pharmaceutical companies want to market mixtures of remedies, they should develop them according to the principles of homeopathy and test the effects of the mixtures on healthy individuals (proving) rather than relying on information about the ingredients used separately. Otherwise, the mixture practice is a dangerous innovation, because it is impossible to predict the action of a mixture based on the action of its constituents. To demonstrate this point even further, Hahnemann says in Aphorism 273:

> In no case of cure is it necessary to employ more than a *single simple* medicinal substance at one time with a patient. *For this reason alone, it is inadmissible to do so.* ... In homeopathy ... it is absolutely prohibited to administer to the patient, *at one time,* two different medicinal substances.

Notice that Hahnemann says "at one time" which means at the *same moment*. This does not mean that two different remedies cannot be given on the same day, especially in acute cases. For example, after a car accident a patient might need Aconite for the fright and Arnica for the bruising, taken at least 15 minutes apart. In my own practice I have occasionally given an acute remedy to take as needed while the patient was on a chronic remedy. For example, an asthma patient taking LMs of Nat. sulph. as his chronic remedy might also have Arsenicum 200c on hand, in case of an acute attack which might otherwise land him in the hospital. And von Boenninghausen often gave his classic croup remedies Aconite, Spongia, and Hepar sulph. within the same day, but not at the same moment.

The homeopath might want to put his own spin on his practice, but he should not deviate from these proven, fixed rules. If the practitioner cannot decide between two remedies in a chronic case, he does not have the true "totality" of the symptoms (see Chapter 6 on Prescribing). Many modern French homeopaths give one main deep-acting chronic remedy in high potency and another in low potency for so-called "drainage" purposes. The drainage remedy is intended to produce a discharge and create an outlet for the exodus of the disease. This approach does not appear in Hahnemann and the old masters like Kent, and the self-styled purists of today (myself included) do not approve of it. In my practice I have always seen that the well-selected remedy is capable of producing such a discharge, indicating an impending cure.

The last thing we want to do is to imitate allopathic medicine, in which many drugs are given at the same time, each with its own side effects, creating such a muddle of symptoms that the original disease picture is lost. We have all seen patients on a dozen different prescriptions, some for the original condition, the rest to counter their side effects, and all creating a jumble which makes our job as homeopaths much more difficult.

Provings

Proving, or experimentation with remedies on healthy individuals, is a *third* principle and *a must for any medical science.* Hahnemann gave detailed instructions for provings in Aphorisms 105-114. He was the first to introduce the concept of scientific experiments on medicinal substances as a basis for prescribing with them. From ancient times until well into the 18th century, much of what was known about drugs was based on pure speculation or symptoms caused by poisonings. In 1666, a dean of the Paris Faculty of Medicine, Dr. Patin, wrote:

> They say that poison is not a poison in the hands of a good doctor. Most of them have killed their wives, their children, or their friends, and yet notwithstanding they go on to speak of a drug they themselves would not dare to touch.

Allopathic medicine has never tested remedies on healthy persons to discover their precise chemical and physiological effects before prescribing them for the sick. This is where Hahnemann's approach was revolutionary. For the first time in the history of medicine, a doctor conceived the idea of testing medicines on himself so that he could observe their properties in detail. Hahnemann proved more than a hundred remedies on himself. And later, under his supervision, his pupils (mostly physicians and family members) experimented with a vast number of substances, noting all their effects. Before Hahnemann's innovation, drug effects were only known from reports of accidental poisonings. These only reveal the most extreme symptoms, which are primarily physical rather than mental/emotional. Later additional but limited information was obtained from laboratory experimentation on animals, organs and tissues, and from clinical verification of symptoms by cure, again only providing information about the full-blown physical pathology.

In homeopathy, however, a vast amount of information is available from the provings about each of the major remedies and its effects, not only on all the tissues, organs and functions of the body, but even on the mind, the emotions and the energy level. Since the same remedies have been used for two centuries, information about the curative effects of the remedies has been confirmed from clinical experience.

Hahnemann started his provings in 1789 with crude medicines in doses that were very small relative to the doses commonly used in medicine then. But even these comparatively small doses, when applied in accordance to the law of similars, caused such a violent aggravation of sufferings that Hahnemann was forced to experiment with ever-smaller doses. At first he simply divided the remedies into ever-smaller crude doses (i.e. still containing measurable amounts of the medicinal substance). Hahnemann had already proved in practice the effectiveness of minute doses of a drug, successfully curing syphilis in 1789 with doses of mercury which were a small fraction of the toxic doses used by the allopaths. Later he found he could actually enhance the effectiveness of the remedy substance, while avoiding the violent reactions, by diluting it until barely a trace remained, while adding to its dynamic or energetic state by succussion (vigorous shaking) or trituration (grinding in a mortar and pestle).

In fact Hahnemann discovered that substances which were inert in measurable quantities, like salt or charcoal, actually took on medicinal properties while prepared this way (a process Hahnemann called "potentization"). He was able to demonstrate this theory of potentization to his followers in a proving of Carbo vegetablis, the remedy made from charcoal. The crude charcoal produced no effects on the provers, and then Hahnemann showed his pupils how to develop its medicinal powers by trituration (see Fig. 6-1). The provers were even more convinced when they found in later clinical practice that the same symptoms developed during a proving of potentized charcoal could be cured in their patients by the remedy. The immediate implication of this discovery was that the process of potentization could bring out curative powers in otherwise inert substances (such as Lycopodium, one of our most powerful remedies, made from a substance so inert that pharmacists used it to coat tablets).

Hahnemann took this discovery one step further: substances such as mercury and quinine, whose medicinal effects were already known from allopathic medicine, were found to have even greater healing powers when potentized (becoming the remedies Merc. sol. and China respectively). Hahnemann found by further experiment that, in general, all substances gained curative power and caused fewer aggravations of existing symptoms after they were potentized. He thus established two principles of dynamization: that the curative power of a remedy (or any drug) is in inverse proportion to their material quantity; and that their medicinal power can be enhanced (or developed in an inert substance) by dilution and succussion or trituration.

The proving of remedies is a great undertaking, a fascinating adventure, for we never know what we will find. It demands the keenest observation of symptoms produced and requires careful weighing of their relative value. A properly-conducted proving produces a living monument of value for all time. The following guidelines for provings are based on those set forth by Hahnemann himself in the *Organon*.

The Prover: Anyone can participate who is in a reasonable (not perfect) state of health and able to observe in himself and report any changes from his ordinary feelings and sensations. A proving ideally should be made by at least 50 people, including all ages and both sexes, to provide the widest and most representative range of responses. The most valuable provers are the hypersensitives (see the Sensitivity Scale in Chapter 5), since they exhibit peculiar symptoms often not experienced by others and are likely to report more mental/emotional symptoms. Kent refutes the idea that provers must be in perfect health with an example of a Lachesis proving (with a dose of 10M!).[2] The prover, who was not in perfect health, showed symptoms for three months. The symptoms were clearly genuine proving symptoms rather than a similar aggravation, because they were entirely new, completely subduing the provers' existing symptoms; and when they subsided, all her old complaints came back.

While it might be difficult to assemble 50 provers, there should be at least a dozen. Fewer cannot provide a valid basis for sorting which symptoms are most frequently-occurring. And a symptom which could otherwise be important for a remedy could be missing entirely if there are only a handful of provers, each of whom happens not to experience it. The susceptibility of one individual toward a remedy may be almost nil; whereas another individual of the same age and type, for some unknown reason, is exceedingly sensitive to the remedy. People who have shown peculiar idiosyncrasies toward certain substances make the best provers (for example, those with severe reactions to poison ivy or bee stings will show the most symptoms of Rhus tox. and Apis respectively; more about idiosyncratic reactions to remedies in Chapter 5). No one prover will produce all the symptoms of a remedy. A symptom well developed in any one of a dozen provers, without being present in the others, may be a very valuable symptom. Therefore we need a great variety of provers to obtain a complete picture of the drug.

To prepare for the task, the prover should have a thorough physical examination and have his case taken by a homeopath as if he were a patient, including such details as the family history, the illnesses to which he and his family have been susceptible, his peculiarities and susceptibilities, and an observation of what is normal for him. Then he should note his daily state of health (including mental and emotional state) in detail for a week before he begins his proving. He will then find it much easier to describe anything that deviates from the normal. The prover should then continue his usual diet and habits throughout the proving. Provers should not use drugs, coffee, heavy perfume, or any other substance which might cancel or interfere with the action of the remedy.

Principles of Provings: Provings must include mental and emotional as well as physical changes; the former are more important than the latter in matching the patient with the remedy. And the record must include all the details of external circumstances and concomitants, without which it is useless for clinical purposes. The prover must not have any preconceived ideas (and thus must not know the remedy name in advance). He should not be frightened by any apparent "wilderness of symptoms" which may arise. His job is to accurately and objectively record whatever comes up in his own words, not in the language of medical diagnosis. Then when we ask patients to express their symptoms in their own words, we find them speaking in the language of the *Repertory*.

No new symptom should be omitted no matter how trivial. It may be of little significance to the medical diagnosis but of the greatest value in choosing the remedy. What can be apparently more trivial than the sensation "of a hair felt in the throat"? Yet this proving symptom later became the deciding factor in selecting Arsenicum by one of our great masters in one of his greatest cures. And an abundance of proving symptoms is no reason to eliminate some of them (although there was an early attempt by Dr. Richard Hughes to simplify the Materia Medica by limiting proving records to five pages).

Hering suggested that the proving symptoms appearing *last* are the most important and most useful for remedy selection because the first symptoms of all drug actions tend to be the most common, e.g. malaise, headache, nausea; the more specific and peculiar develop later. Therefore the time of onset of symptoms must also be recorded (although Hahnemann was the only one of the early provers to do this until von Boenninghausen did in 1840).

Substance of Provings: Homeopathic remedies are made from a wide variety of substances including plants (roots, bark, stems, leaves, juices, gums, oils or whole plants), insects, minerals, chemicals, tissues or secretions from healthy bodies (sarcodes) or diseased ones (nosodes), and vibrational energies (x-ray, sunlight, moonlight, magnets). The following inert media are used to prepare or to administer the medicines in dry or liquid form. They have no medicinal power; a large or small pellet can carry the exact same potency.

- lactose (Sac. lac.) for grinding (triturating) an insoluble substance
- pharmaceutical grade cane sugar for preparing globules of the remedy

- distilled water to prepare and administer medicines
- alcohol (Everclear or vodka), to prepare and preserve mother tinctures and potencies
- glycerin as an alternative preservative
- syrup simplex for syrups such as Chestall®

The remedy substance should be procured in its purest state, with the exact circumstances of collection and preparation recorded in the proving. For example, plants should be collected in the wild at the optimal time (which varies depending on the plant and part used), and not grown in greenhouses. Only the fresh juice should be used, as heat devitalizes the medicinal substances. Neither should we dry the plants, as many medicinal qualities will be lost. If the medicinal substance is taken from an animal, it should be preserved and subsequent supplies can come from the same species. The few drops of bushmaster venom courageously collected by Hering in Surinam sufficed to provide the whole world with Lachesis for a century. Like Hering, we need to collect remedy substances in the wild, as zoo-raised animals cannot be expected to produce the same potent chemicals.

Potency Used and Duration of Proving: In Aphorism 128, Hahnemann specifies using a few pellets of the 30th potency. Other potencies can certainly be used, as they often have been. But the old masters warn us to not use potencies higher than 30c, to avoid unnecessary aggravations, especially in sensitive people.

The proving should begin with a single dose (which will be sufficient for the hypersensitives, with repeated doses possibly causing them discomfort or suffering). However, most provers will feel no effect from the single dose. Then the dose can be repeated daily until some effect is produced. The remedy must be stopped at once when symptoms appear and not be repeated until absolutely all symptoms have ceased. The finest symptoms, as a rule, are those that develop late, months after the remedy has been discontinued. Thus the proving should not be made in haste; the best provings will cover two years, especially with the deeper acting remedies. The question may arise: "How would you know months later that a symptom was due to that remedy and not to something else the patient may have taken or from his environment?" Because by repeating the same remedy, similar symptoms are elicited; and illnesses covering the same symptoms are cured by this remedy. It does not matter whether the symptoms in a proving are primary or secondary, for as long as the remedy can produce them it can cure them. If the remedy stimulates the prover to re-experience old symptoms, these should still be counted among the symptoms associated with the remedy; this just shows that the prover had a special predisposition to them. These symptoms will receive a low rating in any case because only one prover experienced them.

If there is no effect in the prover after five days or so, we will have to *raise the potency* to 200c (just as if giving the remedy therapeutically). If no effects follow, we can make the remedy even stronger by putting it in water. In general the remedy should be left alone after the first dose so that its true character may be fully revealed. It should not be disturbed by any other remedy nor by repetition of doses, until sufficient time has elapsed for it to take effect—which can mean weeks or even months. As mentioned before, the symptoms of the greatest value are those *last* developed. Thus the remedy's most important symptoms can be lost to the record by interfering too soon with the progress of its action.

How long should a proving last? The longer the better, with practicality dictating the limit. Ideally, provings extending over several generations of the same family would show a greater variety of deeply seated chronic symptoms than the short voluntary provings made by Hahnemann and his followers. How can we try to compensate for time? Perhaps by using higher potencies or better yet, with LM potencies (which are fast-acting and deep-penetrating but as gentle as a low potency, as described in Chapter 6). Then we might be able to answer the question of the old masters (who did not know about LMs): How long do we wait and what do we do if the prover does not react to a 1M? Dr. Adolph Lippe said that in such a case he would stop the proving. He believed that if the prover had not shown susceptibility by that point, repetition of the remedy would not induce it. Now that we have LMs available, we could continue the proving with an LM potency (based on my clinical experience that LMs are more powerful than 1Ms).

Pushing Provings to Pathology: Provings are not extended until they cause pathology, only to the point of temporary functional or physiological symptoms. (When remedies are known for their action on a particular pathology, such as Nat. mur. for multiple sclerosis, this is based on clinical experience with cured cases rather than on provings.) In the early history of homeopathy, Dr. Richard Hughes, one of the first homeopaths in England, advocated extending provings until they produced objective pathological signs, which would then be given more weight than subjective symptoms. But this goes against our system of prescribing by the totality, by which method pathological signs have the *lowest* value in remedy selection. And what prover would volunteer to risk a perhaps irreversible pathology?

Fortunately we do not have to conduct this experiment, because it was already done by the Vienna provers in 1848, who demonstrated that massive doses close to the crude substance, frequently repeated, revealed few useful symptoms and caused life-long suffering. Using higher potencies or LMs has since proved safer, as well as more beneficial, by bringing out new symptoms that have been found to be reliable guides for the cure. Symptoms produced by the higher potencies are almost invariably subjective ones, so important in our prescribing (see Prescribing, Chapter 9).

The Vienna provings were the outcome of "logical" reasoning: if we want to make sure that the remedy "did" something, then there must be enough of it (by approaching material doses and/or by frequent repetition) to make itself *felt* so immediately as to give certainty that what is felt *is caused by the drug taken*.

This reasoning is incorrect, however. Drugs act differently in different doses. When the *crude* drug is used, it produces a chemical reaction. We also have the *mechanical* action of drugs, which causes the system to eject the drug before it is absorbed, as it is with large doses of Ipecac. When a remedy is expelled by the violence of its own action, we cannot see its exact specific primary action on the Vital Force of the prover. Symptoms thus produced only represent the poisoning effect of the remedy substance and therefore belong to its *destructive* side, not to its *curative* side.

The remedy must be given in minute doses to show its *dynamic* action, which manifests itself through the Vital Force, producing peculiar reactions of the drug according to the susceptibility of the individual. This dynamic action gives the homeopathic prescriber the best indications for the remedy. Such symptoms are the most valuable part of the provings.

Again, the dynamic doses may be still further divided by the size of the dose (6c or less as compared to 30c). Moderately large potentized doses of remedies produce *generic* reactions which can be used to classify remedies by family with the same action. For example, moderately large doses of Arsenicum produce vomiting, diarrhea, cold sweats and cramps. This is a dynamic reaction, but it is very similar to the reaction produced by Cuprum, Veratrum album and other remedies, so it cannot be used to distinguish among these remedies. Still smaller doses are necessary to make peculiar symptoms of individual remedies stand out.

The Infinitesimal Potentized Dose

Perhaps allopathy is taking a closer look at homeopathic principles:

> Biopharmacy is a science which deals with methods of strengthening the pharmacological action of medicines. It has been established recently that the action of drugs often depends on their method of preparation and in the form in which they are administered. It has been established for instance, that if Aspirin is ground 30 times finer than it is now, its action will be doubled, and consequently, its therapeutic dose could be decreased.[3]

The fourth law of homeopathy is the infinitesimal dose. Hahnemann understood perfectly well that strong doses of a remedy would add unnecessary strain to the patient's body, which was already weakened by illness. In allopathy, the dosage of medications is often increased to obtain a strong physiological response, producing uncomfortable and unnatural reactions. This does not happen when the same drugs are administered in highly diluted, or homeopathic, form. There are no adverse reactions since no residue is left in the body; there are almost no molecules of the original substance in the remedy. And of course the clinical results are better, as is so well demonstrated by the 200 years of clinical research begun by Hahnemann.

The principle of the minimum dose is the same as the Arndt-Schultz Law of bio–chemistry: minimum doses of a drug (or chemical, thermal, or electrical stimulus) *stimulate* cellular activity, medium doses *inhibit* or depress it, and higher doses *destroy* it. Two hundred years ago Hahnemann showed clearly that *much smaller doses of the drug are needed to bring about a reaction in the diseased body*. In fact, he showed that in the chronically ill, the diseased part of the body reacts much more intensely to a remedy than the healthy part does.

Hahnemann, a true scientist, based his laws of homeopathy on experiment and observation. In *Chronic Diseases* he stated:

> It requires quite an effort to believe that so little a thing, so small of a dose of medicine, could effect the least thing in the human body. I do not demand that anyone should comprehend it. Neither do I comprehend it. It is enough that it is a fact and nothing else. Experience alone declares it and I believe more in experience than in my own intelligence. ...
>
> What would men have risked if they had at once followed my directions in the beginning, and had made use of just these small doses from the first? Could anything worse have happened than that these doses might have proved inefficient? They surely could do no harm![4]

In a paradigm which states that patients are cured by medicine, it would make sense that more medicine could bring about a quicker cure. But homeopathy is based on a paradigm of healing that the patient, or more precisely his Vital Force, brings about the cure. Medicine does not cure. All that remedies can do is to *stimulate the patient's curative powers.*

How can we understand the action of a remedy which does not contain even one molecule of the original substance? Modern physics is just beginning to catch up with Hahnemann's vision of two centuries ago: that matter is essentially energy, that remedies based on energy can be more powerful than those limited to mere matter, and that remedies are essentially information which can be conveyed to the body's own healing energy by their vibrational pattern imprinted onto the inert carrier substance. This brings us to the principle of Potentization. The remedies are not active if they are simply diluted; they must be energized by succussion or trituration.

Hering's Laws

Few homeopaths except Kent, von Boenninghausen, Lippe and Gross have contributed as much to the development of homeopathy as Constantine Hering, born in 1800 in Germany. As a young medical doctor, he was sent by a professor to investigate and discredit the "quack" Hahnemann. The rest is history. Because he was objective and had a love of truth in his heart, Hering became not only one of Hahnemann's staunchest supporters, he also left his own legacy to homeopathy: three essential laws of case management. (Strangely enough, the only encounter Hering had with Hahnemann was to see him walking with his family in his gardens, but at that time Hering was still an allopath.) In 1845, two years after Hahnemann's death, Hering published his *Guiding Symptoms,* better known as "Hering's Laws." These same laws—a set of observations on how true healing occurs—have also been an intrinsic part of Traditional Chinese Medicine for five thousand years.

According to Hering's Laws, the disease heals and the symptoms appear:
- From above to below
- From the interior to the exterior
- In reverse order of their arrival

From the interior to the exterior: This law is well-known in Traditional Chinese Medicine as one aspect of diagnosis according to the Eight Conditions: Yin/Yang, Fullness/Emptiness, Cold/Heat, Exterior/Interior.

The well-chosen remedy hastens the natural course of healing by driving the disease out of the body to the surface, where it may temporarily manifest as joint pains, discharges, rashes and itching. The patient knows he is healing because he feels better at a deeper level than these surface symptoms. Examples of this rule occur frequently in the practice. An asthma patient starts breathing better, but now he exhibits more joint pains; or his previous eczema, suppressed by cortisone creams, reappears. The disease went from an essential internal organ to a safer (because less important) and more superficial part of the body—the joints or skin. The strong burning and stinging of vaginitis may give way to a copious discharge. The mental/emotional symptoms may improve while the physical symptoms either exacerbate or reappear from years past (see Suppression, Chapter 13).

The homeopath must explain this to the patient on the first visit or, inevitably, the patient will do what he has learned from allopathic medicine—suppress the new symptoms with ointments, suppositories and creams, undoing the great healing work of the Vital Force under the influence of the remedy. Patients unfortunately want to get rid of rashes and discharges as soon as possible, by any means necessary. Little do they know that they are working against the best instincts of their Vital Force: bringing the symptoms from the most interior (mind, emotions or essential organs) to the most exterior part of the body (joints and skin).

When this exteriorization of the disease occurs, the best thing the homeopath can do is to continue the same remedy, not to yield to the patient's demands to change it. The same remedy will finish off the healing process and relieve the skin symptoms and discharges. To appease the patient, often a placebo (blank pellets, known as Sac. lac.) is given for these "new" symptoms, while the patient is advised to use *natural* (non-suppressive) measures for comfort and pain relief (listed in Chapter 13, Suppression).

From above to below: I have seen this Law the least often in practice, but it certainly exists. Most often I have seen it in skin conditions and joint diseases. For example, a patient with eczema all over the body may have it disappear from the face first, then from the upper extremities, then the trunk and lastly the lower extremities. If the patient begins with the eczema only on the head, it may disappear from the head while appearing on progressively lower parts of the body, moving down to the lower extremities before leaving the body for good. This progression does not necessarily happen, as I have seen a rash all over the body disappear all at once, if the remedy was well-selected.

Symptoms return in reverse order of appearance: Another disconcerting event for the patient, if unexplained, is the healing of symptoms in the *reverse order of their first appearance*. Sometimes called *disease replay,* this phenomenon was first noted by Hahnemann in *Chronic Diseases* (1828). In other words, *the last symptoms to appear are the first ones to disappear, and old symptoms may return in reverse chronological order.* If a patient declares, "Doctor, the symptom I originally complained to you about has improved, but now I have a symptom I have not had for two years," then praise the Lord, you are on your way to curing her.

It is good to keep in mind that this curative replay is *not always in exactly the opposite* order. For instance symptoms appearing in order 1-2-3-4 can disappear in order 4-2-1-3, so that symptom 3 still exists while the other ones are already gone. The most common return of old symptoms are those that have been suppressed. Hence one can easily understand the importance of taking a detailed history about previous medical conditions and their possible suppressive treatments.

Knowledge of this Law by patient and doctor alike will bring understanding rather than confusion. *Do not alter* the remedy at this point, as the same remedy will resolve the patient's problems. Old symptoms should pass through quickly. Mostly they are milder and shorter than their original state if the remedy is given in the proper amount. The last symptoms to develop are always first to yield, and the oldest ones are the most stubborn. There is one exception to this rule: symptoms which have been constant and unchanged, typically the *local ailments* such as a goiter. This is a *one-sided* pathological state and often is the last thing to clear along with the oldest symptoms. This local complaint may linger long after the other signs have disappeared, because it is a disease entity in itself (as explained in Chapter 4, Pathology). As Hahnemann said in *Chronic Diseases:* "The oldest ailments and those which have been most constant and unchanged, among which are the constant local ailments, are the last to give way."[5]

For the practitioner to understand this replay of old symptoms, a timeline of the patient must be constructed from birth (even including intra-uterine influences such as traumas to the mother during pregnancy) to the moment of consultation. Without such a developmental time line it is very hard to understand complex chronic diseases because they are produced by different etiologies at different points in the timeline, creating interweaving layers of disease. This timeline can also help the homeopath caution the patient about old symptoms that may return. As Hering noted:

> In all chronic and lingering cases, the symptoms appearing last, even though they may appear insignificant, are always the most important in regards to selection of a remedy. The oldest are the least important. All symptoms have to be arranged according to the order of appearance. Only such patients remain well and truly cured who have been rid of their symptoms in the reverse order of their development.

Many more old homeopaths have stressed the importance of the last symptoms, as they represent the most recent expression of the symptomatology. They are connected to the most active layer within the Vital Force.

Individualization

Often, in the middle of a busy day, a patient would say to me: "I would think you doctors would get tired of diagnosing and treating those same old cases, day after day, year in and year out." "But, my dear patient," I would say, "the homeopath does not treat diseases, he treats sick individuals, and no two patients with the same disease are ill in exactly the same way. The patient's individuality is present, whether he is well or sick, and this individuality is part of the spice of medical life, which gives it enough variety to flavor it." As Kent expressed it so eloquently, "It is an absurdity to find a tailor's cut which will suit all people, then why and how does a scientific man think of discovering a specific remedy which will suit all men?"

While this seems to be common sense, allopathic medicine treats all patients by the protocol for their diagnostic category. All diabetes patients, for example, receive the same treatment with only minor variations. As homeopaths we see how different all these patients are, not only as people, not only in the grief or humiliation or other trauma which triggered their disease, but even in its specific symptoms. By basing the remedy on all these factors, the homeopath will individualize it to the patient and bring him to a true cure, which allopathic medicine is not able to do in diabetes or any other chronic disease.

I have seen enough examples in my own practice. Often I received a child's chart from a pediatrician with page after page of nothing but the weight, height, what vaccinations were given, a short diagnosis of otitis, pharyngitis, or ADD, and, all too often, what antibiotics were given. Nothing else was noted about the child: his personality, his creativity, how he might have reacted to the divorce of his parents, his best friend moving away, or his pet dying. It was as though the child was nothing but a diagnostic category, so that a standardized protocol could be instituted. But we have to individualize in every case because different individuals develop different symptoms from the same stress or trauma. Following this principle, we cannot possibly expect to find specific protocols for specific diseases; thus we do not automatically treat scarlet fever with Belladonna, nor measles with Pulsatilla, nor malaria with China.

Kent expressed this principle of individuality eloquently in his *Lesser Writings*: "As long as man is capable of believing that diabetes is disease, he will be insane in medicine. His mind is only directed toward the results of disease. So long as he thinks that man is sick because his organs are not doing proper work, just so long he cannot construct a treatment that accords with the *Organon*."[6] If it were possible to remove gross pathology without disturbing the patient's physiology, our work would certainly be easier. But the distribution of our sympathetic and parasympathetic nervous systems is so delicately arranged that no surgery can be done without affecting their harmony and function. We cannot put under a microscope the mental, emotional and functional physical symptoms, which are all expressions of disorder and unnatural forces in the patient's body. Pathology, unfortunately, has become the master, not the tool in modern science. (There *is* a role for pathology in homeopathy, however, as discussed in the next chapter.)

To summarize the laws of classical homeopathy:
- The law of similars
- Single remedy
- Provings
- Minimum potentized dose
- Hering's Laws
- Individualization.

What Makes a Remedy Homeopathic?

Based on these laws, we can see that many products are falsely sold as "homeopathic" in pharmacies and health food stores. More and more pharmaceutical and vitamin companies tout their products as "homeopathic." In fact, most people believe that any medicine sold as an herb or "homeopathic remedy" must be homeopathic. Medical professionals as well as lay people suffer from this misapprehension. The homeopathic community has to take responsibility for educating the public in the real nature of a homeopathic remedy, so that they can easily distinguish a true homeopathic remedy from a pseudo-homeopathic one.

This difficulty arises in part because the same substance (Nat. sulph., for example) can be homeopathic, allopathic or biochemical depending on how it is prepared and used. When Nat. sulph. is used in material doses for its predilected action on the liver and colon, it becomes an allopathic remedy. Nat. sulph. can also be a biochemic remedy when used in a 6x or 12x potency, as one of Schuessler's twelve tissue salts, to correct a deficiency of this salt. But when this same remedy is used homeopathically, its basic principle of application is fundamentally different. According to homeopathic principles, this remedy will cure a patient only when the *totality of the symptoms* of the case is similar to the totality of symptoms produced by proving the remedy. In addition to acting on the organs or tissues (as in allopathy), or a deficiency of a tissue salt, the remedy acts on the whole patient, including the mental and emotional planes.

Because of this fundamental difference in how the remedies are used, differences can be seen among these three systems in the following:

- the use of *combinations of remedies,*
- the *form* of application, and
- the required *dose.*

In allopathy, drugs are expected to act on particular tissues or organs. When several organs are affected in a chronic disease, symptoms are addressed by a number of drugs given in *a mixture.* In the biochemical method also, for a similar reason (the presence of nutritional deficiencies), the tissue salts are often given in mixtures. In homeopathy, since the remedy has to match the whole totality of the symptoms, there cannot be more than *one remedy at one time.*

In allopathy the dose must be crude or material (not energetic or dynamic) since the seat of action is the tissues and organs (i.e. the physical plane, not subtler planes). In the biochemical method, the seat of action is on the level of the tissue salts, which are present in the body as trace elements. So the dose of the remedy must correspond: it must be minute but molecules of the remedy substance must still be present, i.e. the dilution cannot exceed the limit set by Avogadro's law (24x). So tissue salts are given in minute material doses (6x or 12x). In homeopathy, the seat of action is on the deepest and subtlest planes (the mind, the emotions, the Vital Force) which respond even when the remedy is inhaled or rubbed on the skin. And the higher we go in potentization, the more the remedy's intensity and depth of action increases.

A remedy must have the following characteristic features to be in accordance with homeopathic principles:

- It must be based on *the totality of the symptoms: mental, emotional and physical*. No one should take a remedy from a homeopath who does not listen carefully, take note of, and incorporate symptoms on all three levels.
- It must be *a single one, instead of a mixture*.
- It can never have *a substantial material dose*.

Laypeople and professionals alike should remember these three principles of homeopathy in assessing homeopathic physicians and remedies.

Explaining the basic principles of homeopathy to our patients is often helpful in gaining their full commitment and cooperation. Some of the following points may be helpful:

- Each individual reacts to an infection/trauma according to his own nature.
- His symptoms are the result of that reaction, and they represent the body's attempt to get well.
- The body reacts as a whole, each tissue doing its part, and the totality of the symptoms represents a single effort requiring a single remedy for the cure.
- The curative remedy is the one which stimulates a reaction in the body similar to the one the body is already attempting, in other words, it causes symptoms like those already present.
- The curative reaction of the body is a positive effect, i.e. the protective mechanism is stimulated, not depressed; therefore, minute doses of the similar or curative remedy must be used, because small amounts of drugs stimulate while large doses suppress.

Now that we have a good understanding of the principles of homeopathy, we can use them to better understand the action of herbal remedies and vaccinations.

Are Herbal Remedies Homeopathic?

Herbology is often lumped together with homeopathy, but it is actually much closer to allopathic medicine in its principles of remedy action. The herbs are used in a material dose so they can only effect a *crude secondary* reaction rather than the unique *curative* response of the homeopathic remedy. And the material dose of herbs often leads to toxicity, a problem of allopathic and not homeopathic medicine. Most herbal formulas are also mixtures, whose longterm effects are difficult to predict. Whether the result is favorable or unfavorable, we do not know which herb is responsible and thus how to adjust the mixture.

Improving Vaccinations with Homeopathy

It is well known that many homeopaths oppose vaccinations across the board, which is difficult for allopathic physicians to understand since they credit vaccinations with nearly or completely eradicating many previously-epidemic infectious illnesses. There are a number of excellent books devoted to this subject. They demonstrate the dangers of vaccinations and the fact that these diseases had already declined, due to improvements in sanitation and public health, at the same rate in countries which have never had mandatory vaccinations and those that have.[7] I would refer the interested reader to the research and make the case here that instead of condemning vaccinations, homeopathy could show how to improve vaccinations and make them safer. (For example, all known cases of polio in this country between 1980 and 1994 were caused by the vaccine itself).

Right now vaccinations do follow the Law, "Like Cures Like." But other fundamental principles of homeopathy are violated: the minimum dose, refraining from frequent repetition, and administering only one substance at a time. Violating any one of these principles has the effect of knocking down and weakening the Vital Force. No wonder we see that one effect of over-vaccination is a weakened immune system, a reflection of a weakened Vital Force. Another danger is that eventually sensitive people subjected to repeated injections of mixed vaccinations will prove them (i.e. succumb to the disease for which they seek protection). "Live" vaccines and those injected directly into the tissues are the most dangerous since they bypass the body's natural lines of defense.

Now we can understand why polio vaccinations are causing polio cases and why, for instance, a vaccination program against measles in a school in Albuquerque, NM was immediately followed by 58% of the students coming down with the measles. (Public health officials unfortunately concluded that the vaccine did not take, so re-vaccination was ordered.) The latest study of the AIDS vaccine showed that the weakened virus, when tested in adult monkeys, may actually *cause the disease it was meant to prevent*. Dr. Anthony Fauci, head of the National Institute of Allergy and Infectious Diseases, commented, "To me, this confirms that we are not ready to go into humans with a live attenuated vaccine." Now the mood is somber indeed. Dr. Robert Gallo, co-discoverer of AIDS, recently said that if the live attenuated approach failed, it would mean that the AIDS vaccine development is no further ahead than it was fifteen years ago at the dawn of the epidemic. "We have no guarantee that we will ever have a vaccine," Dr. Gallo said.

If homeopathy could offer something to those working on an AIDS vaccine, it would be the suggestion to use of all the principles of homeopathy, not just "like cures like." An AIDS vaccine based on potentization and the infinitesimal dose would at least be totally safe. Remember that Louis Pasteur, one of the great early experimenters with vaccinations, killed thousands of people with his rabies vaccine before he sufficiently reduced the dose. Hering, meanwhile, had already safely cured rabies in 1835, 50 years earlier, with the remedy Lyssin—a homeopathic dilution of rabid dog saliva. If the same proven principle could be used in modern vaccine research, perhaps great suffering could be alleviated.

Chapter Four

Homeopathy and Pathology

Historical Background

Pathology in Hahnemann's time was an undeveloped science. He declared it an unsafe basis for medical treatment and demonstrated that the remedy could never be selected based on pathology alone. Therapeutics based on pathology must of necessity be a system of broad generalizations leading to standardized protocols, instead of the strict individualization of homeopathy. Furthermore, remedy provings were never pushed to the point of pathological changes (as discussed in the Provings section of the last chapter).

This is another reason why Hahnemann did not pay much attention to pathology. Our proved remedies match the beginning of the disease. We never match the remedies with the full-blown pathology only. In homeopathy we do not need to wait until pathology develops; we can prescribe on the prodromi, the subjective symptoms, in many conditions where allopathic medicine cannot. Where sometimes in advanced pathology (the "one-sided diseases," see later in this chapter) it is beneficial to match the disease picture with the physical pathological aspects of the remedy, in less progressed pathological states a remedy covering the totality of the symptoms would always cover the pathology.

Hahnemann did conduct a full physical examination of his patients and included gross pathological findings in his prescription. As one of my favorites among the old masters, Dr. Grimmer, expressed it:

> We study the *Organon* and the writings of Hahnemann. We find that he stresses the totality of the symptoms alone, he included every symptom he could get. Hahnemann went over his patients, he examined them. Everything that he could learn about his patients was recorded. This formed the picture. And so it is with the use of pathology.

The followers of Hahnemann all agree that the totality of the symptoms, including all the pathological signs, form the true picture of the patient's diseased condition. Pathological signs must be duly noted and receive appropriate consideration, as discussed later in this chapter. Dr. Constantine Hering stated:

> No one can be a successful disciple of Hahnemann, who is not well versed, as Hahnemann himself was, in the learning of the medical schools; and it would be just as impossible for him to act judiciously without a knowledge of anatomy, physiology, pathology, surgery, together with chemistry and botany, as for a man, ignorant of navigation and seamanship, to carry a vessel with safety into port.

Dr. Farrington was even more adamant:

> We include all symptoms that we can observe. Then what have we? A mass of symptoms seeming to have no connection at all. They come from a human organism that is all order and perfection, and all the parts of which work in perfect harmony. When even one of these parts is out of order, there must be a certain clue to string these effects together and picture a form of disease; and when you get this form of disease, what have you? A pathological state. I hope that no diploma will be granted to any man in this class who does not study pathology.

In selecting our remedy, he further urges us not to neglect the known effect of certain remedies on certain pathologies, like that of Thuja on warts.

And Nash, the great pioneer in homeopathy, offers his opinion in the debate between those who would choose remedies based on pathological signs and those who prescribe on symptoms alone:

> It requires us to be broadminded to be a good physician. It seems to me like folly to pose as either an exclusive pathologist or symptomatologist. Both pathology and symptomatology are valuable and inseparable, neither can be excluded. Pathology is what the physician can tell (sometimes); symptomatology is what the patient can tell.

In his famous *Repertory* even Kent gives us many rubrics which refer to pathology: abscess, cancer, caries, polyps, angina pectoris, bronchiectasis, inflammation, emphysema, etc. Many of our remedies are known for what Kent called *pathological generals*: for example, Causticum for its gradual paralysis, especially of single parts; Conium for its ascending paralysis; and Plumbum for paralysis with excessive and rapid emaciation.

However, the use of pathology in homeopathy should be *integrated, and not isolated*. Unfortunately in allopathic medical schools the subjects are often taught independently, without an integrated approach. Allopathic medicine may claim to treat the "biopsychosocial" aspects of the patient, but too often it relies entirely on pathology for diagnosis and prescription.

The Value of Pathology in a Homeopathic Prescription

Opinions on this point run the gamut in today's practice of homeopathy, from the lay prescribers who believe that a knowledge of pathology is unnecessary, to allopathic medical professionals relatively new to homeopathy who believe it to be all-important. As we have seen, Hahnemann himself used pathology as a part—admittedly a minor part—in determining the totality of the symptoms. Since each remedy has a typical sphere of action in certain tissues or organs of the body, pathology can sometimes be an aid to prescribing, especially when there is a paucity of symptoms which would normally take priority. For example, I had a patient with localized bronchopneumonia; there were no deciding symptoms, but auscultation and X-rays indicated that the lesion was confined to the left lower lobe. This directed my attention to Nat. sulph., which typically affects this portion of the lung. Further study of the case confirmed the choice, for the patient's mental, emotional and general symptoms did indeed fit Nat. sulph. The remedy—and note that it was not prescribed *on pathology alone*—acted promptly.

But more often, the symptoms leading to the selection of the remedy lie outside of the pathological state entirely. In fact the simillimum (closest match) is the remedy whose *general* symptoms (those affecting the entire person) best correspond to the general symptoms of the patient, even though the *particular* symptoms (those related to a part or an organ, even including the Chief Complaint) may not correspond or cannot be elicited. (More on general and particular symptoms in Chapter 9, Prescribing.) The ideal case would be one where both pathological and non-pathological signs and symptoms of disease and remedy correspond, but does not always occur. As a matter of fact, pathology and the allopathic diagnosis ideally should not influence the homeopath at all in the selection of the remedy, for we want to prescribe for the patient and not for his disease. In reality, when there is a paucity of symptoms, pathology may be a useful guide, as we have just seen.

There is a faction within homeopathy which does prescribe on the pathology of the case; this erroneous approach dates back to Hahnemann's contemporaries, including Dr. Richard Hughes, who was one of the first homeopaths in England and influential in its development there. These would-be pathologists consist of two groups—those who want to make homeopathic prescribing an easy routine affair and those who believe that pathology is the only true basis for a rational science of prescribing. Neither follow the basic laws of homeopathy. The latter may be attempting to defend homeopathy against the criticism leveled by allopathy, that we are not sufficiently grounded in pathology. But if a detailed knowledge of pathology is enough to cure chronic diseases, then surely allopathic medicine would have cured them by now. For we can grant that allopaths are masters of pathology, with all the diagnostic technology at their disposal; yet for all the lab tests, CAT scans, MRIs, and PET scans, allopathic medicine is unable to use this information to effect the cure of even one chronic disease. For example, the pathology of cystic fibrosis is well known in its effects on the pancreas, lungs, etc.; yet allopathic treatment can only palliate the suffering of such patients, not prevent the inevitable fatal outcome.

As the great homeopath Carroll Dunham wrote in his *Homeopathy, the Science of Therapeutics:*

> Physiology and pathology themselves teach us that the science of pathology can in no sense serve as a basis or foundation for the science of therapeutics. ... And those of our school who insist upon pathology as a *basis* of therapeutics, who look upon the single objective symptom and its nearest organic origin as the subject for treatment, and who deride the notion of prescribing upon the totality of the symptoms, and claim to be more than mere symptom coverers, in that they discover and aim to remove the *cause* of the disease—these colleagues are false in their pathology, according to the highest old-school authorities, as they are faithless to the doctrines, and impotent as to the successes of the founder of the homeopathic school.[1]

To the real homeopath every case of pneumonia is unique, though he knows they are all of an inflammatory nature and very similar in their gross features. But he is not satisfied with a superficial knowledge of these gross features; he dives deeper, and then he discovers how each case of pneumonia differs from every other. These minute differences are the true guides to the selection of the proper remedy. The simple, truthful language of the symptoms must never be translated in our repertories and materia medica into the jargon of pathological diagnosis. Pathology might indeed point to the fatty degeneration of the heart, or to a cirrhosis of the liver, or to some other arbitrary classification; nevertheless, the remedy indicated by the totality of the symptoms *will cure the patient whether or not it is known to cause* fatty degeneration or cirrhosis. A pathological basis for homeopathic prescriptions would exclude mental and subjective symptoms, often our surest guide to a proper selection even though they are pathologically insignificant.

Yet there are specific circumstances in which a knowledge of pathology can be helpful to the homeopath, as discussed in the next section.

How Modern Pathology Can Be Helpful to Homeopathy

Prognosis: We must be able to assess the progress of disease in our patients in order to give them an accurate prognosis without false promises. Sometimes pathology is so advanced that homeopathy can only palliate (see Chapter 16, Palliation and Incurable Diseases). Of course, as discussed in that chapter, patients termed incurable by allopathic medicine can sometimes be cured with the right potency selection if the patient's Vital Force is strong enough, but one should never promise this in advance. In cases where only palliation is possible, we should tell our patients so, reminding them that the remedy will enhance their quality of life and support their Vital Force, providing them with the best possible experience while their illness runs its course.

Indicating the active miasm: A knowledge of pathology can indicate to the homeopath the active miasm: for example, a patient with recurrent cystitis, vaginitis, and bronchitis who shows a recurrent tendency to form polyps and warts indicates an active sycotic miasm (see Chapter 21, Sycosis). Hydrocephalus, acromegaly, VSD or ASD and other congenital heart malformations all indicate the syphilitic miasm (see Chapter 22, Syphilis). So pathology helps us to arrive at the miasmatic diagnosis which is one of the main bases of our prescription in chronic diseases. It assists us in eradicating this deep-rooted state, thus effecting a true cure and not mere palliation.

Help in potency, dosage and remedy selection: As will be discussed in the next chapter on Potency, low potencies (LM and 6c) must be used where there is advanced pathology and the case is incurable (such as in advanced stages of diabetes, cancer, and TB). High potencies could cause a severe aggravation from which the patient's system could not rally. High potencies overwhelm the Vital Force, already struggling with the disease state, to such an extent that the Vital Force, in its weakened state, cannot rouse a secondary curative reaction.

Knowing pathology will prevent you from selecting deep-working remedies in conditions where the Vital Force is much diminished. For example, if you have a case of TB with cavernas or cavitations and weakening of blood vessels, a constitutional or miasmatic remedy (such as Silica, Lycopodium or Tuberculinum) could kill your patient. You *can not* give deep-acting remedies at this time. You must choose a remedy for the local lesion chosen by location, sensation, modification and concomitants, matching these indications with a *lesional* remedy like Sanguinaria, Drosera, or Millefolia. After the pathology has been palliated and the Vital Force has been strengthened by these lesional remedies, you can prescribe the deeper working remedy for a complete cure.

The repetition of dose depends also on the nature of the disease, as we will discuss further in Potencies (Chapter 5). A knowledge of pathology can help us determine the acuteness of the disease. The nature of acute diseases is very rapid and violent, requiring frequent repetition of doses. Here the action of the medicine is very rapidly exhausted from the system. But in chronic diseases the onset and progress of the disease is such that a single dose (especially of a high potency) takes a long time to completely exhaust its action, naturally requiring less frequent repetition.

Paucity of symptoms: Pathological signs like fissures, red orifices, warts, skin lesions, nail changes, and herpes blisters may be our only guide to the simillimum in certain cases with a paucity of mental and emotional symptoms, such as in treating comatose patients or animals.

This reminds me of a patient who came to see me after being treated unsuccessfully by several other homeopaths for a complaint of anal pain with a sensation "as if a splinter was imbedded," a classic symptom which normally would guide us to the correct remedy. But numerous remedies like Nitric acid, Ratanhia and Aesculus were tried in vain. But this case showed the importance of a thorough physical examination, even in homeopathy. When I examined the anus, there was actually a splinter present! No remedy was needed, only *tolle causam* (as Hahnemann said): sometimes you just have to "remove the cause."

Recognizing one-sided diseases: Pathology also plays a role when it *threatens the life* of the patient. When *advanced* pathology develops it often becomes the active layer of the case; it even "becomes" the case. For example, systemic lupus erythematosus (SLE) typically affects many different organs in the body, causing widespread symptoms which would all be included in the totality of symptoms. However, when SLE becomes far advanced, kidney failure can become dominant over all the other symptoms, and this life-threatening situation would have to be treated as top priority over all the other aspects of the disease. Hahnemann called such conditions *one-sided* diseases and related them to advanced stages of chronic miasms. When a local lesion becomes dominant it represses the system-wide symptoms and becomes the active layer of the illness, i.e. the one that needs to be treated first. The organic pathology of the case becomes advanced enough to control the symptomatology of the Vital Force and so it becomes the *lesional layer*. Hahnemann observes in the *Organon* that such lesions are usually caused by the chronic miasms (although a pathogen might also be involved).

In lesional prescribing the remedy is chosen by:
- the location and nature of the complaint
- sensations, discharges, color, etc.
- modalities
- concomitant symptoms such as generalities, aversions or desires and the *active* mental symptoms.

Once the one-sided symptoms were treated, Hahnemann said, the remedy would bring out repressed aspects and general symptoms so that a more constitutional remedy could be chosen to complete the cure on the vital level and prevent recurrence. In a one-sided lesion, the pathology takes on a life on its own and breaks away from the main constitutional state. By selecting a lesser known remedy, we bring this isolated aspect back to the rest of the syndrome or annihilate it so that only the constitutional symptoms remain.

Among the one-sided diseases, the so-called *local ailments* (i.e. ailments appearing on the surface, such as goiter) occupy an important place. A local ailment can be caused by an acute trauma, such as a burn, and can then have system-wide sequelae such as hypovolemic shock. According to von Boenninghausen, a grave local injury such as a large contusion, torn flesh or a third degree burn draws the whole body into a sympathetic response with symptoms such as high fevers. In such cases the whole organism demands dynamic assistance from a remedy in order to complete the work of healing. A knowledge of pathology would obviously be helpful in such cases.

Adapting to modern times: I have already emphasized the importance of prescribing for the patient, not the disease. However, in modern times one of the first questions a patient asks of his physician is, "What is my diagnosis, doctor?" (He may want to get on the Internet so that he can check up on your information!) We can't really say, as Hahnemann did, "The name of the disease is of no concern to you." By giving a disease name to the patient's condition we can more intelligently discuss its nature and prognosis. It is best to tell the patient that he has a "kind of depression" or a "kind of arthritis." Besides, in this litigious society, disease names are necessary for the physician's protection; and a diagnostic category is required for the patient to receive insurance reimbursement. A pathological diagnosis is also essential for death certificates or court testimony; you cannot say that the diagnosis was "never well since his divorce."

Management of the case: A knowledge of pathology is essential to determine the period of isolation, diet, rest, exercise and other measures involved in the general management of a case. A perfect prescription is more than just prescribing the simillimum. (See Perfect Prescription, Chapter 9). In case of infectious diseases the physician needs to know the incubation time, the method of transmission, and preventive measures. A knowledge of pathology may also help to make a correct second prescription (discussed in detail in Chapter 9, Prescribing).

We would prefer to rely on the observation power of the patient than on the objective information of pathology, but the modern patient is lulled into a passive reliance on the physician. So we have to depend more than we would like to on our own observations, which include physical assessment, diagnostic tests, and laboratory results. Physical findings could include a lessening of a liver enlargement or a decrease of crepitations in the lung. And if the laboratory tests do improve after a while under your treatment, like blood glucose in diabetes for example, while the patient's condition remains stable, then we know that we should not change the remedy.

Documenting the effectiveness of homeopathy: For many years homeopathy has gained adherents, both lay and professional, through numerous case reports of remarkable cures. While most of these reports were convincing, it must be conceded that many could not bear the light of modern scientific scrutiny due to inadequate documentation. This issue is of secondary importance to the Hahnemannian homeopath, who focuses on curing individual patients rather than diagnostic categories.

However, we now need to demonstrate the value of homeopathy to the scientific community at large. It is not enough for a homeopath to declare that she has cured an asthma case unless she can document both the diagnosis and the cure with pulmonary function tests, lab tests, objective findings in auscultation, X-rays, etc. Without such pathological evidence her cure will not be accepted and homeopathy will lose this opportunity to advance its claims. If homeopathy is to take its rightful place in modern medical practice, we must document our clinical successes and present them in series of hundreds of cases and not as isolated scattered examples. Unfortunately, we don't have homeopathic hospitals to do this kind of work, so the task is up to individual physicians to document each case with all the modern diagnostic technology possible. Each of us must document our clinical successes with pathological findings such as complete analyses of blood and urine, culture-and-sensitivities, X-rays and MRIs. Then we can substantiate our claims. Forward-looking members of the scientific community are reaching out for confirmation of anecdotal cases; it is up to us to meet them more than halfway and convince them of the truth of our claims.

The value of allopathy: There are times when emergencies call for allopathic palliative and even life-saving measures. As Hahnemann said in a note to Aphorism 67:

> Palliatives or antagonistic treatments are only justified in highly urgent cases, in sudden accidents to previously healthy people where danger to life and imminent death permit no time for a homeopathic helping-means to act—not hours, quarter-hours or even minutes. Examples include cases of asphyxiation, apparent death by lightning, suffocation, freezing, drowning, etc. Only in such cases is it permissible and expedient …

To this category we might add major organ failures, antidotes to poisons, overdose, etc. Hahnemann himself approved of allopathic treatment in these drug instances.

Chapter Five

Potencies

The Dilemma about Potencies

The question of potency selection has always been controversial. Students of homeopathy learn very quickly never to enter into an argument about potencies, for this topic will cause more feathers to fly and engender more ill-will than any other subject. But there must be some guidelines for the student. Those in this chapter are based on my readings in the old masters and confirmed by my experience. I was fortunate enough to receive an early introduction to the LM potencies, which are at once the gentlest and most powerful of potencies, as explained in detail in the next chapter. The LM potencies are seldom used outside of India, and through this book I hope to share with my professional colleagues my experience with LMs based on treating thousands of patients.

Some homeopaths claim that if mental symptoms are outspoken, high potencies should always be chosen. Others believe one should always start with low potencies, with some using 6c potencies throughout chronic treatment. Still others believe that a 10M is necessary to cover the totality of a chronic case. Yet others choose the potency based on their confidence in the remedy; the more sure they are of the simillimum, the higher the potency they use. Each of these approaches is based on a single concept rather than on Hahnemann's three-part guideline for potency selection: an observation of the *nature of the disease* (acute or chronic), the *nature of the patient,* and the *nature of the remedy.*

Many modern homeopaths who recommend high potencies such as 1M, 10M, even CM (100,000c) believe that Hahnemann did not recommend them because he never used potencies above 30c. But according to his second wife, Mélanie, Hahnemann experimented with all potencies from 3c to 1M when he thought they were warranted:

> Your inquiry note whether Hahnemann altered his views about potencies in the last period of his life, and whether he made use of high potencies, I can answer this in

this way: Hahnemann used all degrees of dilution, low as well as high, as the individual case required. I saw him give the third trituration, but I also know that he used the 200th or even the 1000th potency, whenever necessary.[1]

Von Boenninghausen confirms this in his *Lesser Writings:*

> In direct contradiction that Hahnemann did not use higher potencies than 30c, I can demonstrate by his letters which I have carefully preserved, that, especially in the last years of his life, he was most zealous and insistent in carrying on the dynamizations higher and higher and to diminish more the materiality of the dose.[2]

Dr. Richard Haehl, who wrote the best biography of Hahnemann, tells us that the most common potencies he used were from 3c to 60c (in addition to LMs, which were still unknown when Haehl was writing). The first time Hahnemann used 60c was in 1825, according to Haehl. But he continued to recommend limiting the potency to 30c: "I do not approve of you potentizing medicines higher than 30c. There must be a limit to the matter, it can not go on indefinitely."[3] The real reason for this limit was that his science was still evolving and still under attack. He wanted all homeopaths to be uniform in the beginning.

However, in examining Hahnemann's case books of his last three years in practice, I have found that Hahnemann frequently used potencies up to 200c. Rima Handley, in her account of Hahnemann's last years based on examining all his Paris case books, explains:

> Around [1838] he began to use a higher range of centesimal potencies ... up to 200c. ... By 1838 ... two great experimenters, Korsakoff and Jenichen, had individually succeeded in producing potencies attenuated up to 100c and 1500c (even higher later). This was way beyond the lower potencies with which Hahnemann had been content for so long. However, although he had apparently tried these very high potencies, he was uneasy with them, probably because he had not made them himself and was not therefore quite sure how they had been prepared. When he began to use higher potencies on a regular basis he therefore restricted himself to those lower than 200c, which he was able to prepare himself, by hand. He used these increasingly often during his time in Paris.[4]

In Hahnemann's day, Korsakoff and Jenichen were the only ones making high potencies, succussing by hand beyond 10M. Both of them were laymen, and at first Hahnemann did not have confidence in their remedies. But Jenichen finally succeeded in sending some of his potencies to Hahnemann through his friend Gross, who was one of Hahnemann's first students. Hahnemann's good results led him to change his mind (temporarily) about the higher potencies; he experimented with them until about 1833, when the aggravations they caused led him to seek a gentler method.

Some homeopaths believe that there *needs* to be an aggravation in order to procure a healing (and many patients think so). Nothing could be further from the truth. Some homeopaths feel that an aggravation lasting several months is acceptable. How does this follow Hahnemann's concept of a gentle cure, which he emphasized by placing it right at the beginning of the *Organon*? Even Kent gave up the exclusive use of high potencies as causing too many strong aggravations and introduced instead the practice of moving upward through the potencies, starting relatively low at a 200c. Practitioners who open a chronic case with a high potency such as 10M attribute to Kent the belief that an aggravation is necessary for good results. But Kent himself states in his *Lesser Writings*:

> There is a wonderful latitude between the tincture and the CM potencies *[remember that he did not know about LM potencies]* and in my judgment the selection of the best potency is a matter of *experience* and *observation* and not a matter of law. The indiscriminate use of one potency is very likely to bring reproach upon our art. They all have their place. Keep the *mild* potency as long as it works. It is not well to jump degrees. The best action is the slight aggravation, the *ideal* one is the one that does *not* aggravate but ameliorate. We do *not* seek to produce an aggravation, that is not the best, not the longest curative effect. You encourage the patient to become oversensitive by using the highest potencies instead of going low to begin again. Whatever potency a physician uses, that one potency is *not* sufficient for *chronic* diseases. It will generally do for *acute* diseases. As a rule two doses in the same plane give the best result. After long observation I have settled on the series of degrees as of 30c, 200c, 1M, 10M, 50M, CM, DM and MM. It is not uncommon that the patient continues to improve *on each potency* for 3 to 4 months.[5]

Some modern-day homeopaths wish they had a 500c available. But here too we can learn from Kent who used all the in-between potencies. He observed for instance that "after a good action of 200c, after waiting till it was no longer active, although I gave the 300c, 500c and 800c, the 1M acted much more strongly and the 300 and 500 usually failed. The same with 80M, 60M, etc." So with his experience he settled on the above sequence. On the other hand, there are numerous examples in old journals of experienced homeopathic prescribers using unusual potencies like 2M and 45M with great success.

High-potency prescribers (or "Kentians", a term used in this book for practitioners who open with a high centesimal potency, administer a single dose, and wait several weeks or months before giving another dose) should heed Kent's own words. An aggravation occurs when the remedy is so strong that it represses the secondary curative response from the Vital

Force, as though it has knocked down or numbed the Vital Force which can then only recuperate sluggishly, if at all. This will obviously slow down the cure. Instead the choice of potency should take into account the three factors dictated by Hahnemann: the patient's *constitutional* sensitivity, the *nature of the disease* and the *nature of the remedy.* In Aphorism 281, Hahnemann also gives us precise guidelines for assessing the sensitivity of the patient: it can be rated on a scale of 1 to 1000. This means a potency which would not affect a *hyposensitive* (such as a Calcarea) will cause tremendous aggravations in a *hypersensitive* (such as Phosphorus). Thus high potencies may work well in relatively non-sensitive patients with a strong Vital Force, but they are dangerous to use across the board, as will be discussed later in this chapter under Sensitivity.

Where does this discord about potency come from? Studying Hahnemann's work in its historical context may provide a deeper understanding which may reunite us as homeopaths.

History of the *Organon* Explains Choice of Potency

The *Organon* went through six different revisions from 1810 to 1843, the sixth being completed just before Hahnemann's death. Homeopaths who call themselves "classical" all practice according to the *Organon*, but differences have arisen because we practice by different versions of it. In fact most homeopaths practice according to the principles of the *4th edition* (except that the potencies—200c and up—are based on the 5th edition). The 6th edition was not published until 1920, with Boericke's English translation appearing a year later. Each of these versions was the result of ceaseless research on Hahnemann's part, based on his practice. He was constantly trying new methods and replacing earlier ones in his tireless search, lasting many decades, for the "rapid, gentle and permanent cure" for his patients. This is the reason why so many think that Hahnemann's teachings are contradictory and that he did not practice what he taught. Nothing is further from the truth! All this bewilderment can be overcome by examining the facts.

We can honestly state that the publication of the 4th edition of the *Organon* in 1828 was the turning point for the history of homeopathy, since it is the basis for most classical homeopathy worldwide today. In 1828 Hahnemann also published his *Chronic Diseases* which included his theory of *miasms*, which was too farfetched for most homeopaths, both Hahnemann's contemporaries and our own. Nevertheless, Hahnemann's most loyal students followed him in his teachings.

In the 4th edition, Hahnemann introduced the use of a single dose of one poppyseed globule of the remedy and taught that as long as symptoms continued to improve, no repetition of the remedy was allowed. Repetition was only done when there was a relapse of symptoms (Aphorisms 242 and 245 of the 4th edition). It was the "wait and watch" method of case management. At that time Hahnemann believed that premature renewal of the dose would lead to a relapse, or that new symptoms of the remedy would be added to the symptoms of the disease, confusing the case. It is easy for us to see that most homeopaths worldwide still practice according to the "wait and watch" method. At this point Hahnemann's disciples were experimenting with high potencies, but Hahnemann himself cautioned against them and limited his potency to a 30c.

High Potencies Introduced

In the 5th edition (1833), followed by the second edition of *Chronic Diseases,* Hahnemann introduced important changes. The 5th edition is called the "Limit Breaker." After much consideration, Hahnemann removed the limit of 30c and supported the use of high potencies on the advice of his first disciples, Drs. Gross and Stapf. But Hahnemann the master pharmacist was careful as to how these high potencies were made. One of his disciples was Julius Caspar Jenichen, Master of Horse for the Duke of Gotha, and recruited by Gross to make the potencies. He was a man of tremendous physical strength. So forceful were his successions that it was said the remedy vials would ring like a bell or jingle like coins as he shook them in mid-air. He worked at his task from 10 p.m. till 3 a.m., keeping himself awake by drinking cold black coffee and noting the time he had created his new potency. Jenichen's high potencies long remained controversial, partly because he did not communicate with Hahnemann about how he was preparing them.

This changed in 1846 when Jenichen wrote to Dr. Staph, one of Hahnemann's most trusted first students: "The words of our Gross: Where is the limit? We can only be enlightened about this by experiment." Jenichen writes about Arsenicum 8000c which was "made by the faithful power of my arm and executed by 165,000 strong strokes." He says it was born at 2:30 a.m. on January 1, 1846:

> And I am very eager to know if this baby will die soon or whether it will reach an age of centuries. The experiment must decide. This triumph I hope does not belong to me but to Hering: "Every year higher!"[6]

Von Boenninghausen commented that he had confidence in Jenichen's potencies because the latter was well known to have the unusual strength and perseverance required to make them according to the Master's strict instructions. Jenichen further says that he wished

> that the preparation of these high potencies would not take so much time; my enthusiasm would give out on me a long time if it was not for the knowledge that I am

> making medicinal preparations for the whole sick world and knowing that no other person can make these potencies; that is what keeps me going and keeps up my courage and continually renews my bodily powers; I do not therefore deserve any particular praise for I do nothing but my duty.[7]

Von Boenninghausen further commented that it did not matter whether Jenichen followed Korsakoff's method (in which the contents of the vial are emptied out between successive potencies and 99 drops of water added to the liquid which adheres to the vial) instead of the more expensive method in which a new vial with alcohol is used at each step. Based on his own clinical experience, von Boenninghausen said that remedies made by Korsakoff's and Jenichen's method were acceptable. He expressed regrets that at that time (1846) the two doctors who had used high potencies for a long time, Gross and Stapf, were unable to try the new potencies because one had passed away and the other was no longer practicing. Von Boenninghausen concluded that many years would be required to fully confirm the value of Jenichen's potencies.

Administration of the Remedy in Water and Repetition of the Dose

Besides the use of higher potencies, other important changes were introduced in the 5th edition: *frequent repetition* of the remedy and administration of *solutions in water* instead of the dry dose. Hahnemann begins his exposition of the new method by describing a situation in which it would *not* be appropriate (Aphorism 245, 5th edition):

> Every perceptible progressive and *strikingly increasing amelioration* in an acute or chronic disease is a condition which, as long as it lasts, completely precludes every repetition of the administration of any medicine whatsoever, because all the good the medicine taken continues to effect is now hastening toward its completion. Every new dose of the medicine would in this case disturb the work of amelioration.

Notice the word *strikingly*. Unfortunately this response does not happen as often as we would hope. What should we do when there is only slow movement in a case? Again Hahnemann guides us in Aphorism 246:

> On the other hand, the *slowly progressive amelioration* consequent on a very minute dose, whose selection has been accurately homeopathic, sometimes accomplishes all the good the remedy in question is capable of performing in a period of forty, fifty days. This is however rarely the case, and besides it must be a matter of great importance to the physician as well as the patient that were it possible, this period should be

diminished to one half, one quarter, and even still less. Firstly, the remedy has to be chosen by the totality of the symptoms. Secondly, the remedy is given in the minutest dose so as not to over-excite the vital force. Thirdly, the remedy must be repeated at *suitable intervals to speed the cure,* if necessarily, but without producing aggravations.

It is the third statement ("the remedy must be repeated at *suitable* intervals to speed the cure") that draws our attention, since it encourages us for the first time to repeat the doses of the remedy as much as needed to speed up the healing of the patient. In fact Hahnemann now had an entirely new concept of what was "suitable" in remedy repetition: whereas before he might wait several weeks or even months for the action of the remedy to be used up, in the 5th edition he was thinking in terms of daily, or every-other-day, repetition of the remedy.

A third change in the 5th edition was the use of the medicinal *solution* (dissolving the remedy in water). In *Chronic Diseases,* Hahnemann wrote:

> Experience has shown me that it is most useful in diseases of any magnitude to give to the patient the powerful homeopathic pellet *only in solution* and this solution in divided doses. In this case we give the medicine, dissolved in seven [3.5 oz] or twenty tablespoons [10 oz.] of water in acute and subacute diseases, every hour or every half an hour, a tablespoon at a time, or with weak persons or children, only a teaspoon may be given as a dose. In *chronic diseases* I have found it best to give a dose of the suitable remedy at least every two days, more usually every day.[8]

In Bradford's *Life and Letters of Hahnemann,* Hahnemann states:

> I have been able to administer Sulphur daily for months at a time with the most astonishingly good effects, as long as they continued to do good.[9]

Contrary to the practice of the many "Kentian" prescribers who still do not put remedies in water, Kent himself advocated giving the remedy in water and in divided doses as he said, "this has at times been favored over the single dry dose." He said further that "this is open for discussion, requiring the testimony of the many, not the few, to give it weight." Of course many great homeopaths did in fact give remedies in water later, their results bearing out Hahnemann's recommendations.

We can conclude that there were three major changes made in the 5th edition of the *Organon*: the use of potencies higher than 30c, repetition of the dose in shorter intervals to speed up the healing, and the administration of the remedy in water. Again, Hahnemann was guided in these changes by his Aphorism 2 of the *Organon*: he was seeking a rapid, gentle and permanent cure, without aggravations.

The 6th Edition of the Organon and LM Potencies

In his last edition (the 6th), Hahnemann rejected "everything" he had written in the 5th edition and told his followers he had now "found his most perfect method," or the LM method (described in detail in the next chapter). In fact, the last 12 years of his life were dedicated to perfecting this method. In a footnote to Aphorism 246 of the 6th edition, Hahnemann explained that with each edition of the book he had presented the best method he knew up to that point, but that his continual experiments forced him in all honesty to replace his earlier methods with the new ones:

> What I said ... in the fifth edition ... was all that my experience allowed me to say at the time. It was written with the purpose of preventing these adverse reactions of the life principle. However, during the last four to five years, all such difficulties have been fully lifted through the modifications I have made since then, resulting in my new, perfected procedure [for fifty-millesimal potency medicines]. The same well-chosen medicine can now be given daily, even for months *when necessary*.

LM potencies, the "forgotten treasure" of the 6th edition (as Pierre Schmidt termed them),[10] require more explanation; at this point perhaps only 10% of practicing homeopaths in the world know how to use LMs, and most of them are in India. Since the entire next chapter is dedicated to this greatest treasure of homeopathy, I want to present now the advantages and disadvantages of the high potencies or "Kentian" potencies.

Advantages of High Potencies

For a high potency prescriber, potencies for chronic cases start at 200c, followed by 1M, 10M, etc. This is an easy method for the practitioner. He sends the patient home with a single dose of one remedy or even gives it right in the office. Compliance is 100%, no mistakes are made. He warns the patient about the most likely aggravations and tells the patient to call back in another month or so. That means fewer phone calls for the physician. If the patient phones because of an aggravation all he has to say is that it is a good sign, that he wanted to see an aggravation, that he does not know how long the aggravation will last, and that the patient should call back in a month.

The advantages for the patient include compliance and simplicity of taking the remedy, since the practitioner himself can dose the patient right in the office. However, the greatest advantage goes to the practitioner, who has fewer calls. He knows that a single dose of 200c will act for at least three weeks, and he does not have to intervene before that (again, this is according to the 4th edition, not the 5th or 6th edition of the *Organon*). In the 6th edition,

Hahnemann himself calls this method "barbaric" as it certainly does not follow his ideal of a "gentle cure." I believe that the main reason most current practitioners still use this method is the unfortunate misperceptions and misinformation about the LM method. I have heard presenters at conferences give out such misinformation: for example that LMs suppress or cause aggravations, or that LMs are unwieldy and take too much time to master and administer. In fact LMs are *easier* to work with than centesimals because the practitioner rarely has to wrestle with the knotty question of when and whether to repeat the remedy. LMs provide much greater clarity at every step of the way.

Another advantage of high potencies is that the patient himself will not willingly or inadvertently overdose himself and bring on an aggravation by taking too much of the remedy. In a way I agree with this concern, and although I generally prefer LM potencies, there are situations in which I would give the patient a single dose of 200c or 1M right in the office. I would do this especially if I see that the patient is so accustomed to taking a drug every day that he will have difficulty following the LM method (which requires adjusting the frequency to every other day, or every third day, and then only as needed as the remedy takes effect). I would give such a patient plenty of Sac. lac. (placebo) and let him take a daily dose.

Elderly patients like taking a remedy every day because it mirrors allopathic medications. To my own despair, even when I told this kind of patient to stop the LM or 6c dose, they refused to do so because they felt "so good" with the remedy and were convinced they needed it every day. As a result, they brought on an aggravation, sometimes discouraging them to the point of abandoning the therapy. I will never forget the little Italian gentleman in his 70s who consulted for vertigo. He was so happy the remedy worked that he insisted on continuing to take it. *"Dottore, dottore!"* he would say. "I feel *so good,* why stop?" I thought I had explained to him the importance of stopping, but he didn't listen, and of course his vertigo came back and was much more difficult to treat this time. I wish now that I had just given him Sac. lac. After a few such experiences I began using high potencies in these cases; at least the practitioner and not the confused patient controls when the remedy is repeated.

Another possible advantage of high-potency prescribing applies more to the beginner than to the experienced homeopath: there is a great temptation to give up on a remedy too soon, from lack of confidence, or upon the insistence of the patient who likes to see rapid changes. The tendency is to change the remedy too frequently, at a time when it would be most disastrous to do so. For instance, with a 1M potency, unless the remedy is canceled, we should not consider changing the remedy for the next six weeks. However, an experienced prescriber will not fall into this trap. An experienced LM prescriber can see patients more frequently, however, and take advantage of the LMs' power to cure in about a third of the time (as Hahnemann said they would, and as my experience of using both centesimals and LMs has confirmed).

Disadvantages of High Potencies

Disadvantages of high potencies can be numerous, beginning with the ever-present aggravation. "This is excellent," some homeopaths will say, "because it shows we selected the right remedy," since it is a *similar* homeopathic aggravation, i.e. the existing symptoms occur in a higher intensity. But with LM potencies there are *many* ways to know whether we have chosen the right remedy, without an aggravation and usually within a few days of the first dose. The guidelines are detailed in the next chapter.

Although an immediate aggravation after the administration of the remedy can occur with low potencies, there is a great difference in the *intensity* of the aggravation. The aggravation after a high potency can be so *acute* that it lands the patient in the hospital (in the case of asthma, for example). Or the aggravation can be *long-lasting* (up to several months or more, based on reports from well-known centesimal prescribers). Either way, the patient is likely to give up on homeopathy forever.

With low potencies, the aggravation will rarely last longer than a few hours, a day or two at the most, if the remedy intake is stopped the moment the aggravation appears. (The aggravation is also usually *milder* than with high potencies.) This is especially important for the hypersensitives, who tend to react so easily to the remedies. Homeopaths show a real lack of compassion for their patients if they fail to individualize the potency as well as the remedy, and do not take into account their patients' sensitivity level (see the guidelines later in this chapter). This is, after all, one of Hahnemann's basic principles of homeopathy.

This continued long-lasting similar aggravation from a too-high potency (of even the well-chosen remedy) is nothing to pass over lightly. Hahnemann warns us that this will even inhibit the cure and—what is even worse—will make the disease picture more complex as this remedy will now superimpose other symptoms onto the natural disease:

> But if these aggravated original symptoms appear in subsequent days still of the same strength as at the beginning, it is a sign that the dose ... was too large, and it is to be apprehended that no cure will be effected by it; because the medicine in so large a dose is able to establish a disease, which in some aspects, indeed, is similar to it. ... [However] the medicine in its present intensity unfolds also its other symptoms which annul the similarity; it produces a dissimilar chronic disease instead of the former, and indeed, a more severe and troublesome one, without thereby extinguishing the old original one. ... I have myself experienced this accident, which is very obstructive to a cure and cannot be avoided too carefully.[11]

Hahnemann considered selection of a too high potency one of the three worst mistakes of the homeopath, the other two being the incorrect choice of remedy and the too hasty repetition of the dose (at least at the time of the 4th edition).

Thus the practitioner should not send his patients into the storm of an aggravation without considering the consequences. Kent himself said: "When the dose is too large to cure, man receives it as a sickness." This should be a caution to those who prescribe high potencies indiscriminately, no matter what the sensitivity of the patient is.

There is another problem with Kentian prescribing: the *fear of canceling* the remedy. Because such prescribers are so afraid that their one-time single dose will be canceled by external factors such as camphor, mint, other medications, coffee, etc., they absolutely forbid the patient to use any of these substances. Some Kentian prescribers give their patients a full-page list of items to avoid, including such modern commonplaces as electric blankets and dental treatments. They are so rigid in their rules that they lose many patients right from the onset of treatment. Take a patient with rheumatoid arthritis or asthma, for instance. Very often these people are on high doses of steroids and other suppressive medications. Some Kentians refuse to treat these patients until they stop their medications. This is often impossible, and when the patient stops her allopathic drugs, she may land in the hospital with an acute attack.

Some Kentians go even further and deny the patient the benefit of other *complementary therapies* (such as acupuncture, Reiki, chiropractic adjustments, Bach flower remedies, hypnosis, yoga, etc.). But acupuncture follows the same laws of healing as homeopathy, and the integration of these two powerful, energetic medicines is beneficial to the patient, not harmful. Some homeopaths claim that Hahnemann was opposed to acupuncture; there is a brief mention in the introduction to the *Organon* as part of a list of suppressive allopathic treatments. Perhaps Hahnemann was misinformed (acupuncture follows Hering's Laws just as homeopathy does) or more likely, acupuncture was being badly practiced in his day (see Appendix 5 on Traditional Chinese Medicine). We know he was in favor of other therapies such as magnetism and Mesmerism which were based on vibrational energies just as acupuncture is. I have treated thousands of patients with homeopathy and acupuncture simultaneously, and I have found that the patient benefitted when treated in combination. Acupuncture or chiropractic done badly, or not in harmony with the laws of healing, *can* interfere with chronic homeopathic treatment, just as superficial, symptomatic homeopathic prescribing can interfere.

Of course it is wise and logical that the patient should not start two different modalities *at the same time*. Whatever reaction the patient would have, good or bad, the homeopath would not know what did what. However, if the patient starts improving on the homeopathic remedy, I might suggest to the patient to stop the acupuncture treatments. Usually the patient does not need any prodding in that direction since it saves him time and money. It is *possible* that an alternative treatment can cancel the remedy (I have seen this happen with an *inappro-*

priate treatment by an acupuncturist or chiropractor which interferes with the action of the remedy by confusing and weakening the Vital Force.) Again, this is a problem for the single dose, wait-and-watch prescriber, not the LM prescriber, since LMs are given daily. Of course, don't let an acupuncturist or chiropractor intervene to treat the return of an old symptom (Hering's Law). A wrong treatment will disrupt the case, a risk you cannot take. And if the patient is worse after a complementary treatment modality, advise the patient not to repeat it. Concentrated *vitamin supplements,* especially multivitamins and B complex vitamins, can increase the energy of the patient and cover up symptoms which would otherwise spontaneously develop, thus making case management more difficult. Therefore the patient should not *start* taking these vitamins at the same time as taking a remedy.

Hahnemann, the first promoter of sanitation, public health measures and preventive medicine in the modern era, dedicated the last five aphorisms of the *Organon* to different complementary therapies including magnets, massage, hydrotherapy, electricity and Mesmerism, of which Hahnemann was a practitioner. Mesmerism uses a combination of hypnosis, magnetic healing with hands, polarity therapy, and psychic healing (Aphorisms 288 and 289). These techniques enhance the Vital Force, which is why we use them.

I might add that psychotherapy as a complementary therapy is of interest in terms of homeopathy's capacity to act as a catalyst and speed the therapy along; in other words, homeopathy has more to offer to psychotherapy than the other way around. Patients who are already in psychotherapy when beginning homeopathic treatment often report that they are more in touch with their emotions and more able to express them. The only limitation I have seen with psychotherapy is that its practitioners are not trained to recognize the physical symptoms of emotional traumas like grief, as homeopaths are; they may prematurely declare the patient healed when only the mental/emotional picture is cleared. In fact I have had psychotherapists come to me as patients claiming that their grief was resolved, while their physical symptoms were clearly manifesting unresolved grief.

In reality, no matter how strict Kentian prescribers are in telling their patients to avoid mint, coffee, black tea, and other medications or treatment modalities, these interfering factors are rarely severe enough to stop the action of the *correct* remedy. If they interfere at all, this will be clear from the weak reaction to the remedy: the patient will show only slight improvement across the board. If this seems to be the case then the interfering substance should of course be removed. If patients can't stop drinking coffee immediately, let them take the remedy *after* the intake of coffee, not before, as there is much less chance that the remedy will be canceled. In practice I have seen that a remedy can be canceled by coffee, but this is not always the case. Hahnemann, Kent, and von Boenninghausen describe cases in which they strongly prohibited coffee only to see that months later, the remedy worked, while the patient confessed he never stopped drinking the coffee. It amazes me that LM potencies are not canceled even by such strong suppressive forces as radiation and chemotherapy, so in reality, I am not too worried about coffee cancelling the remedy. However, I do consider coffee an addictive drug with a harmful effect on the whole body, and for that reason alone I try to wean patients off coffee.

Another difficulty in high potency prescribing, if not the greatest obstacle, is the question with which our famous predecessors like Kent and Lippe grappled: when to repeat the dose? The easy answer is "when the effect of the remedy has ceased," but in practice this point is not so easy to determine. The reaction of the Vital Force tends to go in waves, like the ripples from a pebble dropped in a pond. There is an initial "splash" (the immediate, visible effect of the remedy on the Vital Force), then a period of calm, then there may be repeated ripples of weaker action trailing off apparently indefinitely. There may be an initial improvement from the remedy, then a plateau, then a small further improvement, and another plateau followed by an even slighter improvement … at what point has the remedy stopped working? Because it is difficult to tell, and because the high-potency prescriber fears repeating the remedy too soon lest she cause an aggravation and spoil the case, she often waits too long to repeat the remedy.

The result is needless suffering for the patient and delay of the cure. Kent advocated being on the safe side with high potencies, so "waiting" is the only safe thing to do. He even describes cases in which the finest curative action of the remedy did not even *begin* until two months after the administration of the single dose. Thus the practitioner must wait months before even determining whether or not his remedy has worked; if it appears not to work, was it the wrong remedy, or was it antidoted by any one of a dozen common substances? Since assessing the action of each dose can take several months, the entire course of treatment is of necessity slow. Hahnemann found it too slow two hundred years ago, which was one factor impelling him to develop LM potencies with their rapid action. How much more difficult is this type of wait-and-watch prescribing in modern times, with patients expecting the rapid action they have become accustomed to from allopathic drugs, and threatening to give up on homeopathy if they do not see speedy improvement.

Guidelines for Potency Selection

As we have mentioned at the beginning of this chapter, the three major indications for the choice of a potency are the *sensitivity of the patient, the nature of the disease* and *the nature of the remedy*. In order to understand sensitivity, we must begin by explaining terms such as susceptibility and idiosyncracy, as they are different expressions of sensitivity.

Susceptibility (Predisposition) and Idiosyncrasy: *Webster's* defines *susceptibility* as "having the capacities for feeling or emotional excitement, capacity for receiving impressions; a constitution of the body which disposes it to the action of disease under the application of an exciting cause" and *susceptible* as "responsive to any stimulus or having a sensitive nature." This susceptibility is greatly modified through sickness, environment, emotions, occupation, lifestyle, etc. We all might get sick to some extent when exposed to a severe northeast wind, but when someone gets sick from the *slightest draft,* then he must be especially susceptible to exposure to wind. So that person easily becomes sick with diseases (like tonsillitis, otitis, and fevers) caused by the factor to which he is especially susceptible, in this case wind. Further, everyone seems to have a weak spot in the body, and whatever acts unfavorably upon the person goes at once to that locality. For instance, among people with a susceptibility to wind, one may get laryngitis, another pneumonia, and another a runny nose.

We can use this concept of susceptibility to some degree in selecting our potency. The general rule is: The greater the susceptibility, the lower should be the potency. Of course we do not have a lab test or other objective measure of susceptibility. Yet there are certain rules of thumb we can follow. The susceptibility of children is usually lower than that of adults because of their intact Vital Force. (The only reason children catch more infectious illnesses than adults is that their natural immunity is being developed through these exposures. Adults who have never been exposed are extremely susceptible, like the native Hawaiians who were decimated by a measles epidemic brought by the first white traders.) So high potencies are to be preferred in children (unless they are suffering from advanced pathology, a situation which demands low potencies). The susceptibility of a patient with chronic disease gradually increases as their chronic suffering weakens their Vital Force; thus in those cases we must start with low potencies.

In Western medicine we use the term *idiosyncrasy* for a special hypersensitive state always present in a particular patient: "a peculiarity of the constitution, in which one person is affected by an agent, which in numerous others would not produce any effect." For example certain foods cause urticaria in particular people—strawberries may cause it in one person, while shellfish cause it in another. One person may suffer from unbearable travel sickness, another from headaches or neuralgic pains at the approach of a storm. One patient craves fresh air and must have all the windows open, while another must be sheltered from the slightest draft. Looking at all these examples, it seems that many people have an idiosyncrasy or peculiarity to something.

An idiosyncrasy can even be produced by a remedy, because the remedy induces a state of susceptibility: for example, the provers of Thuja may get diarrhea from onions, while Lycopodium provers cannot eat oysters. These particular idiosyncrasies have also been cured by the corresponding remedies. This marked idiosyncrasy is not always observed with the *crude* material: for instance crude salt will not produce the slightest mental/emotional disturbance, but high potencies (Nat. mur.) can produce severe symptoms in those susceptible to it.

Another interesting example of this idiosyncrasy is that a patient is rendered more sensitive to Rhus tox. after once suffering from poison ivy. But Rhus tox. in homeopathic doses will cure the patient of his sensitivity to poison ivy, whether before or after he suffers from it. It is well understood that the patient is always *highly sensitive to his needed remedy*. We can conclude that a person who has an idiosyncrasy is not healthy; in other words, he needs the action of the similar remedy for the removal of that peculiar state of the constitution.

Sensitivity Guidelines: All individuals do not have the same sensitivity, even if their Vital Force is normal. The real yardstick for the physician to measure the patient's sensitivity is her reaction to the first dose. In Aphorism 281 Hahnemann has already told us 150 years ago how to deal with different sensitivities in patients:

> *[Doses]* should be heightened far less and more slowly with patients in whom one perceives a considerable excitability than with the more unreceptive patients, with whom one can raise the dose more rapidly. There are patients whose uncommon excitability is one thousand times greater than that of the most unreceptive ones.

This paragraph gives us a good idea about the vast differences of individuals to the action of remedies. A *hypo*sensitive patient with a sensitivity rating of 1 would probably not even feel a dose which could cause a life-threatening aggravation in a *hyper*sensitive with a rating of 1000.

Constitutional Sensitivity: Kent noticed that country people could stand more frequent repetition of a homeopathic remedy as well as of allopathic medicine. So homeopaths practicing in the country did not see the sharp aggravations seen in city people (more about this in the next chapter, LM Potencies and in Chapter 15, Management of the Case). The following are examples of specific innate constitutional types corresponding to each of the three sensitivity types:

Constitutions of high sensitivity: People born with the innate constitution Phosphorus or born in an Arsenicum state tend to be highly reactive, whether to emotions, atmospheric conditions, or environmental toxins. They tend to be nervous individuals (they have a *nervous-sanguine temperament),* and may be restless, sympathetic, easily excited, worried and/or obsessive-compulsive. They may be sensitive to perfumes, gasoline, cigarette smoke, etc. Some even react to the slightest amount of vitamins, herbs, remedies, and drugs. Some unfortunate souls have Multiple Chemical Sensitivity and have become "universal reactors": the world becomes a hostile environment for them because they react to everything in it (paint, carpet, fabric, fumes, etc.). Their senses are hyperacute and their symptoms appear and change quickly. Fortunately they can be successfully treated with homeopathy. However, when seeing such a patient for the first time, the homeopath must carefully assess her sensitivity. (For questions to use in assessing sensitivity, see the sample intake form in Appendix 1.)

In addition to the innate constitution, the patient's current state of health can also affect the sensitivity. For example, we have to expect increased sensitivity in cases of *advanced tissue pathology, weakened vitality* (special care must always be taken with the *elderly*), and a history of *prolonged drug use* or drug reactions. The remedies associated with *constitutional* hypersensitivity can also be associated with a *temporary* hypersensitivity in patients who need them *therapeutically*. For example, a Sulphur patient, not normally hypersensitive, can become hypersensitive if he needs Arsenicum to cure his traveler's diarrhea. (Note that this principle does not work in reverse: a patient with a hypersensitive constitution does not become less sensitive when needing a "less-sensitive" remedy like Calcarea, because illness always acts to weaken the Vital Force and make the patient more sensitive, if anything.)

When treating a hypersensitive patient, use lower potencies (LM or 6c) and repeat infrequently. Use one pellet of a dry centesimal potency first as a test dose (even when intending to continue with LMs). When using the LM method we will use a large bottle (8 oz. or even 16 oz.), more cups, more water in the cups, a small dose, etc. If all else fails, use the *olfactive* method or *friction* method (application directly on healthy skin).

Adjustment of LM potencies for hypersensitives is explained in detail in the next chapter on the LM potencies. The *olfactive* method works as follows:

- Take one #10 pellet (poppyseed pellet, 6c or LM) of the remedy and place it in a one dram vial.
- Add one drop of water to dissolve the pellet, then fill the small vial with alcohol, leaving one-third of the vial empty so there is enough air left for succussions.
- The vial is then succussed an average of 6 times or less, depending on the sensitivity of the patient. The remedy should be succussed (given a direct, firm blow against a resilient surface such as the palm of the hand or a leatherbound book) just *prior* to the inhalation.
- The vial is then held under the nose and the vapors inhaled by the patient who inhales once from each nostril.

Hahnemann recommends not using the olfactory method any more frequently than one would give the dose by mouth. In Aphorism 288 of the 5th edition he says:

Should both nostrils be stopped by coryza or polypus, the patient should inhale by the mouth, holding the orifice of the vial between his lips. In little children it may be applied close to their nostrils while they are asleep with the certainty of producing an effect.

We must never underestimate the power of inhalation. Hahnemann as well as von Boenninghausen used the olfactive method successfully to treat one of the worst types of pain, severe acute facial neuralgia (trigeminus neuralgia). Olfaction is first mentioned by Hahnemann to von Boenninghausen in his preface to "Repertory of Anti-psoric Remedies" (1823) by which he treated acute and chronic diseases, and this for several years for all his patients. But this choice was overtaken by LM potencies as is stated in Aphorism 248. Most students of Hahnemann did not follow the olfactive method and considered it a weak point of homeopathy. In my own practice I have found it so effective that some hypersensitives only need one olfaction a month; most need it no more than once a week.

For patients who still aggravate on olfactions, the *skin* method is required: the remedy is dissolved in water and a few drops are applied to any *healthy skin* (the opposite of allopathic medicine in which creams and medications are put on the unhealthy or affected skin). Hahnemann observed that mineral baths taken by patients with certain conditions (arthritis, rheumatism, etc.) were more effective for patients with healthy skin. In such cases, he tells us how much quicker the cure is when the remedy is taken internally and also rubbed on the healthy skin. On the other hand, he says, such baths have inflicted great injury to patients who suffered from ulcers and cutaneous eruptions, because the skin conditions were suppressed and erroneously considered cured. Therefore, Hahnemann cautioned against rubbing the homeopathic remedy on skin which is broken or diseased.

Constitutions of average sensitivity: examples are Sulphur, Lycopodium, and Silica. These types have a fairly stable constitution, good Vital Force, and moderate reactions to food, environment, medicines, etc. As for disease conditions at this sensitivity level, the pure mental-emotional diseases (depression, anxiety, phobias, suicidal tendencies) are in this group since they have limited or no tissue pathology.

Use moderate potencies and dosage: if using the Kentian ("single-dose, wait and watch") method, use 200c and 1M; if using LMs, do 4-6 succussions with one teaspoon daily of the remedy.

Constitutions of the lowest sensitive group or hyposensitives: Calcarea and Baryta carb., for instance. They have slow reacting senses and a tolerance for large amounts of medicines, herbs, vitamins, etc. Sensitivity may also be decreased in patients of *any* constitution who have taken too many drugs, especially tranquilizers and sedatives. They often lack energy and may be in a weakened condition, lacking reactive capabilities. After extensive surgery the Vital Force can also be slow to react, and we must continue repeating the remedy and increasing the dosage/potency until we see a reaction.

In the hyposensitives, Kentians can use higher potencies (1M and 10M) while LM practitioners would prescribe at least 8 to 12 successions, more frequently repeated, and 1 tablespoon instead of 1 teaspoon of the remedy. Personally, if LMs were inappropriate for such a patient, I would consider using 6c in water, a teaspoon or even a tablespoon three times a day.

Nature of the Disease: Here are the questions to consider: Is it acute (needing high potencies) or chronic (low potencies)? Is it in the early (high), middle or late stage (low)? Is it still in the functional stage without much pathology (high) or is the pathology far advanced (low)? Is it a skin condition (low?) Is the disease on the physical (low), mental (high) or emotional level (high)? Is the patient dying and needing to be eased into death (high)?

Nature of the Remedy: Is the remedy fast-acting (Belladonna, Aconite, Arsenicum, requiring high potencies) or slow acting (Thuja or Lycopodium, indicating low potencies)? Nosodes are slow and deep acting. The old masters recommended using them in a 200c potency (I use 30c for hypersensitives). They should not be followed by another remedy for several weeks.

Summary of Potencies and Their Indications

Sensitivity Level	Indications	Standard Starting Potency
Hypersensitive	Hypersensitive constitution (Phos., Arsenicum) Advanced tissue pathology Weak Vital Force Elderly Prolonged drug abuse/drug reactions	**LM:** 8 oz. bottle, 2 succ., 1/2 tsp. **Centesimal:** 6c 1 pellet dry *olfactive method* *skin method*
Normosens.	Normosensitive constitution (Sulphur, Lyc., Silica, etc.) Stable Vital Force Pure mental/emotional diseases	**LM:** 4 oz. bottle, 4-6 succ., 1 tsp. **Centesimal:** 200c or 1M 3 pellets dry or 1 pellet in water
Hyposensitive	Hyposensitive constitution (Calcarea, Baryta carb.) Tolerance for large amounts of meds, herbs, vitamins Lowered Vital Force e.g. from overuse of tranquilizers, sedatives	**LM:** 4 oz. bottle, 8-12 successions 1 Tbsp. **Centesimal:** 1M or 10M 3 pellets dry or 1 pellet in water

Symbols of Potencies

M.T.   mother tincture, the alcohol-based extract from which plant-based remedies are made; not yet potentized at this stage

c   centesimal, a dilution of 1 in 100. CH stands for Centesimal Hahnemannian (made by Hahnemann's method of using a new vial for each potency) and CK for Centesimal Korsakoffian (made by the Korsakoff method mentioned earlier)

x   decimal, a dilution of 1 in 10, also written D in Europe

LM   a dilution of 1 in 50,000, also seen as Q, short for quinquagesimillesimal (from the Latin for 1/50,000th), abbreviated as LM1, LM2 or 0/1, 0/2 or Q1, Q2, etc.

Recommended Usage for Some Common Potencies

The following guidelines are based on my readings in the old masters and have been confirmed by my own experience.

6x   This is a very low potency which I use in specific instances: cell salts such as Calc. phos. 6x chronically for osteoporosis (2 pellets dry or 1 tsp. twice a day, one month on and one month off; or if using for a fracture, keep taking continuously until the fracture is healed); Thyroidinum or Folliculinum 6x for certain conditions involved the thyroid or ovaries respectively (for glandular support); Graphites 6x to prevent adhesions after abdominal surgeries; and Staphysagria 6x to prevent mosquito bites.

6c   This is a relatively low potency, somewhat comparable to LMs (*only* in that it can be used daily for chronic cases). I recommend it to my students when they are first working with chronic cases, until they have mastered case management well enough to work with LMs. (LMs require some expertise because the remedy works so quickly and the situation can change so fast.) Even for the experienced LM practitioner, there are still scenarios in which 6c is preferred:

- Prescribing for someone long-distance who can only get a 6c
- A patient so sensitive that they can't take LMs no matter how reduced the dose
- An elderly patient living alone who is so confused and forgetful that she can't observe changes in her symptoms as necessary to make adjustments in the LM dose
- Any patient who may not be able to remember or follow the instructions for LMs (although you are also giving written instructions). This may not necessarily be an elderly patient; it can be a patient in a brain fog needing Thuja or Sepia, for example.
- Elderly patients whom you would like to take LMs prn (on an "as needed" basis), but they are so accustomed to taking medication every day that they are likely to take the LMs daily and run into an aggravation; they may be able to take a 6c daily.

30c This is a potency commonly used in acute cases, although I have found better results with 200c and 1M in *intense* acute situations. It is easily available in health food stores and is safe for lay people and students as they begin to learn homeopathy. The concern I have with 30c is that it may not be strong enough in acute situations, leading to frustration and discouragement, even giving up too soon on the well-chosen remedy. I encourage my patients and students to start using the higher potencies for acutes as soon as they feel confident and comfortable with them.

200c This is the beginning of the high potency series recommended by Kent for chronic cases. (Ironically enough, the old masters said that it can cause aggravations *worse* than the higher potencies when used in chronic cases, as Kentians often do.) 200c is preferable to 30c in acute infectious diseases or other strong conditions such as emotional or physical traumas. I also always use the 200c potency first for nosodes (repeating at 200c or 1M), except I use 30c for hypersensitives. Many prescribers use 200c in chronic cases, in the "single dose, wait-and-watch" method, but the old masters recommended great caution with 200c because of the aggravations they experienced with it.

1M This is the same as 1000c and paradoxically, it can be gentler than 200c in terms of aggravations in chronic cases. Kentian prescribers commonly use it in chronic cases. I use it in specific chronic cases (elderly or forgetful patients) and when something stronger than 200c is needed in acute cases. Also, after having used 200c two times, Kent would use 1M twice, as part of the series 200c, 200c; 1M, 1M; 10M, 10M; 50M, 50M; CM, CM; MM, MM; after which he would start at 200c again.

10M The same as 10,000c. I usually use a 10M potency for giving the constitutional remedy, i.e. to strengthen the innate constitution, to strengthen the patient physically, mentally and emotionally and prevent recurrence at the end of a case when the symptoms are cleared up. The constitutional remedy in a 10M potency can also be given during a period when the patient is generally healthy, to "polish the diamond," in other words to bring out the best qualities and mitigate the weaknesses of the innate constitution. Many prescribers use 10M in chronic cases, whether to follow 1M or to open a case (for example, when the case is mostly mental/emotional or when the prescriber is very sure of the remedy).

CM is 100,000c. Other high potencies include 50M (50,000c) and MM (1,000,000c). I use CM only rarely, in a life-or-death situation that demands a really intense, powerful dose. For example, I have used Pulsatilla CM to turn a breech baby. The old masters had many uses for

CM, for example Pyrogenium CM, one dose, for near-fatal septicemia and for victims of overdose of vaccinations. (The early experimental doses of vaccinations were so high that thousands of people died from overdoses.)

LM   This is the miracle potency which Hahnemann discovered in the last years of his life: it is has the amazing property of working very powerfully, like a high potency, but with very little aggravation, like a low potency. It comes before 6c in the number of steps needed to make it, but it acts more like a 1M or higher. The patient can customize it to her own individual situation by changing the number of succussions and the amount taken, even on a daily basis if necessary.

Specific variations on the above indications:

- **Sports injury** or other acute trauma to a basically healthy person: 30c, then 4 hours later 200c, then 4 hours later 1M (in each case 3 pellets dry). This method was used by the famous Swiss homeopath Dr. Pierre Schmidt from Geneva with spectacular results. In my practice I have seen great success with this method in sports injuries.

- **Acute mental and emotional pathology:** In this case the higher potencies can be used immediately, depending on the urgency of the situation. For example, an elderly person has lost his wife of 50 years and is so depressed he is suicidal. This situation is serious. Aurum CM can be given, or the highest potency available. If you only have 10M, put it in water and repeat it every 10 minutes while you hospitalize the person.

- **When you don't have the right potency on hand:** If you are traveling, or have a sick child in the middle of the night, you may not have the correct potency on hand. Or you may be advising a patient over the phone in an emergency situation, and the patient only has 30c of the indicated remedy on hand. An acceptable substitute for 200c, when only 30c is available, is to put one pellet of 30c in a small bottle of spring water, succuss it several times before each sip; instead of taking a teaspoon, take a tablespoon or more at once. The remedy can be made more potent with more succussions. I ran into this situation so frequently in my practice, when I answered acute calls after hours, that I encouraged my patients to buy a kit of 100 remedies in a 200c potency to have on hand when I prescribed an acute remedy. Most health food stores do not carry this potency.

  On the other hand, if you have a chronic case and only have the remedy on hand in a high potency, do not attempt to adjust the potency downwards. In a chronic case you have time to order the LM or 6c potency you need, since you can usually have it delivered in two days. As a professional, you should have a full range of remedies in LM, 6c, 200c, 1M and 10M potencies. To give patients a few pellets to take along in urgent situations, I use "white block" bags, 2" x 4" clear plastic ziplock bags with a white patch on which I write the name of the remedy and any instructions. (These bags are available inexpensively from commercial packaging suppliers.)

Potency Selection in Acute Disease Incident to Chronic Treatment

Patients under correct chronic prescribing for a long time show fewer and fewer acute diseases. In other words, their susceptibility is eradicated (they are truly cured). However *explosions of latent psora* do occur sometimes, particularly when the Vital Force is increased by the proper chronic remedy, as though the Vital Force is trying to clean house. What to do? First, the prescriber should determine whether acute symptoms arising during chronic treatment are a result of the remedy, and if so, whether it is a healing crisis or a similar aggravation (see Chapter 12). If it is a healing crisis or a mild aggravation, no remedy should be given, merely Sac. lac. (placebo). If the aggravation is life-threatening or unbearably painful it may require an antidote. Another option is to give the indicated acute remedy in a low-to-medium potency (30c or 200c), and this will probably not interfere with the chronic treatment. (In acute exacerbations of active chronic disease you can often give the acute complement of your chronic remedy; for a list, see page 209.) In very severe acute diseases, during the course of chronic disease it will sometimes be better to give the acute remedy in high potency while halting the intake of the chronic remedy. After the acute condition has subsided, the previous chronic remedy is usually indicated, but be on the lookout for a change in the symptom picture which will require retaking the case and prescribing a new remedy.

Dosages and Methods of Administering the Remedies

Dry vs. in water: When the remedies are given in water, it enhances their effectiveness. This discovery of Hahnemann's has been borne out in my experience. Diluting the remedies in water enables them to touch more nerve endings, thus transmitting their energy more effectively to the body. (Usually, of course, the remedies are given in the mouth, but they will work when put anywhere on the skin and especially on sensitive skin like the lips, for example if the patient is unconscious and you can't open the mouth.)

But giving *high* potencies in water is too intense, so potencies of 200c and up are generally given dry, except for *acute* infectious diseases, acute traumas (physical and emotional), or emergencies. In these cases the high potencies *should* be given in water to make them more powerful and fast-acting.

Three pellets is usually the dose for administering the remedies dry, and I recommend one pellet in 4 oz. of water when giving the remedy in water. (Give the remedy a teaspoon at a time except in really acute situations, when you can give it by the tablespoonful.)

Situations in which giving a 6c or 30c dry is better than putting it in water:
- You may not have water available, for example if you are traveling, so you need to know how to convert the dosage in water to the "dry" dosage.
- You are following the "sports trauma" protocol of 30c-200c-1M mentioned above and you take the 30c dry. This is an exception to the general rule.
- 6c in water in chronic cases can be too strong for hypersensitives (Phosphorus, Arsenicum, Mercury).

General principles for giving remedies dry and in water

Dry: Three pellets (only one for hypersensitives)

In water: One pellet (or one teaspoon of an LM solution) in 4 oz. of pure water (distilled water, spring water, filtered water; anything is preferable to tap water, although the remedy will still work if that is all you have). Stir to dissolve. (A poppyseed pellet will dissolve quickly; a larger pellet may need to be crushed between two pieces of clean paper to dissolve.) For LM potencies in chronic cases, take one teaspoon and discard the rest of the water.

For *6c in water* (in chronic cases), take one teaspoon three times a day. Hypersensitives can adjust the dosage downwards by taking only one teaspoon daily, or one pellet dry daily, or may even need to take only one pellet dry once a week.

For *centesimals in water for acute situations,* take one teaspoon as needed, as often as every 10 to 15 minutes (see below). In strong acute situations, take by the tablespoonful. In my experience, Kali bich. for thick, sticky mucus always needs to be taken by the tablespoonful to dislodge the mucus.

Frequency of administering the remedies

These factors determine how frequently you give the remedy:
- The potency of the remedy, as described in the next section.
- The purpose of the remedy, therapeutic or constitutional: constitutional remedies, because they are high potency (10M) only need to be given 2 or 3 times a year (adults) or 4 times a year (children), as needed (when the person is out of balance or needs extra resistance to disease).

- How fast the remedy is used up in the patient's body. This in turn depends on:
  - The patient's constitution (strong, hyposensitive constitutions like Calcarea use it up more quickly so you give it more frequently; you give it infrequently to the hypersensitive patients, Phosphorus, Mercury and Arsenicum). Note that the word "constitution" refers to the patient's innate constitution, not the therapeutic or layer remedy.
  - The patient's layer or current remedy needed for treatment. (Patients who need Sepia, Nat. mur. and Arsenicum may be hypersensitive no matter what their innate constitution.)
  - The patient's Vital Force (children generally have a strong Vital Force and use up remedies more quickly than adults; patients with a weak Vital Force will use them up more slowly and need them less frequently than healthy patients, in chronic cases).
  - The virulence of the disease. An acute disease with a sudden onset, like a sudden raging fever, will use up the remedy more quickly than an acute condition with a slower onset (and of course more quickly than a chronic disease). For example, in an already weakened patient with a chronic obstructive pulmonary disease, who is hindered by a severe, spastic, cramping cough, you could give Cuprum 1M or even 10M every 10 minutes. High potencies in acute situations can be given frequently (for example, a remedy for a suicidal patient). The rule about frequent doses in acute situations overrides the rule about high potencies being given only once a month or less frequently. For example, if you are giving Aurum to a widower who is suicidal, you may need to give CM not just once but several times in one day. In this case the person's life is at stake so you do not hold back.
  - If there are maintaining factors the remedy will have to be administered more frequently: for example if the patient continues to take allopathic medication and your remedy is trying to work despite its effects; or if you are treating a patient with Staphysagria for the effects of suppressed anger related to abuse, and she stays in the abusive relationship.

The higher the potency, the more long lasting each dose, in chronic cases: a single dose of a 200c potency or higher potency can last for weeks, months and even years. In emergencies and acute cases you can give 1Ms several times a day, because the remedy is being used up quickly by the trauma. The old masters gave high potencies very frequently in life-threatening acute cases, such as a 10M every 10 minutes or a CM every four hours.

Specific Applications of Centesimal Potencies

(LM potencies are covered in the next chapter.)

1. Chronic Cases

In general: 1 pellet of 6c in 4 oz. of water, based on Hahnemann's principle of dissolving the remedies in water and dividing the dose. Because 6c is much slower acting than an LM, take 1 tsp. 3 times a day for at least 4 weeks before you even think of changing the remedy (unless there is a dissimilar aggravation, which *requires* a change of remedy). After this, slow down if there is a successful result (at least 50% improvement). Slowing down means going to 1 tsp. per day. Then go down to 1 tsp. every other day, then less frequently. Then stop and wait and see what happens. See Chapter 15, Management of the Case, for specific scenarios.

For sensitive patients: start with 1 pellet dry for 2 days. If no aggravation or noticeable effect, try 2 pellets dry for 2 days; if no reaction try 3 pellets dry for 2 days (i.e. one pellet 3 times a day). (If the patient can take 3 pellets per day, it means the patient is not actually hypersensitive to the remedy, and the LM practitioner can safely use LM potencies. For the practitioner working with 6c, if the patient has no reaction at this dosage level, continue until there is a reaction or consider retaking the case and rethinking the remedy, or look for obstructions to the cure.) Once the remedy starts working, continue at the same dosage, and follow the rules above for general cases. Just keep in mind that it is better to go too slowly than too quickly with hypersensitives.

LM potencies are always my first choice for hypersensitive patients, unless there are specific reasons not to use them, such as an elderly, confused, or forgetful patient who may not be able to follow the instructions.

2. Acute Cases

1 pellet of 200c in 4 oz. of water, take 1 tsp. as needed. Stir before taking *each* teaspoon. Do not repeat before 10 to 15 minutes have passed. Hahnemann says that the remedy should be repeated every 10 to 15 minutes until a perceptible improvement takes place (such as a fever going down). Then he recommends using the "second best remedy," Sac. lac. (placebo). Look for any change (especially mental/emotional) after 3 doses within one hour. Mental/emotional changes may well happen first, such as a change from an anxious to a calm mood. They are a sign that the remedy is working, even if the physical symptoms have not changed. Also if a patient with a high fever falls asleep, it is a sign that the remedy is working and the body is healing, even if the fever is still high. Do not wake the patient to repeat the dose. (If a patient has gone into a coma, on the other hand, put the remedy on the lips.)

If there is no change on any level after three doses in an hour, you most likely have the wrong remedy and need to find the simillimum. Three doses of the simillimum within one hour will definitely have a noticeable positive effect (if you are using a 200c; if you only have a 30c on hand and are confident of the remedy, try to make it stronger by putting it in a small bottle and succussing it many times between doses; also give tablespoons rather than teaspoons). You will have even faster results if with hypersensitives in acute cases, because they will react more quickly to the remedy. Be careful with hypersensitives: "repeat as needed" means only when the improvement has stopped and either there is a worsening of the symptoms, *or* they have stabilized at a point of less-than-desired health.

If you use up all 4 oz. of the water in less than 24 hours and want to make another cup, it probably means it was the wrong remedy. Do not make another cup of the same remedy. Try to find the simillimum. (An exception would be if you have a very intense, highly acute situation or the patient's reactions are extremely dulled, in which case you might need more than one cup of the right remedy.)

If no water is available, use 3 pellets dry as a substitute. (For sensitive patients, start with 1 pellet dry, as above under Chronic Cases.)

3. Constitutional Remedy

In children, administer when the acute phase is over, to prevent recurrence, for example a child with a Calcarea constitution, who keeps getting Belladonna ear infections. Once you have cleared an ear infection give Calcarea 10M to strengthen the child's Vital Force and prevent recurrence (presuming that there is no other underlying disease layer to treat, as you would expect to find in adults.) In adults, when all the disease layers and miasms are cleared, finish the course of treatment with the constitutional remedy. Give a 10M potency *once*, 3 pellets dry (1 pellet dry for hypersensitives). Adults 2-3 times a year, children 4 times a year. Your guideline is the patient: as long as there is improvement, do not repeat the constitutional remedy. Or as long a they remain on a good plateau, do not repeat. If some mental/emotional symptoms start coming back, it is time to repeat. For example, if a Sulphur patient starts getting short-fused and losing patience with others, it is time for his constitutional remedy.

4. Nosodes

The old masters recommended giving nosodes in a 200c potency because they are deep-working remedies and that potency is needed to reach the deepest level. If you need to repeat after several weeks, you can give the 200c one more time and then go to 1M for the third dose or go right away to 1M for the second dose.

Give 3 pellets dry (30c for hypersensitives). *Do not repeat for at least* 3 weeks or as long as the remedy holds. In most cases, you will follow the nosode with its complementary remedy (Medorrhinum followed by Thuja, for instance) rather than repeating the nosode a third time (see more about this in Chapter 17, Nosodes).

In the case of epidemics, you should use the nosode of the epidemic more often: once a week (once a month or so for hypersensitives) for the duration of the epidemic (for instance, Influenzinum 200c during the flu season).

5. Epidemic Prescribing

When one member of a family has an acute illness like a flu and is taking a remedy (1 pellet in 4 oz. of water, 1 tsp. as needed, as listed under Acute Cases), give each member of the family one teaspoon per day from the same cup as a preventive. Also, if you know an epidemic is coming and has not hit your area yet, if you can find out the cardinal symptoms and determine the remedy, you can have everyone take 1 tsp. per *week* as a preventive (or if the preventive remedy is a nosode, take 3 pellets dry). If someone in a family has it, everyone else takes 1 tsp. per *day* as a preventive (i.e. take it more frequently because the exposure is greater).

Epidemic prescribing will be described in more detail in Chapter 9, Prescribing.

Adjusting the Remedy

- In acute cases, you will adjust depending on *how acute the condition is.* Is it just a little sniffle? Then you do not need a high potency. In fact you may not need a remedy at all. Is it a life-threatening emergency? Time for 1M, 10M or even CM.
- In chronic cases, you will adjust depending on *the hypersensitivity of the patient.*
- In acute cases, you will generally be trying to make the remedy *stronger.*
- In chronic cases, you will generally be trying to make the remedy *less strong.*

Making it stronger in acute cases

If the remedy is well indicated but does not seem to be working:

First, do you have a stronger potency on hand? Can you go from 30c to 200c, or from 200c to 1M? This is the simplest way. Do not change the remedy before you have used the stronger potency of the same remedy (if you feel sure of the right remedy).

If you do not have a stronger potency on hand, you can make your existing potency stronger by putting it in a small bottle and succussing it between doses, by giving tablespoons instead of teaspoons, and/or by administering it more frequently. You can also put several pellets in the bottle; this will make it *slightly* stronger.

Adjusting the potency in chronic cases

We do not usually adjust by the nature of the disease. It is in the nature of all chronic cases that we want a slow, steady, gradual amelioration. So I recommend starting with LM1 or 6c.

First determine if the person is a hypersensitive (which you determine by asking them about their sensitivity level to homeopathic remedies, allopathic medicines, environmental chemicals, anesthesia, vitamins, etc.) Also, be aware that there is a tremendous *range* of hypersensitivity, from a mildly hypersensitive who says, "I usually cut my aspirin in half and that's enough" to the extreme hypersensitive who has to live in total isolation (a universal reactor). The difference in magnitude of sensitivity between these two is *much* greater than the difference between a normosensitive and a hyposensitive patient. In other words, one hypersensitive might be able to take only 5% as much as another, while a Sulphur might need 75% or 80% as much as a Calcarea. In a way you need to think of hypersensitives as having their own sensitivity scale. If we use the analogy that finding the right potency is like tuning the dial on the radio to the right frequency, then it is as though hypersensitives are on the FM dial and all others are on the AM dial.

Just to illustrate how extremely sensitive some patients can be, I am reminded of a patient whose Chief Complaint was tachycardia which would wake her with strong palpitations in the middle of the night. She had to experiment a lot to find the exact right dosage for herself: if she took too little of the remedy, it was not enough to stop the palpitations from waking her up. But if she took too much, she had an immediate similar aggravation: the palpitations would occur right after she took the remedy in the morning. She found she had to dilute the remedy in five successive cups of water, measuring a drop from an eyedropper at each step!

Making it stronger in chronic cases

While this situation is rare, sometimes you do need to make the remedy stronger (for example in one-sided diseases), in which case you can increase the succussions, increase the quantity (to one tablespoon) or even have the patient take their dose directly from the bottle without diluting it. You may also have incorrectly assessed the patient's sensitivity. If the patient is less sensitive than you thought, you will find her reporting no reaction to the well-indicated remedy after a week. In this case, increase the succussions.

But you will almost invariably be adjusting down, not up, in chronic cases. If the remedy is too strong, the patient can suffer; but if it is not strong enough, it just means the process will take a little longer. Thus it is better to err on the side of caution. In this the LM prescriber agrees with the Kentian, but the LM prescriber has the advantage of daily adjustments.

Adjustments for hypersensitives:

6c: Instead of one pellet in 4 oz. of water, 3 tsp. a day, they can either:
- Take one tsp. a day
- Take one pellet dry per day
- If even that is too much, take one pellet dry per week

LM: this will be covered extensively in the next chapter, but to summarize:
- Reduce the number of succussions to two (this is done before other adjustments)
- Reduce the quantity taken from the remedy bottle and from the dosage cup, from one teaspoon to 1/2, 1/4, 1/8, or even measuring drops from an eyedropper
- Dissolve the remedy in two, three, or even more successive cups
- Take the remedy less frequently, perhaps only once a week or once a month
- If the above still cause aggravations, administer by olfaction. If that is still too strong, give in the form of skin applications on healthy skin.

Other adjustments for hypersensitives

Instead of 3 pellets dry (for a constitutional remedy, nosode, etc.) start a hypersensitive with 1 pellet dry. If they do not react, you can increase to 2, then 3.

In acute cases, you do not need to adjust for hypersensitives. You can give a 1M to a hypersensitive in an intense acute condition, which you could never do in a chronic case without causing a severe aggravation.

Learn to Be Flexible

Strangely enough, in my experience some patients even in acute situations will react better to 30c than to 200c or to 5 pellets dry rather than 1 tsp. of the remedy in water. This is the exception, not the rule, but as you will see in practice, every patient resonates to a particular potency, like every radio station with its own frequency. Listen to the patient and make note of his own peculiar sensitivity or idiosyncrasy. Fortunately, once you have determined the best dosage level for the patient for one remedy, you can usually use the same dosage level for all subsequent remedies.

In general, as you can see, you have to be able to work with all potencies. A practitioner who does not use all potencies fails to use homeopathy to its full potential. The potency as well as the remedy must be individualized to the patient. As your experience and expertise grow, you will know when to change from one potency to another. Until then, you may want to refer to the guidelines above.

Dose and Potency Are Two Different Notions

Often I see a major misunderstanding in modern homeopathy regarding the nature of the potency and the *amount or dosage* of the remedy ingested. Most practitioners do not relate the *minimal or infinitesimal dose* to the *number* of the pellets ingested. Some practitioners teach that the size of the dose (one or many pellets) does not make a difference. This has caused many side effects and aggravations which could easily have been avoided if Hahnemann's suggestions were followed.

Hahnemann states in Aphorisms 275 and 276:

> The appropriateness of a medicine for a given case of disease does not rest on its apt homeopathic selection alone, but also on the *necessary, correct size (or smallness) of its dose*. A medicine given in an *all-too-strong dose* for a given case of disease, even if the medicine is completely homeopathic to the case and in itself of a beneficial nature, will still damage the patient as a result of its size and the too-strong impression it makes on the life force and (due to its similar homeopathic action) on precisely those parts of the organism that are already the most sensitive and the most attacked by the natural disease.

For this reason, a medicine that is homeopathically appropriate to a given case of disease, but that is given in too large a dose, does much more damage than an equally large dose of a medicine that is allopathic to the disease. ... As a rule, *all-too-large doses of an apt, homeopathically-selected medicine give rise to great misfortune,* especially if these too-large doses are frequently repeated. Not seldom, they endanger the patient's life or make his disease almost incurable. Too-large doses certainly do extinguish the natural disease ... but the patient is then more strongly sick from the quite similar, only far more violent medicinal disease which is very difficult to expunge.

So we see that the correctly chosen remedy in too high of a dose *(this does not mean potency)* can cause a medicinal disease which is most difficult to destroy. (Of course this is also true if the potency is too high, but here we can see that too high a dose has its own effect separate from potency.) The *more perfect* the remedy is—in other words, the closer to the "bull's eye—the *more control* is needed over the potency, the dosage, the medium it is given in, and the repetition. It is better not to tell your patients to open their mouth and swing in as many pellets as happen to roll out of the tube. With this method the *size* of the dose *as well as its potency and repetition* can become a source of aggravation even if the remedy was perfectly chosen.

Some homeopaths are convinced than when Hahnemann referred to the *size* of the dose, he meant the *potency*, not the *number* of pellets. But why would he have made all those changes in his successive editions of the *Organon*, why would he continually have reduced the amount of the dose, if his experience had shown that it did not make a difference? He also says in *Chronic Diseases:* "I have myself experienced this accident … when I gave Lycopodium and Silicea in the billionth dilution, giving four to six pellets."[11] And anyone in practice has seen this frequently: one teaspoon of the remedy might aggravate a hypersensitive while a tablespoon might be necessary for a curative effect in a hyposensitive. In Aphorism 248 Hahnemann mentions giving "one *or increasing more* teaspoons of the remedy when needed" (he was talking about the doses of LM potencies again). By gradually increasing the amount of the dose from one tsp. to two or three *when needed* (and *not* if the case responds to 1 tsp.), the cure often progresses when it is stuck. So the amount *does* count.

In this context the reader might wonder how to respond to an anxious mother telling you that her child just swallowed all those sweet little pellets in her homeopathic remedy tube. Do we need to summon the ambulance and call the poison control center? Not at all. This situation usually does not pose a danger at all because the remedy is not homeopathic to the child, for whom it was not prescribed. The real danger is when the remedy is perfectly homeopathic and the patient is sensitive, has an advanced disease and/or hidden tissue pathology, which (thank God) is usually not the case.

Timing of Administering Remedies

Periodic symptoms: In treating periodic symptoms (every third day, every two weeks, every new moon, premenstrual, etc.) or occasional recurring symptoms like a headache or asthma attack, one should give the chronic remedy *after the latest attack has subsided*. The aggravation can be intense if given before or during an attack. If the "root" or corresponding chronic remedy is given immediately after the attack, the next one should be less intense. For a headache or dysmenorrhea attack itself, use an acute symptomatic or "weed" intercurrent remedy to help the patient. Once the attack is over you can work on the root of the problem and avoid or lessen the next attack.

Time of intake: In general, it is best to take the remedies *at bedtime* so that they can start working while the person is resting. The next day, the patient can observe his reactions (aggravations, improvements, no change) and communicate them to you. There are some exceptions to this rule: Phosphorus, Ignatia, and Bellis perennis, for example. If given at night, the patient may be awake all night with a restless, hyperactive mind. As a general rule, if possible, we will administer the *remedy away from the aggravation time*. For example, Nat. mur. is given away from its aggravation time of 10 a.m. Remember also that Phosphorus may have an aggravation 36 hours after it is taken.

The menstrual cycle: It is better to wait at least 3 days after the beginning of the menstrual period before taking a chronic remedy for the first time. In addition, the patient should not start taking a new remedy less than one week before the menses, especially if there are menstrual symptoms in the complaints. Otherwise, the menses can delay the action of the remedy or produce excessive aggravation. This is especially important with LM potencies, in which we carefully observe the reaction to the first dose to assess whether the potency is correct.

Chapter Six

LM Potencies

LMs: a Unique Potency, a Unique Method

Many homeopaths have not yet taken advantage of the great power of LM potencies, and those who do may only use them for hypersensitive patients. But our main goal is to accelerate the cure for *all* our patients while minimizing the aggravations. Hahnemann developed LM potencies at the end of his life (the last ten years) for this specific purpose, because he felt that the aggravations caused by centesimal potencies caused too much suffering for the patient. Being a master pharmacist, he developed a technique for making the remedies deeper and faster acting while at the same time more gentle. My own experience treating thousands of patients with centesimals and with LMs has borne out Hahnemann's assertions.

The LM potencies are made by diluting the remedy in a ratio of 1 to 50,000 at each step instead of 1 in 100, while still keeping the succussions at 100. (A detailed explanation is provided below under How to Make the Remedies.) The high number of dilutions raises the power of the remedy very high, while the relatively low number of succussions keeps the aggravations low. The result is that the remedy action quickly penetrates very deep, to the mental-emotional level and far back in the patient's timeline. This allows a cure in much less time than Hahnemann's previous centesimal method, which is exactly what he was looking for: the rapid, gentle and permanent cure. At the same time, any aggravation wears off quickly, usually in 24 hours or less, thereby allowing immediate adjustment. By reducing the intensity and duration of action through a high degree of dilution, we can now regulate the homeopathic aggravation, something that was impossible before the invention of this potency.

LMs* are also called Q potencies, both of which refer to the 1 in 50,000 dilution. (L and

---

*Sometimes the notation LM is used to mean 50M in the progression 1M, 10M, LM, 100M. In that case LM means 50,000c, which is entirely different from LM or Q potencies, as will be explained in detail below. In brief, LM potencies are diluted 1 in 50,000 times but succussed only 100 times at each step. A 50,000c would be diluted 100 times and succussed 100 times at each step, and the process repeated 50,000 times—a much higher dose, especially in terms of succussions.

M are the Roman numerals for 50 and 1000 respectively, while Q is an abbreviation for "quinquagesimillesimal," derived from the Latin *quinquagesimus* [50th] and *millesimus* [thousandth]). The specific potencies are notated 0/1, 0/2 or 1/0, 2/0, or Q1, Q2, etc. in which the 0 stands for the tiny poppyseed granules on which they are prepared.

I would also like to point out that the LM potency cannot be compared with a 3c or 6c potency, as many practitioners believe. LM potencies have a much deeper action than the centesimal scale. LMs give us the best of both words: *they are as gentle as the low potencies and as powerful as the highest centesimals.* Far from being a low potency, the LM1 has actions equivalent to a higher potency even though it is the lowest end of the LM scale. It is a much higher potency than 30c. In practice I have often seen that a hypersensitive would not react to 30c but would have an initial aggravation to a standard dose of LM1. (Of course we have many ways of adjusting an LM, tailoring the remedy to the patient.)

The Myth of Aggravations

Why do we advocate using LMs to avoid aggravations? Some homeopaths believe that an aggravation is *necessary* in order to procure a healing. Nothing is further from the truth. And some homeopaths feel that an aggravation, even lasting days or weeks, is acceptable.

Most homeopaths practicing today treat chronic diseases with high centesimal potencies such as 200c, 1M and 10M and actually look for an aggravation to demonstrate that the remedy is working. As I have mentioned in Chapter 5 on Potencies, they attribute this approach to Kent, which is why I refer to this method as Kentian prescribing. But in fact Kent himself did not approve of bringing about aggravations, as we can see in his *Lesser Writings:*

> Keep the *mild* potency as long as it works. It is not well to jump degrees. The best action is the slight aggravation, the *ideal* one is the one that does *not* aggravate but ameliorate. We do *not* seek to produce an aggravation, that is not the best, not the longest curative effect. You encourage the patient to become oversensitive by using the highest potencies instead of going low to begin.[1]

An aggravation is the primary action of the remedy which is so strong that it represses the secondary curative response from the Vital Force for a longer or shorter period. This will slow down the cure. I advise the readers to investigate carefully the definitions of *primary action and secondary action* expressed in Aphorisms 63 and 64 of the *Organon* (see Chapter 3, Laws and Principles). The primary action is the action of the agent (like our remedy) which shocks the Vital Force and causes an alteration in the health of the individual for a shorter or longer period (in the case of low and high potencies, respectively). The secondary action is the opposing action from the Vital Force with a net result of improved health.

The historical background of potencies given in the last chapter explains the source of discord in potencies. The LM potencies are teachings of the 6th edition, which Hahnemann completed in 1842. Some modern homeopaths write that the 6th Edition has almost nothing new to offer. How mistaken they are! The last edition represented a major advance in Hahnemann's thought: 60 new aphorisms were added, 49 partial additions, and 40 aphorisms were obsolete in comparison with the 5th edition of the *Organon*. But Hahnemann could not publish it that year because of the bungling of his publisher, and he died the following year.

According to von Boenninghausen, who corresponded with Hahnemann within two months of his death,* he had received word from him about the latest, yet unknown potency (LM) which he referred to as "our highest potency." In von Boenninghausen's *Lesser Writings*, the Baron wrote about the use of high attenuations:

> The immortal Hahnemann had in the last years of his life, arrived at a profound conviction of the efficacy of high attenuations, and had accordingly for some time followed in the preparation of his remedies, a method different from what he had recommended to the public in his former works. The modifications then introduced he intended to publish to the world in the last edition of his *Organon*.[2]

This last letter was drafted a scant "two months before his death." As you can see the Baron says the LM acts like our present high and highest potencies, which means like 30c and higher.

Hahnemann's wife Mélanie, in spite of many promises, never released the 6th edition. She wrote to the English Homeopathic Association that she was willing to send it for a sum of $50,000, which would be equivalent to the income she derived from practice. She said it would take her two years to read and transcribe Hahnemann's handwriting, and that she had fallen on hard times because the allopaths turned on her when she was no longer protected by Hahnemann. Unfortunately her request was refused and the 6th edition remained unpublished in her lifetime. Others like Hahnemann's grandson, Dr. Suss-Hahnemann, tried to publish a "6th Edition" but Melanie warned them not to do so, threatening them with a lawsuit: "I beg to inform you that the exclusive rights to publish the 6th Edition belongs solely to me and I possess the 6th Edition of the *Organon* written by my late husband's hand. Dr. Suss' work can have no claim whatever to be genuine."[3] (Suss saw Hahnemann only twice

---

*"I am otherwise enabled by a correspondence carried on with him since the middle of the year 1830 up to May of this year, thus within two months of his death, which correspondence was carried without interruption and with diligence, that Hahnemann even up to the last continued to diminish the doses."

in his life, first as a child and afterwards as a young man the day before Hahnemann's death. It is therefore understandable that Suss was not considered a close associate of Hahnemann, nor a great expert.) When Melanie died in 1878 (from bronchial catarrh like her husband), her adopted daughter, Sophie von Boenninghausen, was given the manuscript to continue to work on it. She herself asked $25,000 but no offers were forthcoming.

The manuscript remained hidden in an attic in Germany and was not discovered until after World War I. It was finally published in 1920, with the first English edition appearing in 1921 (translated by William Boericke, nephew of the co-founder of Boericke and Tafel). But by the time it was published, the practice of homeopathy was already well established based on the single centesimal dose, "wait and watch" method of the 4th edition. Thus the guidelines of the 6th edition were not truly put into practice until 1950 by Dr. Charles Pahud of France and then by the famous homeopath Dr. Pierre Schmidt of Geneva in 1954. Dr. Schmidt published a small booklet, *Hidden Treasures of the 6th Edition of the Organon,* and stated: "The main points which I wish to raise here are either entirely new and somewhat revolutionary when compared with accepted notions divulged and applied in the five earlier editions of the *Organon,* or points already stated but re-drafted and re-examined. They are, as a rule, barely known or not known at all by homeopaths."[4] The Choudhury family began using LMs in India in 1957, and to this day most of the world's LM practitioners are in India. LMs were not introduced to America until recently, because homeopathy in this country is dominated by the legacy of Kent, who unfortunately never knew of LMs because he died five years before the 6th edition was published.

How LMs Are Made

To fully understand the differences between centesimals and LMs, it is helpful to compare how they are made. Most centesimals are made by diluting one part of the remedy mother tincture in 99 parts of alcohol (such as Everclear or vodka) and succussing it 10 times to make a 1c; repeat for each successive potency.

Remedies which begin as solids (such as most minerals) go through the process of *trituration* which Hahnemann developed. (Liquids like snake venoms are dropped onto lactose and triturated. A milliliter of liquid is equal to a gram of solid in this case, so 1 ml of a liquid remedy would be poured over 99 grams of lactose and then triturated.) The goal is to grind one part of the remedy substance with 99 parts of lactose in a mortar and pestle, but Hahnemann found it unwieldy to grind the whole batch at once, so he would divide the 99 parts of lactose into three batches. He would grind and scrape the remedy with the first batch for 20 minutes, then add the second batch and grind and scrape another 20 minutes, finishing with the last batch for a total of 60 minutes grinding and scraping. When Hahnemann first developed this method he declared it equivalent to diluting and succussing in a 1 in 99 ratio; i.e. he said it was an alternative way to make 1c. By the time a solid remedy substance has been triturated up to 3c, it is soluble and can then be diluted and succussed like a liquid remedy. (See Fig. 6-1, Hahnemann's Directions for Trituration.)

LM potencies begin the same way as centesimals, except that they are made by trituration up to 3c no matter what the original substance. Plants are crushed with lactose instead of being made into a tincture. Remedies which begin as a liquid (like sepia ink, snake venoms, and Petroleum) are dropped onto lactose pellets in a 1 to 99 ratio. Apparently as Hahnemann worked with triturated remedies he found that this process released the dynamic or energetic properties of the remedy better than dilution and succussion.

To understand the vast difference between LMs and centesimals it helps to understand Hahnemann's line of reasoning and why he began experimenting with the LMs. His students and homeopathic colleagues around him were experimenting with very high potencies (up to 16M) and skipping many steps between potencies administered to patients, thus jumping thousands of succussions between doses. The result was what Hahnemann called the violent energy of the higher doses. Hahnemann was looking for a way to increase the dilution without so much violent succussion, and a way to progress more gently from one potency to the next in the course of treatment.

Hahnemann, one of the master pharmacists of his era, came up with a simple and ingenious solution for *increasing the dilution,* thus making the remedies ever safer (especially considering that some were made from poisons) while *holding back on the succussions,* thus keeping the energy at a gentler level. Instead of succussing 10 times for each 1 in 100 dilution, the LMs are only succussed 100 times for each 1 in 50,000 dilution.

Administered in water (a development of the 5th edition, as we have seen), the LMs became a truly revolutionary tool—within a healing system which was revolutionary in itself—for healing at a deep level while controlling aggravations. Putting the remedies in water accomplished several things at once:

♦ It enhanced the effectiveness of delivery, since the teaspoon of water could touch many more nerve endings than a tiny pellet.

♦ It allowed a single dose to be split into many administrations; a single pellet of a potency would be "spread out" into an entire bottle.

♦ Succussing the bottle allowed minute upward adjustments of the potency (finer tuning than the 10 succussions between centesimal potencies) in keeping with Hahnemann's 6th edition dictum never to give the same potency twice.

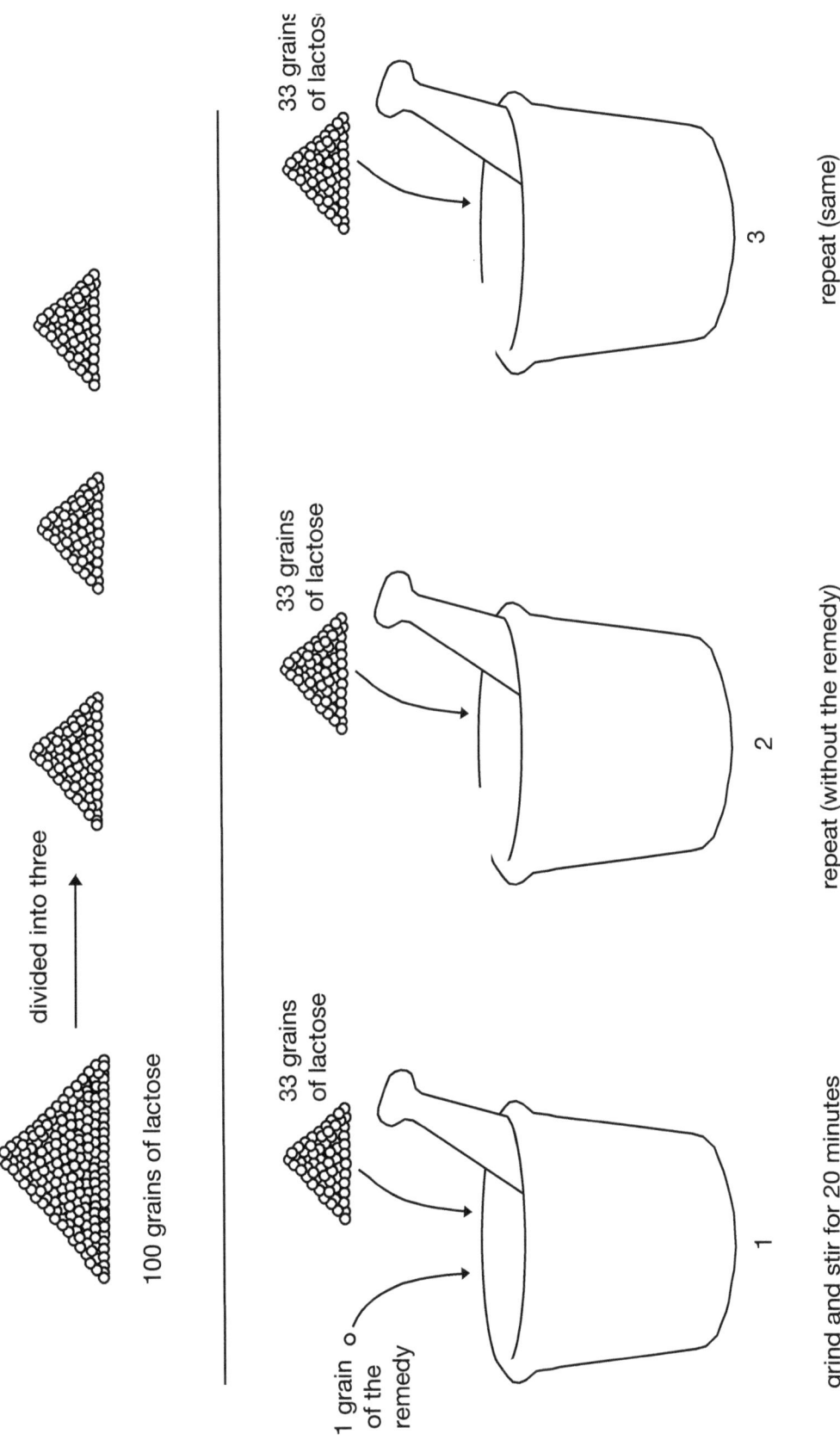

Fig. 6-1: Hahnemann's Directions for Trituration

♦ It thus allowed for highly refined adjustments to respond to aggravations and to the individual temperament.

Putting LMs in water allows for many ways to adjust both the potency and the dose, thus allowing these as well as the remedy itself to be individualized to the patient. The practitioner can adjust the size of the remedy bottle (usually 4 or 8 oz.), while the patient can adjust—on a daily basis if necessary—the number of successions, the number of cups it is dissolved in, and the quantity taken (1 tsp., 1/2 or 1/4 tsp., etc.). The patient can take the remedy once a day (chronic) or several times a day (acute) and can "plus" the remedy when the bottle is nearly finished. (All these adjustments are described in detail below.) The simple fact that the remedies are gentle enough to be taken daily allows much more freedom for adjustments.

In sum, to make LMs, start with a 3c made by trituration:

	Remedy in Plant Form	**Liquid Form**	**Mineral / Solid Form**
1c	Triturate the whole plant	Start with the liquid (sepia ink, venoms, petroleum, etc.). Drop onto lactose with 1 in 100 parts of the liquid, e.g. 1 ml to 99 g lactose, then triturate.	Start with the mineral in powder form. Triturate 1 part in 99 parts of lactose
2c	Triturate 1 part of 1c in 99 parts of lactose.		
3c	Triturate 1 part of 2c in 99 parts of lactose.		
LM1	Take 1 grain (0.062 grams) of 3c and add 500 drops of a mixture composed of 1 part alcohol and 4 parts distilled water (i.e. 100 drops alcohol and 400 drops water). Take one drop (note that you *have not succussed* this mixture) and put it in 2ml of alcohol. Succuss 100 times. Now you have the **LM1 stock bottle.** Pour 1 drop from your LM1 stock bottle onto 500 poppyseed pellets (#10 pellets). These are your **LM1 pellets,** which you will use to make your patient's remedy bottle.		
LM2	Take 1 pellet of LM1 and dissolve in 1 drop of water. Add 99 drops of alcohol. Succuss 100 times. Now you have the **LM2 stock bottle.** Pour 1 drop from your LM2 stock bottle onto 500 #10 pellets. These are your **LM2 pellets.**		
LM3	Take 1 pellet of LM2 and dissolve in 1 drop of water. Add 99 drops of alcohol. Succuss 100 times. Now you have the **LM3 stock bottle.** Pour 1 drop from your LM3 stock bottle onto 500 #10 pellets. These are your **LM3 pellets.**		

The tedious part of this process is making LM1. Practitioners usually purchase an LM1 kit and make the LM2, LM3 etc. by hand as patients need them. Making the higher LMs only takes a few minutes to make enough to last for years. If your 500 pellets run out you just use a drop from the appropriate LM stock bottle to impregnate another 500 pellets.

Read Aphorisms 269 to 271 in the 6th Edition to follow Hahnemann's advice in his own words. As to the precise method of trituration, I refer the reader to *Chronic Diseases*, Vol. I, pp. 147-148.

Details of Making LM2 from LM1

You will need to order 1/2-dram bottles (regular cap, not dropper bottles), one-dram dropper bottles, blank poppyseed pellets (#10 pellets available from homeopathic pharmacy suppliers by the pound or quarter-pound) and empty bullet boxes to hold the LMs you make. Scientific precision tweezers with a fine point are also helpful to handle the tiny pellets.*

First take one pellet of LM1 and put it in a one dram dropper bottle. This will be your LM2 stock bottle. Add one drop of distilled water to moisten it. Keep a special dropper labeled just for water and a different one for alcohol; be sure not to measure either with the dropper belonging to the stock bottle.

After it has dissolved, add 99 drops of alcohol (Everclear or unflavored vodka). Succuss the stock bottle 100 times.

Now fill a 1/2-dram bottle 1/3 full with poppyseed blank pellets. When full, it holds 1500 pellets. When 1/3 full it will be close enough to 500 pellets.

Put 1 drop from your LM2 stock bottle in the bottle with the pellets. Immediately cap it and start rolling it around to coat all the pellets. This is your LM2. (See Figure 6-2.)

Be sure to label all your bottles; I use 1/4" round labels for the caps and 3/8" x 5/8" labels for the sides, taping them so they don't peel off when inserted into the bullet box.

Making the Remedy Solution Bottle

To make a remedy solution bottle for the patient, take a new 4 oz. bottle like a cough syrup bottle (an "Rx bottle" ordered from a pharmacy supplier). Put in one LM poppyseed pellet of

---

*The pellets which are commonly referred to as "poppyseed" pellets are technically not the same size that Hahnemann specified. "Poppyseed" pellets are the common name for #10 pellets, meaning that 10 of them laid end-to-end are 10 mm long (i.e. each has a diameter of 1 mm). Hahnemann specified lactose pellets of which 100 would weigh 1 grain. According to information kindly forwarded by Julian Winston, such pellets would have a diameter of 0.92 mm rather than 1 mm.

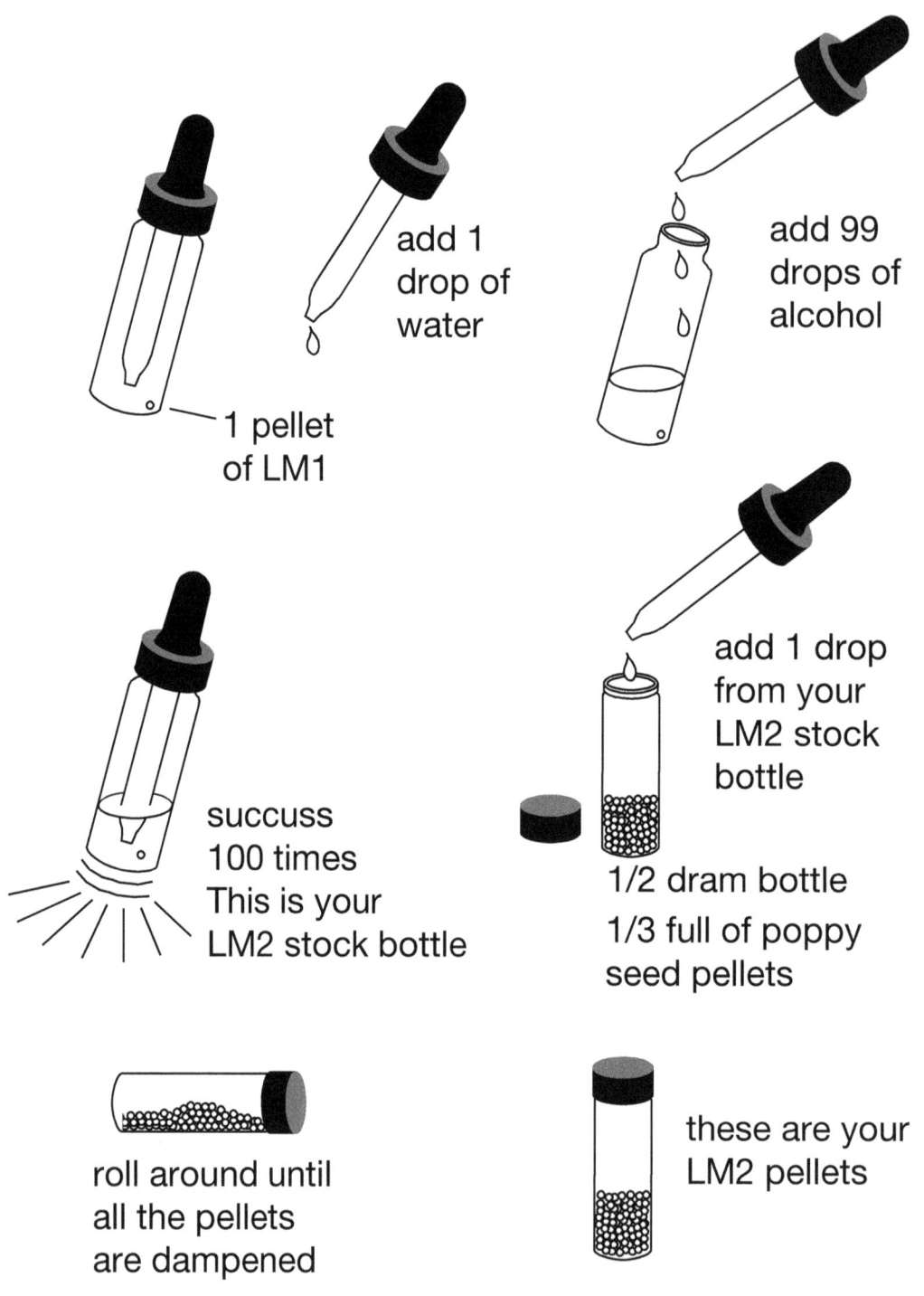

Fig. 6-2: Making LM2

the remedy (you can shake the closed bottle and listen for the rattle of the pellet if in any doubt whether the tiny pellet is in there). Fill the bottle with distilled or purified water (no tap water except in emergency) up to the line halfway up the neck of the bottle (space has to be left for the succussions). The size of the bottle is adjusted for hypersensitive patients to 8 oz. or occasionally 16 oz. As a preservative, add 15 drops (one dropper-full from a one-dram bottle) of Everclear or vodka to a 4 oz. bottle. If you use an 8 oz. bottle for a hypersensitive, you should more than double the alcohol, perhaps using as much as 1 oz. of alcohol, because the bottle will last more than twice as long. (Hypersensitives often take 1/2 or 1/4 teaspoon instead of a teaspoon, and towards the end of the first bottle, they may be taking the remedy only as needed.) The alcohol should be vodka or Everclear, not methyl or rubbing alcohol. I use vodka because it is the only kind of alcohol that can be tolerated by patients suffering from yeast overgrowth and fermentation (based on my extensive experience in treating this population).

Some patients in recovery from alcoholism may object to even a few drops of alcohol as a preservative, even if you explain that the amount is so small that it will not have a noticeable effect. (They may object because they have taken a vow not to take even a drop of alcohol, or because the odor of alcohol when they open the bottle can be a trigger for them.) For these patients you can use glycerin instead, doubling the amount because it is not as effective a preservative as alcohol.

A 4 oz. bottle will be finished in about three weeks if the patient is taking a daily dose of one teaspoon. If the bottle needs to be stored for a longer period because the patient is taking the remedy prn, more alcohol is needed as a preservative. Be sure to label the bottle with your name and the patient's name, the date, the name of the remedy, the potency (LM1, LM2, etc.) and the number of succussions to start with.

Standard Succussions (for the Non-Sensitive Patient)

Hahnemann introduced a new concept with the LMs: the patient succusses the remedy each time he takes it and thus can control his reaction to it. Demonstrate succussions to your patient with a demo bottle (not the actual remedy bottle) and ask for a return demonstration. Strike the bottle firmly against the palm of the opposite hand from a distance of about two feet. A leatherbound book can be used instead of the palm. Emphasize to your patient the importance of using a firm, resilient surface. A tabletop, for example, is not an acceptable substitute.

Also emphasize to your patient that the remedy bottle *must be succussed before each dose.* Why? After the first dose (assuming that the remedy is working), the patient will be less ill.

The second dose must consequently be *adapted to the less morbid condition*. As the patient needs less and less of the remedy, you are speeding up the process of healing by giving the remedy more penetration power through the succussions. Consequently, Hahnemann recommends giving the same remedy, but more highly dynamized. He cautioned against repeating the *same* LM potency even once (in *chronic* cases), this being detrimental and even possibly leading to incurability (the same meaning without succussions in between). "Before proceeding, it is important to observe, that our vital principle cannot well bear that the same unchanged dose of medicine be given even twice in succession, much less more frequently to a patient."[5] (I have never seen this happen, however; I have had patients make the mistake of not succussing, and the remedy still worked.)

The practitioner tells the patient how many times to succuss the bottle at first, based on the patient's sensitivity. The average, normosensitive adult starts with 8 succussions. The hypersensitive, as well as infants, the elderly and patients with severe tissue pathology, succuss it 2 to 5 times. The hyposensitive (i.e. a Calcarea constitution) succusses it 10 to 12 times. After the initial dose the patient can adjust the number of succussions according to his reaction, as described below.

After the patient has succussed the bottle, he takes one teaspoon from the bottle and stirs it into a cup of 4 oz. of distilled or filtered water. Then he stirs vigorously with a plastic spoon and takes one teaspoon from this cup (*the dosage cup*) as his dose. (Infants receive 1/2 tsp. from the dosage cup.) The patient throws the rest of the 4 oz. away. (Be sure to tell them never to drink the whole cup. I encourage patients to give the "remedy water" to their plants and have heard remarkable stories of supposedly dead plants returning to life and even to bloom.) To avoid mismeasurement, give your patient a small plastic cup with teaspoons marked on the side (the standard med cup used in hospitals, available inexpensively from pharmacy suppliers). Emphasize to your patient the importance of designating a different cup to mix each remedy. To increase compliance, you can give the patient a clear 9 oz. plastic cup from the supermarket, with the 4-oz. line marked and the remedy name noted in indelible marker. (Once patients start using many remedies, e.g. for acutes, it will avoid confusion if they keep a separate cup for each remedy and label the cup.) The patient can keep on using the same cup for the *same remedy*. A sample instruction sheet for patients is included in Appendix 1.

Dosage and Administration of LMs for a Non-Sensitive Patient

The patient succusses the remedy and takes a teaspoon from the dosage cup every day *if necessary*. Typically the non-sensitive patients will take it daily in the beginning of their treatment. Sensitive patients may only need it once a week or even once a month, and non-sensitive patients taper off to a similar schedule over the course of several months of treatment.

The patient is taught to stop taking the remedy at the slightest hint of an aggravation, which usually nips the aggravation in the bud. The patient waits for the aggravation to disappear, the subsequent improvement, and then another downturn before starting the remedy again. This usually happens in a couple of days. When resuming the remedy, the patient permanently reduces the number of succussions (usually by 2, e.g. from 8 to 6) to avoid another aggravation. When the number of succussions has been reduced to 2, the patient starts reducing the amount of liquid instead, since the remedy always has to be succussed. (In practice I never go to 1 succussion because I have not found any noticeable difference between 2 and 1.) The curative action of the correct remedy should be so rapid that you will rarely need to go higher than LM10 before a new remedy, if any, is called for. In my experience chronic cases are usually resolved by LM5 or 6, and often by LM 2 or 3. Hahnemann's own LM pharmacy contained many remedies from LM1 to LM10 and only a few up to LM30, such as Sulphur and Merc. sol. (for the treatment of syphilis, so rampant in his time).

Adjustments for the Hypersensitive Patient

The first way to adjust for hypersensitives is to reduce the amount of liquid at each step to 1/2 teaspoon and have them dilute it in two different 4 oz. cups of water: they take 1/2 teaspoon from the remedy bottle, stir it into a 4 oz. cup, take 1/2 teaspoon from that cup and stir it into a *second* 4 oz. cup, then take 1/2 teaspoon from the second cup as their dose (called "making a second cup"). Extremely sensitive people can reduce the amount to 1/4 or 1/8 teaspoon at each step and dilute it into 3, 4 or 5 different cups. The frequency can also be reduced. Sometimes one dose every 7 or 14 days is enough to avoid aggravations. You may wonder how you decide among these different methods. Fortunately hypersensitives are so sensitive to the remedy that they can easily tell you, based on a little experimenting, what works for them. It may also be a matter of the patient's convenience and preference: some may find they can save time by taking the remedy every other day, while others may be too sensitive to the slight start-and-stop effect of this method and need to take it daily at half the previous dose. One patient may find it difficult to measure 1/16 of a teaspoon in two cups and may prefer 1/8 of a teaspoon in three cups, while another may find it too tedious to make three cups. With LM potencies the treatment is patient-centered: we explain how to adjust and then empower patients to take the adjustment process into their own hands.

If the patient is still aggravating on the liquid LMs no matter how much you adjust it downwards (which happens rarely, and only in the case of extreme hypersensitives), go to the *olfaction* or *friction (skin)* method, described in Chapter 5.

Advantages of LM Potencies vs. the Centesimal Scale

These are the advantages I have found for LMs in my own extensive experience with both types of prescribing. They apply to all patients, but especially to hypersensitives who suffer too much from the aggravations caused by high centesimal potencies. I have had other practitioners tell me that LM potencies aggravate, or that they do not notice a difference between LMs and centesimals, but invariably I have found that these practitioners are administering LMs by a method different from Hahnemann's method outlined in this book, which I have found to work extremely well.

- LMs are quicker and deeper in action with less aggravations. Aggravations are minimized and can be regulated more easily (see Aphorisms 245 and 246). Normally, in skin diseases and serious chronic cases, the homeopathic aggravation of the centesimal scale can give rise to immense suffering of the patients. As Kent himself expressed: "I should rather be in a room with a dozen people slashing with razors than in the hands of an ignorant prescriber of high potencies. They are means of tremendous harm, as well as of tremendous good."[6] It is evident that while high potencies are consistent with the first and third ideals of cure, i.e., rapid penetration and permanent restoration, they frequently violate the second ideal, a *gentle* impression.

- There is no leap or jump in this method. The patient starts with LM1 and goes up to LM2, then LM3 and so forth after finishing each bottle. By succussing the remedy bottle each day, the patient gradually raises the potency so that it is closer to the next remedy bottle, making a very smooth progression of potencies. It is in the nature of chronic diseases that they do not aggravate suddenly, but progress gradually and slowly. So the potency of the medicine should not be increased suddenly. The cure also comes slowly and gradually. *It is the nature of the real cure, the homeopathic cure.* Kentian prescribers administer remedies with large gaps, from 200c to 1M, to 10M, etc., hence strong aggravations are possible. The issue of *similar aggravations* is a serious one, as the suffering caused by long aggravations leads many patients to abandon homeopathy and return to the suppressive methods of allopathic medicine.

- If there is any aggravation with LM potencies, it will disappear within two days at the most when the remedy is stopped, usually much faster—several hours to half a day (although in *extremely* sensitive people the aggravation *occasionally* lasts longer).

- While many LM prescribers might consider centesimals more appropriate for acute situations because their nature is somewhat similar (quick onset, early aggravations, and strong primary action of the remedy), LMs can also be used in unusual acute situations where high potency centesimals have not helped. Make LM1 in a 4 oz. bottle and take one *tablespoon* at least twice a day and as often as every hour from the *same cup,* stirring vigorously before each dose. I have used this in an acute situation (a tennis elbow) when I knew I had the simillimum (Bellis perennis) and the condition was responding only very slowly—even to high potencies in water and to Dr. Pierre Schmidt's favorite method (30c-200c-1M each one dose with 4 hours inbetween). There was a dramatic response due to the great penetration power of LMs.

- Deep acting remedies like Lycopodium and Calcarea can be used daily and repeated for months.
- Long standing chronic diseases can be cured *more quickly* using this scale, at least in my experience. For instance longstanding illnesses like asthma can be cured in a matter of months rather than years. This is also the case for numerous other serious chronic illnesses. The repetition of the dose with Kentian potencies is not possible if there are remnants of disease, so the patient suffers longer. (This method requires waiting until the practitioner is sure she can repeat, which means waiting until the patient is suffering again.) So it requires longer periods of time to effect the cure. The LM method hastens the process of cure by frequent repetition.
- It can be seen within two to four days whether or not the remedy has been selected correctly. After a single dose patients typically report a sense of well-being and improvement on a deep level, such as having more energy or being able to sleep better, whether or not their chief complaint has improved. With 6c we often have to wait several weeks or months (3 weeks at least) before we can notice any changes. With 200c and higher potencies we may see a change quickly—but often at the cost of an unwarranted similar aggravation. Any improvement with centesimals may come so much later that the patient often does not attribute it to the remedy. The homeopath ends up taking the blame for the aggravation while receiving no credit for the improvement.
- Because of the quick and clear action of LMs, disruption of the case by the wrong remedy is quickly noted and also wears off much more quickly than a disruption created by high potency centesimal doses.
- In mental illness, where even a low centesimal potency can aggravate, LMs can cure smoothly.
- In cases of longtime suppression (and it is hard to imagine any chronic disease in our present time that has not been suppressed), this potency works very effectively. LMs can *revive suppressed symptoms* better than centesimal potencies, in my experience.
- LMs are excellent in palliating incurable diseases (where there is great pathological damage) without the danger of aggravation.
- In other *apparently* hopeless cases of advanced pathology (according to allopathic prognosis), LM potencies may not only palliate better than any other potency, it may even cure

them. Where Kentian prescribers have to be extremely restrained in treating advanced pathology (because an aggravation could be fatal), LM potencies can be used more aggressively and often "cure the incurable" because of their gentleness. This is especially true in what Hahnemann called one-sided diseases, as described in Chapter 4, Pathology).

- Practitioners who give a single dose every few weeks or months may be concerned about their remedies being canceled by coffee, camphor, mint, dental interventions, etc. This is not the case with LMs, which are rarely canceled by any of the above; and if they are, it does not matter because the patient repeats the remedy the next day.
- Practitioners of the "wait and watch" method may find it necessary to forbid their patients to use nutritional supplements or receive other treatments such as acupuncture, chiropractic or massage for fear that these will muddy the picture and make it difficult to tell whether the remedy is working. With LM potencies, it is clear from the first day or two whether the remedy is working, so that patients can then be encouraged to do everything they can to support their vital energy.
- It is not necessary for the patient to discontinue prescription medication. LM potencies are more effective than centesimals, again in my experience, in working through the patient's Prozac, Albuterol, insulin or any other medication which patients are reluctant to give up, and which in fact would be dangerous for them to give up before the remedy has had time to act.
- The patient understands this method more easily because of its resemblance to the allopathic method of daily dosing. (Although not always taken daily, LMs are administered more frequently than centesimals usually are.)
- Patients are taught to observe their own symptoms and adjust their own dosage, which gives them a much greater sense of participating in the healing process and leads to greater patient satisfaction.
- A homeopath can easily make LM2, LM3 and so forth from LM1, so that he only needs to buy an LM1 and then he has a complete pharmacy at his disposal.

Looking at all these advantages, I feel that Hahnemann has given us his greatest gift in the LM potencies. It is unfortunate that by a historical accident only perhaps 10% of the homeopaths in the world (and fewer in the US) have been trained in using this potency. The new O'Reilly translation of the 6th edition has stimulated renewed interest in LM potencies, but there has been a dearth of adequate instruction available for practitioners sincerely interested in learning how to use them. In addition, many who would otherwise want to try LMs have been deterred by misinformation passed around at conferences: that LMs are too difficult and too unwieldy to use, or that patient compliance is poor. In my own experience, I have found that the majority of patients can understand and correctly follow the directions for LMs; not only that, they enjoy the sense of actively participating in their own healing. I always tell them that they are the pilot and I am only the co-pilot in their healing journey. The sense of empowerment they receive from observing their own reactions daily and making their own adjustments is healing in itself.

As for difficulty of use, LMs require a modicum of additional study in the beginning, but they more than make up for it in the ease of practice which they provide. I have worked with both centesimals and LMs, and I found a remarkable difference when I converted my practice to using LMs almost exclusively: the pace of cure was so speeded up that I felt my entire practice had been put in a VCR on "fast forward;" and the patients' reactions were so highlighted and clarified that it was like switching from black-and-white to color TV. I no longer needed to spend time puzzling over the patients' reactions and how to proceed because LMs made the picture dramatically clearer.

I hope that this book can serve as a guide for students and experienced practitioners alike so that Hahnemann's last and most remarkable achievement receives the wide publicity and extensive use it deserves. Yes, the practitioner will receive more phone calls from patients than when treating with high potencies. LMs change the clinical picture so fast that often the patient needs to consult with the practitioner again within the first week. But as healers we must not deny our patients the benefits of LMs because of a minor inconvenience to ourselves. The gratitude of your patients and your sense of fulfillment in your practice will more than make up for it.

Practical Advice for LM Prescribing

Adjust for hypersensitives: Ascertain the sensitivity of the patient by asking them whether they have previously aggravated on homeopathic remedies; whether they are sensitive to environmental chemicals, fumes, or weather changes; whether they have difficulty coming out of anesthesia; whether they typically reduce their dosage of allopathic medicine to 1/2 or 1/4 the recommended amount; and/or whether they tend to have allergic reactions to vitamins and herbs. If you suspect the patient is hypersensitive, it is better to be conservative and give her an 8 oz. bottle with 2 succussions. The worst that can happen is that the cure takes a little longer than it otherwise would. For example, you tell the patient to do 2 succussions and it turns out she needs 4. If you err in the other direction, and tell a patient to use 4 succussions when they really need 2, the resulting aggravations will slow down the process of cure much more.

Remember that an LM is much more powerful than 30c (which is why I have often seen that a hypersensitive could tolerate 30c but not an LM1, 2 succussions). So if the vitality and sensitivity is such that one would be concerned about giving a 30c, then *do not give LMs* in a normal dose. Use 8 or 16 oz. bottles with 2 succussions, dilute in several cups if needed, give one dose as a test dose and repeat *only if necessary*.

Giving an initial test dose: When starting a new remedy, give a test dose by asking the patient to take one dose and then *skip the following day* so that he has a full 48 hours to observe the effect. Make sure that the patient does not interfere with this first dose (by avoiding coffee and not starting any other new modality or a new diet at this time) and see how the reaction compares to the three scenarios in Figure 6-3. Assuming that you have chosen the right remedy, the first possibility is a strong positive reaction such that the patient feels an extra amount of nervous energy (taking off like a rocket). Much as the patient might like this, stop the remedy for several days and reduce the amount of succussions because it means that the dosage is too strong and will lead to an aggravation. Normally the number of succussion is reduced by two (e.g. from 8 to 6) if there is an aggravation. But in this case you can consider reducing much more, e.g. from 8 to 4 or even 2, depending on how intense the reaction is.

A second scenario is a similar aggravation: stop the remedy until the aggravation is over and adjust the succussions and/or the amount given. (Consider adjusting the succussions down to 2 if the reaction is intense, as in the first scenario.) The third scenario is the ideal one, the "Driving Miss Daisy" response: a gentle beneficial reaction (a sense of well-being, sleeping longer and deeper, etc.). There may or may not be any improvement in the Chief Complaint at this point. The patient can then resume the remedy at the same number of succussions. A fourth possibility (not shown) is a *striking* improvement in the patient's chief complaint. In this case, Hahnemann said *do not repeat until the improvement stops,* which can take several days or even weeks. (A final scenario is not a reflection on the potency but on the choice of a remedy: a dissimilar aggravation indicates that the remedy is the wrong remedy and the case must be re-analyzed.)

Our general rule is that if an aggravation occurs we adjust down; if the dose is not strong enough, we adjust up. We suspect the dose is not strong enough if the patient fails to react to the well-chosen remedy in a week or so, which is rarely the case if no other obstructions are present (see Chapter 14, Obstructions to the Cure). There are several ways of adjusting, by decreasing or increasing the following:

- the number of succussions
- the amount of water in the solution bottle, by using an 8 oz. or 16 oz. bottle
- the dilution (number of tsp. taken from the bottle and put into the 4 oz. cup of water)
- the quantity of the dose from the cup itself (1/2, 1/4 or 1/8 tsp.; 2 tsp. or 1 TBS., etc.)
- the number of cups used to dilute the remedy
- the days of intake (every day or skipping days).

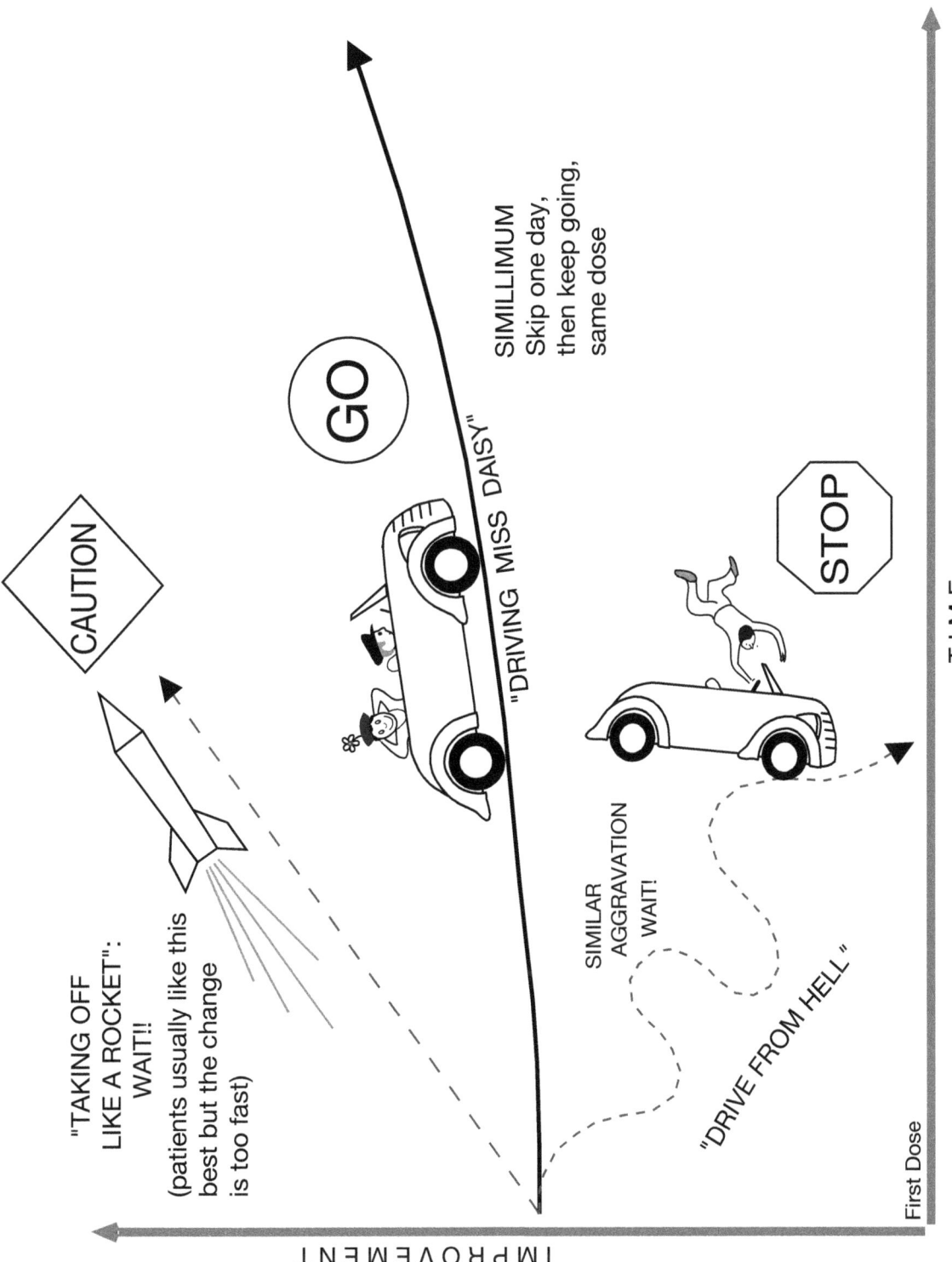

Fig. 6-3: Possible Scenarios Following the First Dose of LM1

Normally I adjust the number of succussions first, down to the minimum of 2 before applying the other measures.

Reduce succussions between LM potencies: When the patient goes from LM1 to LM2 she reduces the number of succussions by 2, e.g. from 8 to 6, then when going from LM2 to LM3 from 6 to 4. When the number of succussions has been reduced to 2, you cannot go any lower so the patient starts taking 1/2 teaspoon from the bottle and from the cup (written 1/2-1/2).

Ending with 200c or 1M: Depending on the compliance of the patient, after LM2 or LM3 I sometimes give the same remedy (if still indicated) in a 200c or 1M potency. This has certain advantages. First, some patients get tired of taking a dose prn, which becomes especially confusing when the remedy is needed less and less often. There is a real danger that they will overdose themselves because they do not pay attention. At the same time, as we progress with our LM potency, with each dose slightly stronger than the previous one, the natural disease grows smaller while the artificial disease created by the remedy grows larger.

Therefore, there is a growing danger of accessory symptoms of the remedy, unhomeopathic to the case, if the dose is repeated too soon (see the discussion of accessory symptoms in Chapter 12). A 1M has less penetration power than LM3 (which has built in all the succussions of LM1 and 2). This "lesser" potency therefore might correspond more closely to the diminished natural disease, keeping accessory symptoms to a minimum. Of course, when you

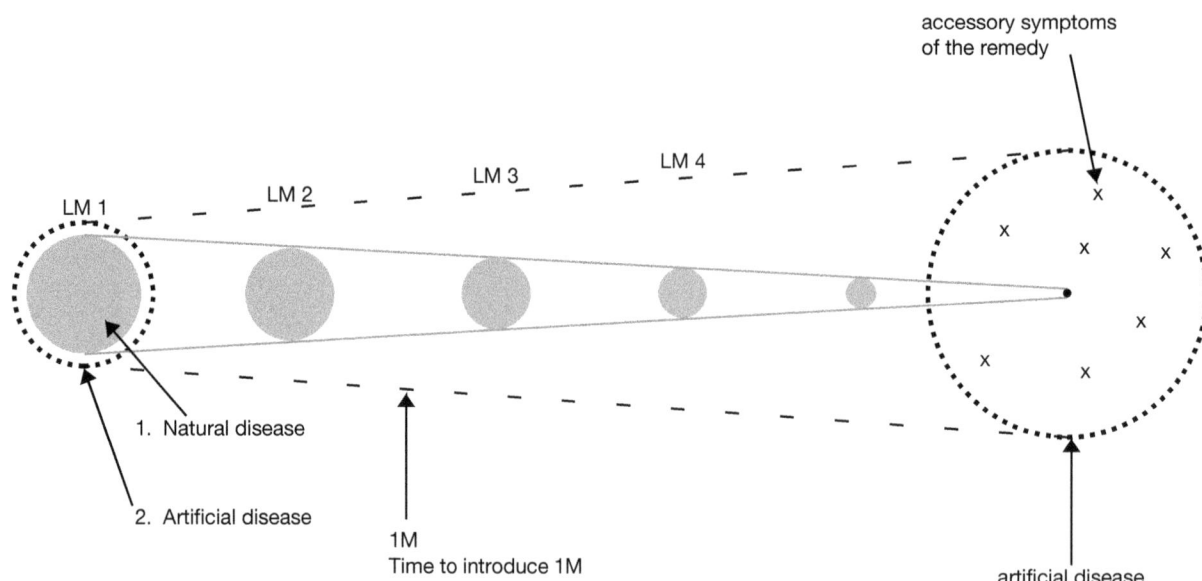

Fig. 6-4: Administration of 1M after LM2

have an intelligent and diligent patient, you certainly never need to use another potency but LM. A very sporadic LM dose prn when symptoms resurface speeds up the healing process. But the above method can be applied if the patient is too busy and does not pay attention to his progress (which happens more often than one would think), or the patient becomes confused as to when to repeat the LM potency. (See Fig. 6-4, Administration of the 1M Dose after LM2.)

Plussing the bottle: For sensitive patients, in order to dull the possibly aggravating step from LM1 to LM2, I would tell them that when the LM1 bottle has only one teaspoon remaining, to fill it with purified water halfway (2 oz. for a 4 oz. bottle, 4 oz. for an 8 oz. bottle), and then continue with the same number of succussions (this is the *plussing* method). Since the last teaspoon of LM1 contains all the added succussions, it is the strongest teaspoon of LM1 and is therefore the ideal one to be diluted. This way, when the patient finishes this plussed bottle and takes the first teaspoon of LM2 (if still needed), any aggravation will be minimal or non-existent. This is only necessary when going from LM1 to LM2, not from LM2 to LM3 etc., and only for sensitive patients.

Plussing is also a good way to test whether a patient still needs the remedy. I might do this when I think the patient is at the end of the remedy. If the patient is about to finish LM4 and I am not sure if she will need LM5, I might have her plus the bottle. If her symptoms return slightly, she needs the added stimulus of LM5. If not, the plussed LM4 might coast her gently to a complete cure. Another situation in which I might do this is a practical one: if the patient is about to run out and cannot get a refill in time, I tell her to plus the bottle. If she continues to progress, then I know I can definitely reduce the succussions and maybe the frequency or dosage for the next LM bottle. If there is no progress she definitely needs the next LM and possibly at the same number of succussions. I usually don't do this deliberately, but if the situation comes up, the information is useful to me.

Nosodes: Nosodes are sometimes found in LM potencies, but as a rule, I would advise using nosodes in a 200c potency, as the old masters did. 200c is more appropriate for their deep-working and slow-acting nature. (I start with a 200c and then if I need to repeat it I have the options of repeating 200c or going directly to a 1M.)

When not to use LMs: Exceptions for the use of LM potencies are few, but they exist. LM potencies are *not indicated* in the treatment of the three great miasms *as long as their external manifestations are present*: recently erupted itch (scabies), or syphilitic chancre, or figwarts. These situations require large doses of the remedy from the beginning with *higher and higher potencies* daily or even more often. This procedure has no danger of causing medicinal aggravation since the practitioner can observe the progress of treatment day by day until the disappearance of these local symptoms signal a perfect cure. (As modern practitioners we are not normally confronted with these situations. By the time patients come to us, the condition has usually been suppressed and we see it in the chronic miasmatic state. It was a very common occurrence in Hahnemann's time, however. And American homeopaths may see it if they volunteer to work in Third World countries, because suppressive treatments are not so widely available there.) LMs may also be contraindicated depending on the patient's temperament or forgetfulness. Sample Case 6 in Appendix 4 provides a good example of a situation inappropriate for LMs.

In ascending order: Some Indian practitioners start with LM6, for example, giving it for three days, stopping for a month, then giving three doses of LM12, waiting another month, giving three doses of LM18, and so on. This method may work in the hands of a very skilled and experienced practitioner, but I would not recommend it to a beginner and I have not found it necessary in my practice. I always start with LM1 and proceed to LM2, LM3 etc. without skipping potencies. The only exception was that Hahnemann advised sometimes starting with LM3 in *very hyposensitive* individuals. But practitioners should follow the basic rules until they are thoroughly familiar with the phenomenal power of LMs before they start experimenting with different methods of administration.

Other Indian homeopaths give the remedy in *descending potencies*. Dr. Choudhury introduced this method in India, giving sensitive patients first a few doses of LM1 and then, when the patient regained his vitality, raising the potency to LM3 or 4 and after that gradually descending the scale again. We can understand the reasoning. After application of the simillimum the disease state becomes weaker, the patient feels improved on all planes, yet by going to LM2 the remedy becomes stronger. So he preferred the descending method, going down from LM4 to LM3, etc. But we can adjust for this by reducing the succussions, giving the remedy less frequently and in smaller amounts. Also, as a practical matter, it seems difficult to judge how far to jump with a particular patient once the initial doses of LM1 are given, whether to LM3 or LM6, etc. Like the ascending potencies, this method may give very good results in the hands of an experienced practitioner but is not recommended for the beginner. Hahnemann did use descending potencies at one point in the beginning, but later, he used ascending potencies throughout his cases, which Choudhury attributes to his senility and the heavy burden of more important assignments. But we know from historic accounts that Hahnemann remained mentally sharp and able to do his best work up to the time of his death. In my own practice, I always use the ascending scale Hahnemann recommended, with excellent results.

Overreaction by hypersensitives: A few hypersensitives can be so sensitive that they seem to react to *any* seemingly well-indicated remedy with many new symptoms. The accessory symptoms can even overshadow the patient's clinical picture, giving the practitioner the false impression that the remedy is wrong. After several false starts, the practitioner realizes that the problem is not his choice of remedy but the patient's extraordinary hypersensitivity. (If they were truly accessory signs, the remedy wouldn't have to be changed, only the potency.) I would not use LMs in this case because they will react to even the smallest dose due to their deep penetration power. I would first try 6c dry, one pellet per day, adjusting up if necessary by putting it in water and giving 1, 2 or 3 tsp. a day, or adjusting down if necessary by going to the olfactive or skin method.

Administer in water: The famous Indian homeopath Patel tried giving LM potencies dry on the tongue, claiming they worked that way too. But he admitted that the medicines in liquid worked better. *One should never use the LM potencies dry,* only in water as Hahnemann prescribed.

Always start with LM1: In a footnote to Aphorism 246, Hahnemann states: "Use begins with the lowest degrees [i.e. LM1]." He did not say, "Start with LM6 or LM10." "Imitate me, but imitate me well" is Hahnemann's motto.

When we finish a layer, for instance with an LM3, and new symptoms requiring a new remedy show up, what should be the potency of this second prescription? For instance we finish a layer of Sepia at the end of a bottle of Sepia LM3. Now the totality of symptoms of Nat. mur. appears, representing an earlier layer in the patient's timeline. We have to start again with LM1 of Nat mur. This is a new layer, the patient has no Nat. mur. in her system, so it is logical that we start over again. However, if returning to the same remedy after a lapse of time (the patient seemed to be cured but symptoms recur later), resume where you left off that remedy. If she is halfway through a bottle of LM3, she must start at the same place. If the remedy has spoiled (flecks are floating in it), she will have to take a new bottle of LM3 and pour half of it out, also succussing it approximately the same number of times as the accumulated succussions in the previous bottle.

End at LM30: Hahnemann made LMs up to LM30, because as he stated, "everything has to come an end." In fact when his medicine chest was discovered, it had all the remedies proven at that time in potencies to LM10 with only Sulphur and Merc. sol. up to LM30. He had about 1700 LM potency remedies in this chest versus about 500 C scale remedies (which indicates his preference at the end of his life)! Most chronic cases are cured by the time we reach LM10. (Occasionally a hyposensitive with a disease layer of many years' duration will need more.) An exception occurs when palliating incurable diseases. I used Arsenicum in a cancer patient whose oncologist gave her two months to live. She lived another three years and reached LM16, enjoying good health, energy and moods to the very end. Some practitioners like Patel in India have reached LM50 (especially in Nux vomica and Sulphur) but Patel started his cases with LM10 and jumped potencies from there.

Administer correctly: Many modern homeopaths think that LM potencies are a type of low potency remedy that can be repeated daily "because they don't aggravate." Nothing is further from the truth. We already know that LMs are not repeated automatically, day after day. And it is mainly the incorrect use of the LM potencies (starting with LM5 instead of LM1, giving the pellet dry, giving a dose directly from the bottle, etc.) that gives the mistaken impression that "LMs also aggravate," as I have heard some Kentian prescribers say. As we have seen in previous sections of this chapter, a very small aggravation is possible and easily corrected through the various means we have of adjustment of the dose. But that is not what these homeopaths refer to. Some of them even claim, "I used the LM potency and my case aggravated. Then when I used the centesimal scale, I had no aggravation and my patient was cured." If this were true, why would Hahnemann in the 6th edition declare LMs his greatest achievement and encourage his readers to discard his previous discovery, the centesimals? I believe that many of the problems reported with LM potencies stem from an unfortunate lack of training and textbooks available for LMs. For example, I have heard of homeopaths giving the LM pellet dry on the tongue, or starting with LM6, or giving a teaspoon directly from the remedy bottle, or jumping from one LM to the next after only a few days. Almost every time *improper application* was the sole reason for aggravations from LMs.

Do not automatically give the remedy daily: It bears repeating that an LM potency is not repeated indiscriminately day after day just because, as many believe, "it is such a gentle potency." In Aphorism 246 Hahnemann said: "Every noticeably progressing and conspicuously increasing improvement … excludes any repetition of the medicine." Cases with such "conspicuously increasing improvement" are of course the most wonderful reactions we can have, and if the patient is sensitive enough I have seen a layer resolved with a single dose of LM1.

Alas, as Hahnemann said himself in the same paragraph, these cases are rather rare, and he continues in a footnote to the same paragraph, "The same well-chosen medicine can now be given daily, even for months when necessary." We need to pay great attention to each word Hahnemann said, particularly to the words *when necessary*. We need to educate our patients as to the different outcome scenarios so they know how to adjust on a daily basis and when to stop taking the remedy. In addition to the patient instruction handout in Appendix 1, I give them a copy of "Driving Miss Daisy" (Fig. 6-3) and a basic rule of thumb: "When in doubt, stop the remedy and call me."

Administering in eyedroppers: Most homeopaths who tell me that they use LMs seem to administer them in eyedroppers rather than 4 or 8 oz. bottles. This is not the method Hahnemann recommended, and I am not sure where it started. It is definitely more convenient for the patient, and I am open to the possibility, although I have never tried it this way myself. I do have several concerns about giving LMs in this way. It makes sense to me that the wave forms of the succussions (and thereby the power of the energetic imprint of the remedy picture) would be altered if almost the entire volume of the bottle is penetrated by the dropper. Most practitioners who use LMs in eyedroppers tell me that they aggravate or that they are no better than centesimals, which tells me that eyedroppers may not be as effective a method as the remedy bottles. David Little's research with hundreds of patients in India over the past 12 years indicates that the size of the remedy bottle has a significant impact on the effectiveness of the remedy. Also, one would think that measuring with an eyedropper would give the sensitive patient more control over the size of the dose, but the opposite is the case. We have some patients so sensitive that they need to measure the remedy by drops from an eyedropper when taking it from an 8 oz. bottle. They would lose flexibility if they were measuring from the much smaller volume in an eyedropper.

I would like to hear from practitioners who get results from LMs in eyedroppers comparable to my results with remedy bottles, since eyedroppers would certainly be more convenient to the patient. Again, I would like to encourage other practitioners to try LMs by the method described in this chapter, especially those who have had discouraging results with LMs in eyedroppers or LMs administered by any variation on what I have described here. I believe we owe it to our patients to try different methods until we find the one that will be the most rapid and gentle for them. As Hahnemann said, *aude sapere* ("dare to know").

Chapter Seven

Case-Taking

The Scope of Homeopathic Case-Taking

Hahnemann explains homeopathic case-taking in Aphorisms 83 to 104 of the 6th edition of the *Organon*. I want to present in detail what Hahnemann meant in these paragraphs and how we can adapt them to modern times for a candid, unbiased, and thorough examination of the patient.

To the homeopath, the patient's symptoms become a living portrait of the symptoms of a remedy. Remember that for the purpose of prescribing, the *name* of the disease is of little importance. We do not have a specific intake form for epilepsy or diabetes because these are simply the results of chronic miasms. Hence the homeopathic dictum that "there are no diseases, only sick people."

Taking a case does not just consist of noting symptoms as the patient recounts them to you. One of our first concerns is try to find out *where the energy leaks are.* If we are not sealing these leaks, we are losing Vital Force due to a trauma, a poor diet, a continuous stress factor, bad habits, etc. The homeopath needs to consider *why* the patient is behaving in a particular way. What motivates him to continue bad habits, even though he is aware of them? Sometimes it is overambition, as in the case of the Nux vomica person who is an executive and has a million things to do, finds no time for relaxation or proper nutrition, and neglects every aspect of a balanced life. Ulcers might be a result of this life-style. Sometimes it is humiliation leading to low self-confidence and great performance anxiety, which are common in the Lycopodium patient. As will be explained in Chapter 9 on Prescribing, the Never Well Since is the object of our detective work.

The homeopath must take her case with much greater detail and sensitive observation than most other practitioners do. Most tend to brush aside any unusual symptoms as if they were purely imaginary; even more so if the patient says, "I think I got sick because my mother died [or I lost my job, or I found out my husband was having an affair]." But these represent the essence of the case, the Never Well Since, and thus are the most important symptoms to the homeopath. Allopaths put more faith in the results of diagnostic tests, whereas homeopaths rely primarily on what the patient says about her condition.

Throughout the previous century, prescribing for chronic patients in homeopathic clinics was based solely on their report of their symptoms and not on objective data. An allopathic diagnosis was not made unless the pathology was so far advanced that the prognosis was poor. This method was so effective that conditions were routinely cured in homeopathic clinics which are considered incurable today (such as cancer, for example, and the great infectious diseases of the last century).

The success of your first prescription depends largely on how you take the case. In casetaking, you always have a puzzle to solve; the more pieces you find, the more easily you can see the picture. Dr. H.C. Allen, one of our famous homeopathic forefathers, said that a case well-taken is nine-tenths prescribed for.

The object of the homeopathic consultation is to find out why the individual was susceptible to a disease, to explore the details of its evolution, and to discover precisely how this patient differs from all others bearing the same diagnosis *(individuality)*. The process of case-taking is usually lively and exciting. People may be difficult to understand, contradictory, strange, and secretive, traits we encounter every day in our practice; but there is always a person to unify the whole picture. The patient has an internal consistency even if the pieces do not seem to hang together at first.

Half of the cure is established by being present for the patient, who must feel your attention focused only on him. Establishing a rapport with the patient is essential. The homeopath must be sympathetic, calm, and receptive, like a photographic plate ready to receive the image of the patient without preoccupations, preconceptions, or prejudice. Silence *is* golden, especially in the beginning of the inquiry. Sympathetic listening comes most naturally to practitioners of certain constitutions (Phosphorus and Calcarea especially), but every homeopath can listen empathetically and establish a good rapport with the patient.

Observation

It is often said that case-taking starts when you meet and greet your patient in the waiting room. You have to be a Sherlock Holmes in order to understand who your patient is.

In the waiting room: When you meet your patient in the waiting room, one patient will be calmly waiting for you, reading a book or maybe knitting some socks for Christmas (Calcarea). Another one will be fuming at you for being five minutes late, telling you in no uncertain terms that you are wasting his precious time (Sulphuric acid, the "time is money" guy). Then there is the one who is chatting away with your receptionist or anyone else willing to listen—easy to find because of her vivacious and sympathetic nature (Phosphorus). The only one who avoids her is the Nat. mur. person who wants to remain incognito.

Another one is pacing around while stretching his limbs and cracking his fingers (Rhus tox.), but he is no match for the child running around like a VCR on fast forward (Tarentula hispanica).

Does a child interact with others, or anxiously hold mommy's hand or even hide behind her (Baryta carb.)? Maybe the child is cautiously watching the other children, sitting close to mom and waiting for an invitation to join the play (Calcarea). Does it look like the ostentatiously dressed lady wants nothing to do with the rest of the patients, powdering her nose, making it clear to everyone that she should not be approached (Platina)? Or can you tell that your visitor just wants some peace and rest because she is nodding off with all that commotion around her (Sepia)? Is there a man checking out all the women and undressing them with his eyes (Lycopodium)?

When you shake the patient's hand, is the handshake firm and the hand dry and hot (Sulphur, Nux vomica)? Or is the handshake limp and the hand cold and clammy (Calcarea)? Or is the patient inclined to hug you (Phosphorus, Pulsatilla)? You should also note the patient's complexion. Are there cracks in the skin (Sulphur, Graphites)? Is the skin dirty looking (Psorinum, Petroleum)? Is the hair limp (Nat. mur.) or prematurely greying (Lycopodium)? Note any skin rashes, warts, or cysts, and whether the hair is greasy or thinning. As you lead the patient into your examining room, many more clues reveal themselves before a word is uttered.

In the examining room: Watch how closely the patient sits to you in her chair. Does she sit with her legs crossed, as if worried that her uterus will fall out (Sepia; fortunately it hasn't happened yet!). Does she sit with her arms folded as if to guard against your questions (Nat. mur., Lachesis, Thuja)? Is she leaning towards you, as if visiting an old friend, ready and willing to share all the information she has? A Phosphorus might do this because she is overflowing with sympathy and friendliness and already considers you one of her good friends. But of course, everyone is her "best" friend. She might ask how you, the practitioner, is feeling that day. A Pulsatilla might be equally eager to tell her life story, but you have the feeling that she wants to be reassured. She tries to touch you, pleading, "Do you think you can help me, Doctor?" At your positive response, tears instantly give way to a radiant smile.

Is the patient sitting stiffly (Rhus tox.) or withdrawn and still (a depressed Pulsatilla) or pacing slowly about the room (Aurum)? Is she a guilt-ridden Kali bromatum, wringing her hands? Or is he an Arsenicum who comes with a suitcase full of all his vitamins and supplements and his entire medical record—all six volumes? Is her speech stuttering (Causticum) or hasty and incoherent (Lachesis)? Does he repeat the last word of each sentence (Thuja) or keep repeating what he just told you because he can't remember if he told you or not (Causticum)? Does he keep changing subjects, his speech revealing a jumble of disconnected thoughts (Cannabis indica) or does he forget what he is saying in the middle of a sentence (Thuja?)

Your first question, "What brings you to me?" can elicit quite a variety of responses or lack of them. Maybe you have "Mr. Know-it-all" in front of you (Sulphur) who tells you in no uncertain terms that he has researched his case on the Internet, and therefore he feels qualified to tell you his diagnosis while proposing a plan of treatment. He wants to be in command of the interview because he knows the facts ("Ideas, abundant," K53; "Theorizing," K87; and "Haughty," K51).

He is not the only one, though, with a controlling and superior attitude. In others it reflects a desire to control the situation out of a sense of pain or shame. Think about the proud Nat. mur., who at first is only willing to share the minimum of information with you until she feels she can trust you. But this is merely a self-defense mechanism because she has been hurt too many times. Her pride is certainly different from that of the haughty Platina, who would not even give you the time of day were it not for her unbearable facial numbness. With a condescending attitude, she even says, "Look, I am not just a regular patient. I want your undivided attention because I have a very special case." She really believes herself to be superior, not to be considered on the same level as anyone else ("Delusions, does not belong to her own family," K21; "Delusions, body, greatness of, as to," K22; and "Delusions, diminished, everything in the room is, while she is tall and elevated," K24).

For some patients you will only find out later why they were so controlling. Think about the dogmatic and rigid Kali carb. person ("Obstinate," K69) who always suppresses his emotions, no matter what. But the emotional suppression is expressed on the physical level: "Back pain, lumbar region," K909, and "Back, stiffness," K946. And the self-confident, controlling behavior of Lycopodium is a front for his great lack of confidence, even cowardice (K17). He is afraid you will find out that he is truly not the person he is presenting. Couple that to his love for power (K69) and you understand that it might be difficult to recognize his constitution at first. Often, however, his prematurely grey hair or his sexual complaints ("Genitalia, male, erections, too quickly," K710 and "Sexual passion, without erection," K711) are clues to his true personality.

Maybe the patient answers your questions slowly or not at all. Is the patient "mulling" it over, as a ten-year-old Calcarea solemnly explained to me? Maybe you can tell the patient is suspicious from his half-closed eyes and the way he asks *you* questions. He never gives you a straight answer, but rather a cautious, incomplete one, and he does not trust your remedy either (Lachesis). "This isn't going to hurt me, is it?" ("Delusion, poisoned, medicine being," K31, Lachesis). Yet another patient is unwilling to answer you because when you smiled at him, he thought you were laughing at him ("Delusion, laughed at," Baryta carb. and Ambra grisea, K28).

Alternatively, there might be a waterfall of words to your first question, reflecting a hurriedness on the mental plane in which the patient makes one statement after another, often not even finishing the previous thought ("Thoughts, rapid, quick," K88 and "Thoughts, intrude and crowd around each other," Nat. mur. and Cannabis indica, K87). Or this may reflect his perfectionism (Aurum) even to the extent of a delusion ("Delusion, neglected his duty, that he has," K30). Or perhaps is it the great anxiety and perfectionism of the Arsenicum patient? His tongue is the only thing that never gets tired and you wish it would. He is always trying to fit in more details of his case, afraid of leaving out the most important symptom.

Most of the time, anxiety and restlessness will be seen on the physical level: tapping the feet or constantly moving them (Zincum, Graphites, and Lycopodium), biting the fingernails (Baryta carb.), wringing the hands (Kali bromatum), or twitching (Causticum, Staphysagria). And who can forget the Tarentula hispanica child, who (his mother sighs) only settles down when he listens to music ("Sensitive, to music, amel.," K79)?

Look at how your patients are dressed: flashy, with many colors according to the latest style, sometimes too young for her age (Phosphorus); in very elegant and subtle colors (Carcinosin); in black, white or purple (Nat. mur.); or in very loose clothes, more like a formless dress, or baggy pants held up by suspenders (Calcarea)? While Phosphorus enjoys wearing sparkly jewelry, Platina is more likely to wear enormous gold earrings and flaunt a huge diamond. Do none of the clothes match and you have the impression he threw on the first ones he could reach from a rumpled heap on the floor (Sulphur)? Or is the patient a woman in her forties dressed like a little girl in a sailor suit (Pulsatilla)?

Does the patient want the windows open because she is "suffocating" (Pulsatilla), does he bring his own blanket even when your office is well heated (Nux vomica, Silica), or does he wants the air-conditioning turned off because he is very sensitive to drafts (Hepar sulph.)? I have had patients so environmentally sensitive that they walked into my office wearing masks that looked like they were straight out of *Star Wars.* Immediately I knew what remedy to prescribe (Phosphorus or Arsenicum) and even the potency and dose (the smallest possible dose, prn).

If you have a receptionist to schedule your appointments and collect payments, she can also provide you with a wealth of information. Some patients demand an immediate appointment, whether because they think they are more important than anyone else (Platina), or they are going to die on the spot if they can't see you right away (Arsenicum), or they have important business to take care of and they want to get it over with (Sulphur, Nux vomica). Some insist on speaking directly to you, the practitioner, instead of having a message conveyed by the receptionist; this may reveal the egotism and haughtiness of a Sulphur or a Platina. If a patient consistently forgets his checkbook, it may be a sign that he is having financial problems. Then again, it could be a shrewd Sulphur who has calculated how much interest he can make on the money he owes you if he pays you later. Some patients want to be close to the receptionist, whether out of an overflowing sense of friendship (Phosphorus) or clinginess (Pulsatilla). Others might try to make a date with her (Lycopodium). I will never forget the Lycopodium patient who remarked on my "gorgeous" receptionist and told me privately he wanted to ask her out. I had to break the news to him that she was not available: my receptionist was also my wife! Still others want the music in the waiting room changed to something more subdued, more in tune with their emotional vibration (Nat. mur., Aurum).

What jewels for your prescription. You have hardly asked your first question, yet you have an abundance of useful information. Be sure to note all your observations, as they will not only help you find the remedy, but they will also provide benchmarks for how your patient improves (improved behavior, disappearing of tics or twitches, clearing up of the skin, etc.).

The Rules of Inquiry

Write down key points *exactly* in the patient's own words and you will be surprised how the patient often expresses herself in the exact language of the Materia Medica. Allow the patient to have her say, if possible without interruption, unless she goes off the subject. Unnecessary interruptions break the continuity of the patient's thoughts and she will forget symptoms or state them differently than if encouraged to spontaneous expression. Remain silent and observe the patient's facial expression, body language and manner of speech. Just advise her in the beginning to speak slowly enough for you to record what she is saying.

Only retain what is applicable to the case, which will come with experience. Margaret Tyler said that the longer she practiced the less she wrote down. This was not a sign of laziness. What she meant was that she only wrote down what was useful for her prescription: the unusual symptoms and the essence of the case. As Hahnemann states in Aphorism 153:

> In the search for the homeopathically specific remedy ... the more *striking, exceptional, unusual* and *odd* (characteristic) signs and symptoms of the disease case are to be especially and almost solely kept in view. ... *These, above all, must correspond to very similar ones in the symptom set of the medicine sought.*

As will be discussed in Chapter 9 on Prescribing, a single symptom of this kind usually weighs far more in remedy selection than a long series of common symptoms. Speed and discrimination will come with experience.

During the intake some patients, especially hypochondriacs (Arsenicum), present their ailments in too glaring color and exaggerated expressions. Many of these suggestible patients are convinced that they have diseases, or will have them, which they definitely do *not*. No amount of reassurance avails with some. For other patients, a simple statement that "You just do not have the symptoms of that disease" will do wonders. (Never tell such a patient what the symptoms *are,* though!)

The loquacious patients (Phosphorus, Lachesis) will try to take you on an elaborate tour of their lives. But others withhold essential information, whether from fatigue (Sepia, Phosphoric acid), or because they don't want to bother you (Staphysagria) or because they have been so deeply hurt they do not easily trust anyone for fear of being hurt again (Nat. mur.). These types have to be prodded into saying anything at all. But never hurry a patient or suggest symptoms to him. A suggestible patient trying to impress you will respond positively to all your questions about symptoms.

Begin a new line for each symptom, so that you can go back and fill in details later when it is your turn to ask questions for clarification. When you feel satisfied with the patient's spontaneous rendition, you can and *must* ask questions to clarify and differentiate.

Finally, note your observations of the patient's behavior, appearance, facial expressions, etc. and inquire which features were peculiar to the patient when he was well (to establish the innate constitution, discussed in the next chapter).

Sometimes if the onset of the condition was disgraceful or shameful, the line of questioning must be delicate, tactful and skillful. Among the "disgraceful" causes are the secret errors of youth (STDs, one-night-stands, rapes, unwed pregnancies and abortions) which occur more frequently than one might suppose. The experienced practitioner can often infer these causes when the totality of the symptoms indicates remedies like Platina, Lycopodium, Staphysagria, Conium, Thuja, Medorrhinum, or Sepia (in a young woman). Sending out a questionnaire in advance is helpful, for a patient may give more complete answers in writing while at home, in her own environment, than in talking to a new practitioner.

Another way to put patients at ease is to allude to the topic indirectly, in a way that makes it seem commonplace, and see if the patient picks up on it. "It's interesting, I've noticed that many of my patients who have these same symptoms also report that they had problems with an abusive relationship at some point in the past." Or "Lots of times we find that women who need this remedy find it helpful for whatever problems they may have had as children with inappropriate touching by an older male figure." If this scenario applies to the patient, she will almost always leap to confirm it. The objection might be raised that this is a leading question. It is not, because it is not a question. If it does not apply to the patient, it sounds to her like idle chitchat. If it does, the vehemence with which she responds to it proves that she is not merely being suggestible.

If your patient is a secretive type (Nat. mur., Lachesis), you cannot always ask directly about emotional problems. But you can ask them "innocent" questions like "Where do you like to travel," "What kind of people do you like," and "What do you like to do at parties?" Their answers will give you the same kind of information as you would get from direct questions such as "What do you do when you are upset?" or "What makes you jealous?"

Psychotherapists, psychiatrists, physicians, and lawyers as new patients tend to hide their emotions. When asked about their feelings, they will often deny any problems. They may report physical symptoms and mental ones but not emotional ones. They may also need to be questioned indirectly.

Sometimes the patient will reveal her inmost soul indirectly. An opera singer who was one of my patients invited me to a recital. The songs she chose were all an evocative expression of her Nat. mur. state, for example:

> My dear love, at least believe me,
> That my heart languishes without you.
> Your faithful lover ever sighs,
> Cruel love, put an end to this anguish.

Through her choice of songs she was pleading to receive Nat. mur.!

Another young patient, suffering from Chronic Fatigue Syndrome, brought me the following poem which he had written:

> *Dark Light of the Soul*
> Dear God, are you there?
> Can you hear me, do you care?
> I know you are busy, but this won't take long.
> I need to find out why, what I've done wrong
> And to let you know I'm hanging on.
> Should I keep on writing you this song
> Or should I tear it up and throw it all away?
> Sometimes, it's hard to have faith in something I can't see.
> When I'm weak and scared and all alone
> It's my faith that comforts me.
> I just wish sometimes I could hear you say
> That you'll make it all just go away
> Or to feel your arms holding me tight
> Where I'm safe and everything's allright.
> With the sunrise will come a brighter day
> In your warm and everlasting light.
> Can you tell me how to ease the pain?

> Can you tell me when the rain will end?
> Can you tell me, will it be the same?
> Will the friends I've lost still know my name?
> Can you tell me if I'll ever live again?
> Dear God, are you there?
> It's me again, in case you care.
> I know you're busy, so I won't delay.
> Will you help me face another day?
> When I get down on my knees to pray
> Can you hear the whispered words I say?
> Or should I tear them up and throw them all away…

It is not difficult to see the despair and anguish this young man was going through. But he has not given up all hope (a clue to his psoric miasmatic background).

We can also put patients at their ease by mentioning our own weaknesses. I always try to be humble to encourage the patient to speak more freely. For example, in asking about fears, I would always begin my mentioning my own fear of heights (Sulphur!). Macho men might be otherwise reluctant to admit to any fears.

When the patient is a teenager I would always spend time with the teenager alone, being sure to tell the teenager that all information is confidential (unless I feel he is in danger of harming himself or someone else). I might also lead into some difficult topics by saying something like, "A lot of my patients your age are dealing with some really tough issues and they feel that their parents and teachers don't really understand them."

Be sure to watch your patient carefully, especially his *emotional reactions:* the intonation of his voice and his expressions, especially his mouth and eyes. Is he looking you straight in the eye? The eyes are the windows of the soul and will reveal much about the patient. Are the eyes dull and lifeless (Syphilinum)? Does the patient wear sunglasses even when it's not sunny out (Nat. mur.)? Does a child turn to her mother for the mother to answer for her when you ask a question (Pulsatilla)?

Notice how the patient describes his favorite food to determine whether it is a real craving: sparkling eyes and delighted intonation reveal a genuine crush. But if he mentions supposed desires and aversions with a flat intonation and no change in expression, you hardly have symptoms worth noting.

Pierre Schmidt used to say, try to make your patient laugh once and cry once during the initial consultation. Then you know you have really touched the patient and created an atmosphere of trust. So often patients told me at the end of the consultation: "Doctor, I already feel so much better, and I haven't even taken the remedy."

The Questions

I send my new patients a written intake form, a sample of which is in Appendix 1. (This intake form is not meant as the universal intake; other practitioners will want to modify it for their patient population and the information they find most useful. I have revised it many times over the years.) I ask patients to return it at least one week before the appointment. This gives me time to review the case at my leisure over the weekend before they come, so that I already have several remedies in mind and can do a differential diagnosis when they come. Of course sometimes I change my entire interpretation of the case when I meet them in person! I remember one woman who described herself as a grandmother and had very fine, spidery handwriting, which made me assume she was an elderly lady without checking her date of birth. I was ready to give her Arsenicum for her environmental sensitivities and fear of being poisoned by toxic chemicals. Much to my surprise she was a beautiful, self-assured, blonde Phosphorus who looked ten years younger than her 42 years (typical of a Phosphorus). She was extremely sensitive, even for a Phosphorus. Like the canary in a mine shaft, she had been stricken by toxic fumes at her workplace months before everyone else in the office came down with the same symptoms. The toxic chemicals had caused neurological damage, leading to her wavery handwriting. Phosphorus turned out to be a better remedy for her, covering the chief complaint as well as Arsenicum did and strengthening her hypersensitive constitution.

Other advantages of the written intake are speed and accuracy. You don't have to waste precious time during the interview recording simple data like age, height and weight. Information like past medical history and family medical history is recorded directly by the patient, reducing errors. The patient may also be more willing to divulge personal information in writing, although this can go both ways; sometimes a patient will answer a sensitive question by saying, "I will discuss this with you in person." But at least she knows what information is important and can think about her answer.

I usually begin by asking, "What brings you to see me today?" This open-ended question starts the patient talking and allows for a wide range of concerns, not just physical symptoms. Ask the patient to tell in her own words how she became ill and exactly how she feels. If she seems to hesitate, just say, "And what else?" This is especially important when you ask the patient to recount the history of her main complaint, as you want to get the picture from the beginning and how it has changed over the years with or without treatment. Continue this system of interested listening until she seemingly has exhausted her history. As you record symptoms, distinguish their *relative importance*, placing poorly marked symptoms in brackets. Underline the important ones with 1, 2 or 3 underlines or follow with the numbers 1, 2 or 3, representing increasing intensity or importance to the patient.

How Not to Ask Questions

Direct questions: Avoid questions which the patient can answer with a yes or no, such as "Do you crave sweets?" Instead, ask "What do you crave?" (or better yet, "If you didn't have to think about fat or calories or any books you've read about proper diet, what foods would you most want to eat?") Don't ask, "Are you thirsty?" Instead, ask "What are your drinking habits?" A patient might say, "Yes" to being thirsty, thinking about his morning coffee and his soup at noon, even if he doesn't drink anything else all day. Other patients deny being thirsty because they associate thirst with plain water, while they drink sodas or tea all day long. And others drink 8 glasses of water a day because they have read this is healthy, but they never have an actual sensation of thirst (which would be of significance to us).

Leading or suggestive questions: Never ask a question which puts the answer into the patient's mouth: "Are you anxious about your new job?" "Are you chilly?" "When you are upset, do you feel better if someone comforts you?" You will bias the patient's answers. Some are so anxious to please the practitioner that they will confirm whatever they think she wants to hear. This can actually be more of an issue for experienced homeopaths who think they know the right remedy early on in the case and then start skewing the questions to confirm it. Your patient needs to feel that you are listening to him and taking the cues from his answer, not imposing your own interpretation. And as we have said, such an experience is healing in itself.

Alternative questions: Avoid questions which require the patient to choose between two different alternatives: "Do you prefer sweets or salts?" or "Are your menses clear or dark?"

Changing the subject: While you are dealing with one symptom confine yourself to that one instead of skipping around, which can confuse the patient.

Ideally, the intake interview should satisfy the following criteria:
- succinct enough to fit in the allowable time frame,
- oriented towards finding the therapeutic diagnosis (the remedy) rather than the pathological diagnosis, and
- providing information corresponding to that available in the repertory or Materia Medica.

Sequence of Questions for the Best Intake Interview

The hierarchy of symptoms in Chapter 9 on Prescribing must be kept in mind so that you are sure to inquire about causality and mental/emotional symptoms. In practice, however, it is best to start with the Chief Complaint and all its modalities. In my early days of practice,

I used to follow the theoretical teachings strictly, always asking the mental/emotional symptoms first, but I soon realized that this was a mistake. In fact, a first-time patient, knowing nothing whatsoever about homeopathy, can feel hurt or resentful of this interrogation about his character when he comes to see you for a headache, an asthma attack, or some form of rheumatism. He may think you have mistaken him for a mental case and are making a disguised psychoanalysis. On the other hand, asking about mental symptoms at the end is also a mistake because by then the patient is tired, and thinking the questions are irrelevant, he may answer curtly, impatiently, or without detail.

I find it works best to begin with the Chief Complaint, even though it comes last in our hierarchy, because that is after all why the patient has come to you. This naturally leads into asking about the Never Well Since. Even though both subjects have already been covered in the written intake, they are so important that you should go over them in person, keeping in mind any differential diagnosis you need to make based on your analysis of the written intake information. Any general symptoms not covered in the written intake come next, then mental and emotional symptoms sandwiched in the middle. As a good observer, you can also note many Mind rubrics without having to ask: timid, loquacious, easily offended, embarrassed, restless, haughty, laughing immoderately or inappropriately, etc.

End the interview by clarifying or extending the written intake questions related to food cravings and aversions, sleep, and (for women) the menses. (The general aggravation of symptoms *before, during or after menses* is of greater importance than such questions as early, late and excessive menses.) Questions about sexuality may not be comfortable in the first interview (although I am amazed at how often patients, especially women, volunteer this information right away). And for men the Chief Complaint may involve sexual function (impotence, erection disturbances, etc.)

After the patient has had time to express his main complaint without interruption, you may say: "I have listened carefully to you; let's change roles and I would like to ask you more precise questions. I might interrupt you when I have the information I need. This just means that a longer explanation is not necessary." This will allow you more control over your time. Otherwise, you might be able to see only one patient a day, which is not very practical. Next, you start formulating various questions to fill in the gaps. You cross-examine the patient to clarify, verify, and amend the information she presented.

Above all, I focus on clarifying the Never Well Since: not only the "facts" of what happened when the Chief Complaint began, but even more importantly, how the patient reacted. Be sure to ask how she *felt* while the particular stress or trauma was happening. Different people can have very different reactions to the same event, and you should never assume. For example, one child may react to being abused with suppressed anger, trying to become a sweet, good little girl (Staphysagria). Another may fight back and start cursing (Anacardium), while another may feel guilty and feel as though it is her fault (Aurum), and yet another may be stimulated to precocious sexual feelings and start masturbating (Platina, Staphysagria, Origanum).

I also try to anticipate different obstacles to the cure, described in Chapter 14. If there are life-style factors which might impede the patient's recovery, I would help the patient explore options for improving the life-style and removing the obstacles.

Finally, I would ask the patient to clarify or expand on the written intake information about the past medical history and family medical history, including diseases and causes of death of family members. The patient often does not provide complete answers, which are of utmost importance for determining the active miasm.

Be sure to obtain enough information to make the following four diagnoses:
- *Etiologic diagnosis*: determining the true triggering cause (the Never Well Since) and possible maintaining causes; keep in mind the words *why, when* and *how.*
- *Chronic miasmatic diagnosis*: using the past medical history and family history to determine the active miasm and other possible miasms present, to ensure eradication of the miasm.
- *Personality diagnosis:* the patient's constitution and temperament. The constitution is especially important for determining dosage.
- *Therapeutic diagnosis:* The current remedy and also the remedy anticipated for each layer in the timeline (which the patient submits with the written intake; see Appendix 1). I look for the layers created by emotional or physical traumas (see Figure 14-2) and also indicate suppressive medical treatment with a *. This helps me to see the direct consequences of such suppressions and to anticipate the return of old symptoms.

The Physical Examination

The role of the physical examination depends on what kind of practice you have. In my own practice I rarely need to conduct a physical examination of the patient, as my patients treat me as the healer of last resort rather than as their primary care physician. With the limited time available for each patient, I prefer to spend it asking questions. A homeopath would make an ideal primary care physician, however, and in this situation should conduct an examination.

In certain situations I would always do a physical exam, especially if the Chief Complaint is a skin condition. The dermatologist's diagnosis of eczema, psoriasis or acne is not helpful. Instead I would note any crusts or scales, the color of any discharge, indurations and ulcerations, vesicles, bullae and furuncles. A bluish-purple boil would indicate the need for Lachesis;

a boil that is just forming, with the skin still hot and red and tight but without a pus pocket would indicate Belladonna, while a ripened boil that had come to a head would be ready for Hepar sulph. or Silica.

If you do acute prescribing you will need to do physical exams more routinely, for sore throats and ear infections for example. It is helpful to listen to the lungs in cases of asthma and pneumonia: are crepitations and rhonchi at the right lower base (Kali-c.) or left lower base (Nat-s.)? Is the patient drowning in his mucus (Ant-t.)? Abdominal palpation is important in case of liver and spleen disease as well as colon disorders and appendicitis, to name a few. With the increased frequency of prostate cancer in men, a rectal examination will be necessary if the patient complains of slow urination, dribbling, frequency, urgency, or hesitation.

Without doing a formal physical exam, you can certainly note what you observe about the physical appearance. Is the patient lean, obese or muscular? Do you see the picture of a chronic miasm in their physical structure: the thin chest and clear translucent skin of the tubercular miasm; the warty, hairy appearance of the sycotic miasm; the scaly, "dirty" skin or skin eruptions of the psoric miasm; the defective bone structure, congenital deformities and dental abnormalities of the syphilitic miasm.

It is a good idea to let the patient point to the area of discomfort. You will be surprised that the stomach disorder is really a liver problem, or a heart problem is an intestinal disorder. Don't assume that your patient's knowledge of anatomy is the same as in your textbooks! A child will always say, "My stomach hurts," no matter where the condition is located. And even adults tend to say, "My stomach hurts" about any pain between the diaphragm and the pelvic floor. Elderly people may be especially self-conscious about mentioning the colon and may use "stomach" as a euphemistic substitute. We know that each remedy has a typical sphere of action in certain organs and tissues, so knowing the location (regardless of diagnosis) can indicate a certain remedy.

Tongue diagnosis was once a part of the family doctor's assessment, but most practitioners nowadays (except acupuncturists) never examine the tongue. But this organ can give invaluable, objective signs which will draw the attention of the homeopath to a certain organ. What do we look for in the tongue? A "normal" tongue found in a healthy individual is neither plump nor thin. It has a moderate red color, is relatively wet and has no coating ("fur") or else a thin, white coating. In illness there is a change in the coating: when toxins accumulate, the fur becomes thick, oily and yellow. The tongue is divided into areas which correspond to the different organs in TCM (Fig. 7-1).

The easiest aspects of the tongue to learn for a non-acupuncturist are the changes noted in the color of the tongue and the tongue coating. Always refer to the location of these changes on the tongue, as they will indicate the organ where the stress takes place.

Color of tongue: A red, dry tongue with many cracks indicates intense heat in the body, creating dryness of the mucosae, constipation, thirst, offensive urine, etc. A "black" tongue relates to an illness of the kidney or a depletion of Kidney energy due to fear, phobias, frights, loss of seminal fluids, bone diseases (arthritis, arthrosis, RA), etc. A pale tongue demonstrates a deficiency of the Vital Force in general, with chilliness, prostration, and lack of appetite, as we would see in cachectic situations such as advanced cancer, diabetes, or lupus.

Tongue coating: A normal tongue coating is thin and even, covering the entire tongue, or just the center, because it originates from the Spleen/Stomach unit. The thicker the coating becomes, the stronger the invasion of excessive energy (from climate factors, food intake, emotions). A very dry tongue indicates excessive heat (constipation, strong smelling urine, scanty urine). If the coating goes from thick to thin under the influence of the remedy, it indicates that you have the simillimum, the prognosis is favorable, and the treatment is correct. Thickening of the tongue coating indicates that the simillimum has not been chosen and the case is progressing in an unfavorable direction. (A *temporary* thickening could represent a cleansing reaction under the action of the simillimum, but in this case the coating would thin within the next few days).

Color of the tongue coating: A thin, white fur is normal and shows that there is a good balance in the Spleen/Stomach unit. A greasy, white, thick coating reflects the invasion of Dampness in the body (whether from a wet climate, raw foods, or deficient digestion). A yellow color always represents Heat in the body. When the fur changes from yellow to white, the simillimum is doing good work, and the prognosis is favorable. A change from white to yellow shows that the disease is going from the exterior to the interior (against the direction of Hering's Law).*

---

*For more information on the "tongue picture," see my book, *Acupuncture for the Practitioner.*

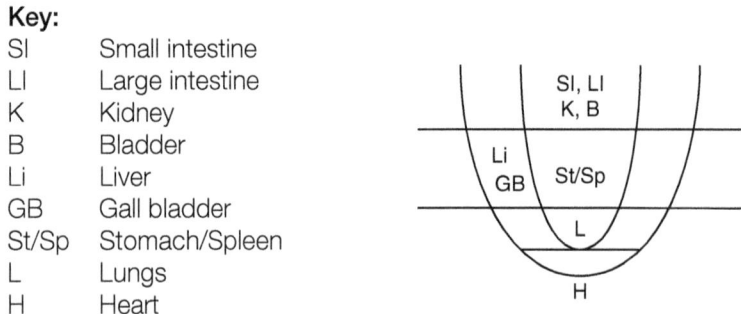

Key:
SI — Small intestine
LI — Large intestine
K — Kidney
B — Bladder
Li — Liver
GB — Gall bladder
St/Sp — Stomach/Spleen
L — Lungs
H — Heart

Fig. 7-1: Area of the Tongue Associated with Each Organ in TCM

Occasionally I have found it necessary to do a physical examination when the indicated remedy did not work. A 23-year-old woman consulted me for a condition diagnosed as rheumatism in the legs, for which she had been treated allopathically for several years to no avail. She found herself increasingly weak, with vague pains and great weakness in the legs. All my questioning indicated Lycopodium, but Lycopodium did not work even in increasing potencies. On giving her a complete physical, I found a curious condition of the throat: it looked as if painted with a yellow-orange varnish. A lab culture found a large number of Klebs-Loeffler bacilli, the signature of diphtheria. Evidently she had paretic sequelae of un-diagnosed diphtheria; apart from a faint dryness of the throat, she had no other local symptoms. Allen's *Nosodes* has the following comment on Diphtherinum: "Painless diphtheria, symptoms almost entirely objective, patient too weak to complain, patient apathetic, prostration, post-diphtheric paralysis, remedy suitable when the most careful selected remedy fails to relieve or permanently improve."[1] Diphtherinum 200c cured her and two weeks later a second culture showed not a single bacillus.

Taking an Acute Case

Case-taking for an *acute* disease will be easier because the symptoms will be fresh in the patient's memory and still new and striking, except that patients are so accustomed to peremptory doctors' visits that they are likely to just say, "I have a cough, give me something." Sometimes for convenience we may abbreviate the disease image with a *collective name*, i.e., flu, measles, rubella, etc., but we know we are referring to the specific symptom picture of the current epidemic. If one homeopath asks another about "this year's flu" the answer may be "It is a Gelsemium flu" or "an Arsenicum flu." But we never forget that we are talking about a *kind* of flu.

In taking an acute case, first ask whether the illness is a simple acute one or part of an ongoing or recurring picture (which needs to be treated with a chronic, miasmatic remedy). Do not assume it is a one-time, short-lived occurrence. Many patients come to you as their last resort after months of OTC or prescription drugs. You may need to give Nux Vomica or Thuja to clear the drugs out of their system before the indicated remedy will work.

If your appointment schedule is booked months in advance with chronic patients, as mine was, most of your acute cases will be tacked on at the end of another consult, or left on your answering machine: "By the way, Doc, my wife just came down with a sore throat. Anything you can do?" Or: "My child kept us up coughing during the night. Please help us get a good night's sleep." With no time for lengthy interrogation (and without the patient present, which of course would be preferable), you will have resort to the *"three-legged stool"* method. At least three sound symptoms are sought and used in the selection. Most important are the Never Well Since and mental/emotional changes, if available. If not, inquire about the *location, sensation, modality and concomitants* of the Chief Complaint (described below).

Of course, if the patient throws you a keynote symptom of a remedy, you are fortunate indeed. It is a challenge to solve acute cases quickly with a minimum of information; it helps keep your mind sharp and also proves to the patient the power of homeopathy.

Often you will not have a Never Well Since or mental/emotional symptoms in acute cases. When you do, however, remember that they rank higher than the physical symptoms. Here are some examples of etiologies which are so typical for acute events that they almost certainly point to a particular remedy (confirmed, of course, with the rest of the case):

- a finger smashed in a car door: Hypericum
- a hangover from too much beer: Nux vomica
- overstraining from lifting heavy furniture: Rhus tox., Calcarea
- exposure to northeast wind: Aconite
- becoming chilled while wet e.g. from perspiration: Rhus tox.
- being struck by lightning: Phosphorus

A complete list is provided in the Never Well Since list in Appendix 2.

Typical mental/emotional symptoms in acute ailments pointing to a particular remedy include:

- extreme clinginess and weepiness, wanting to climb on mommy's lap: Pulsatilla
- neediness for consolation: Phosphorus and Pulsatilla
- wanting to keep busy, feeling better when preoccupied: Sulphur, Sepia
- restlessness and fearfulness: Arsenicum and Aconite (with the former tending to pace around and the latter predicting that he will die at a particular time)
- grouchiness, wanting to be left alone: Bryonia
- crankiness and contrariness: Chamomilla

Also, keep in mind that an acute illness will temporarily cause chronic symptoms to abate or disappear, following the law that two dissimilar diseases cannot coexist: the stronger one suppresses the weaker one. The chronic picture often completely retreats, only to reappear after the acute illness has run its course. This will be the best time to deal with the chronic picture. In fact, there is no time when we can see the chronic picture so plainly and clearly as *at the end of the acute attack*. The condition following acute illnesses is much more apt to show the chronic condition than the lingering effects of the acute, as is so often mistakenly believed.

To find the "three legs of the stool" in acute prescribing, we can use some elements of the mnemonic known as Von Boenninghausen's Seven Levels of Case Taking: *quis* (who), *quid* (what), *ubi* (where), *quibus auxiliis* (with what), *cur* (why), *quomodo* (how) and *quando* (when).*

- *Quis* (who) means taking into account who our patient is; even in acute conditions, patients of certain constitutions are likely to need certain acute remedies.
- *Quid* refers to the etiology: a physical trauma, an emotional shock (grief, hearing bad news, fright, indignation, etc.), a weather influence (exposure to dampness, dry cold northerly wind, storm, etc.). Don't forget allopathic drug actions or side-effects.
- *Ubi* (location) means considering factors such as the location of the pain, right or left sided complaints, and what systems are affected: the nervous, gastrointestinal, urinary, respiratory, etc. Let the patient point to the location rather than trusting their knowledge of anatomy.
- *Cur:* What affects the complaints for better or worse? (cold, heat, dryness, dampness, positions, pressure, walking, standing, lying, menstrual cycle, movement, rest, sleep, etc.).
- *Quando* (when) refers to the appearance, aggravation and amelioration of the Chief Complaint. Only the sharp and definite return of complaints (i.e. 3-5 p.m. of Sepia, 4-8 p.m. of Lyc.) is important to us. Remember to look for *periodicity* in the symptoms (q. third day, q. fourteenth day, every spring, etc.). In this modality, we should also pay attention to whether the onset and disappearance of the symptoms are fast or slow.
- *Quibus auxiliis* (with what) refers to concomitant symptoms, such as diarrhea with vomiting, headaches with nausea or vision disturbances, vertigo with nausea and ringing in the ears. The sensation of the Chief Complaint can also be included here: ask the patient to describe in his own words what the discomfort feels like, "as if ..." Let him give an adjective for his pain: stitching, burning, sore, lancinating, boring, etc.

---

*At the great homeopathic congress in Brussels in 1855, von Boenninghausen offered a prize for the best essay on the topic "the greater or lesser value of the symptoms occurring in a disease, to aid as a norm or basis in the therapeutical selection of the remedy." Several years later, however, the question remained unsolved, so von Boenninghausen proposed his own answer in a treatise called *A contribution to the judgment concerning the characteristic value of symptoms*.[2] Hahnemann had already determined that the striking or unusual symptoms bore the most weight; the question was how to judge what is striking or unusual. Von Boenninghausen used a medieval Latin mnemonic for theology students: *Quis? Quid? Ubi? Quibus auxiliis? Cur? Quomodo? Quando?* (Who? What? Where? With what? Why? How? When?) The baron felt that these seven questions contained all the essential areas for proper case taking.

Pediatric Case-Taking

Case-taking for a child depends on whether the child has reached puberty, not only because of the great difference in symptoms which appear in the pre- and postpubescent child, but also because of the role of the young patient and patient's mother in providing the necessary information. Obviously after puberty the child can fill out her own questionnaire, and younger children may want to participate in the process, whether by writing out their own set of answers or by having the mother ask them the questions. (This should not be the sole source of information, however; one or both parents should definitely contribute their observations for young people up until the time the young person leaves home.) I might need further information from the parents regarding the mother's pregnancy and the young patient's childhood diseases and vaccinations, but I find it extremely important to create a good rapport with the young patient. After all, changes have to come from them, and when the practitioner treats the child as an equal, often a good compliance can be expected both in terms of remedy intake and any changes in life-style.

I always ask even the younger child what they like to play with. If they play with dolls, I ask what kind of games they like to play with them. (Lycopodium likes to play school and boss them around, Calcarea and Silica play house with the dolls as their babies, Phosphorus plays theater or takes them on a stroll, always in different outfits). What kind of movies do they like? Do they like violent games with a lot of shooting, killing and horror (syphilitic miasm)? Or are movies and games all about action, speed, and thrills (sycotic)? Ask the child why they are interested in what they are doing. Ask them if they are animal lovers (Nat. mur. adores dogs and horses, Arsenicum loves cats, Calcarea dotes on all pets, as does Carcinosin. An adult Carcinosin will fight for the survival of all animals, donating her precious savings to "save the whale," the wolf, or a bird). Ask them what they like in school and at home, how they get along with parents and siblings, etc.

Here are some other "innocent" questions which can open a floodgate of information: "What did you see while mummy was driving the car to the office? Who do you like to play with? How do you get along with other kids at school and at home? Who is your best friend? How many friends do you have? What kind of games do you play with your brothers and sisters? How are you doing in school? Anything there you don't like?" And at the end of our questions: "Is there anything *you* want to tell me?" Never underestimate children's insight.

After puberty I want to speak to the adolescent alone (unless she prefers her mother to come along, which I would expect of a Calcarea or Pulsatilla). But I want the youngster to be able to speak freely, to see her perspective on her condition and to what extent it interferes with her daily life. Afterwards I always ask the adolescent's permission to speak to her parents to clarify things. If the situation is shameful or secret (problems at school, difficult relationships with peers, abnormal sexual behavior) I would of course question the parents out of earshot of the youngster. I don't want to add to the young person's embarrassment and shatter his confidence in his parents and physician. Treat the teenager as an adult, if possible, and you will be surprised how he will consider you his friend and give you the information you need.

I find that normally young people want to speak to me alone, and when I find a 20-year-old (or older) bringing her mother along, I have to ask myself why: is she very close to her mother (Phosphorus) or in a Nat. mur. state and needing her mother's support to face a "stranger" with her most intimate problems. Maybe she has the psoric nature ("looking for support") of a Calcarea, or she is a Pulsatilla looking for her mother's approval.

Returning to younger children now, I have in my office toys and coloring books as well as blank paper for drawing. I encourage them to draw something while waiting and bring their creation in for their appointment. I am astonished at what young children draw and how artistic they are. I have seen children draw a figure entirely made up of fruits, others draw religious symbols and figures, and others draw colorful pictures of my secretary. Do they draw a happy family with mummy and daddy (Calcarea, Phosphorus)? Or is one of the family members left out (Nat. mur. might leave out a parent, or a jealous Pulsatilla youngster might leave out a sibling)? Do they draw only knights in armor with their limbs severed and blood dripping all over, or do they like drawings with skulls and crossbones (all expressions of the syphilitic miasm)? Or do they pay attention to detail, precision, and symmetry (Silica)? One little girl diagnosed with autism, the patient of one of my students, drew only in black. After several months on Nat. mur., there were not enough colors in the rainbow to satisfy her (reflecting her innate Phosphorus constitution).

I like to see what books and toys the children choose, and it gives me another topic to talk to them about. A visit to a doctor is traumatic enough for a child. I never wear a white coat (avoiding the "white-coat syndrome") and I keep a little refrigerator full of healthy snacks and drinks from which the children soon learn they can help themselves. Since I never give shots or bad tasting medicine, nothing but "sweet little balls" as the children call the remedies, I have been the hero of many of my little patients.

In taking the case of a child you will need information from the mother about her pregnancy and labor, the family history, and any changes in her child (reactions to vaccinations, illnesses, injuries, emotional events in the family, etc.). And as practitioners we must know what is normal behavior for a child at each stage of development so that we can discern what is abnormal. Don't use the rubrics "Picking the nose," or "Desire to be held" indiscriminately as these are normal behaviors in many young children.

In my office, I would allow the child to be free and observe his behavior. Is he the timid or shy type, hiding behind his mother's skirt (Baryta carb., Silica); does she respond to patting and talking (Phosphorus, Pulsatilla; the Pulsatilla will climb on your lap and want a kiss, the Phosphorus will want to do a little dance and show off for you); does the child watch every gesture you make (Calcarea)? Does the child jump around and destroy things (Tuberculinum)? Is he nervous and alert, watching your every move (Argentum nitricum), dirty (Sulphur, Anacardium) or jumpy at the least noise (Borax)?

Food cravings and aversions: Ask the mother if there is any food the child likes that other kids don't like. How long can the child be without food? Children so often crave sweets that we cannot use it as a symptom, but if a child refuses sweets it is worth noting. Aversions for vegetables is a given for children, unless they are raised in a vegetarian family. The family's food preferences must be taken into account especially if they are from a different culture. Children's natural inclinations are for bread, potatoes, vegetables, milk (mother's milk or goat's milk should be given by preference over cow's milk), and ripe fruits of all kinds. But in our society these natural instincts are drowned out by food ads and cultural habits, so that most American children like pizza, pasta, ice cream, and soft drinks. I have even seen mothers put cola in their baby's bottle! Giving children junk food, sweets and soft drinks instead of more natural foods creates children whose palate is trained to be stimulated by ever-increasing amounts of (let's face it) garbage. Whatever does not taste sweet, salty, fatty or junky is soundly rejected by these children as "yucky" and "gross."

Of course by asking about certain foods we might have certain remedies or constitutions in mind. Cravings for milk yet with an intolerance for it indicates Calcarea; other examples include strong cravings for soft boiled eggs, which most children dislike (Calcarea), cravings for bacon and milk (Tuberculinum), cravings for soups (Carcinosin), or constantly drinking cold water and chewing on ice cubes (Tuberculinum and Phosphorus). Cravings for oranges, unripe fruits, green apples, and salt will indicate Medorrhinum, while cravings for fats might guide our prescription to Nitric acid or Nux vomica. Food cravings and desires can help us understand the active miasm: a strong aversion to meat denotes the syphilitic miasm, a desire for meat the tubercular and psoric, a desire for oranges can confirm the sycotic, etc. (see Chapter 19, Miasms).

Mentals: As usual we don't ask mentals first, knowing that most mothers are very protective of their children. Even when the Chief Complaint involves their children's behavior, mothers tend to tell me how "nice and good" their child can be. It is difficult for parents to discuss children's disturbed or even perverted behavior, which is becoming more and more common. The parents feel the behavior is their fault or want desperately to believe that their child is good and normal, just misunderstood. When a child continually disrupts the class by calling out without raising his hand, the mother will say he is "so spontaneous" (a euphemism for "impulsive") and that the teacher should just pay more attention to him (never mind the 35 other kids in the class). When a teenager put his feet on my desk, practically right in my face, his mother, instead of remonstrating him, was quick to point out, "He already feels at home with you." (Maybe she meant he was challenging me and seeing how far he could go with me, just as he did at home with his parents!) Another mother told me she could not understand why the coach did not let her little boy play more often in his team's football games. "I know he's not a star, Dr. Luc, but he should still get a chance to play." Looking at the little chubby fellow with the thick glasses, I sensed he was probably the worst fumbler on the team!

A good question to start with is how much the child needs *affection* (except when sick, when most children want consolation). Pulsatilla and Phosphorus can never get enough, with the difference that Phosphorus receives *and* gives while Pulsatilla seems like a bottomless pit who never receives enough. Make sure to ask about change in their behavior if other children are born after the little patient. (Jealousy after the birth of a younger sibling is a strong indicator for Pulsatilla). On the other hand, Nat. mur. children, although longing for affection, will never show this, as though an inner voice forbids them to ask for it. This turns them into loners, misunderstood by parents and peers. Parents will shower more affection on the kissing, hugging Pulsatilla child than on her aloof Nat. mur. sister, which only makes the situation worse. And little Mr. Sulphur has to be forced to give his grandma a kiss because that is "girlie" behavior. He would rather give a firm handshake, because saying "I love you" is difficult for him.

The next emotion is *sympathy* which can be expressed at an early age. I ask the mother how the child reacts to someone who is sick or handicapped. We think of Phosphorus first, but also Calcarea, Staphysagria and Causticum (the latter out of sensitivity to injustice and cruelties). The child's sympathetic reaction often leads to physical symptoms such as tic nerveux, muscle twitching, and head movements. I had a pretty eight-year-old girl who presented with facial tics. It was the hardest thing for me to find the Never Well Since. Neither the mother nor the child could help me. But the formation of styes, headaches, stomachaches, and lower abdominal pains made me think of Staphysagria, which promptly relieved (K145, headache from grief, vexation; K515, stomach pain after vexation; K561, abdominal pain after vexation). Upon further questioning the mother finally told me that she had taken in her niece who was condemned to a wheelchair because of MS. Shortly after that her child's behavior started. And when my own Calcarea son was four years old, I saw him putting a blanket on his 6-year-old brother who had fallen asleep on the sofa. I certainly would never expect my Sulphur son to do the same for his little brother!

Next I ask about their *reaction to music*. Of course most children react positively, unless they are sensitive to noise. But do their symptoms improve with music (Tarentula), do they dance to it like a crazed clown (Stramonium, Tarentula)? If they like classical music, this is unusual in a small child, but we see it in Aurum and Nat. mur. by age 10 to 12. Do they have a strong sense of rhythm (Sepia)? Sepia dances with her body while Nat. mur. dances with her mind! Or do they dance with great flair and a total lack of inhibition (Phosphorus)? I never had to ask twice for a Phosphorus girl to show me her dance steps. She might complain of being tired and not interested in a visit to the doctor's office, but she will never be too tired to show off her latest routine, under the proud eyes of her mother. Next would come an invitation to her dance recital where (as one little girl was quick to point out) she would be dancing in center stage, where a star was painted on the floorboards!

Next comes *obstinacy*. We all know the terrible twos when the child starts to assert itself. But sometimes the temper tantrums are abnormal (Tuberculinum, Calcarea, Stramonium). Stramonium children are the head-bangers. The more obstinate the behavior, the more Tuberculinum will be indicated. If you can confirm this behavior with a history of recurrent colds and swollen glands, Tuberculinum is likely to be the simillimum. A Calcarea keeps on kicking and banging for a while even when you have left the room (a Phosphorus gives up as soon as she does not have an audience!). Or he steadfastly refuses to come out of his room when called (while a Pulsatilla will leave the door open, hoping you will come in and reassure her in her flood of tears).

The Tuberculinum has more malice and destructiveness. He breaks something which might be the favorite possession of his parents or another child. I had a beautiful toy parrot in my waiting room which would repeat words when spoken to. But the first Tuberculinum child that came in managed to break it into many pieces, to the consternation of my other little friends. He showed no remorse, just a grin, while the mother tried to reassure me that he was "a good boy." I was not fooled, however; I put "malicious and destructive" in his chart and prescribed Tuberculinum!

Fastidiousness is something we don't expect in children. Most mothers have to beg and plead with their children to clean up their room. We see complaints from parents in Anne Landers' column about the hurricanes that seem to strike their children's rooms. But sometimes we see a child fussing over the smallest thing. If everything has to be neat, if he does not want to wear clothes with a little spot, if certain colors have to match, or if he always puts his toys away neatly arranged, then we should consider this a useful symptom. Arsenicum, Anacardium, Nux vomica, Graphites, and Carcinosin have this symptom. I had a patient in Belgium who was germ-phobic and a neat freak to the point of being obsessive-compulsive; my mother, who was the village kindergarten teacher, remembered this same man from thirty years earlier as a four-year-old coming to school, the only one in a little suit and tie! Arsenicum helped this man to return to a normal life; he no longer had to wash the phone after each use or get up in the middle of the night to wash his car.

Fears are quite common and should not be used unless they are very unusual or very marked. When a child is suddenly fearful of an older child or adult, we must try to reassure the child until she feels comfortable telling us why. One of my patients left his three- and five-year-old sons in the care of his father, who was visiting for the first time from overseas. He noticed how they shrank from their grandfather afterwards and refused to see him off at the airport. Their fearfulness and crying fits continued for weeks afterwards until they finally told him what had happened: the alcoholic and abusive grandfather (i.e. with a strong syphilitic miasm) had "played" with them by holding a lit cigarette lighter close to them and threatening to burn off their penises. The patient felt terrible; he knew his father had been abusive to his mother but never imagined he could turn his destructive impulses towards these innocent children.

Sometimes a child expresses a great fear of one of the parents (another reason to talk to the child alone). I remember an 8-year-old girl who came with her mother for behavioral disturbances (at school she was diagnosed with ADD, but her mother complained bitterly of the bad treatment she received there). When the mother told me that this girl grew up during a time when her husband was a fullblown alcoholic and she saw her parents fighting all the time, I had a clue to her remedy. Young children in such a terror situation learn very quickly to "be good," in fact too good. They do not take any initiatives, out of fear of incurring the parent's wrath, and the parents make every decision for them. This girl became violent in both language and behavior and very rebellious towards the safer, more caring parent, the mother. When I talked to the young girl by herself, she told me that "someone makes me do it, I can't help it." This expression of her struggle to gain some independence and still be a good girl could be translated as "a devil on one shoulder and an angel on the other," the classic keynote of Anacardium. And in fact Anacardium brought great relief to this innately sweet and gentle girl.

Strict parents and overparenting can be almost as harmful to children as emotional neglect. Remedies such as Carcinosin and Staphysagria (which complement each other) should always be in the differential diagnosis for children with emotional or physical symptoms due to an authoritarian or domineering parent.

The older the child the more we will value their fear as a symptom, of course. (Never include any doubtful symptoms in your case-taking.) The younger the child, the more fearful of noise, so use this symptom only when the child shudders at the slightest noise. Fear of the dark is common, with many children requiring a little night light, but the Stramonium fear of the dark should get your attention because of the intensity of the symptom. And if the child is ten years old and still can't be in his dark room alone, definitely use it. Other diagnostic fears can include fear of strangers (Baryta carb.), of downward movement (crying when being put down in crib, Borax), of animals, especially dogs (Belladonna, Tuberculinum) or harmless animals like cows and horses (Bufo and China). Often most fears disappear or diminish when we administer the constitutional remedy. Children as well as adults of a Calcarea or Phosphorus constitution are likely to have the most fears.

Sensitive to reprimands: One of the mental characteristics of sycosis is shame. Sensitivity to reprimand—the child being very sensitive to being scolded, even mildly—is a related one and confirms Medorrhinum or Nat sulph.

Environment

In these modern times children are exposed to situations and stimulations never available to earlier generations. How many children come into my office with a video game, nervously clicking away in search of the next highest level of the game! No time for anything else; worse, no desire for anything else, such as exploring nature, interacting with other kids, getting some fresh air, and getting some much-needed physical exercise. (It is shocking that my children and their friends, in comparison with my generation, are in much worse physical shape. Calcareas tend to stay chubby or flabby, often prone to viral infections because of a lack of fresh air and physical strength.) Computers have changed the landscape not only for adults but for children as well. In fact, the child now seeks constant stimulation through video games; reading is something of the past. (And you can certainly see this in the quality of their spelling!) One can only wonder if the computer just fuels the fire for an ADD child who cannot sit still while doing his homework (Lycopodium) or needs constant stimulation, trying to incite other children to misbehave while cunning enough not to get into trouble himself (Tarentula).

Unfortunately, with the birth of the Internet, the floodgates have been opened for the possible pollution of our children. You can try to monitor what your child accesses on the Internet at home, and if you are successful they can just go to the library and download all the pornography they want, not to mention the pedophiles who haunt the chat rooms. The numerous sycotic teenagers will be attracted to risk-taking, even criminal behavior, while the less-common syphilitic youngsters will be lured with the fascination of sexual perversions. Danger seems to lurk everywhere for our children, and the Internet, which could be a great source of information for them as encyclopedias were for us, puts some of our children on the wrong track.

Despite glowing reports about the strength of our economy, in most families both parents have to work, leading to the new phenomenon of latchkey kids who are forsaken, abandoned and desperate to belong somewhere. We think of Nat. mur. for griefs and losses like the death of a parent or a divorce, but for children I often find myself using it for simply "lack of emotional nourishment," which is a grief situation in itself for these neglected children.

I have the typical sycotic teenagers as patients who like to stay out until all hours of the night and sleep late in the morning. Dressed in black leather, with rings piercing everywhere and their hair in fluorescent colors, school and jobs were out of the question for them. Their parents did not care or could not control them, and the result was that the night became the day for them. Any drugs they might use would only stimulate the sycotic miasm further. The world has certainly not become a better and safer place for our children, and I am afraid that something more than a homeopathic remedy (God forbid, Prozac or Ritalin) is needed to restore the balance in these children.

Clinical Case: One of my patients, a 12-year-old boy diagnosed with ADD, was often left alone after school and would often leave home, unbeknownst to his parents, looking for some action (a real sycotic expression). One night he and a friend found a motorboat on the river and decided to take it down to Atlantic City (where the action is!). Once they loosed it from its moorings they were unable to start it and drifted downriver, finally drifting ashore. They were picked up by the police walking along the highway at 3 a.m. And now a homeopathic remedy was needed to fix all this! I took a real liking to this young fellow, who boasted in my office (another sycotic expression), "No one will control me!" I even took him out to buy him a birthday present, for which he drew me a very beautiful picture (of course of an action figure). To my great disappointment, his mother sent him away to a school for incorrigible children. Is he a future criminal? I hope not, since I could see the goodness in him, but I fear for him nevertheless.

The family and personal history

The younger the child, the more interested we are in the intra-uterine experience, labor and postnatal state (see intra-uterine prescribing in Chapter 10).

Labor: If there is slow or induced labor, the use of forceps or suction cup which can all possibly induce a "kind of" head trauma, think of Helleboris, Cicuta (especially if seizures), Nat. sulph. and Thuja as chronic remedies, Arnica as the acute. A recent investigative television program highlighted the dangers of vacuum-assisted delivery, which has increased the frequency of subdural hematomas, skull fractures, and even neonatal deaths. Eleven babies died in six months because of vacuum extraction, usually because it was used for longer than the recommended 30 minute limit.[2] Arnica or Bellis perennis could be a savior for both newborn and mother in this situation.

Postnatal state: Record reactions after vaccinations (Thuja, Silica, or the nosode of the vaccination itself), and the severity of childhood diseases (which might require the nosode to "antidote" this action and clear the terrain). According to Elizabeth Wright-Hubbard, one of my favorites:

> Basically, children should have the childhood diseases. They throw off certain impurities and clarify the constitution. Cases properly handled should leave the child with no sequels and in better health. The patients who come to the doctor in adulthood saying they never have been ill and boasting how they had no childhood diseases are often those with serious, incurable troubles. For instance, many cancer patients and many who die from sudden heart ailments and who were in vigorous health give no history of childhood disease. Aside from the fact that you should have these illnesses, another point in *[preventing or]* suppressing them at an early age when they are suitable is that, when skipped at an early age, they often occur later in a far more serious form, such as mumps with complications in testes in men. Furthermore, these preventatives, given in good faith in the name of perfect health, introduce through the normal protective skin elements completely foreign to the human body.[3]

A Typical Child's Picture Nowadays

Theoretically if we could have the child under homeopathic treatment from conception (treating the parents' miasms before conception) and control the environment, diet and hygiene as well, we would end up with very few adult patients. Unfortunately, a typical case in our modern world progresses like this. The baby is often born with a rash due to the mother's medication intake during pregnancy. Or there are feeding problems at a very early age: the mother's milk disagrees, she has no time for nursing, etc. Formulas are prescribed to make the baby "plump and healthy." Then a rash appears either from sweating or from an allergic reaction to the formula; then cortisone is prescribed. If the suppression is successful, the next step may be bronchial colds (remember that the lungs and skin are connected in Traditional Chinese Medicine). Then comes a succession of nose colds and ear infections with never-ending rounds of antibiotics. By the age of two the child can be a candida sufferer, asthmatic and weakened. By the time the child is school-age he may be so asthmatic that he is dependent on inhalers. (School nurses report drawers full of inhalers to be given to the children at break time, something unheard of and unnecessary a few decades ago.) The ever present inhalers make the children speedy, absent-minded, foggy and impulsive. Next, ADD and ADHD are promptly diagnosed with the inevitable prescription for Ritalin. When this does not work any more, we have Cylert. When the side effects become too much, the doctor throws in the towel and turns her attention to the numerous children at the earlier end of the scenario. This is when the child is likely to come to us, after "everything else has been tried" and the side effects of the medications have compounded the original problem. And of course the parents will expect instant results or else they will leave you, claiming that homeopathy does not work!

Puberty adds to the chaos, because the child's changing hormones kick up latent miasmatic activity. This picture is not an exaggeration but unfortunately all too common. Most of the children I saw as patients came because their parents were fed up with the monthly intake of antibiotics for recurrent colds, with the side effects of cortisone and inhalers in asthma and eczema, with the increasing ineffectiveness of Ritalin for ADD/ADHD, and with the constant syrups and antibiotics to clear the ever-present mucus in their darlings' throats. And how proud those same parents were when they told me, "Dr. Luc, since I started with you two years ago, my child has not needed a single dose of antibiotics!" I can only shudder at how, next to our heavily-overmedicated elders, our children are the target for an ever-increasing assault of medications. Our children already receive 20 vaccinations by the age of two, beginning with Hepatitis B at birth; and children are now being prescribed Prozac and Zoloft! We need to teach the parents the dangers of suppression and the true cure which is only possible with homeopathy: preventing the recurrence of ear infections, colds, and flus.

Prescribing for Pets

While you have to be a licensed veterinarian to *charge* to treat pets, your patients will definitely be asking you to treat their little furred or feathered companions as a *favor*, once they see the power of homeopathy. You will give great joy to your patients and also prove beyond a shadow of a doubt that homeopathy does not work by the placebo effect! Just as the veterinarian uses the same antibiotics and cortisone for pets as physicians do for humans, we use the same remedies in homeopathy for pets as for their "parents." Case-taking is a bit of a challenge, since we cannot ask the animals their mental/emotional symptoms, but you will be surprised how observant their owners can be, and if they bring the pets to see you, you can sharpen your own powers of observation by examining them. A sample intake form for pets is provided in Appendix 1. Here are some hints for adapting casetaking to pets.

First, encourage your pet-owning patients to establish a baseline by carefully observing their pets' normal behavior. This will help determine the constitution (see the next chapter, which applies to pets as well as humans) and also clarify any changes in behavior which could point to a remedy.

How does the pet behave when the owners have been away for a while? Jumping all over them with friendly licks, or acting aloof, as if hurt? How is the pet with strangers? Reserved, overly friendly, hostile? Does he tremble with fear when going to the vet? How is he with other animals? With children? Does he like to eat all the time? Does she like to walk or is she a couch potato? Is she sensitive to being scolded? Is he more of a coward or does he never back off to protect his territory? Is he playful or is the pillow his best friend? Does she want closeness to you? Does she follow you around everywhere? Does he stick to your side when you take him out on a walk, or is he constantly tugging at the leash and wanting to explore? Does she tend to gain weight, or is she a nervous "race horse"?

These questions refer to the nature and temperament of the pet. If we see a sudden change in temperament, we should pay attention. A pet who goes from being very docile and submissive to being aggressive and irritable should be examined to find out what caused this sudden change, and to ward off a possible physical illness from developing. A pet may display jealousy of a new member of the household, indicating the need for Pulsatilla or one of the other jealousy remedies. Or a pet whose owner is usually around most of the time and then suddenly changes routine and spends all day at work may show the signs of an abandonment remedy, by sulking and distancing (Nat. mur.) or being constantly underfoot, wanting to sit on the owner's lap and continually offering a paw (Pulsatilla). If a dog refuses to relieve himself when walked and saves it up until he comes back home, this can be a sign of needing Nat. mur.

If a dog crouches with his tail between his legs, pulls his ears down and back, and opens his mouth with the lips pulled back, these are the fear signs for a dog, who may need Gelsemium (especially if he seems paralyzed by fear). Argentum nitricum is another great fear remedy for pets, especially if the pet seems very restless, nervous and trembling, and if the fear is accompanied by urination or defecation (just like the Argentum nitricum person who gets diarrhea when nervous!). A Phosphorus dog is likely to be fearful in general, and especially cowers when there is thunder and lightning; these dogs are easy to recognize because they love massage, tickling, attention and company in general and are usually very friendly and feminine. They loved to be groomed and perform at shows where they are the stars of the show with a nice bow in the fur. A pet who runs and hides under the sofa when a stranger enters is likely to need Baryta carb. A dog who is very sensitive to noise but is otherwise rather bossy, aggressive and wanting to get ahead of the others in getting food or attention from the owner is likely to need Nux vomica. Pets who become very submissive, almost to the point of cowardice, because they have been abused verbally or physically, even emotionally, may need Staphysagria to keep them from wilting at any approach. As you can see, there are many ways to observe pets' behavior and deduce indications for the same remedies that humans need.

In addition, encourage the pet owners to observe physical characteristics which are normal for the pet, so they can report any changes: what is the normal thickness and texture of the fur? What do the tongue, gums and oral mucosa usually look like? They should feel the paw pads occasionally so they can tell when the pet is unusually hot or cold (and when one paw is hot, the other cold, it can be a sure sign of Lycopodium, as it was for one of my bullmastiffs). What kind of food does she like, and how much? Is she very particular? Is she very thirsty or hardly at all? Is she messy in her eating habits or does she clean out her bowl to the last particle? How is his stool, and where does he do it? Three times a day, or once every other day? Does she like to lie in the sun or is she always looking for fresh air in the house, lying under the fan? Does the dog like to stick his nose out the window when riding in the car? Does he jump up early in the morning for his morning walk or do you have to drag him out the door? All of these factors can indicate the pet's innate constitution (if they are normal) or the therapeutic remedy needed (if they have changed at the same time as the illness).

I have included the case of my female bullmastiff, Ali, in Appendix 4 because it is an excellent example of a veterinary case as well as of miasmatic diagnosis.

CHAPTER EIGHT

Constitution, Timeline, and Temperament

> No knowledge is perfect unless it includes an understanding of the origin—that is, the beginning; and as all man's diseases originate in his constitution, it is necessary that his constitution should be known if we wish to know his diseases.
> —*Paracelsus*

What Does 'Constitution' Mean?

The term 'constitution' has different definitions in modern homeopathy. Some authors use it to mean the remedy that matches the patient's totality of symptoms for a chronic condition, with particular emphasis on the patient's personality and temperament. In this usage, the constitutional remedy is the *currently*-needed *chronic* remedy, in contrast to an acute remedy. The patient may have needed different constitutional remedies at other times of her life, depending on the circumstances.

Others use the term to mean the remedy that matches a patient's individual type and which is *unchangeable for life*. This lifelong remedy can be any one of the hundreds or even thousands of remedies available. Some homeopaths believe that this same life-long remedy will cure any acute condition that arises for the patient, if given in an acute potency.

The constitution can also mean the *innate* constitution, the underlying "stuff" of which the person is made on a mental, emotional, and physical level, but which is *not* necessarily the *curative remedy* for the patient's current condition, whether acute or chronic. In this view, the patient will need different remedies at different times of his life, depending on the different layers formed by traumas or Never Well Sinces. These remedy layers form on top of the innate constitution, like the layers of an onion.

To clarify the terminology which will be used in this book, 'constitution' will follow the third definition, that of innate constitution. The remedy needed for a particular layer can be called the 'temporary constitution,' in keeping with the first definition, but I have found this to be too confusing, so I call it the therapeutic remedy, the layer remedy, or usually just the remedy. In this system of working with the constitution, the patient receives the remedy for each layer in her timeline, working backwards from the present, and when all the layers and miasmatic states are cleared she receives her constitutional remedy in a 10M potency, 3 pellets dry. The constitutional remedy will strengthen the patient, prevent recurrence of acute conditions, and help "polish the diamond" by bringing out the best qualities of the constitution and minimizing any weaknesses.

The main difference between this definition of 'constitution' and the second one is that in this model there are only seven possible innate constitutions, with any number of possible remedy states imposed on them. At the time of conception a person can be a Sulphur, Phosphorus, Calcarea, Calc. phos., Silica, Lycopodium, or Baryta carb. Most of these are minerals involved in basic physiological processes. Lycopodium and many other polychrests contain a high percentage of one or more essential minerals.

It is the life experiences which impose a pattern such as Pulsatilla, Nat. mur., or Sepia. If the developing child is strongly influenced by a trauma in utero, she can be born with all the qualities of one of these layer remedies. For example, I have often seen in my practice that when a pregnant woman receives a terrible heartbreak or shock, her child is born needing a grief remedy like Ignatia or Nat. mur. The child of parents with active gonorrhea can be born a Medorrhinum. In these cases, the symptom picture of the acquired remedy is stamped on the baby so early, so profoundly, that it is "as if" the patient is a Nat. mur. or a Medorrhinum.

Clinical Case: I saw a baby at age 4 months whose Chief Complaint was tachypnea (attacks of rapid respiration, more than 80-100/min.). Her parents had consulted many specialists to no avail. Since the child was born in this condition, I knew the trauma must have happened intra-utero. I asked the mother if anything had happened in pregnancy. She told me that when she was three months pregnant, the doctors told her that she would probably miscarry the baby (although the mother could not tell me what test this prediction was based on). The Never Well Since was the all-too-common "hearing bad news." I asked the mother exactly how she felt at that moment. She said she felt an enormous sense of loss and lamented, "Why did this have to happen to me?" She sighed and wept for many days until finally she was told that her baby was safe. But the damage had already been done to the baby (and also to the mother, who became very anxious about her baby). The remedy which the mother needed at that point—Ignatia—was also the one the baby needed when she was born. After one month on Ignatia LM1, prn, the baby's breathing became completely normal. Her allopathic specialist simply said, "She must have grown out of it."

Clinical Case: I had a patient, a man in his forties, all of whose symptoms pointed to Nat. mur. He had had them his entire life, as far back as he could remember. I asked him if he might have had an experience of abandonment in infancy. He promised to ask his mother and found out something he had never known before: she did not want to be pregnant with him, had decided on an abortion, and was already in the stirrups in the doctor's office when she changed her mind. The unborn child took this as an abandonment and was born a Nat. mur. Nat. mur. resolved his Chief Complaint (recurrent herpes simplex attacks) and brought out the qualities of his innate constitution (Sulphur).

We find that no matter how many Nat. mur. qualities a patient has, for example, we can always see the innate constitution peeking through. A Nat. mur. who is a Phosphorus underneath will be different from one who is innately a Sulphur or Calcarea. One important difference is in the sensitivity level. A Phosphorus will need the smallest possible dose of Nat. mur. or else she will aggravate. A Sulphur will need a moderate-to-strong dose, and a Calcarea may not react at all unless we give her an extra-strong dose of Nat. mur. Thus it is essential to determine the constitution in order to adjust our dosage correctly to the patient.

The constitution will show through in many other ways like the energy level and body type. A Phosphorus, no matter what her current remedy layer, will tend to have an initial flare-up of enthusiasm and energy at the beginning of a project, then quickly run out of steam, while a Calcarea will always be slow to get going and then be persistent once he has some momentum built up. A Phosphorus will tend to be willowy, a Calcarea stocky or even chubby.

It is also helpful to know the constitution because each constitution is associated with certain typical acute remedies and layer remedies. Phosphorus patients, being the most emotionally sensitive and impressionable, are the most likely to develop states such as Nat. mur., Staphysagria, Causticum, Pulsatilla, and others related to emotional traumas. The high-energy, hard-working Sulphur is likely to develop a Nux vomica state and even a Sepia state. Calcareas are the least likely to develop a layer, because they have a sturdy, solid strength which makes them resilient in the face of most life-experiences. However, they have a weak spot: they are so devoted to their home and family that a loss in that area can lead them to a Nat. mur. state, Pulsatilla state (more often seen in girls and little boys), or Stramonium state (more often seen in older boys). Calcarea also has a physical weak spot: lax ligaments, leading to sprained ankles and lower back strain which require Rhus tox., one of the acutes of Calcarea.

While each constitution has *typical* chronic remedies it needs, a strong traumatic blow can impose a layer on a patient of *any* constitution: for example, a high-impact car accident with a resulting blow to the head can create a Nat. sulph. layer in any constitution.

This understanding of the innate constitution and remedy layers should become more accepted as homeopaths become aware of the concept of etiology, layers, stresses, vaccinations and other complex diseases repressing the true innate constitutional state. I am not alone in this opinion, as I have seen many of the old masters (Compton Burnett, Pierre Schmidt, Margaret Tyler, Foubister, and Shepherd) taking these facts into account in their therapeutic approach. Figure 8-1 illustrates how a patient's timeline can be used to determine the series of remedies which will be needed, ending with the constitutional remedy (Phosphorus, in this case) in a single 10M dose.

While the innate constitution usually does not change, there is one exception: many children are born Calcarea (about 50% among my American patients, by rough guess) and of those a certain percentage will change into Sulphur, Lycopodium or Calc. phos. (Many patients are born Sulphur, Lycopodium or Calc. phos without going through a Calcarea stage.) Dr. Douglas Borland, whose *Children's Types* has contributed so much to our understanding of constitutional prescribing for children, has noted a *change in type* in children as they develop. For instance, according to Borland, he often saw typical Calcarea children among 2 and 3 year olds, but rarely after age 3. There was a second period, he said, from about 2 to 8 or 9 years old, during which the child's type remained fairly constant, although it might have changed from that of the previous period. A third period lasted from about 9 to about 15 years of age,

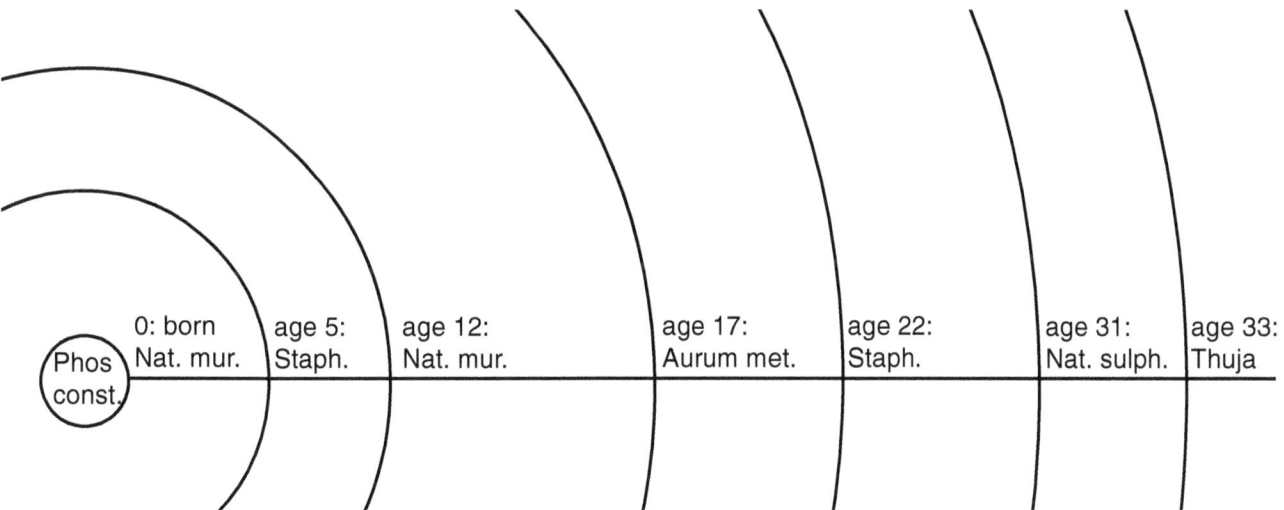

Fig. 8-1: Layers in a Patient's Timeline

(see explanation on following page)

Key to Fig. 8-1:

Julia, a 35-year-old divorced woman, presents with a chief complaint of recurring yeast infections. She has had them since she was 33 and was given several rounds of antibiotics for the flu.

Current layer: NWS antibiotics. *Remedy:* Thuja.

In addition, she has had headaches, backaches, memory loss and unexplained crying fits since she was in a serious car accident at the age of 31.

Previous layer: NWS head/spine trauma. *Remedy:* Nat. sulph.

She has also had recurring urinary tract infections. She traces them to a failed marriage; she says she got married too early, and to the wrong person. He turned out to be abusive to her, mostly verbally (putting her down a lot) but also occasionally physically (slapping her) and sexually (forcing sex on her). She developed recurring UTIs about this time and has had them on and off ever since.

Layer: NWS humiliation, abuse. *Remedy:* Staphysagria.

Actually, she says, she used to get them a lot when she was a little girl. This man she married kind of reminds her of her babysitter's boyfriend who used to come over with the babysitter and "fool around with her." She has no actual memories of abuse but she has a "creepy feeling" when she thinks about him now. Since UTIs are such a typical expression of Staphysagria (one of the top abuse remedies, covering sexual abuse in particular) you suspect that in fact she was sexually abused as a little girl.

Layer: possible sexual abuse. *Remedy:* Staphysagria.

She got married at a time when she was very depressed and was even thinking about taking her own life. Her mother died when she was 17, leaving her with no relatives and no money for college, which had been a lifelong dream of hers.

Layer: loss of everything important. *Remedy:* Aurum.

She was anorexic as a teenager. She describes herself as very lonely, emotionally withdrawn, perfectionist, self-critical. She was like this ever since she was born (her mother thinks it's because Julia's father left when her mother was pregnant with her). Her emotional withdrawal became much more severe when she was a teenager, because she moved when she was 12, leaving behind her only friend; also she was not able to bring her dog to her new home.

She thus has two *grief/loss layers:* one prenatal, and one from age 12. *Remedy:* Nat. mur.

Note: remedies are given for purposes of illustration only. Each layer has more than one possible remedy. The point is that the patient will probably need each of the remedies in reverse order. Then, to strengthen her, you give the remedy for her innate constitution, which is Phosphorus.

during which the child again remained fairly constant, but a type different from the previous one. After the age of 16, according to Dr. Borland, children gradually developed their permanent adult type.

Looking at my own practice, I see a slightly different phenomenon. I would see the first changes at around age two, and the next big change definitely around puberty when the lifelong constitutional change is achieved. Many Calcarea children remain Calcarea throughout life; of those who change, the majority become Sulphur, some become Phosphorus, and a few become Lycopodium. Again at puberty some of the stocky or even chubby Calcareas shoot up and become Calc. phos. (see Fig. 8-2). Of course, times have changed since Dr. Borland was practicing: different mental and emotional stresses, foods, and disease expressions, among other factors, may well account for the changes. The important thing for the practitioner is to know that these changes do take place. They do not indicate a mistake in the homeopath's original assessment of a young child's constitution.

Two Sides of the Coin

The constitutional types, like all the polychrests, have both a light and a dark side. Depending on the circumstances and life experiences, the same quality can have positive or negative effects. For example, a trait such as *boldness* may add to an individual's business success but hinder a relationship with a sensitive, private individual who might consider him an uncaring clod ("too pushy, too business-like"). The role or mood of the observer can also determine how the trait will be received.

And the innate or true constitution contains traits which in themselves are potentially positive but may turn more negative under the stress of illness and disharmony in the system. For instance, a stubborn individual may achieve his goals in business, but this stubbornness may turn into an obstacle when he falls ill and disregards the advice of his well-meaning spouse and physician. So there is an interaction between the constitution and the influences which act upon it.

To take another example, Nux vomicas have courage, drive, competitiveness, and decisiveness. But they are also prone to anger, frustration, and the tendency to dominate others. These qualities can be pathological, depending on the situation and the intensity of their expression. This is true of all the polychrests. Sulphur has a tendency to political, metaphysical, and scientific speculation. These tendencies can be healthy, leading to great accomplishments, but when perverted they can easily become extreme radicalism (as in terrorists), impractical philosophical rationalizations, and fruitless pseudo-scientific theories which lead nowhere.

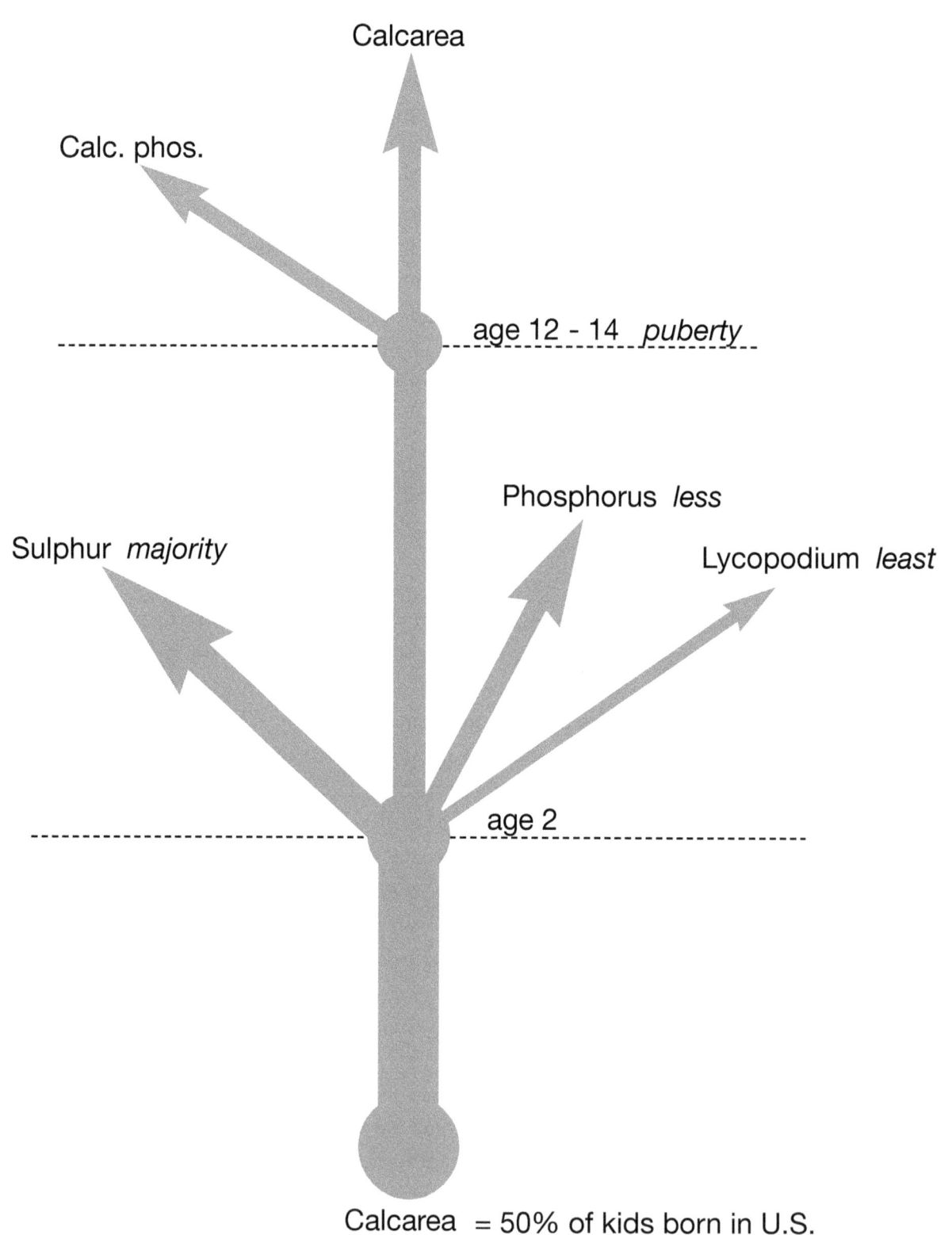

Fig. 8-2: Changes in the Constitution of a Child Born Calcarea

A particular constitution with a particular temperament has a tendency to develop certain pathological symptoms (or morbid signs, as Hahnemann called them). For instance, if a young child suffers from a grief or loss leading to a Nat. mur. state, a constitutionally Sulphur child will tend to move on and grow out of it while a sensitive, sympathetic Phosphorus child could remain a Nat. mur. for the rest of her life. Once a Phosphorus becomes a Nat. mur., she tends to set up situations for herself which reinforce the Nat. mur. state. (I call it "taking the Nat. mur. road" instead of the Phosphorus road which is her birthright.) The Nat. mur. road is predictable: a Nat. mur. will not open to others easily, and a Nat. mur. child may only have one close friend, setting herself up for another grief if the friend moves away or they are assigned to different schools. Or she may pour all her affection into a pet (typical for a Nat. mur., who trusts the unconditional love of a pet), then suffer a grief when the pet inevitably dies or is run over. As a teenager, she will be overly sensitive and easily offended, even more so than her peers, leading to more isolation and suffering. She may suffer from anorexia or bulimia, whose etiology so often shows a grief such as the parents' separation or divorce.

She will often begin a pattern as an adolescent which she will continue throughout life: choosing an unattainable or unsuitable partner. As a teenager she may get a distant crush on a teacher or on a boy who is unlikely ever to notice her, because this is safe: she cannot be hurt if the relationship never gets beyond the fantasy stage. As a young woman she may choose men who are unsuitable because they are recovering alcoholics or drug addicts or otherwise seem like "good causes" (one of the Nat. mur. "theme songs"). But she will treat these men as "fixer-uppers," trying to reform and perfect them until they inevitably grow tired of her nagging and leave her.

Years of repeated griefs and heartbreaks will make her try to protect herself emotionally, walling off her heart and making it ever more difficult for her to get close to a partner, a friend or even a co-worker. Since she tends to think that these losses are her fault, she will overcompensate by trying to perfect herself, usually by working much too hard, leading her into a Sepia state. She can also get into a Sepia state by crusading to reform something or taking on too many responsibilities as a way to forget her own misery. (Nat. murs. tend to become crusaders because they try to reform the world just as they try to perfect themselves and those around them. Members of MADD, Mothers Against Drunk Drivers, provide a perfect example: women whose children have been killed by drunk drivers and who try to channel their enormous grief into a constructive attempt to keep drunk drivers off the road.) We often see Nat. mur. and Sepia states alternate in these patients. Unless treated homeopathically, they never have a chance to return to the outgoing, upbeat, vivacious and social nature of their innate Phosphorus constitution. This scenario is illustrated in Figure 8-3.

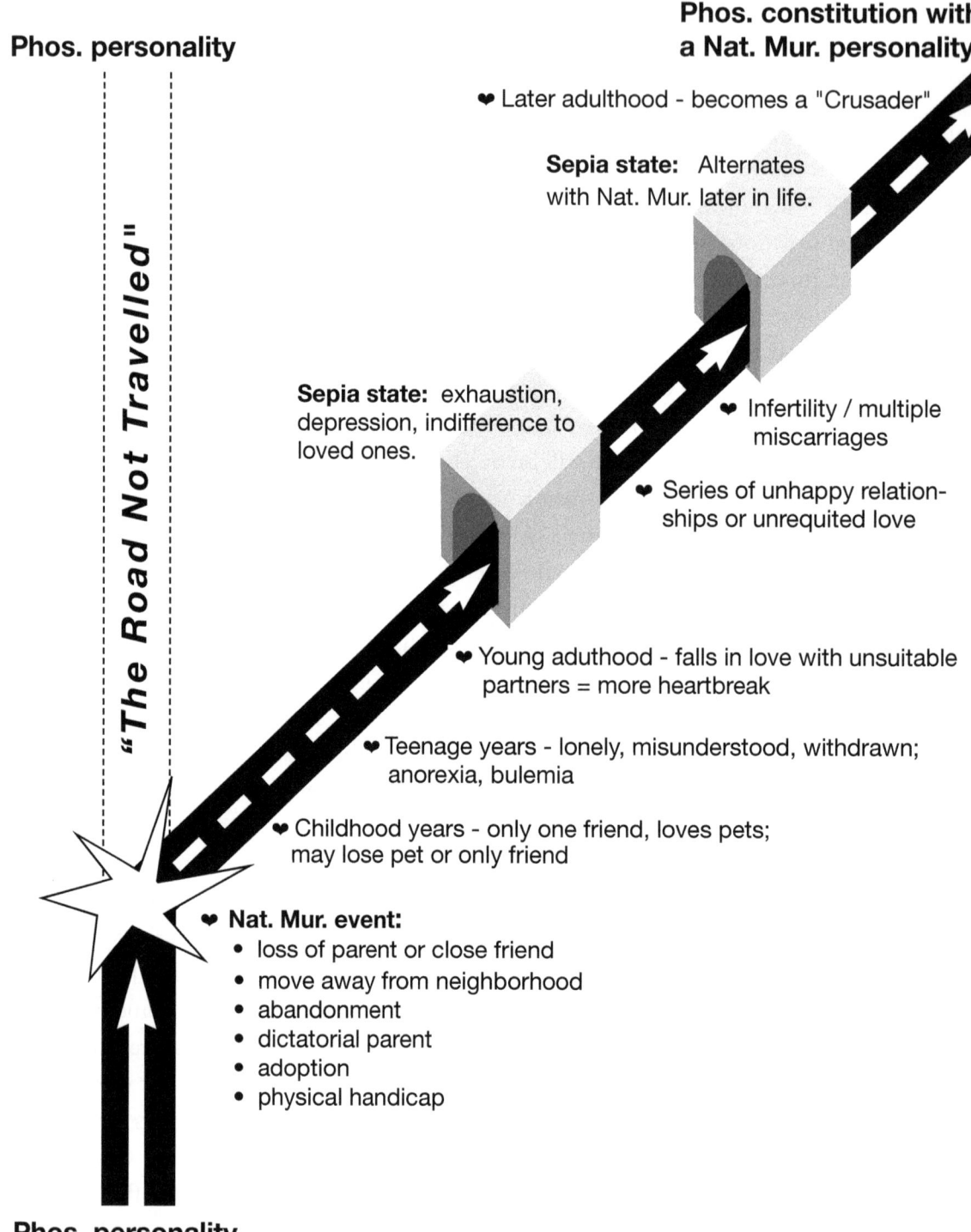

Fig. 8-3: Lifelong Effects of a Nat. mur. Event on a Sensitive Phosphorus Constitution

Indications for Constitutional Prescribing

Protection in childhood: Homeopathy will do more to restore children to health when they are sick, to overcome their inherited weaknesses, and to prepare them for a healthy and useful life than any other system of medicine. Patients who have had the benefit of good homeopathic prescribing since childhood incur fewer chronic diseases later in life. The best protection comes when the child's constitutional remedy is given, after removing all the layers. Children usually have far fewer layers than adults, of course, since they have not received as many buffets from life. We can remove the layers relatively quickly and give the child her constitutional remedy (always 10M, 3 pellets dry) to protect her from childhood diseases and bring out the best qualities of her constitution.

Preventing recurrence: When the appropriate acute remedy cures but fails to prevent recurrence of the illness (as in recurrent otitis media in children), the constitutional remedy will strengthen the Vital Force and prevent recurrence.

Ending the treatment: After treating the patient's layers, in order to reinforce his health, we give the constitutional remedy as our last therapeutic gesture.

Acute diseases: In acute diseases presenting different symptoms in each patient but resulting from the same morbific agent (childhood diseases); or in acute diseases presenting similar symptoms, but resulting from different morbific agents (such as allergies), the constitutional remedy can *prevent recurrence*. It is not usually used as the acute remedy. (Occasionally, of course, a Phosphorus will need Phosphorus for her cough out of the dozens of possible cough remedies, or a Sulphur will have a skin condition requiring Sulphur acutely. In these cases the remedy is prescribed by its indications just like any other acute remedy.)

Avoiding aggravations in hypersensitives: While we usually work from the most recent layer to earliest, an extremely hypersensitive patient might react to every remedy, even in the slightest amount and potency, with an aggravation.* While there are many more options like adjusting the LM potency downwards or using the olfactive or skin method, another possibility is to strengthen the Vital Force with the patient's constitution in an LM potency prn (see Fig. 8-4).

---

*This discussion applies to the treatment of *chronic* cases, not acute. I have often found that my students hesitate to use a higher potency in a sensitive constitution such as a Phosphorus. However, if we deal with a strong, acute miasmatic state, we have to counteract with a strong potency of the indicated remedy, even in hypersensitives. If a Phosphorus has a heartbreak or bronchitis, do not hesitate to give her a 200c or 1M of the indicated remedy. You do not need to use a 6c for fear she will aggravate.

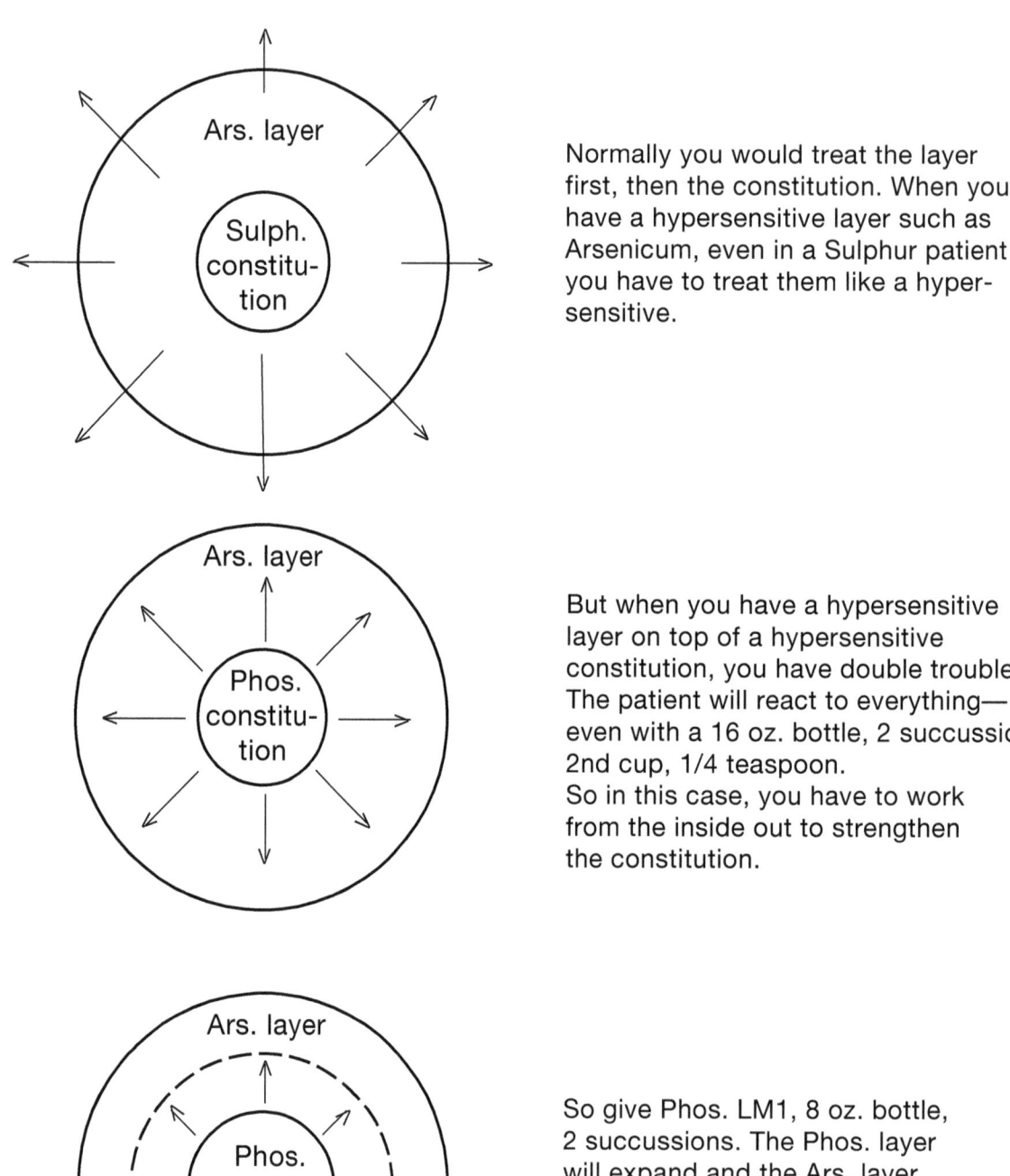

Fig. 8-4: Constitutional Treatment for Hypersensitives

When Constitutional Prescribing Is Not Indicated

Some homeopaths use only the constitutional remedy, even for an acute attack. (By 'constitutional remedy,' they may mean the currently-indicated chronic remedy which was acting before the acute situation arose, rather than the innate constitution.)

Using the current chronic remedy may in fact work in acute events. The question is why it works sometimes and other times not at all. It will work when the acute disease is not too intense and thus creates a relatively small layer. In these circumstances, the chronic remedy strengthens the patient's Vital Force so that it can annihilate the acute layer. (Of course, we may not forget that acute conditions often disappear on their own without any help from our remedy.)

But if the acute incident is more serious or long-lasting, it takes on a life of its own (creates a bigger layer), dominating the Vital Force and creating uncomfortable or even life-threatening symptoms. For example, a patient who has acute traveler's diarrhea for several weeks will obviously need acute remedies such as China or Arsenicum while the chronic remedy is suspended.

While it may be true to a certain extent that a patient who needs China or Arsenicum chronically is more susceptible to an acute attack requiring the same remedy, this notion of inherent susceptibility is not enough to explain why people come down with acute illnesses. When the "morbific force" (as Hahnemann called it) of an acute illness is strong enough, people of all constitutions and temperaments are susceptible. For example, when I went to China on a group tour, everyone except me came down with traveler's diarrhea, and they were definitely not all China and Arsenicum remedy types.

Since giving the chronic remedy in an acute attack may not work, precious time can be lost while waiting to see how the patient responds. At the very least, the practitioner should first assess the strength of the Vital Force and the intensity of the acute event to see if this method is likely to work. If it doesn't, precious time will be lost, the patient will suffer, and as a result he may resort to suppressive drugs. My own preference is simply to give the indicated acute remedy while suspending the chronic treatment, if any.

Some homeopaths believe that prescribing the innate constitution will treat all the patient's acute conditions *and* remove all the layers. Experienced professional homeopaths who follow this system know that there are obvious exceptions to this approach (as in a car accident, for example). But beginners who follow the advice too literally can endanger their patients. For instance, a Phosphorus patient could die from being given his constitutional remedy in a case of acute TB. He will probably need a small lesional remedy like Sanguinaria. Unless the constitutional remedy happens to match the specific acute symptoms, it will take a different and sometimes small remedy before we can use the constitutional remedy to complete a lesional case like this. The strong, even life-threatening, acute layer needs to be separated from the chronic state of the patient. In fact in some advanced states of chronic disease (the "one-sided diseases" described in Chapter 4, Pathology), the constitutional remedy is completely contraindicated. Terrible aggravations can come from *ignoring the layers* of disease in advanced cases. Even giving the "layer remedy" can be contraindicated during an acute attack. For example, Margaret Tyler said not to give Nat. mur. during a crisis headache because it can cause a strong aggravation. Instead give Bryonia, the acute, complementary remedy of Nat. mur.

Further Remarks on the Constitution

We can make a distinction between four different remedies:

1. The *constitutional* remedy reflecting the mental, emotional, physical, and miasmatic foundation of the person, usually unchanging throughout life (except for the changes noted in the Calcarea constitution).

2. The *miasmatic* remedy determined by the inherited miasm.

3. The *functional, therapeutic, or layer* remedy needed to cure the current Chief Complaint.

4. The *disease* remedy which is needed only in cases of advanced pathology, addressing the symptoms of the pathology.

In choosing rubrics to prescribe on, try to differentiate between those that reflect the patient's lifelong state (probably belonging to the constitution) and those that date from the same time as the Chief Complaint (probably belonging to the therapeutic remedy). Sample Case 3 in Appendix 4 illustrates how to separate the rubrics reflecting the constitution from those reflecting the layer. However, we must not forget that the constitution often is also the therapeutic remedy, especially in the case of Calcareas, because these types are so non-reactive that they do not tend to form layers.

We have primarily used Phosphorus, Sulphur and Calcarea as examples of constitutional remedies because they are the most common remedy types in this country. They will not be discussed at length in this chapter because portraits of these common polychrests are so easily available elsewhere. *

---

*My students have found Catherine Coulter's *Portraits of Homeopathic Medicines* especially helpful. My personal favorites are Margaret Tyler's *Homeopathic Drug Pictures* and Kent's *Lectures on Homeopathic Materia Medica*.

The Hippocratic Temperament

One important aspect of the patient's constitution is the temperament, which could be considered his "emotional climate." However, unlike the constitution, the temperament can change as different layers are formed. In fact, if the patient displays a temperament which is not in keeping with his constitution, it is a strong indication of the remedy needed. For example, a Nat. mur. layer can make a normally upbeat and outgoing Phosphorus brooding and withdrawn. If a Calcarea child's parents are involved in a painful divorce, the normally calm, gentle, and docile child might go into a violent Stramonium state.

The word 'temperament' has been used in different ways in homeopathy, just as 'constitution' has, leading to some confusion. Kent used it to mean an aspect of what we call the innate constitution:

> Temperaments are not caused by provings, and are not changed in any manner by our remedies, however well indicated by symptoms found in persons of marked temperamental makeup. To twist these temperaments into our pathogenics, or symptomatology, is but a misunderstanding of our homeopathic principles.[1]

In our understanding of the word 'temperament,' the patient's temperament *can* change and *can be changed by the remedy.* Giving Stramonium to the violent Stramonium child can change his temperament back to his naturally phlegmatic Calcarea.

More than two thousand years ago, Hippocrates made a classic four-fold division of human temperaments: *sanguine* (optimistic, outgoing, loquacious), *melancholic* (sad, taciturn, cautious, anxious), *choleric* (angry), and *phlegmatic* (calm, mild, slow-going). These temperaments correspond to Fire, Water, Wood, and Earth in TCM respectively.* The old masters found these Hippocratic temperaments very useful in analyzing their patients, and I have found them useful in my own practice. The rest of this chapter will be devoted to these temperaments since their descriptions is much less easily available than descriptions of the seven basic constitutions.

---

*It is interesting that the Chinese added a fifth element, Metal. The Metal person is dogmatic, rule-oriented, rigid, and self-controlled to his own detriment; he strives to create a life of routine, devoid of surprises. Kali carb. is a perfect example. The correspondence between homeopathic remedy types, the Hippocratic temperaments, and the Five Element types in TCM is discussed further in Appendix 5 on TCM and in my book, *What About Men*.

In my student days we used to act out a humorous pantomime which depicts the reaction of four different people upon finding a hair in their soup. The first one flies into a rage and throws soup and dish at the waiter (choleric). The second one makes a face, shrugs it off, picks up his coat and walks out whistling a tune (sanguine). The third one breaks into a crying fit because the most awful things always happen to him (melancholic). The fourth one looks at the hair, leaves it right there, goes on eating and after finishing the dish, orders another portion (phlegmatic). This skit illustrates how different people can have different reactions to the same situation, and that these reactions are spontaneous, not a matter of conscious choice. The choleric cannot respond in a phlegmatic fashion, nor can the melancholy force himself to be cheerful. A vitriolic Nitric acid personality with its vitriolic response pattern cannot be turned into a placid, agreeable Pulsatilla.

The Greeks believed that the body is composed of four elements: earth, water, fire, and air, which gave it the four qualities of dry, cold, hot, and moist, and which generated the four humors: blood, phlegm, yellow bile, and black bile. While the humors literally represented fluids thought to circulate in the body, metaphorically each became associated with a prevailing emotion: blood with joy, called the sanguine temperament (from the Latin *sanguis*, blood); phlegm with worry and contemplative calm, the phlegmatic temperament; yellow bile with anger, called the bilious temperament; and black bile with sadness, called the melancholy temperament (from the Greek roots *mela* and *choler*, meaning "black bile"). These four temperaments became known as the Hippocratic types or temperaments. Equilibrium of the humors and moods was necessary for health, and disequilibrium meant disease. Hippocrates' concept of health and disease may be represented by the following diagram:

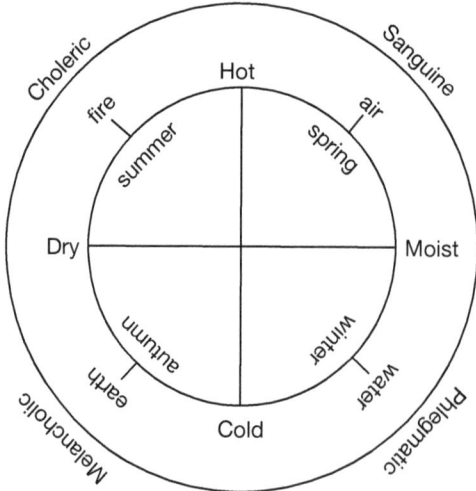

Fig. 8-5: The Hippocratic Temperaments

Hippocratic types were included in our Materia Medica by Hahnemann, Hering and Allen among others. For instance, Hahnemann says Pulsatilla is suited to the "slow, changeable, tearful, phlegmatic temperament." On the other hand, he said, quick movements, rapid resolutions and a cheerful mood are more often found in the sanguine temperaments like Phosphorus. This classic division of human nature into four temperaments is based on over two thousand years of astute observation of human nature. However, most people have a *mixture* of the four temperaments; none of them are found in their pure form in individuals, any more than all the characteristics of a Sulphur would be. Nevertheless, in most people one or two temperaments predominate.

In practice, assessing the temperament is most useful when noting *changes* in the temperament different from the *basic* disposition. For example if a phlegmatic type like a Calcarea becomes more aggressive, angry and violent, then he has taken on a choleric temperament *temporarily*. This change in temperament must be given high priority in prescribing. Hippocrates taught this over two millennia ago: "There are basic states of the constitution but there are also temporary temperaments and humors." If a sweet Pulsatilla girl is raped, we would expect her temperament to change temporarily. Of course the innate constitution cannot change, especially the physical characteristics such as a stocky or lean build. (Some prescribers incorrectly use physical characteristics like hair and eye color, the shape of the eyebrows, etc. These are not considered morbid symptoms and cannot be used to prescribe on; also, they are lifelong characteristics and not characteristic of the disease layer.)

The following are descriptions of the four temperaments with their associated remedies.

Sanguine
- Extremely happy by nature and openly emotional.
- Wants to capture every possible enjoyment in life. This desire sometimes makes her restless, even flighty and dissatisfied.
- Never feels that life is boring; oversensitive mentally and emotionally to her surroundings.
- Emotional life is usually the best developed, more active than the mind and the will (ability to follow through on plans and goals).
- Does not spend a great deal of time in thought or reflection. The attention is usually centered on the present moment: "*Carpe diem,* tomorrow is another day and I'll decide about it then."
- In sad circumstances is able to express her sympathy fully in a way that others would find comforting (this is the most sympathetic type). Easily demonstrates her own feelings and experiences others' losses deeply.

- Has no problems making decisions or resolutions, but has great difficulty taking positive action (great beginners, bad finishers). Forgets plans unintentionally since she so easily becomes involved in something new.
- Does not think about her goals in life because she is so much involved with the present (forget tomorrow, the excitement is today); therefore goals can be rather hazy and un–defined.
- Her immediate and abundant enthusiasm for a new project and her ability to communicate it is infectious to other people and can be responsible for the project's popularity.
- Can snap back from failures and setbacks quickly. They do not embarrass her because people know of her good intentions, so she accepts them as due to circumstances beyond her control; besides, she is quickly interested in another new project.
- Can work rapidly but is not always concerned about the quality of her work; easily distracted so tasks are left unfinished; postpones unpleasant jobs in favor of doing what she enjoys.
- If not busy with a project, looks for small, effortless but pleasant little tasks; greatest desire in life is enjoyment.
- Has "millions" of friends and enjoys them all, calls them all her "best" friends and close confidants; wins friends easily and effortlessly because she is very affectionate and pleasant. However, she rarely thinks about a friend when away from her (even tends to forget about a friend until she meets her again); and when she loses one friend she soon finds another one.
- Does not like people whose lives and schedules are so planned and premeditated that they are never spontaneous, "let their hair down" or enjoy exploring on a trip or an outing.
- In crisis situations can express her views freely and eloquently, with much conviction and feeling, even loquacity; yet while others seem to agree with her, her suggestions are often not followed by the group.
- When people are rude to her it upsets her at the time but she quickly forgets an insult or offense; it does not continue to bother her nor does it affect her future relationship with that person.
- When she gives advice, it usually comes from the heart; she enjoys giving suggestions and helping people with their problems, even volunteering advice when not asked because of her sympathetic nature.
- It is not important to her to size people up; she is able to enjoy them and accept them as they are.
- She can lose her temper and say what she thinks but she gets over it very quickly and is very apologetic; she soon forgets the whole matter, moving on from such unpleasantness.

- Loves talking, especially engaging in gossip and chitchat ("if no news, send rumors!"); the conversation is probably not of world-shaking importance.
- Today's problems can upset her a bit but she does not worry about tomorrow.
- Needs a profession in which she can be creative, free from the limitations and routines of a 9 to 5 job. She enjoys work involving beauty, travel, and/or entertainment, or perhaps her clairvoyant abilities, such as being an artist, hairdresser, cosmetician, dancer, interior designer, actress, tour guide, stand-up comedian, astrologer, singer, musician, or model.
- *Characteristics:* hopeful, sentimental, affectionate, passionate, playful, openhearted, optimistic, restless, compassionate, adventurous, intuitive, forgiving, enthusiastic, friendly, loving, gentle. *Weaknesses:* can be careless, restless, dissatisfied, wasteful, impulsive, weak-willed, shallow, inconsistent, unreliable, unstable, fragile, dreamy.

Constitution most frequently associated: Phosphorus

Frequently encountered remedies: Lachesis, Ignatia, Aurum (restores the joy of life)

Five Elements: Heart/Fire/Joy

Choleric

- Has a lot of drive, very practical and not very sentimental or emotional, to the point that his partner will complain of "insensitivity."
- Struggles with his surroundings because of the constant drive within him to change existing conditions out of boredom. Since a change, even for the better, is always resisted, there is occasional friction or misunderstanding with others. But he always plays an active part in the world.
- Impatient, always on the go and thinks everyone else is lazy because they don't think, move and act as fast as he does.
- Will-power and decision-making ability are better developed in this type than in others. He is the "general of the troops" or the CEO of the company who must turn to another type for advice (his chief of staff will be a thinking Earth type) as well as to a partner who is more emotionally developed.
- Thinking is clear but can be influenced by the urge to do something or get something done ("straight ahead, top speed" and there is no reverse gear in his car!).
- If a friend is suffering, he would not say much or feel the sorrow too deeply; but he would find something he could do to show his sympathy through actions rather than words; he would also encourage them to go on, using logical arguments ("there is a business to take over, you have two children to support, make some new goals in life, go to school again," etc.).

- He can grasp a situation instantly and see at once what has to be done, then does it. He enjoys making decisions and deliberately puts himself in that position. Although he does not want others to make decisions for *him,* he has no qualms about making decisions for *others;* in fact he enjoys and thrives on it.
- He has very clearly defined goals in sight and seems to know instinctively the best path to reach them; nothing stops him from making definite progress in spite of obstacles. He almost always accomplishes his objectives.
- In new projects he is the *driving force* behind them. His energetic will and practical thinking give fire and inspiration to his employees or coworkers.
- He has very few failures or setbacks in life but is very hard on himself when they do happen, as he feels they are a mark of weakness. Wants to avoid embarrassment and loss of face at all cost and is therefore determined to see each project through to success.
- Works very rapidly without sacrificing quality, can handle many things at the same time and do them all well; work is so important that his whole life centers around it; restless when he is not doing something; feels he must "earn" his rest after working to exhaustion; does not allow his feelings of dislike to keep him from doing a job which needs to be done; believes that those who allow their feelings to influence them are weak.
- When he is not working you can find him doing something constructive involving physical exertion (exercise machines, sports); his greatest enjoyment in life comes from opportunities and successes.
- Independent and self-sufficient, which keeps him from having close friendships; most of his friendships come from business or work; besides, his friends have to conform to the high standards he sets for himself, with no place for those he considers "lazy," "dumb" and "superficial" people; his friendships change with circumstances and he must resist the temptation to use friendships for status or goal purposes; he is usually only interested in people with whom he is working on a goal, sport or project; feels he is too busy to acknowledge others; does not want to waste time on idle chitchat or spending time with others merely for the sake of friendship.
- People who are slow or can't make up their mind irritate him.
- In crisis situations, he does not hesitate to take a public stand; he sees immediately what the problem is and how to resolve it; if one or two people have their feelings hurt a little in the process, he feels that this is the price that must be paid to get things done right, so they should just get over it.
- Often does not note an offense since he is too busy, but if he is humiliated or offended he is tempted to pay the offender back in some way.
- Usually too busy with his own projects to give advice but if he does, he expects it to be

followed; if not, don't come back for more! His time is too valuable to waste on those who don't appreciate it.
- He has a special ability to evaluate others' abilities and talents, especially when they are useful to him in accomplishing a project.
- Has a volcanic temper, touchy and hot-tempered; when he loses his temper he can get violent; usually finds it very difficult to apologize, is more tempted to get even with the other person or simply to move on and not "waste any more time on that moron."
- Talking has to be purposeful; he is too busy to engage in small talk or idle chatter; prefers to act upon a problem rather than to talk about it; is interested in worldly things and philosophical matters, especially when they relate to his business.
- Problems are not worries but rather challenges; his only worry is providing for his family, but that is usually not a problem for someone of his drive and acumen.
- Professions in which he excels involve leadership, business acumen, and practical realities: attorney, physician, CEO of a company, army officer, inventor, non-fiction writer, realtor, car salesman, broker, high-powered executive, reporter or TV news anchor.
- *Other characteristics:* daring, enterprising, aggressive, forceful, confident, decisive, determined, leader, witty, creative, logical, great memory, ambitious, faith. *Negative qualities:* stubborn, self-centered, careless, insensitive, inconsistent, temperamental, cruel, sharp-tongued, authoritarian, bossy, cocky, crafty, impetuous.

Constitutions most frequently associated: Sulphur, Lycopodium

Other frequently associated remedies: Nux vomica, Chelidonium

Five Elements: Liver/Wood-Wind/Anger

Phlegmatic
- Slow, calm, steady, and rather unemotional.
- Prefers a placid uneventful life devoid of inner and outer turmoil. Tends to stay on the sidelines rather than in the hustle and bustle of life ("my home is my castle").
- Rarely gets excited about anything, except when her home is threatened: this home by extension means her family, pets, house and little neighborhood.
- Her mind and willpower tend to be equally well developed: she may surprise everyone with exceptional insight and common sense as well as an excellent ability to handle calculations, whether in schoolwork or a profession such as accounting; while her willpower can go to the extreme of stubbornness, the emotional part is the least developed. The willpower is as often negative as positive, i.e. resistance to change rather than creating something new.

- Can think clearly and to plan ahead but does not become emotionally involved in plans nor does she feel the drive to act quickly; the mind is not influenced by emotions or will.
- Being sensitive to "hearing bad news," she reacts to a catastrophic sad event in a friend's life with discomfort, not knowing exactly how to deal with it or help; does not feel the sorrow deeply enough to feel that her words would be very helpful; can even feel embarrassed at not expressing more sorrow, but at the same time thinks, "Thank God my own family is safe."
- Has no trouble making decisions but takes his sweet time about it. Stays calm even in emergencies, weighing all the options and then choosing the simplest, safest and most common sense one. Ponders for a while, than acts.
- Slowly but steadily makes progress towards goals, in fact some of them have already been achieved; his calm, keen eye enables him to see the goal clearly and pursue it with great perseverance while temporary setbacks do not cause him to be discouraged; he is like an unstoppable tank, moving with great weight and momentum and deliberate speed, crushing all obstacles to the goal; refuses to be rushed. Because he is resistant to change and comfortable where he is, he needs to move to the goal one step at a time, becoming familiar with each new phase so that it becomes his familiar "home" before moving on.
- In new projects he will make a good *chief administrator*. His level-headedness, steady disposition, perseverance, patience and ability to remain cool and collected in times of personality clashes and conflicts will see the project through when others would be ready to give up.
- Setbacks and failures do not bother him since they are viewed as temporary conditions in his certainty that everything will work out all right. Although he moves slowly, his spirit will persevere until he reaches his goal (his stubbornness will help him with that).
- Works slowly but very thoroughly and dependably, but don't pressure him or he gets upset; he likes to mull over his work; it takes a great deal of motivation to start a new task, especially an unpleasant one, simply because he would rather not put the effort into it, but if forced to, he does it thoroughly.
- When not occupied by a job, avoids strenuous effort and usually prefers to do something sitting down (eating, reading, playing cards, knitting); his greatest desire in life is contentment.
- He enjoys his friends and is very faithful and accepting of them; but his happiness and contentment in life depend on his immediate family, not his friends; as contented alone as with friends; tends to observe people from a distance.
- Usually gives advice when specifically asked and is very good at it because she is objective and impartial and usually sees both sides of the coin; makes a great psychotherapist.

- Is able to size people up if necessary but is not much interested in it; other people's motives and weaknesses do not bother her.
- Does not like people who are in a hurry or those who are always fussing about something.
- In a crisis situation acts as a peacemaker, calmly and tactfully behind the scenes trying to patch things up; everyone will be quite satisfied and no one offended by the compromise she proposes.
- Thick skinned (not disturbed by offenses), although she notices them; she will not allow herself to become upset right away by the rudeness of others. Sensitive to teasing, though this will take a long time to show.
- She hardly ever loses her temper, more because of her docile, placid nature than because of any great self-control, even in the face of injustices or wrongs committed against her.
- Tends to be a quiet person yet cheerful and pleasant even if she does not have much to say; does not often originate a conversation but enjoys conversing if someone else engages her.
- Avoids worries by striving for simplicity in life.
- Preferred professions involve the earth, children, or accounting: computer programmer, geologist, park ranger, forester, mathematician, accountant, school administrator, teacher, farmer, veterinarian, landscaper.
- *Other characteristics*: pleasant, passive, serene, calm, cheerful, comforting, diplomatic, diligent, home-loving, efficient, virtuous, gently humorous, peaceful. *Negatives:* selfish, lazy, indecisive, faint-hearted, follower, dull, indifferent, self-righteous, meekness, procrastinator, introverted.

Most frequently associated constitutions: Calcarea, Baryta carb.

Five Elements: Earth/Stomach-Spleen/Worry

Melancholic
- Somewhat sad, deeply emotional.
- Senses a conflict with the world around him, hence tends to withdraw into a world created by his hopes, dreams, and aspirations.
- Rarely free from concern and care; there is always the eternal worry, "What if?"
- Possesses deep emotions and the ability to think deeply, but decision-making (will power) is poorly developed; procrastination and indecisiveness (irresolution) are marked.
- His mind probes deeply to the point where too much time is spent thinking; his emotional involvement often tends to influence his thinking.

- In sad events, can express her sympathy better by writing a note rather than by using spoken words to convey the depth of sorrow felt in her heart.
- Usually carries decisions out once they are made but often gets stuck in the process of mulling over a problem, weighing all the pros and cons; the more sides he sees of the problem, the harder it becomes to decide.
- Has very idealistic goals (strives for perfection) but has great difficulty in deciding how to get there; therefore is often frustrated because her goals seem so far off and her progress so slow.
- A perfectionist in his job and very conscientious; while others might approve of his work, he is apt to criticize himself and find fault with it; he often puts off an unpleasant job because he can't decide how to do it; but if forced, does a good job because of the high standards he sets for himself.
- When not busy doing something, his mind stays restless and busy (constantly asking, "What if?" and worrying about the future); his greatest desire in life is perfection.
- In new projects, tends to be the inventor, the thinker; he had the vision for it, saw the need for it and drew up the ideals, goals and overall philosophy which gave birth to the project.
- Setbacks and failures discourage her and when experienced, she is ready to throw in the towel; often feels unable to cope with life's problems; in fact her fear of failure often keeps her from entering areas where she might experience it; failures are often the result of her unrealistically high standards for herself.
- Always has a few close friends who mean the world to her; she does not make friends easily but she is exceptionally loyal (to a fault!) once she does; she maintains friends over the years and when she loses one, it leaves an empty spot in her heart.
- Does not like people who are shallow and superficial; prefers serious conversation about subject that stimulate her, rather than chitchat, when she talks at all; if not, she is bored, although she would try not to show it for fear of hurting others' feelings.
- In crisis is too reserved to express her feelings publicly, but she tells several people privately what she thinks should be done; hates to get involved because she is afraid to hurt people or make the situation worse.
- She feels insults deeply (oversensitive, easily offended); does not seek to get even with the person offending her but finds it hard to forget and stop brooding over it (persisting thoughts) and most of the time an offense will permanently affect her relationship with that person.
- Although she feels she has good advice to offer, she often hesitates to give it for fear that if it is acted upon, and does not work, it would reflect badly on her; sometimes she sees so

many facets of the problem that she is overwhelmed.
- Has an unusual ability to evaluate people, with insight into their personality and character; she easily spots a fake or sees other people's faults.
- She allows her anger to build up until eventually it surfaces in a big blowup; she tends to bear a grudge for a long time.
- Her preferred professions involve helping others and/or her perfectionist eye for detail: psychotherapist, social worker, librarian, book editor, graphic designer, inspector, private investigator.
- *Other characteristics:* reserved, introspective, contemplative, self-controlled, strong-willed, patient, concrete, elegant, proud, resourceful and analytical. *Negatives:* pessimistic, gloomy, cold, revengeful, bored, self-centered, critical, suspicious, frugal, phobic, taciturn, arrogant.

Associated remedies: Nat. mur., Arsenicum

Five Elements: Water/Kidney/Fear

Part Two

The Healing Process

Prescribing

The Second Prescription

Special Forms of Prescribing

Chapter Nine

Prescribing

The Value of Symptoms

We often see cases presented in journals and at conferences in which a remedy is selected based on no observable or elucidated principles, only by matching one or two uncommon or peculiar symptoms with a remedy. The result for the student is bewildering and overwhelming; it seems that an encyclopedic knowledge of Materia Medica is necessary before even beginning a homeopathic practice. Even live cases or video cases, in which the student can watch the instructor examine the patient and select the remedy, are not instructive unless the student has first learned solid principles of case-taking and symptom analysis.

Yet the old masters, beginning with Hahnemann, have given us these solid principles for finding the simillimum in an orderly, logical way. I have used these principles with great success in my own practice, and I have passed them along to my students. Most of my first-year students, without having memorized much Materia Medica, have been able to solve difficult cases by good case analysis and repertorizing. In this chapter I will undertake to share this legacy from the old masters in the hopes that others will find it useful. This method will provide the homeopath with a consistent chance of finding the curative remedy (and let us remember that unless tissues and organs have degenerated beyond all hope of recovery, *there is a remedy that will cure*).

Incorrect prescriptions may confuse the case by ameliorating some of the symptoms and preventing others from manifesting, thereby muddying the overall picture. Thus one important rule of prescribing is that if the remedy is not clear at the end of the initial consult, the patient should receive Sac lac. or nothing. If you *believe* you have found the simillimum, you can go ahead and prescribe it; if it later turns out to be the simile, it may throw up symptoms which will guide you to the simillimum. However, if you are really not at all sure, it is better to give Sac. lac. if you feel pressured by the patient to give a remedy. Then you must study the case further if you have enough information, or complete the intake later if you do not. *It is safer to do nothing than to do wrong.*

The Search for the Simillimum

Modern homeopathy, with several thousand remedies available, needs to simplify the labor of finding the simillimum, especially in complicated cases. Some homeopaths tend to take the path of least resistance, finding an easy way out like keynote prescribing. Others have made the process overly complex, I feel, by focusing on small remedies without relying on the classic principles of prescribing. The mountain of intake information often seems to indicate more than one remedy, but the laws of homeopathy demand that we cover each case with just one. Figure 9-1 illustrates how the simillimum covers the totality of the case, while the simile covers only part of it.

Finding the simillimum depends first on the evaluation of symptoms. Different master homeopaths, beginning with Hahnemann, have contributed their own ways of valuing the symptoms. Even in longstanding chronic cases with many apparently diverse disease conditions, *there always is method and order running through the case* if only we can find the clue. (Sometimes, of course, the clue is the patient's timeline; the diseases arise from different traumas at different stages of the patient's life and have no more internal logic than that.) At the end of this chapter I describe my own way of weaving through the maze of symptoms, entirely based on Hahnemann's teachings. It will give the reader a universal method of case-solving: it has worked so well in my practice and in my school that if I give a patient's case to 65 students, the majority of the students arrive at the same remedy which cured the case. I give all the credit to Hahnemann and the strength of his teachings. This gives further support to the notion that homeopathy is founded on scientific principles.

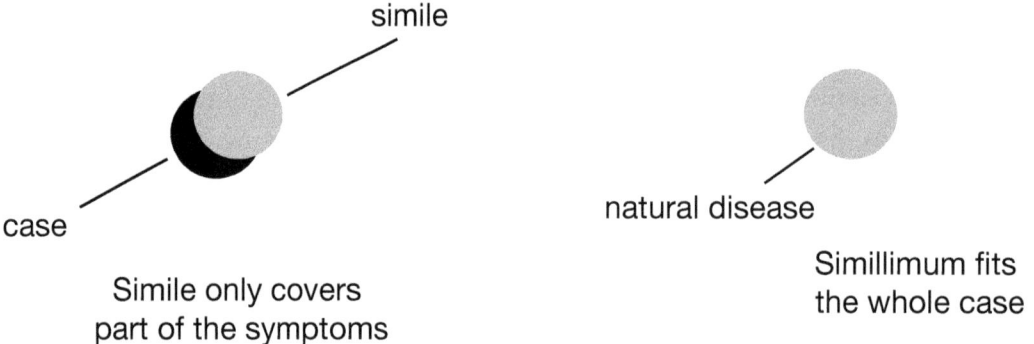

Fig. 9-1: Simile and Simillimum

General Principles of Remedy Selection

Similarity and difference: First, the selection of the remedy is based on both *similarities* and *differences:* determining which remedies have a similar symptom picture to that of the patient, then differentiating among these similar remedies. The beginner confronts the problem of *similarity*: after finding the totality of symptoms he tends to find too many remedies which seem similar, and he cannot tell which is to be chosen above the others or why. The experienced homeopath sees the *differences:* for instance, a fever with lack of thirst points to both Apis and Pulsatilla, but the emotional symptoms such as the jealousy of Apis versus the gentle, easygoing nature and weepiness of Pulsatilla will easily help us to differentiate between them. A knowledge of Materia Medica will obviously make this process faster for the experienced homeopath, although the beginner can do the same thing by repertorizing.

Symptoms produced by the simile: The simile does not fit the symptom picture exactly, does not strike the Vital Force properly, and requires more repetitions and more time to move the case along. The simillimum fits the case exactly, its action goes right to the bulls'-eye, and the cure is speedy, gentle, and effective. The effect can be so remarkable as to seem miraculous, as we have all seen, such as excruciating pain or profuse hemorrhage ceasing within moments after the remedy was given.

Should we despair if we do not hit the simillimum every time? Not at all. Even the best prescribers in homeopathic history such as Drs. Adolph Lippe, Constantine Hering, and later Pierre Schmidt, Margaret Tyler, and Elizabeth Wright-Hubbard would often struggle to find the ideal remedy for their patients. But there is a consolation: *when you give the simile, it can give you the answer for the simillimum.* The simile can stimulate the Vital Force enough to throw other symptoms to the surface. This is especially helpful when the original symptom picture was obscured by a paucity of symptoms. While some of the symptoms produced by your remedy belong to *its* symptom picture, there should be at least one symptom which *belongs to the symptom picture of the simillimum.* For example, in one case, Nat. mur. was the second choice for the remedy; the first choice made little vesicles break out all over the patient's fingers, a clear indication for Nat. mur. In another case of a small child with eczema, the parents' divorce when she was very young pointed to Nat. mur. but there was a paucity of other indications in the case. After the first remedy palliated for a while and then stopped working, the mother observed, "You know, she seems glum, she just keeps to herself and won't talk to me any more," pointing to Nat. mur., which cured. Henny Heudens-Mast recently presented a case in which the action of the simile led the patient, a little girl, to start eating sand (which is made of silica), clearly pointing to Silica, which matched the totality in her case.[1] Thus similes are detours on the way to the cure; the journey can take longer but we do arrive at our destination, as illustrated in Figure 9-2.

As mentioned in the section on provings, one of the obstacles to finding the simillimum is the lack of proven remedies. When a new remedy is proven, homeopaths often see it as a shortcut where two or more remedies had been needed to obtain the same result (as Lippe said when Apis was first proven). Another obstacle is that all the characteristics of a given remedy are not yet known, even for our favorite polychrests. If indications for our remedies were fully known, the prescriber's burden would be considerably lightened and their healing power would be more universally available.

Chronic symptoms persisting in acute disease: As a rule, in *acute* diseases there is little difficulty in determining the totality of the symptoms, for the deviation from normal health is usually sharp and well-defined (by the location, sensation, modalities and concomitant symptoms). As seen before in Laws and Principles, the chronic disease is suspended while the acute disease prevails. However, *all* the symptoms of the chronic disease do not necessarily give way to the acute symptoms. Kent noted that *some symptoms of the chronic disease may persist and are active during the acute disease.* Such symptoms are considered *peculiar* and thus belong at the top rank of our hierarchy (described later in this chapter). Prescribing for such an acute illness often presents us with the opportunity to address chronic and acute conditions together and strengthen the Vital Force at the same time.

True chronic diseases: Chronic diseases are more complicated, for the present symptoms often show only a partial picture of the disease, while many former symptoms are now inactive or suppressed. Even if we can trust the patient's memory, old symptoms must be used with caution, for they may have arisen from an unhealthy environment, drug suppression, or an acute miasmatic state caused by a vaccination or acute infection.

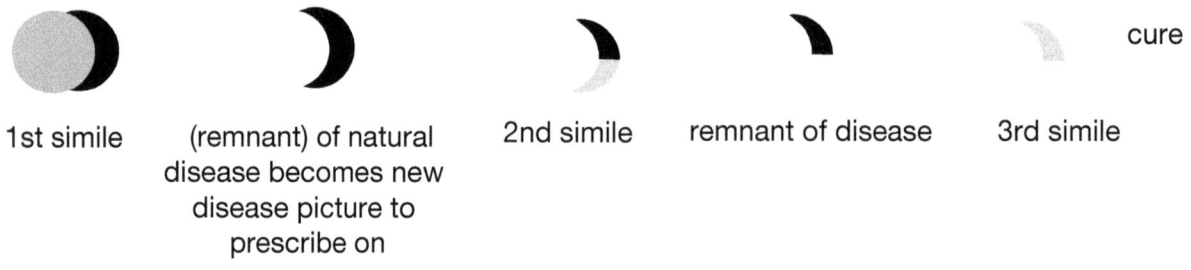

Figure 9-2: Similes Leading to the Simillimum

In chronic cases, theoretically we try to find a remedy whose symptoms correspond "exactly" (as regards to intensity and character) to those experienced by the patient. This can rarely be done in practice; in fact, if it were necessary always to select a remedy that corresponds perfectly to every one of the symptoms, our already vast Materia Medica would be utterly inadequate. But then, who among us has made finer cures than the old masters in homeopathy (Hahnemann, von Boenninghausen, Hering, Lippe, Kent, Farrington) with their very *limited* number of fully proven remedies? They *knew each remedy through and through,* in a way that very few among us do nowadays, because they proved the remedies on themselves. In their hands, comparatively few remedies were sufficient in the majority of cases. So new provings, although indispensable, are not the only answer. We must comprehend the spirit of each remedy *and* those symptoms that characterize the patient.

Symptoms of the patient, the disease and the end-pathology: In every case of disease, there are at least two and sometimes three classes of symptoms:

♦ First, common and pathognomonic symptoms of the disease (such as polydipsia, polyuria, and glycosuria in diabetes).

♦ Second, the peculiar or characteristic symptoms of the patient.

♦ Third, in cases of advanced pathology, symptoms belonging to the end-pathology such as kidney failure in advanced lupus.

Basing the remedy selection on the first and third class is a recipe for failure. Too many remedies will be found for the first class, the common symptoms of the disease (fatigue, edema, pain, inflammation, constipation). Waiting for the third class of symptoms to develop is cruel and unnecessary since the patient's Vital Force will be greatly weakened by then (and of course few if any remedies were proved to the point of pathology). The second class, the symptoms characteristic of the patient, are the ones to which Hahnemann directs us for a successful prescription.

Subjective and objective symptoms: We can also divide symptoms into subjective and objective: the subjective symptoms are those of the patient's own consciousness, those not knowable to the practitioner except as the patient describes them (such as pain). The objective symptoms are those observable and measurable, whether in diagnostic tests or by the practitioner observing the patient. (In allopathic medicine the word 'signs' is used for objective symptoms, but in homeopathy the word 'symptoms' is used for both objective and subjective ones.) The patient's description of her symptoms is more valuable to the homeopath than blood work and diagnostic tests. The objective symptoms are mostly useful in the absence of mental/emotional symptoms and the patient's report of her sensations (whereas allopathy prizes objective symptoms).

One of the great advantages of homeopathy is that it can diagnose and treat while the disease is still in the functional stage, preventing organic pathology from developing. This is *true* preventive medicine. Nature is giving us these subjective symptoms to reveal the internal disturbance while there is still time to effect a cure.

It is not easy to separate the symptoms peculiar to the patient from those common to the disease in complex chronic cases. In many long-standing chronic cases (is the homeopath not always the last to be consulted?), especially those that have been long under allopathic treatment (and which ones have not?), these peculiar and characteristic symptoms have been so completely suppressed or lost in the jungle of drug side-effects that our difficulties are increased tenfold. But we can begin by analyzing the different classes of symptoms in their hierarchy of value.

Strange, Rare and Peculiar Symptoms

In Aphorism 153 Hahnemann states:

> In the search for a homeopathically specific remedy ... the more *striking, exceptional, unusual and odd* (characteristic) signs and symptoms of the disease case are to be especially and most solely kept in view. ... The more common and indeterminate symptoms (lack of appetite, headache, lassitude, restless sleep, discomfort, etc.) are to be seen with almost every disease and medicine and thus deserve little attention unless they are more closely characterized.

Even after many years of experience, Kent stated that he regarded this as Hahnemann's greatest teaching. These words reflect different aspects of the same concept. *Striking* stands for surprising, forcible, impressive, very noticeable, a prominent feature. *Exceptional* stands for what is out of the ordinary. *Unusual* means infrequent in such a case; rare, hence remarkable. And *odd* or *characteristic* is what belongs solely or especially to the patient as distinct from other patients with the same disease. We will call these symptoms 'strange, rare and peculiar,' as they are customarily called based on earlier translations.

As Hahnemann explains, common symptoms have no place in the selection of our remedies. In fact, *the greater the value of a symptom for allopathic diagnosis, the less its value in the remedy selection*. For allopathic diagnosis is based on standard criteria which must be present, as listed in the ICD-9 diagnostic manual, while the opposite is true in homeopathy. We do not choose a remedy for a patient with diabetes based on symptoms such as polyuria and polydipsia. "Fatigue" is useless for remedy selection (the rubric in Kent lists over 200 remedies), unless (as Hahnemann expresses it in Aphorism 153), it can be made more characteristic of the patient. For example, "weariness after mental exertion" or "after talking (K1421), or "lassitude after stormy weather" (K1370) narrows down the remedy choice to a few.

Headache is another example: "Head, pain" in Kent starts on page 132 and continues for 90 pages! Unless the prescriber can link the headache to an unusual modality, causality or specific sensation, the hundreds of remedies found in the general rubric on page 132 are of no use in finding the simillimum. But "headaches from blows" (K137) limits our choice to five remedies. From a general symptom, it then becomes a more characteristic symptom, singular to the individual patient and therefore an important piece of the puzzle.

While Hahnemann seems to combine characteristic and striking/exceptional/unusual symptoms in the above aphorism, in practice we find a continuum between symptoms which are typical of the patient and absolutely unique (thus belonging at the top of our hierarchy) and those which are typical but common to many patients (and thus belonging lower down if indeed they are useful at all). For example, I had a patient whose hands constantly dripped with perspiration; water continuously flowed from her hands, day and night, like little fountains dripping onto the floor. This is a symptom which I have never seen in any other patient, have never read about, and have never heard about from another practitioner. Thus it is truly strange, rare and peculiar, deserving top rank in the hierarchy of her symptoms. Another patient might sweat easily on the head, which is *typical* of a Calcarea person (and certainly not typical of all patients), but is very *common* because the Calcarea constitution is so common in our society. Thus this symptom should not go at the top of the hierarchy. If you are not sure how common or rare a symptom is, an easy way to tell is to look in the *Repertory:* if the rubric has only a few remedies listed, it is uncommon and useful; but if it has many listed, it is common and not useful. An exception would be the delusions, which are always uncommon and peculiar no matter how many remedies they have, e.g. "sees spectres, ghosts, spirits," K32 (see Chapter 11, Delusions). The point is that a symptom should only go at the top of the hierarchy, above the causality and the mental-emotional symptoms, if you are certain that it is both very unusual and strikingly expressed in the person.

The more prominent *strange, rare, and peculiar features* of the case should be noted carefully. For these in particular should bear the closest similarity to the symptoms of the remedy. It is a common mistake of the novice to take a case and find fifty symptoms. To his amazement, his preceptor will throw out all but three and match these with a remedy. The totality of symptoms is *not* merely an indiscriminate *numerical sum* of all the symptoms. I remember that when I began studying homeopathy, we had to write up a case for homework. I proudly handed in 20 pages of symptoms. To my chagrin, my teacher threw it out, but he taught me a lesson I never forgot: "You have no case," he said. Not quantity of symptoms but quality (those individualized to the patient) will lead to the simillimum.

So we must begin by looking for *peculiar, characteristic or uncommon* symptom in the case. Remember that they must be peculiar to the patient rather than common to the disease. Dyspnea, edema, palpitations and albuminuria are common symptoms of many kidney diseases, so they will not help us find the simillimum. However, if the patient also has a strong craving for fat, strong-smelling urine, and a sensation as if the urine were cold when voiding, these symptoms would be peculiar to the patient and point to Nitric acid as the remedy. In spasmodic asthma, an aggravation from lying down may be characteristic of the patient, but it is so common that it is useless in finding the remedy. However, if the patient can *only* breathe when lying down (a keynote of Psorinum, which is the only black-type remedy for this subrubric), or in the knee-elbow position (typical of Kali carb.), then these will be invaluable because they are *peculiar* and not just characteristic (which of course they are as well). Asthma attacks between midnight and 5 a.m. would be another characteristic symptom which is less useful because it is not peculiar; many asthma patients have attacks at this time. If the attacks *always* occur at 3 a.m., this information would be useful because it is more unusual.

Remember that the more peculiar a symptom is, the more valuable. When an infant cries because he is hungry, this is normal. When an eighty-year-old has plenty of food and still cries from hunger, this is childish and a peculiar symptom. If a patient cries after her best friend dies, is this normal? Yes. But if she is still crying after ten years, she needs a remedy. The crying has become peculiar. We all remember our first love at age 14 or 15. We felt we could not live without her, fantasized running away with her, and were absolutely sure we would love her forever. This romantic behavior is common for teenagers, a normal symptom that does not need treatment. But when an 80-year-old patient tells us that she cannot live without the man of her dreams, she will be considered childish or even hysterical, possibly needing Helleborus, Baryta carb. or Ignatia. It is not what happens in somebody's life that matters, *but how they react to it*. The more the prescriber knows her Materia Medica, the more alert she will be to peculiar symptoms *spontaneously* expressed by the patient. We agree with Kent: "That which is common to the disease is never peculiar. What is common to the disease will never lead the physician to perceive what is peculiar in any individual."[2] Remember our guiding principle: "Treat the patient, not the disease." That is why Kent would say that a particular patient had "a *kind* of arthritis" or "a *kind* of pneumonia."

There are exceptions to this rule, of course. In epidemics the disease force is so powerful that it strikes a broad spectrum of the population regardless of their individual susceptibilities; thus the typical symptoms of the epidemic can be used to find one or two universal remedies for it, as will be described in the next chapter. And sometimes several members of a family need the same remedy because of peculiarities shared by the family, even though their disease conditions are different. This can happen with a strong active miasm: for example, the syphilitic miasm can express itself in different family members as hereditary alcoholism, compulsive gambling and manic depression, all of which could be treated with Lachesis. Finally, certain remedies have such a strong affinity for particular organs that they are used as a supporting, adjunctive organotherapy in a wide variety of diseases for that organ, such as Ceanothus for the spleen, Crataegus for the heart, and Carduus for the liver. But in all these cases, the peculiarities of the individual patient still must not be forgotten.

So how do we find the *uncommon* symptoms? By keeping in mind what is *common*. Being chilly is common for many people but if it occurs only during urinating, it becomes uncommon. Or if a patient was always hot until he became sick and is now chilly, that is uncommon. Many people can feel faint for different reasons, but fainting from hunger after fasting has only two remedies indicated, Phosphorus and Sulphur (K1360). In a community of people living in similar circumstances, most healthy normal individuals react in similar ways. They laugh at something funny; they perspire and feel thirsty during a heat wave. But when someone laughs at something sad or perspires when it is cold, we can conclude that his natural defenses deviate from the norm. Other peculiar symptoms include fever with thirstlessness, improvement of pain upon pressure, relief from headaches after urination, and symptoms recurring at the exact same time every day. Our *Repertory* and Materia Medica are full of such indications.

The "uncommon" symptoms may be very peculiar at times. I remember a little patient of mine, a 10-year-old girl, who came down with a severe nervous condition of unknown origin. Although normally very independent, once she became ill she could not go to sleep unless her mother sang to her. This "relief from music," being such a prominent symptom, indicated Tarentula hispanica, which in fact matched the totality and cured the little girl. Another of my patients, a young boy, had been sick for a week with a loose, watery stool which nothing seemed to help. He mentioned in passing that he felt sick and even had to leave the table if he saw or heard water running from the faucet. This peculiar symptom made me think of Hydrophobinum, which in fact matched the totality and cured him in one day.

Homeopaths must be disciples of Sherlock Holmes. As this master detective said, "That which is out of the common is usually a guide rather than a hindrance, and that which seemingly confuses the case is the very thing that furnishes the clue to its solution." Those of us trained as allopathic physicians must relearn our case-taking methods because this is exactly the opposite of what we learned in medical school: fit the standard disease description, then treat with the standard protocol.

While emphasizing the peculiar symptoms, of course we cannot entirely neglect the typical symptoms of the disease. But they will be subsequent to, and *of much less value* than those belonging to the patient. In most of our cases, no one remedy has *all* the peculiar or characteristic symptoms, but four or five remedies seem to have *equal numbers* of them. In those cases, the top choice will be the remedy that has these common symptoms in the highest grade (black type or italic in the *Repertory*). Remember that there must be a general correspondence between all the symptoms of the patient and those of the remedy. However helpful peculiar symptoms may be in leading us to a remedy, they are not the sole guides.

Another warning to the student: Remember that to be useful, peculiar symptoms must be *equally well marked in the patient and in the remedy*. In other words, a prominent symptom of the patient must be covered by a correspondingly prominent symptom in the remedy. For example, take a case of rheumatism, markedly aggravated in dry weather and better in damp (which is unusual, since most arthritic complaints are worse in dampness). In such a case, Phosphorus could not be selected based on this modality, for while Phosphorus has it, it is only in the lowest degree (see K1357, "*dry* weather aggravates": Phosphorus is only a 1). Causticum would be more strongly indicated since it is black type (3). While Phosphorus may ultimately be chosen for *other* reasons, it would not be chosen *solely* based on this rubric. In a case with eight peculiar symptoms of which one remedy has six but they all rank (1), while another has only three but they all rank (3), the second remedy is much more likely to cure the case.

Another hint for finding a peculiar, uncommon symptom is its *prominence* in the sufferings of the patient. Does he spontaneously list it as an outstanding cause of his distress? It may be unimportant for the allopathic diagnosis, but clinical experience has shown that any troublesome symptom, whether nausea, sweating, thirst, weakness or fear takes on added therapeutic value when it is *unusually prominent*. For my patient who constantly dripped perspiration from her hands, this was the sole focus of her physical complaints and probably led to social isolation as well. (She was one of my first patients when I started practice 30 years ago, and her case was one reason I explored alternative modalities. How I wish I could treat her now; she was most likely a Silica case.)

Keynotes: A keynote of a remedy is a symptom which is typical of it, so much so that it makes the experienced homeopath think of that remedy. (Sometimes two or three remedies share a keynote, like the pain at the lower angle of the right scapula which is so typical of Chelidonium but also occurs in Bryonia and Carduus). Usually a keynote means the remedy is by far the most frequently associated with it (even though there may be other remedies listed in the rubric). Keynotes are often truly exceptional and rare. They must be at least fairly uncommon or else they would not be so strongly associated with one particular remedy. Depending on how exceptional and rare it is, a keynote may become the #1 rubric in your hierarchy of symptoms.

Following our priority of symptoms (explained later in this chapter), a mental/emotional keynote will be more valuable than a physical one. A physical keynote like Ipecac's nausea with a clean tongue would not be automatically placed above the Never Well Since as if it were strange, rare and peculiar. If I saw a keynote like that in a case, however, I would be on the lookout for an Ipecac etiology and Ipecac mentals.

Study of the Materia Medica allows you to recognize these keynotes which distinguish the remedies from each other: the thirstlessness with fever of Apis and Pulsatilla, the desire to curse and swear of Anacardium, the clean tongue with nausea and vomiting of Ipecac, the strong desire for open air of Pulsatilla, the improvement of pain by laying on the painful side of Bryonia, the pasty white tongue of Antimonium crudum, and so forth.

Many homeopaths prescribe by keynotes: they find something peculiar in the case that points to a certain remedy, then they see whether the totality confirms or disapproves the choice. But a word of caution here. This system of prescribing is very attractive, as it seems so much easier than the tedious comparison of remedies using the numerical method (unless you use a computer program to add the scores). Depending *solely* on this method is very wrong and doomed to failure because it ranks one or two symptoms very high while practically ignoring the others. And remember to rank mental/emotional keynotes higher than physical ones: examples would include the Aconite tendency to predict the time of his death, the Calcarea fear of going insane and of others observing it, and the Phosphorus predilection for séances, channeling and vibrational healing.

A remedy found through a keynote must be confirmed by the totality afterwards. A keynote is a symptom so characteristic of a remedy, that whenever we meet with it we usually find the remainder of the symptoms under that remedy also. The *keynote leads to the remedy, the totality confirms or rejects the choice.* The other symptoms should be in harmony with it like the notes of a chord.

Do not overuse keynotes: they are meant to *shorten* our research, not to *suppress* it. The keynote is a sharp-edged tool requiring the most consummate skill in its legitimate use. This method was invented by Hahnemann, improved by von Boenninghausen, Stapf and Hering, and perfected by Guernsey and Lippe. But I have too often seen cases presented at conferences in which a remedy is prescribed based on a keynote which was merely a particular physical symptom, while the higher-valued symptoms pointed to another remedy. For example, a patient presented at a recent conference was given Kali ferrocyanatum on the basis of "painless menorrhagia," one of its keynotes, when the rest of the case pointed to Nat. mur. As I have mentioned before and will explain in detail below, the remedy which matches the miasm and highest-ranked symptoms (the Never Well Since and mental/emotional) will cure *even if it does not match the Chief Complaint.*

Hahnemann condemns prescribing on one symptom only (even if it is a keynote) as an allopathic way of practicing homeopathy. "The simple symptom is no more the disease, than a single foot is the man himself."[2] Hahnemann was very careful to tell us to look for the striking, uncommon and peculiar *symptoms (plural)*, not the *one most peculiar symptom*. Dr. H. N. Guernsey, the so-called "father of the keynote system," explicitly states that keynotes should not form the *sole* basis of a prescription, which would indeed be simply prescribing for a single symptom. On the contrary, he declared, "all keynotes must be in harmony with and confirmed by the totality of the accompanying symptoms before we have sufficient reason for prescribing."[3] The proper use of keynotes reminds me of the Advent calendars with a little numbered flap for each day before Christmas; children open the little door for each day to see a picture of a toy or an ornament. The keynote is the little door you open, but if the remedy picture inside doesn't match the patient, you have to shut it again!

This fatal error of prescribing for single symptoms led to Lux's heresy of isopathy (prescribing the dynamized nosode for each disease), a practice completely at variance with Hahnemann's method of prescribing. While it may effectively palliate the Chief Complaint, it will not address the patient as a whole person and thus risks the dangers of palliation covered in Chapter 16. To give an example, I do not prescribe Syphilinum for acute syphilis (because I have not found it to work) and only in chronic syphilis if the symptoms match the totality—including mental and emotional—of Syphilinum. (If I see syphilis or gonorrhea in the past medical history, I certainly would *expect* to use the nosode and would be on the lookout for other indications, but I would not give it *unless indicated*.)

So we must select the *most* peculiar symptoms without forgetting the others. Especially when the most striking symptoms point to several remedies at once, we must seek corroboration from the others. In such cases, one remedy can generally be found whose picture most closely matches the patient's symptoms, although it may differ in a few features. Thus (to give an example of where keynote prescribing can lead you), copious eructations of gas suggest Carbo veg.; great weakness suggests Arsenicum; general irritability indicates Nux vomica; sensitivity to cold points to Hepar sulph. One case presented all these symptoms, but the patient also felt worse from talking about his symptoms, expressed fears of incurable diseases, and reported sour rather than burning eructations. Calcarea was the simillimum.

Delusions: The delusions are a special class of peculiar symptoms, with many pages of the *Repertory* devoted to them. They are so important that a separate chapter is devoted to them (Chapter 11).

In conclusion we can say that a strange, rare and peculiar symptom and/or a delusion, if you can find one, takes first place in the hierarchy of symptom value.

Other Types of Symptoms in their Order of Value

Miasmatic States: I have found that diagnosing the patient's miasmatic state is *so essential* to the cure that I have devoted the entire next section of the book to it. The curative remedy must be effective against the active miasm, which becomes an important way to differentiate among possible remedy choices. When analyzing a case, I simultaneously scan for symptoms of the active miasm and for the hierarchy of symptoms, like having two programs running at the same time on a computer. I look up the top remedies in Banerjea's *Miasmatic Diagnosis,* choosing the one *most* effective against the active miasm (even preferring it to ones more strongly indicated by the rubrics). If the patient has a sycotic condition and I have a choice between a remedy which is a 3+ against sycosis, like Arsenicum, and one which is 1+ like Argentum nitricum, I would start with the stronger antisycotic. (This is assuming the patient has what Hahnemann called a true chronic disease, one with a miasmatic background, i.e. not arising from drug toxicity or lifestyle factors.)

The Never Well Since (NWS): The second most important group of symptoms is the "Never Well Since," the answer to the all-important question, "Why did the patient get sick in the first place?" All systems of medicine appreciate the significance of etiology, but homeopathy's understanding of causality is fundamentally different from that of any other except TCM. While allopathy explains most illnesses as caused by a microbe or genetic defect, homeopathy probes more deeply: given that certain microbes are ubiquitous, why are some people more susceptible than others? And why do some people with a genetic marker develop a particular disease while others do not, and still others *without* the marker *do*?

To a homeopath, saying, "The patient got sick because he caught a virus" does not answer the question—it merely restates it. In searching for the answer, homeopathy explores terrain familiar to the allopath, from the long-term effects of physical trauma (even including birth trauma) to diet, environmental toxins, and drug side effects. But homeopathy more often finds the answer in territory unfamiliar to allopathy, in mental and emotional trauma such as grief or loss (of a parent, a spouse, a business, even the loss of emotional nourishment in childhood), financial worry, jealousy, humiliation, and abuse. Homeopathy even acknowledges the possibility of illness from excessive happiness: I had a patient who became ill immediately after marrying her sweetheart, moving into a new house and getting a better job all at the same time. The "positive stress" was too much for her system, and Coffea was her remedy.

To the extent that allopathy recognizes causative factors in the patient's lifestyle and environment, it does not look for those *unique* to the individual, as homeopathy does, but to factors so *common* that the individuals can be lumped together into groups with "known risk factors" for the disease. And it is true that allopathy is beginning to recognize the role of mental/emotional factors such as the death of a spouse after 50 years of marriage. A history of being abused as a child and other measures of a dysfunctional family history were strongly correlated with risk factors for several of the leading causes of death in adults, according to a recent study.[5] But allopathy still lacks the perspective and knowledge base to use this information. How can it protect the grieving widow, as homeopathy can with Aurum? Of course emotional trauma can be addressed with drugs such as Zoloft and Prozac, which rank among the top ten pharmaceuticals prescribed in this country. But such medications merely suppress emotions to allow the patient to function rather than giving the patient the strength to truly process the grief and then let go of it, as a remedy can.

Homeopathy recognizes the importance of life-threatening physical trauma in which allopathic intervention is essential to re-establish vital signs. If a patient is in hypovolemic shock following severe hemorrhage, she will need IV fluids and blood transfusions. But the homeopath will not stop there. Recognizing the dangers of "never well since blood loss" (which we frequently see from abundant menstrual bleeding), the homeopath will give China, Ferrum met. or Phosphoric acid as indicated. I have seen patients suffering from Chronic Fatigue Syndrome for years after such an episode, in which the medical establishment successfully restored vital signs and hemaglobin/hematocrit, but the patient's Vital Force remained chronically weakened.

Acute physical trauma can also become a "Never Well Since": a 25-year-old patient of mine suffered for years from gastric troubles including flatulence, eructations, pain after eating and constipation. Antacids were of no help. When asked the all-important question, she said it started from the day she was struck hard in the stomach with a tennis ball. She almost fainted with the pain, and that night she vomited blood. Based on the Never Well Since, I gave her Arnica LM1, of which a few doses cured her from her long ordeal.

Similarly, in recognizing the role of climate, allopathy may acknowledge the role of dampness in aggravating rheumatism or of heat in aggravating the condition of a cardiac patient, but it offers little suggestion for dampness except recommending that the patient move to Arizona. In TCM, climatic factors play a great role in etiology; in homeopathy, even more so. The *Repertory* lists the influences of climatic factors in all the anatomical sections and especially in Generalities: "Air, change of weather aggravates," as well as cold air, wet weather, dryness, storm, heat, sun exposure, and wind; and in Chill: "Exposure, after," (exposure to a draft, from living on water courses, during rains, residing at the seashore, sleeping in damp rooms, standing in water, exposure to heat of the sun, swamps, from becoming wet, from working in clay or water, K1267). Each rubric, of course, indicates remedies addressing that factor. Likewise under Foods in Generalities we find remedies for diarrhea from fats, for example, differentiated from those for diarrhea from eating fruits.

For the past 20 years scientists have been laboriously mapping all the chromosomes of the human genome. But how useful is this information? A defective gene does not necessarily predict the corresponding disease, and genetically-linked diseases often appear in people who lack the defective gene. All this effort does not answer the real questions: why was the gene damaged in the first place? how can we repair it? and how can we prevent it from happening again? Homeopathy has answers to all these questions in its analogue to gene therapy: miasmatic prescribing, described in Chapter 19. By addressing the active miasm, homeopathy has been successfully treating genetic diseases and preventing birth defects for over 150 years.

So we can see the importance of finding the Never Well Since. This is often the top of our hierarchy, since not every patient has a delusion or a strange-rare-peculiar symptom, but nearly every condition has a trauma that triggered it. The patient may not remember the onset, or may not make the connection, or (as I have often seen in my practice) may have forgotten the connection because his doctor was dismissive of it. To help the patient remember, I ask, "What was going on in your life when you became ill?" (or immediately before, sometimes up to a year before). I also have the patient construct a timeline (see the sample patient intake in Appendix 1). Patients often tell me that constructing the timeline is a healing experience in itself: they start to put things together, to see the patterns in their life, and realize for themselves why they were vulnerable to illness at a crucial juncture.

If we still cannot find the Never Well Since, no harm. We have many pieces of the puzzle and can still see the pattern even if one piece is missing. Sometimes the other pieces point so clearly to a remedy that we can guess the associated causality even if the patient can't remember. If we suggest the causality to the patient, sometimes the memories come back in a flood (often with a flood of tears!). Most notably we may see the unmistakable physical signs of a past history of child abuse, and if a remedy like Staphysagria cures the complaint, that is all we need to know. The memories can be left undisturbed. (Psychotherapists will say that the patient must remember in order to heal, but the remedies seem to help the patient process on a deeper, unconscious level, or through dreams, allowing the patient to grow in well-being and self-confidence without necessarily having to consciously face the pain of the memories.)

In Appendix 2, I have outlined the more common Never Well Since factors which we encounter in practice. The *Repertory* should also be consulted for "ailments from" (which are conveniently grouped together in the Mind section of the *Synthesis Repertorium*). While the *Repertory* may list many more remedies for each etiology than are listed in the appendix, the ones in the appendix are the ones I have found to resolve the great majority of cases in my practice.

Mental and emotional factors: Among the general symptoms (i.e. those symptoms pertaining to the whole person), the mental/emotional symptoms rank higher than the physical generals. Hahnemann and Kent recognized over 100 years ago the high place they take in our hierarchy of symptoms, right after the rare/peculiar and the Never Well Since. (Prescribing *only* on mentals can be palliative, however, just as prescribing on local physicals can be palliative.) The mental state, reflecting the inner core of the being, is bound to be of the utmost importance. These symptoms are naturally the most difficult to elicit, for people tend to shrink from revealing their inmost thoughts and motives, their hatreds, jealousies, desires, and aversions. It requires the greatest tact and full knowledge of human nature to win the confidence of our patient and so understand her deepest thoughts. Of course, the homeopath is well aware of the more common mental states. We all recognize the fastidiousness of Arsenicum, the irritability of Nux vomica, the haughtiness of Platina, the easily offended pride of Nat. mur., and the ever-varying moods in the soap opera life of Ignatia. Their value to us is inexpressible.

Illness starts first on the mental/emotional/energetic plane (with the obvious exception of physical traumas), with physical or anatomical changes coming later. Should we wait for those physical symptoms to appear before we prescribe? Of course not. It is one of homeopathy's strengths that it can prescribe on the slightest emotional or mental factor, forestalling the development of subsequent pathology.

Within this important group of symptoms, some are more important than others. In order of importance, they are:

The will to live: Disease starts from the core of the being, and the will to live is nearest to the innermost self. The most fundamental instinct is self-preservation, and suicide is the deepest aberration. Loathing of life, complete indifference, and self-destructive behavior (alcoholism, eating disorders, drug use) will gain top priority in our hierarchy.

Intellect: This group includes *memory* (short and long-term), *mistakes* (in localities, in writing, reading, spelling, etc.), *confusion* (as to own identity, on attempting to concentrate, as if in a dream, loses his way in well-known streets, etc.) and *concentration*. It is sad to see so many children now with ADD or ADHD, which indicates the strong miasmatic force in this latest generation of children, who show deep mental symptoms rather than physical ones from an early age.

Emotions: These include loves and hates, apprehension, the desire for or aversion to company, weepiness, tidiness, low self-confidence and self-worth, loquacity, taciturnity and hypersensitivity to offense, among others. Also included here are recurrent dreams, such as amorous dreams and dreams of the dead or of accidents. Dreams, especially repetitive ones, reveal the subconscious state of the mind, because in sleep we let down our guard and the deeper states of consciousness can surface. (Interestingly, dreams often change when a patient starts a remedy, often helping the patient process a trauma. The patient may dream of saying goodbye to long-deceased loved ones or expressing anger towards someone who is inaccessible in real life.) Dreams have to be *regular* and *persistent* to be useful. Kent gives us a marvelous array of dreams in his section on sleep. The dreams I have most often encountered among my patients are those about dead loved ones, the body being disfigured, accidents or drownings, misfortune, being chased, being naked in public, being unprepared for exams, events from the previous day or events that have not taken place yet, and frightful dreams (nightmares).

General Physical Symptoms: The general symptoms are those that affect the patient as a whole and thus rank higher than the particular symptoms, which affect only one organ or function. General symptoms are those that can be expressed as statements beginning with "I" (for instance, "I am, I feel, I hate, I love, I crave, I feel better from or worse from"). Physical general symptoms are next in line after mental and emotional generals.

In fact, a general symptom, if it is well-marked, *can overrule any number of even strong particulars.* Let us take an example of gastritis with semi-lateral headache, roaring in the ears, a greasy taste in the mouth, aversion to butter and fat which aggravate, fullness of the stomach after eating, flatulence, and vomiting of food. So far, with generals and particulars, Pulsatilla and Cyclamen compete equally. If we have in addition, diarrhea only at night, nausea from hot but not from cold drinks, and palpitations when lying on the left side, then the balance would turn towards Pulsatilla (particulars only). But what if we find that the patient has the greatest aversion to cold open air? We know that Cyclamen is averse to and worse from open air, while Pulsatilla has a strong amelioration from it. This one strong general symptom would outweigh Pulsatilla's marked particulars and tip the scales towards Cyclamen. So if you have two competing remedies with many particulars in common, but only one of the remedies has the strong general, the choice is obvious.

On the other hand, a number of *strong particulars* must not be neglected because of one or even more *weak generals*. Let us take another example of gastritis with severe pain over the right eye, bitter eructations, pain in the stomach, worse from cold and better from warm drinks, and one foot cold, the other hot. So far Chelidonium and Lycopodium are about equal. If there is in addition constant pain under the inferior angle of the right scapula, a yellow-coated tongue with indentations, and clay-colored stools, no one would hesitate to prescribe Chelidonium. If we then find that the patient feels slightly worse after meals and somewhat better when moving about, these generals would tend to indicate Lycopodium. But they are *only weak and not strongly marked generals,* and consequently they should not be allowed to outweigh the *strong particulars* that indicate Chelidonium.

The following are some significant categories of general physical symptoms:

Internal temperature: Whether the patient tends to be chilly or hot might not be very important in finding the simillimum directly, because the rubrics are too large ("Generalities, heat, lack of vital," K1366 and "heat, sensation of," K1366). In fact I would never "waste" one of my 10 rubrics on it, unless the patient was strikingly different from others on this point. (Remember the classic Hyoscyamus rubric, wearing furs in the summer!) But it can make the difference when you hesitate between two remedies, with one a hot and the other a cold remedy, if the patient is noticeably one or the other. You really have to be precise in your questioning: if the patient says, "I can't stand the heat!" he may really mean he cannot stand a stuffy closed place, no matter what the temperature. So don't ask simply, "Are you a chilly or hot person?" Always ask more questions to clarify. "Are you the first one to put a jacket on, when you go outside with friends? Do you tend to ask for the windows to be shut, when you are in a group? How many blankets do you use? Do you sleep with the window open, even in winter? Do you stick your feet out from under the covers? Do you dislike cold wind?" Remember to be observant if your patient comes in wearing a T-shirt and shorts in the winter or bundled up in warm weather. And if the patient tells you she is neither hot nor cold, as many will, then do not keep pressing her to choose one, because this modality is only useful if it is outspoken.

Temperature modalities: Another frequent error is that a tendency to perspire does not necessarily mean that heat aggravates. (Calcarea can perspire while chilly, resulting in the typical clammy handshake). And an undue readiness to catch colds does not necessarily mean that cold aggravates or that the patient is chilly. Temperature modalities are most valuable when the body as a whole is markedly affected by one temperature and a particular part by the opposite. For example we find in Arsenicum a general aggravation from cold but improvement from cold applications for a headache. Another unusual and useful temperature modality is the exquisite sensitivity to both extremes of Mercury and Nat. carb., finding comfort only in a very narrow range of temperature (i.e., between 70° and 75° F).

Weather conditions: The effect of various *weathers* can give both positive and negative clues. For example, we expect as a rule that rheumatism will aggravate from changes in weather (temperature, humidity, and barometric pressure). The *absence* of such an aggravation is so peculiar that it enables us to eliminate whole groups of remedies. If a *change* of weather does not influence a rheumatism, we can safely discard Dulcamara, Nux moschata, Phosphorus, Ranunculus bulbosus, Rhododendron, Rhus tox., Silica, and Tuberculinum (K1347, "Change, weather aggravates"); if *wet* weather does not affect it, we can eliminate Calcarea, Dulcamara, Mercury, Nat. carb., Nat. sulph., Rhododendron, Rhus tox., and Ruta (see K1421, "Wet weather").

Positions: General symptoms can include the influence of the *various positions,* such as Sulphur's strong aggravation of most symptoms by standing and Lycopodium's aggravations from lying on the right side (and Mercury's even more so). Phosphorus has aggravations from lying on the left (K1373, "Lying, side, on") but ha*s* an aggravation of head symptoms when lying on the right (which is so unusual a combination as to make it *peculiar*). To be of any value as a general symptom, the patient as a whole must be *markedly* influenced by the position, and if only one part (head, an organ) is affected, it takes only low rank, being a particular and not a general anymore.

Sides of the body: The tendency of the disease to affect *particular sides* of the body is often well marked. If the right side is mainly affected we think of Belladonna and Lycopodium; if the left side, Lachesis, Phosphorus and Argentum nitricum. And who can forget Lac caninum's movement of symptoms back and forth from one side to the other (K1400, "Sides, alternating").

Time of day: We often find symptoms aggravate at certain times of day or night. This is a great general symptom which often points us to the right remedy. In fact aggravation at a particular time of day is so specific to certain remedies that it becomes a high-priority general rubric. Think about the asthma attacks between 2 and 4 a.m. of Kali carb., the morning diarrhea of Sulphur at 5 a.m., the twilight aggravation of Pulsatilla, the 4 to 8 p.m. aggravation of Lycopodium, etc. We also have a *periodic return* of symptoms (K1390, "Periodicity") with hay fever returning every year at the same time in Psorinum, neuralgia every day at the same time in Kali bich., the aggravations at new and full moon of Calcarea, and the monthly aggravation of Nux vomica and Sepia. Make sure, though, that the periodicity of a symptom is peculiar to the patient and not typical of the condition (such as the monthly return of menstrual symptoms or the every-third-day fever of malaria), which would make it a common symptom and thus not useful.

Food Cravings, Aversions and Aggravations: These are of great importance in adults, of utmost importance during pregnancy (when they denote the miasmatic state brought from the father to the mother, as explained in the chapter on miasms), and less useful in children. Food cravings and aversions are usually *general* symptoms (even though Kent lists them under "Stomach, desires," an error corrected in the *Synthesis Repertorium*) and can be used if outstanding.

Aggravations are correctly listed in Kent in Generalities under Food and must be distinguished from aversions. An aversion means that the person dislikes the taste of or is repulsed by a food; aggravation means that the patient feels worse after eating the food. If human beings were entirely rational, we would always avoid the foods that make us feel worse, but in real life people often crave foods (like sugary, fatty, and fried foods) and then feel worse after eating them (typical of Nux vomica and of the tubercular miasm). An aggravation can be a general symptom (the whole person is affected, e.g. feels tired and sleepy after a certain food) or a particular (e.g. he gets a headache from a food). If a patient gets diarrhea from fruit (an indication for China: K613, "Rectum, diarrhea"), this is considered a particular, while if she feels worse overall from eating fruit this would be a general and much more useful symptom.

The special senses are often so closely related to the whole being that many of their symptoms are general. For example, when the patient states that the smell of food sickens him after a food poisoning (Arsenicum) or during pregnancy (Sepia, Colchicum), this is a *general*. But if he experiences an offensive smell only in the nose (Asafoetida), this would be a low ranking particular.

Sleep and Sexuality: In this day and age, men's Chief Complaint often has to do with sexual performance (we have at least 30 different "homeopathic Viagras") and women's with menstrual disturbances, both found in the Genitalia section of Kent. Even if the Chief Complaint does not include PMS or the menstrual cycle, the rubrics covering these conditions are important for the female patient in determining both the remedy and the constitution.

Other generals include the effects of sleep such as the aggravation *after* sleep of Lachesis, the aggravation from *loss* of sleep of Cocculus and Causticum, and the great *relief* from sleep of Sepia and Phosphorus (who feels better from a nap, even a short one). The preferred position of sleep can allude to a certain remedy: for example, Medorrhinum's knee-chest position with the head bored into the pillow, Phosphorus' inability to sleep on the left side, and Pulsatilla's tendency to sleep with her arms over her head.

Particulars and Other Important Classes: While general symptoms as a rule rank higher, we must not undervalue particulars. In the unlikely event you had a case with mostly particulars and few or no generals, you would focus on the *most peculiar* particulars, like a headache above the left eye, radiating to the neck (Spigelia). (However, remember that a peculiar *general* outranks a peculiar *particular.* For example, a high fever of 105°F with thirstlessness is peculiar because we expect thirst with such a high temperature.) I have included this scenario for the sake of completeness, but I have never seen a case with few or no generals. I wonder if it would mean poor case-taking or else possibly a comatose patient (but then even simple observation would tell you many things about the patient).

There are still other examples where the particulars and common symptoms might be raised in value:

- Two *common* particular symptoms become valuable when *associated,* for example the coryza with perspiration of Mercury (K328)
- A common symptom becomes valuable when associated with a peculiar *modality,* such as Pulsatilla's chilliness worse near fire, or Asarum's chilliness which warm covering does not ameliorate.
- A common symptom can become valuable if it occurs in a particular *location,* such as aching pain at the inferior angle of the right scapula of Chelidonium (also Carduus and

Bryonia to a lesser degree), at the inferior left angle of Ranunculus bulbosus, and in between the scapulae of Phosphorus and Lycopodium.
- The mere *intensity* of the common symptom can raise its rank, such as the overwhelming sleepiness or narcolepsy of Nux moschata.

The Chief Complaint: The greatest mistake we can make as homeopaths is to fall into the allopathic trap of prescribing for the Chief Complaint. Beginning homeopaths are surprised that when they find a simillimum based on the hierarchy of symptoms, it can cure the Chief Complaint even if the chosen remedy in its proving *does not contain the Chief Complaint*. This demonstrates how important the Never Well Since and the mental/emotional factors are. I force my students to put the Chief Complaint in the last place in the hierarchy of rubrics (see the end of this chapter). Following Kent, I tell my students that one way to check their remedy selection is to ask themselves, "Would this remedy be equally applicable to this patient if the allopathic diagnosis were entirely different?" If so, the selection was a good one, and if not, it was a poor one. As we said before, the greater the value of a symptom for diagnosis, the less its value in choosing the remedy. If by chance our selected remedy does contain the Chief Complaint, even better, but it is not necessary. Of course if we hesitate between two remedies and one of the two has the Chief Complaint, we might be inclined to choose that remedy, but we often have better ways to differentiate. And as a rule, the symptoms of which the patient complains the loudest are not always indicative of or important in selecting the simillimum. There is no need for rubrics indicating diseases by name such as Lyme's disease or Hodgkin's lymphoma. In fact, this can mislead the budding homeopath into "allopathic" prescribing.

The location, sensation, modalities and concomitants of the Chief Complaint will be asked for, as described in the section on taking acute cases in Chapter 7.

The Order of the Symptoms: In sum, we can rank the symptoms as follows in order of decreasing importance:
- Strange, rare and peculiar symptoms (including delusions and *strong* keynotes)
- The Never Well Since
- Mental/emotional symptoms
- Generalities
- Food cravings and aversions
- Sleep and sexuality
- The Chief Complaint, with its location, sensation, modalities and concomitants.

This hierarchy is illustrated in Figure 9-3.

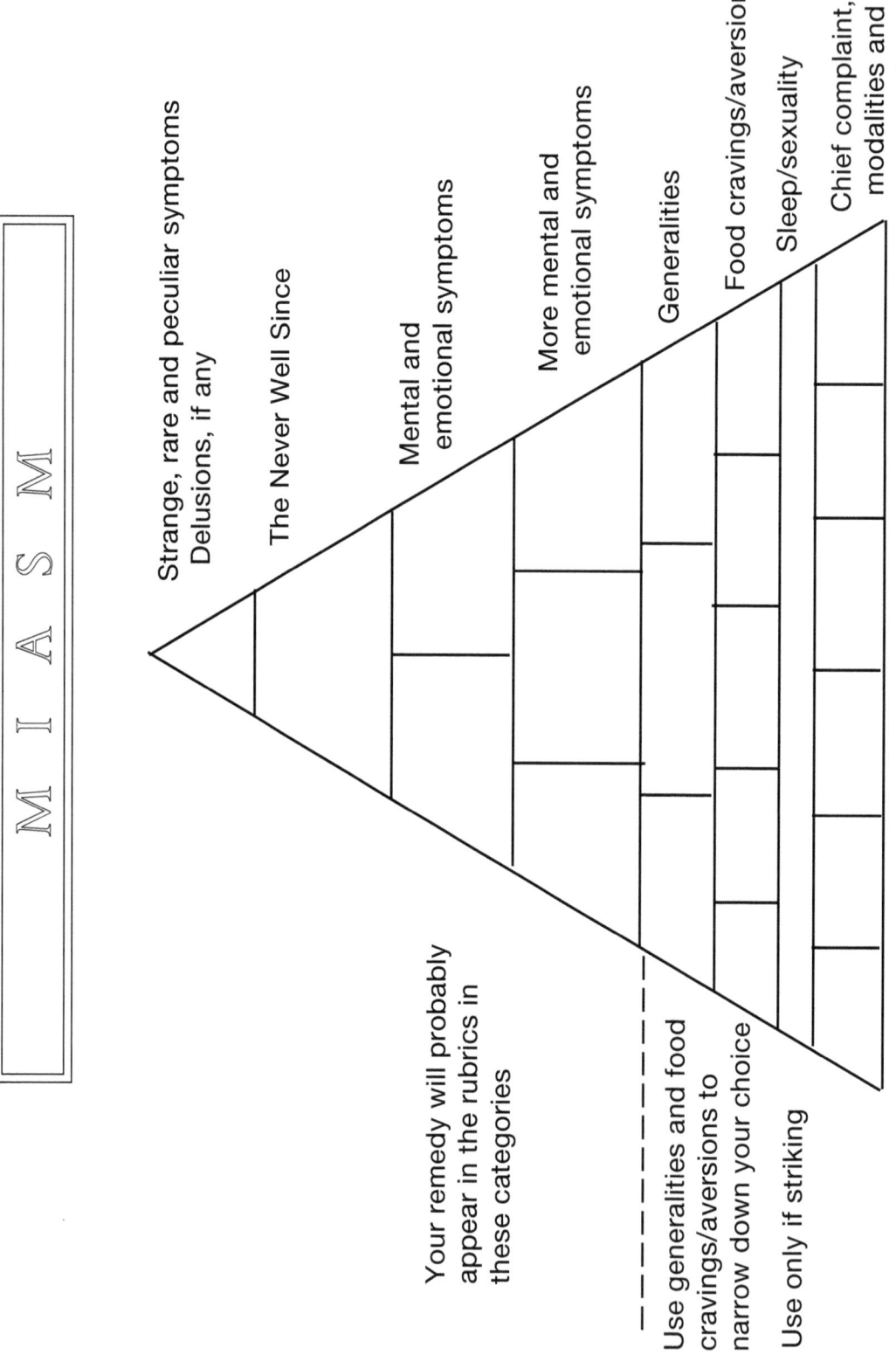

Fig. 9-3, Prioritizing the Levels of the Rubrics

My Own Clinical Method Based on Ten Rubrics

This is how I teach my students to prioritize the rubrics and add the score to find one or more possible remedies (which are always checked in the Materia Medica). The scoring chart is a learning tool, like the training wheels on a bicycle. In practice I rarely need to use it any more, but it is very useful for students to get in the habit of being discriminating and prioritizing the rubrics. I occasionally use it when I am really stuck on a case or the indicated remedies are not working.

Using the scoring chart (Figure 9-4): You will be choosing 10 rubrics covering representative symptoms of your case, in order of the hierarchy. Remedies are listed in the left and given a score of 3 for bold type, 2 for italic and 1 for roman.

In the left hand column, list and score all remedies which appear in your strange, rare and peculiar rubric (if any) in the first column, then in your Never Well Since rubric in the second column. (Place the Never Well Since in the first column if it is empty.) There should not be many remedies here; a strange, rare and peculiar symptom by definition will not have many remedies; and likewise the Never Well Since should not have many remedies. Remedies in the Never Well Since list should be given a score of 3. Then go through the mental/emotional rubrics, scoring each of the remedies you have *already* written down and *adding* any remedies which appear in bold type (if you have *many* remedies already; if you only have a *few,* you should *also add* remedies which appear in italic). For each new remedy you add in the mental/emotional section, go back and *add* the score it would have received in the *previous* mental/emotional rubrics you scored. (In this way you don't have to worry about which mental/emotional rubric should be number 2 or number 5.)

Choice of rubrics: Avoid rubrics with only a few remedies (especially if they are in roman type) or a hundred remedies, because they are not useful. Exception: as just mentioned, if you have a delusion, a strange-rare-peculiar symptom, or a Never Well Since you need to use the rubric even if it only has a few remedies in it. Most of these delusion rubrics have a limited number of remedies. If a rubric in any other category is a large one, try to use a subrubric instead. Another possibility is to use black type and italic remedies only. If a rubric is too small, try to find another rubric for the same symptom (using a thesaurus or a computer program).

Try to think in terms of the language of the *Repertory* when interviewing your patient. You may find it helpful to use the *Repertory* in questioning your patient: if you find an appropriate rubric, you can skim through the subrubrics in your questioning. The more you work with the *Repertory,* the more Kent's phrasing will become second nature to you.

If you have a favorite remedy, or if you think you know the remedy intuitively before you start, be careful not to "stack the deck" by consciously or unconsciously choosing rubrics to support it. Look for a variety of rubrics to cover all aspects of the case. For example, if you have an intuition that the remedy is Staphysagria, you might find yourself choosing from the many rubrics that have "worse from humiliation/indignation," which will skew the score towards Staphysagria even if it is not the simillimum.

The order of importance: First comes a delusion or strange-rare-peculiar, if present. Next is one or two rubrics for the Never Well Since (two if there seem to be two *clearly different* possible etiologies); four or five for mental/emotional symptoms; perhaps two for generalities; one for food cravings and aversions (only if strongly marked and/or unusual) and ending with one for the Chief Complaint. If the Chief Complaint is mental/emotional (e.g. anxiety or depression), include it with the mental/emotional rubrics rather than as the tenth rubric. Use one rubric for sleep or sexuality *only* if a symptom in these areas is strongly marked and/or unusual. If that is the case, it may be part of the Chief Complaint, such as insomnia or impotence, and can be listed as the tenth rubric instead.

These guidelines will be flexible depending on your case: for example, if the case has no mental/emotional information at all, you will need to depend more on the generalities. (This rarely happens, except with a new patient in a coma! Even with infants and pets you can deduce so much from observing the behavior, as described in the chapter on case-taking.) Whenever information from one of the levels is missing, go to the next one in order of importance. If the Never Well Since is missing, start with Mental/Emotional; if that is missing (which should be extremely rare), go to Generalities, etc.

The Never Well Since list in Appendix 2 is not exhaustive: it only includes the top remedies which I have found most useful in my practice. Try to find the Never Well Since as a rubric in the *Repertory* as well and use all the remedies in black type or italic there, because your remedy is likely to be among them. You want your Never Well Since rubric to be as inclusive as possible since everything follows from that. For example, the Never Well Since list has "grief or death of a beloved one" with Nat. mur. as the top remedy. But if you look up "grief, ailments from" in the *Repertory,* you will find many others.

Including alternate rubrics and subrubrics: You may find you have two different rubrics for the same symptom (as in the grief example above), or two different unusual food cravings which are about equally outspoken. In this case you can look up both rubrics and give each remedy the higher of the two scores. If your Chief Complaint has many subrubrics, pick the most distinctive ones (for example, by picking rubrics with relatively few remedies listed). The scoring chart allows for three subrubrics, but of course this is flexible, and in any case you are only confirming the remedy and narrowing down your choice by the time you reach the tenth rubric.

Analyzing the results: When you have completed the mental/emotional rubrics and are halfway done, stop and analyze the results. Keep the remedies which appear in all or most columns and eliminate those appearing in only one or two columns. Do not add any new remedies after this point; just continue to score the ones you already have. (Common sense will prevail when there is an exception to this approach. It applies to true chronic diseases and may not apply when the condition comes from a physical trauma, for example, like the young woman who was Never Well Since a blow to the abdomen.)

So in the *first half* of your scoring chart, *your simillimum is probably already included* and in the *second half*, you will be *narrowing down your remedies.*

Adding up the scores: Put the score for each remedy in the last wide column on the chart. First, add up the number of columns it appears in, then a slash, then the cumulative point total.

Deciding on the remedy: Even if one remedy is the clear winner, you should always read about the top two or three remedies in the Materia Medica to see which one best matches the patient. Here are some additional ways to discriminate among the remedies:

- Perhaps the most important is determining which remedy is more effective against the active miasm. Look up the score of your remedy in the chart in the back of Banerjea's *Miasmatic Diagnosis.* For example, if the patient has an active sycotic miasm, and the choice of remedies is between Arsenicum (+++) and Argentum nitricum (+), this is a great argument for Arsenicum, since it guarantees a deeper-acting remedy, removing the substantial sycotic background of the patient.
- A remedy that gets higher point scores in the *first* half of the chart wins over one that gets higher points in the *second* half, because the Never Well Since and mental/emotional symptoms are more important than which one matches the chief complaint the best.
- Use elimination points, e.g. is the patient markedly chilly or hot?
- Use the association of each remedy with one of the Five Elements in TCM: a patient with many Liver symptoms will need a Liver remedy (see Appendix 5 on TCM).

Remember that the top-scoring remedy is not necessarily the right remedy. See the sample cases in Appendix 4 for examples of how the rubrics are chosen and how the scoring chart is used.

Hierarchy of Symptoms: **Symptoms:**

Delusions/Rare-peculiar   1.
Never Well Since   2.
Mental/Emotional   3.
     4.
     5.
Generalities ("I am, I feel")   6.
Food Cravings/Aversions   7.
Sleep and Dreams *(optional)*   8.
Sexual Symptoms *(optional)*   9.
Chief Complaint   10.
   Modalities of CC   a.
     b.
     c.

Remedies	1	2	3	4	5	6	7	8	9	10	a	b	c	Score

Essence of the Case (NWS):
Constitution:
Miasm:
Therapeutic Remedy: Dosage:
Layers:

Figure 9-4: Sample Scoring Chart

Summary: Prescribing for Chronic Diseases

Hahnemann laid the ground rules 200 years ago for the perfect prescription in Aphorisms 5 and 7:

> It will help the physician to bring about a cure if he can find out the data of the most probable *occasion* of an acute disease, and the most significant factors in the entire history of a protracted wasting sickness, enabling him to find out its *fundamental cause*. The fundamental cause of a protracted wasting sickness mostly rests upon a chronic miasm. In these investigations, the physician should take into account the patient's:
> 1. discernible body constitution (especially in cases of protracted disease),
> 2. mental and emotional character,
> 3. occupations,
> 4. lifestyle and habits,
> 5. civic and domestic relationships,
> 6. age,
> 7. sexual function, etc. ...
>
> In cases of disease where there is no obvious occasioning or maintaining cause to be removed, we can perceive nothing but the disease signs. Therefore, it must be the symptoms alone by which the disease demands and can point to the appropriate medicine for its relief, along with regard for any contingent miasm and with attention to the attendant circumstances.

Figure 9-5 shows how homeopathy, more than any other healing modality, covers every possible influence: the patient's constitution, life-style, and different triggering factors, *besides* the totality of the symptoms. Unfortunately many homeopaths today do not take full advantage of our wonderful healing modality: they practice by the totality of symptoms (Aphorism 7) but not the all-important knowledge of miasms, the patient's constitution, and the Never Well Since (Aphorism 5). Without this the homeopath has assessed only half of the information necessary for a diagnosis, a prognosis, an appropriate remedy, and a clear management plan. The information covered in Aphorisms 5 and 7 form a complete case. *Cause and effects (symptoms) must be united in case taking.*

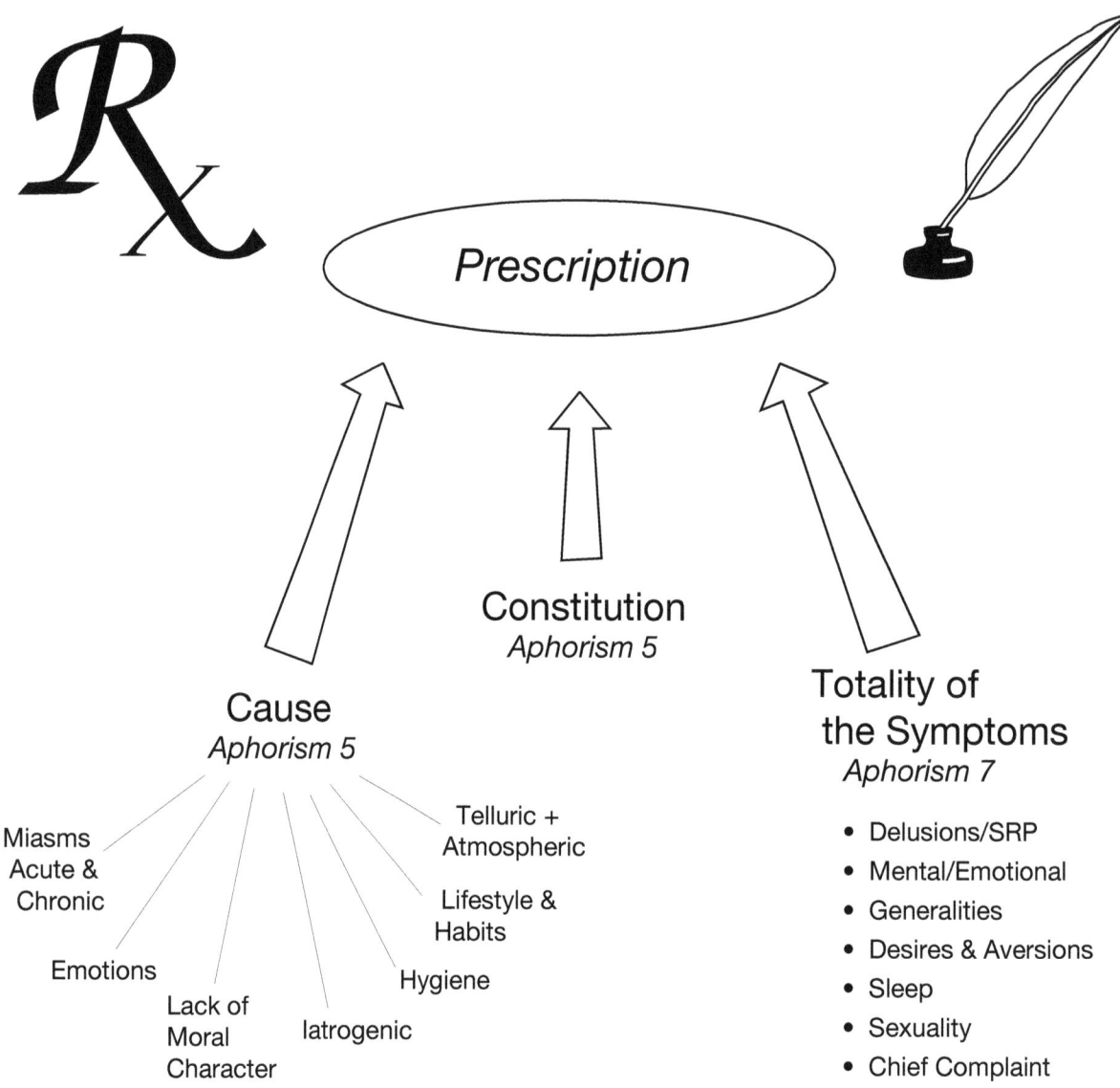

Fig. 9-5: The Perfect Prescription

Prescribing for Acute Disorders

The perfect prescription for acute cases obviously will not necessarily require *all* the elements of Aphorisms 5 and 7. If someone comes for an acute sprained ankle, you need not check his family history, his own past medical history, or his preferences for food or sex. It is also important for homeopaths to realize that patients need to be helped for such acute events. Some homeopaths today do not treat acute illnesses, perhaps believing that it will interrupt the long action of their chronic remedy in a centesimal potency. (I have found this to be another good reason for using LM potencies, because they can be suspended for a few days while the acute condition is treated, then picked up where the patient left off). This attitude towards the patient does not reflect Hahnemann's compassion. If anything, an acute event like a sprained ankle gives us the opportunity to demonstrate how fast homeopathy can work. Some patients will tell you, "Homeopathy is great but it takes time." (Of course they are referring to chronic diseases which *do* take time, especially if suppressed.) But acute disorders are healed in a fraction of the time when remedies are used. We have all used remedies many times with stunning results in traumas, flus, ear infections, etc.

However, if the patient consults you for a *recurrent* sprained ankle, you must recognize this as a chronic condition based on an underlying constitutional weakness or miasmatic condition. In Aphorism 73 of the *Organon* Hahnemann explains for us the different acute disorders:

> An acute febrile disease that befalls a person *individually* is occasioned by malignities to which *just this person* has been particularly exposed. Examples of occasions of acute fevers are excesses in pleasures or their deprivation, violent physical impressions [i.e. physical traumas], becoming chilled, becoming overheated, fatigue, strains from lifting, etc.; or psychical arousals, affects *[emotional traumas],* etc. Fundamentally, however, individual acute fevers are mostly only transient flare-ups of latent psora which spontaneously returns to its dormant state if the acute fevers are not too violent and are soon dispatched.
>
> *Sporadic* acute diseases attack *several* people at the same time, here and there, sporadically, occasioned by meteoric or telluric influences and malignities. Only a few people possess the receptivity to become disease-aroused at the same time.
>
> Bordering sporadic diseases are those acute diseases that seize *many persons* with very similar complaints from a similar cause *(epidemically).* These diseases tend to become contagious when they spread over thickly congregated masses of people ... *[often]* engendered by the calamities of war, floods and famine.
>
> Some acute epidemic diseases are particular acute miasms that recur in the same manner and are therefore known by a traditional name. They either befall a person

only once in a lifetime (such as smallpox, measles, whooping cough, mumps …) [or] recur often in a rather similar way (such as … cholera).

The *first* type of acute diseases are the ones that attack *individually*, brought on by exciting causes such as physical traumas and emotional stress (first part of Aphorism 73). Hahnemann found that in some patients acute disorders did not yield promptly to remedies which seemed indicated and which quickly cured them in others. On examining more closely, he found in these patients the presence of an active miasmatic state. By applying remedies matching the indications of these chronic miasms and acute conditions combined (the antipsorics), he was now successful in these acute cases which were nothing else than acute exacerbations or flare-ups of the chronic miasmatic state.

The *second* type of acute disease attacks are *sporadic,* caused by meteoric (weather) influences like cold dampness, which stimulates the sycotic miasm, or telluric (earth) influences like light, sun, moon, and electromagnetic fields. They affect only a *few* people at a time. They are true acute conditions and should be treated with acute remedies chosen according to location, sensation, modalities, and concomitant symptoms.

The *third* type are the *acute miasms* (infectious illnesses triggered by microorganisms in susceptible individuals) which are self-limiting, tending to form quick crises and ending with death, healing or complication. *Epidemic* prescribing will be covered in the next chapter.

CHAPTER TEN

Golden Rules and Special Forms of Prescribing

Epidemic Prescribing

An epidemic could be considered a mass expression of an acute miasm, affecting a large number of people. Homeopathy is very successful in epidemic prescribing, whether for a known illness such as measles or for an "unknown" one (as it is termed in allopathic medicine when the microbe has not yet been isolated). A classic example of an unknown microbe was the "first" epidemic outbreak of chronic fatigue and immune dysfunction syndrome (CFIDS) in California in 1981. Even when the pathogen is isolated, as in the recent Hantavirus epidemic, modern medicine is helpless to prevent the spread until a vaccine can be developed, which is difficult, costly and not always effective, especially against viruses.

If Hahnemann had done nothing else except treat the great epidemics of his era, he should still be considered one of the greatest healers of all time.* He brought relief to

---

*In his *Lesser Writings,* von Boenninghausen gives us Hahnemann's prescription for the cure of Asiatic cholera. The remedies are still among our top remedies for cholera:

> The chief remedy is Camphor and not one out of hundred patients would have died if Camphor alone would have been used and used immediately at the start; for it is only so useful if used alone and at the beginning of the disease. Therefore everyone must use Camphor at once as soon as any of his family is taken ill with cholera, and must not wait for the help of the physician, which, though it might be good, would yet be too late. If there is not very soon a striking improvement we must not hesitate a moment to at once proceed to the remedy for the second stage, i.e. two or three pellets of refined Copper (Cuprum metallicum). A like good effect will be obtained from white hellebore (Veratrum album in the 4th potency), but the preparation of Copper is far preferable and more effective.[1]

thousands of children stricken by scarlet fever (or in danger of it) with his great remedy Belladonna; he saved Napoleon's army from typhoid fever with the two remedies of that epidemic, Bryonia and Rhus tox.; and he cured the Asiatic cholera that ravaged Europe in 1831 (see footnote on preceding page). Whereas more than 50% of patients treated with allopathic measures died from the cholera, only one out of ten homeopathically treated patients died, and in some instances far less. Note that Hahnemann had already figured out the cholera remedies from accounts he heard from Eastern Europe. By the time this plague hit Germany, Hahnemann could advise his patients what to take preventively, saving thousands of lives. This feat alone should have given him eternal praise, but alas, his jealous colleagues persecuted him even more.

Hahnemann put the ground rules for epidemic prescribing in Aphorisms 100-102:

> In the investigation of the symptom complex of epidemic or sporadic diseases, it makes no difference if something similar has ever appeared before … Each reigning epidemic *[in many regards deviates]* greatly from all former epidemics (which have been falsely labeled with certain names). This is true of all contagious diseases except those that stem from an *invariable* infectious tinder, such as smallpox, measles, etc.
>
> It may well be that the physician does not get a perception of the complete image of the epidemic disease with the first case he encounters since each such collective disease only brings the complex of its symptoms to the light of day with the closer observation of several cases. Meanwhile, the carefully investigating physician can often come so close to the true state, even with the first or second patient, that he becomes alive to the characteristic image of the disease, and then finds a fitting, homeopathically commensurate remedy for it. …
>
> The entire extent of such an epidemic disease and the totality of its symptoms … cannot be perceived in a single patient, but can only be completely abstracted and gathered [inferred] from the sufferings of several patients of different bodily constitutions.

For the classic yearly flu epidemic, allopathic medicine can only make a vaccine from the previously-known virus strains—which of course will not work if the current virus is different or has mutated, as frequently happens. Despite the possibility of side-effects (even of fatalities), vaccination is still encouraged for the weakest members of our society: children, the elderly, and the chronically ill.

For the homeopath, prescribing for a new flu variety is simple. After seeing ten to twenty cases, he records the symptoms common to all of the patients. These are the *cardinal symptoms* of the epidemic, the basis for selecting the remedy. Sometimes he finds that one group of patients have one clear symptom picture, indicating one remedy, and another group needs another remedy; I have never needed more than two remedies for a given flu epidemic. Sometimes there is one main remedy and one or two minor remedies. The main remedy for an epidemic is called the *genus epidemicus*. For example, the Spanish flu of 1918 responded mainly to Baptisia, while the Beijing flu of 1993-94 responded well to Gelsemium first, then Bryonia and Kali bich. These remedies helped my patients overcome this fearsome flu strain in two to three days, while others were in bed for three to four weeks on one futile course of antibiotics after another.

If there are two remedies, it would be easy to create a simple differential diagnosis so that anyone, nurse or parent or public health worker, could tell which to give. For example, if the two remedies are Bryonia and Pulsatilla, the differential diagnosis would be as follows: if the patient has a high fever and is thirsty, give Bryonia; if the patient has a low fever and is thirstless, give Pulsatilla.

Does Oscillococcinum work? This homeopathic remedy is the top-selling flu remedy in France and is now widely available in this country. Some classical homeopaths say that routine prescribing (pathological prescribing) is suppressive. On the other hand I and others have seen it work provided it is given *early* enough. It must be given right at the onset, and it works better for a flu characterized by muscle aches and fever (in other words, a Gelsemium-type flu) rather than a stomach "flu" or flu with head cold. In my own experience it is better for preventing the flu than for treating it. I have also found it effective to use a single pellet dissolved in 4 oz. of water rather than taking the whole tube at once.

As you can see, the homeopath has no fear of a flu epidemic. It provides a great opportunity to prove the effectiveness, the speed and the preventive power of the *single* indicated homeopathic remedy.

Preventive Prescribing

Once you find the *genus epidemicus,* it is easy to act prophylactically, especially for high-risk cases and children. Let's assume one child in a family of four children comes down with a flu corresponding to Gelsemium. Put a 200c Gelsemium pellet in a 4 ounce cup, and as long as the child is ill, each person in the family should take a teaspoonful from the same cup as his daily dose. If the exposure is not so close (for example, someone in the neighborhood or at work has a flu) the remedy can be given once a week in a 200c potency. Cost: one cent a dose, and no side effects! No one else will come down with that particular flu. This method will work even in an outbreak of an unknown virus. Concentrate on the symptoms common to all the victims, look for the simillimum, and give a teaspoonful a day to each possible victim.

The flu and other epidemics are acute miasms which capitalize on the susceptibility produced by the chronic miasms and a weakened Vital Force. The best preventive treatment for an epidemic is the *constitutional* treatment which is best done *away* from the flu season or *before* an epidemic comes to the neighborhood. Give the remedy for the innate constitution in a 10M potency, 3 pellets dry, in a one-time dose. In general we do this for adults only when all their layers have been treated, although we can do it for young children at any time assuming that they have no layers. But even while a patient is still under treatment for a chronic condition, if a flu epidemic is threatening you should not hesitate to give the constitutional remedy with a good chance of strengthening the Vital Force. Someone who is actively responding to his constitutional remedy will be very little affected by the epidemic or will not succumb at all. And someone who has a recurring tendency to catch the flu has a chronic underlying state that must be treated either through constitutional or anti-miasmatic treatment.

Retrospective Prescribing

If you prescribe the indicated remedy for the current clinical picture and it does not work, you may need to go back to the remedy the patient needed at the onset of the illness, even if it does not cover the current symptoms. For example, if a patient comes with a diagnosis of Chronic Fatigue and tells you it all started with a flu or mononucleosis, he may need a remedy such as Gelsemium, Carcinosin or Arsenicum even though he no longer has the original symptoms. Retrospective prescribing is thus a form of prescribing for the Never Well Since. You should always ask the patient the original symptom picture of the illness and then how it evolved over time, whether through treatment or the natural evolution of the disease.

Intra-Uterine Prescribing

Unlike allopathic drugs, which must be given with extreme caution during pregnancy, remedies are ideal treatments for the pregnant woman.

Not only does a woman manifest the remedy she needs most clearly while pregnant, but also her miasmatic condition can be treated, creating a much healthier child. Ideally we would address the miasms of both parents before conception, but few couples come for preconceptional homeopathic treatment.

Carroll Dunham, a famous turn-of-the-century homeopath, described several cases in which women bore children with harelips and cleft palates; one had four such children and another one eight. Dunham went back to his embryology books and found that this abnormality occurs prior to the third month of gestation. He found it was a bone deficiency and surmised it represented a calcium deficiency. The question was whether to give Calc. carb., Calc. phos., or Calc. sulph. The woman with eight such children was very clearly a Sulphur patient, so he tried Calc. sulph., giving it for seven months of her gestation. She bore her next child normally. He repeated this in three other cases while the baby was in utero, and the children were born normal. This type of prescribing opens up possibilities still unknown in allopathic medicine.

If a family has four children and only one was born with a particular problem, we can guess that either at conception or during the pregnancy, one or both parents were in an altered state of physical or emotional health. Either they were ill, took drugs, or more often we find that they went through emotional turmoil which decreased their Vital Force. The mother's emotional state affects the unborn child directly, while the father's emotional state can affect the child by its effect on the mother. If the father is severely depressed, the mother can feel unloved and abandoned, leading to the child at birth needing one of the remedies listed under "forsaken."

For example, if the child has speech problems (delayed or unintelligible speech, typical of children needing Nat. mur.) and has had no griefs or losses in its short life, look for an intra-uterine grief trauma. Always consider the mother's case first. The remedy she needed during the pregnancy usually indicates the remedy now needed by the child. For example, if the mother went through a separation from her husband in the fifth month of pregnancy, this heartbreak situation could call for Nat. mur. The child would then be born a Nat. mur. type, with all the possible symptoms of this remedy: delayed speech or disturbed speech, emotional isolation, anger and over-sensitivity (easily offended).

I remember a case of an 8-year-old boy with a Chief Complaint of incomprehensible speech. Only his mother could understand what he said. The child had undergone three different operations (frenulectomy, tonsillectomy, creation of a pharyngeal flap) to correct his speech and had been in speech therapy for three years, to no avail. But when I asked about possible trauma intra-utero (the inevitable Never Well Since), his mother told me that her husband died suddenly in a car accident when she was six months pregnant. Imagine the shock, the grief, and the sense of sudden abandonment. The mother clearly needed Nat. mur. then and so did the child now. In less than two months on Nat. mur. LM1, the boy was speaking normally. A miracle? No, a proof that the laws of homeopathy work.

I had another patient with two children both diagnosed as autistic. Her husband was a physician and adamantly opposed to her consulting a homeopath, even if I was also a physician. The mother persisted and brought me the more severe case, the younger one, first. Not only did the lack of speech in this two year old child hint at a Nat. mur. etiology, the child's behavior confirmed it (he was thirsty for large gulps of water, he craved salty foods, etc.). I felt

I had to find a grief trauma, but in this little child's life there had been no losses. I inquired about the mother's emotional state while pregnant. She went through an emotionally wrenching divorce, including sitting in divorce court, while pregnant with the child. Amazingly enough, she had had the same experience while pregnant with her first child (i.e. she was now on her third marriage). The second child's "autism" was worse than his four-year-old brother's because the grief of the second divorce was added to the mother's grief state from the first one. I prescribed Nat. mur. LM1 for both mother and child. At the three-week follow-up the mother told me that the two-year-old was already saying a few words for the first time in his life, and even singing little songs with his brother. Unfortunately I never saw them again; the father was the obstruction to the cure!

Prescribing for Birth Trauma

Of course conditions like a "blue baby" are quite obvious. Anytime the baby is born hypoxic, a dose of Carbo veg. will do miracles. Carbo veg. should be given immediately to every baby with a low Apgar score. (The old masters called it the "corpse reviver" and Kent called it one of the "reactive remedies" because it stirred the Vital Force to react.) Chelidonium is an excellent remedy for neonatal jaundice (in a 30c or 200c potency and/or tincture) and will save the baby from the "lightbox" treatment in the hospital—which is probably not physically harmful but extended separation between the mother and newborn can be emotionally damaging for the infant.

Every obstetrician should be trained to give Arnica 200c (or better yet, Bellis perennis 200c) to every woman who has just delivered, to counteract the soft tissue trauma, soreness and tendency to bleed. Arnica can be given to the baby as well to counter the trauma of passing through the birth canal (especially traumatic to the head, with Arnica the top remedy for head traumas of all kinds) and for bruising, e.g. from a shoulder dystocia.

When a schoolchild comes with problems such as lack of concentration and decreased memory, we should never forget to ask about the delivery process. Was it long and strenuous? Were forceps or suction cup needed? Arnica should have been given acutely for such head traumas; chronically, remedies such as Helleborus, Nat. sulph., and Thuja are indicated, while Cicuta stands out if convulsions are present since birth.

As you can see, prescribing for the birth process is two-fold. The homeopath will always prescribe acutely during the delivery, avoiding possible complications for both mother and child. The other aspect is prescribing retrospectively if the patient was not treated homeopathically at the time of delivery.

Lesional Prescribing

As discussed in Chapter 4 on Pathology, lesional prescribing is used when a vital organ is so compromised by an illness (e.g. the kidney in advanced lupus) that it becomes a one-sided pathological manifestation. This imbalance develops serious tissue pathology which represses the symptom totality of the case. This situation usually arises in an advanced miasmatic state or at the end stage of a chronic disease, usually when the patient is weak and the Vital Force is unstable. At this time the symptoms of the local manifestation become the *active layer*, the focal point of the disease.

Usually when we prescribe, we look at the patient's mental and emotional state to understand the ground or terrain which helped to create the Chief Complaint; but in lesional prescribing the whole pyramid of symptoms is turned upside down. All the symptoms, including the mental/emotional ones and even the delusions, are created by the pathology instead of helping to create it. For example, if a patient presents with a few episodes of blurred vision and some mild neuropathies and is shocked to receive a diagnosis of MS, he may become depressed at the prospect of deteriorating function and loss of quality of life. The depression follows the diagnosis, it did not help to create it; if we permanently reverse the symptoms of MS with homeopathy (as my colleagues and I have done many times), the depression will resolve. Or if someone has malignant cancer, their emotional state may become dominated by their (understandable) fears about their illness, possible death, and who will care for family members if they pass away (see Cancer Case 4 in Chapter 24). In other words, the cancer may induce an Arsenicum state in someone who may not have needed Arsenicum at the time of onset. Or if cancer has metastasized to the bones and is causing unbearable pains, the patient may sink into a deep despair and even consider suicide. The pathology has induced an Aurum state and not the other way around. If the pain can be alleviated, the despair and then the suicidal ideation will be resolved as well, so in these cases our priority becomes the local pathology. Fortunately Arsenicum and Aurum will address both the pathology and the mental/emotional state; they are two of our top remedies for advanced cancer, as discussed in Chapter 24.

Remedies chosen by von Boenninghausen's formula become very valuable in lesional prescribing. If the location, sensation, and modalities of the one-sided pathology match with the concomitant general symptoms, a remedy acting directly on the pathology can be chosen without the risk of suppression. If the remedy is successful in stimulating the process of healing in the severely compromised Vital Force, there will be an improvement in the lesion as well as in the general health. The local lesion will gradually recede, leaving a clear symptom picture for the choice of a simillimum for the chronic condition. This is one of the secrets of curing *advanced pathological states*. Often a remedy chosen according to the totality of the chronic condition (as we usually would do) is not the best starting point as the vital organs of function and elimination are too compromised. In this situation we are not using a local treatment first (which could suppress) but rather treating the advanced pathological state in such a way that it moves the case forward without suppressing the symptoms. This situation is one of the exceptions to my preference for polychrests over small remedies.

Zig Zag Prescribing

In cases of incurable disease, the homeopath needs to prescribe on the dominant clinical picture. He will change remedies much more quickly than usual, "putting out fires" as they show up in order to support what is left of the Vital Force by using acute remedies. For example, in treating a patient with AIDS, the practitioner might first address night sweats and fear of death with Arsenicum iodatum, then treat thrush with Borax, then use Bryonia for pneumonia. In terminal cancer, the practitioner might first help the patient breathe with Carbo veg., then take the anxiety away with Arsenicum, then palliate the deep bone pain and depression with Aurum, etc. (see Chapter 16, Palliation and Incurable Diseases). This is basically acute prescribing, except that you never win the battle; you just win a skirmish and then something else inevitably pops up.

Golden Rules of Prescribing

Of course there are no shortcuts or protocols in homeopathic prescribing. But some valuable hints from the old masters will often simplify and shorten your task and make your prescription more successful. I have found many such "Golden Rules" by reading old books and journals; in this chapter are the ones I have found most helpful in my own practice.

Last-appearing symptoms: The *last appearing symptoms* of a case, if outstanding and definite, may not lead us to the simillimum but often they unearth the case and show the way for other remedies. (By last-appearing we mean the last to appear *before* homeopathic treatment was instituted.) New or last-appearing symptoms *after* homeopathic treatment may actually be old symptoms which disappeared years ago and now resurface through the action of your remedy. Never change the remedy as long as your case is following Hering's Laws.

Complementary remedies: A great time-saving rule of Hering's is that the second remedy is likely to *bear a complementary relationship* to the first one. Complementary remedies are listed in the back of the *Repertory* and in many Materia Medicas. (Obviously we are talking about working within the same layer; if one layer is healed and symptoms of a previous layer emerge, caused by an entirely different trauma, the two remedies do not need to be connected. Also in the case of a miasmatic block we move to the nosode, not the complementary remedy.) The last remedy that *acted* is one of the most important guides to the next remedy. (Keep in mind that remedy which is acting should continue to be prescribed, in increasing potencies or successive LM potencies, until it stops acting). The symptoms of the complementary remedy will appear in the patient under the action of the first remedy, and the complementary remedy is needed to complete the picture. (In other words, you do not have to follow this rule on blind faith; the complementary remedy really will be indicated.) If a patient comes to you from another homeopath and tells you that the last remedy that worked for her was Sepia, then you should consider Nat. mur., the complement of Sepia, and see if Nat. mur. symptoms are present in the patient. If Staphysagria acted for a while and then stopped in spite of potency increase, Causticum or Carcinosin will be indicated, both complements of Staphysagria.

After a strong remedy that works well, a *strong complementary remedy* is especially indicated.

Clinical Case: A young person reacts well on Hyoscyamus for quite some time. After some time he develops a rash, itches at night, wants to uncover his feet and he loves sweets. At this point many homeopaths would prescribe Sulphur. However, after one month of Sulphur he has a relapse of his original psychiatric symptoms with a strong fear of being alone in the dark. Sulphur was basically given at the wrong moment leading to an obstruction of the case. In fact, the appearance of a rash after a remedy should never necessitate the need for another remedy since we followed Hering's Law, going from the inside to the outside. If we need another remedy after Hyoscyamus, it has to be another violent, strong remedy such as Stramonium, Belladonna, Veratrum album, or Anacardium. In the above case the body tried to produce the Stramonium picture (the top remedy for fear of the dark and of being alone, K43).

Remedies in series: The prescriber's work is again made easier by looking for symptoms of the next remedy in a series. These series have been compiled from the old masters, and I have used many of them successfully in my practice.

    Aconite-Spongia-Hepar sulph. *(the croup remedies of von Boenninghausen)*
    Allium cepa-Phosphorus-Sulphur
    Arnica-Bellis perennis-Ruta
    Arnica-Rhus tox.-Calcarea
    Arsenicum-Thuja-Tarentula
    Bryonia-Sulphur-Calcarea-Tuberculinum
    Colocynth-Staphysagria-Causticum
    Ferrum phos.-Sulphur-Tuberculinum
    Ignatia-Nat. mur.-Sepia-Sulphur
    Kali bich.-Sulphur-Tuberculinum
    Kali carb.-Sulphur-Kali phos.-Tuberculinum
    Kali iodatum-Lycopodium-Sulphur-Tuberculinum
    Lachesis-Lycopodium.-Sulphur-Tuberculinum
    Nitric acid-Syphilinum-Tuberculinum-Sulphur
    Nux vomica-Sulphur-Lycopodium
    Psorinum-Tuberculinum-Silica
    Psorinum-Tuberculinum-Syphilinum
    Pulsatilla-Kali sulph.-Silica-Tuberculinum
    Pulsatilla-Silica-Fluoric acid
    Sulphur-Calc. sulph-Tuberculinum
    Sulphur-Calcarea-Lycopodium
    Sulphur-Thuja-Tuberculinum.
    Thuja-Medorrhinum-Sulphur

Note: the series of remedies in which Tuberculinum is mentioned are very effective in the treatment of TB cases. And note that Tuberculinum is often the last remedy to be administered in a series.

Antipsoric nosodes: What if the symptom picture definitely and unequivocally points to an antipsoric remedy, which, when prescribed, proves ineffective in the long run? The true simillimum must be among the antipsoric nosodes. Surprisingly, Psorinum is not the most powerful antipsoric nosode. In order of importance and usefulness, the old masters recommended Tuberculinum or Bacillinum, then the bowel nosode (see Chapter 18), then finally Psorinum or Streptococcin.

Acute and chronic remedies: The rule of thumb here is: *Know the acute remedy and you will know the chronic.* For instance, if the patient keeps on having acute events like sore throats and colds responding to Aconite, you can deduct that this patient needs Sulphur, Aconite's chronic, to stop the recurrence of colds and dramatically improve the patient's health. And in case you were looking for the chronic simillimum all along, now you know it!

Here are some examples of acute and chronic remedies:

Acute	**Chronic**
Aconite	Sulphur
Allium cepa	Phosphorus
Apis	Nat. mur.
Arsenicum	Thuja
Bacillinum	Calc. phos.
Belladonna	Calcarea
Bryonia	Phosphorus, Alum. and Nat. mur.
Chamomilla	Mag. carb., Sanicula
Colocynthis	Thuja, Staphysagria, Kali carb. and Lycopodium
Hepar sulph.	Silica
Ignatia	Nat. mur.
Kali bich.	Thuja
Nux vomica	Sepia, Sulphur
Pulsatilla	Silica, Calcarea, Medorrhinum, Thuja
Rhus tox.	Calcarea
Stramonium	Calcarea

Why Nux vomica and Sepia? Nux vomica is concerned with business, with tremendous irritability and has similar symptoms to Sepia (chilly, irritable, constipated, etc.). In an acute situation of business failure, the Sepia person is apt to need Nux vomica acutely.

Note that some chronics have more than one acute and vice versa, because each applies to a specific situation: e.g., Allium cepa is the acute of Phosphorus in an allergy/hypersensitivity situation while Bryonia is the acute in a cough or bronchitis situation; Ignatia is the acute of

Nat. mur. in a grief situation, while Apis is the acute in a water-retention situation and Bryonia for headaches from bright sun.

Another rule of thumb: If you know the *chronic* remedy of the patient, you have a good clue to her *acute* remedy when needed (using the same diagram above). For example, Calcarea is likely to need Belladonna for ear infections and Rhus tox. for sprained ligaments and lower back pain, all of which are conditions that Calcarea constitutions are susceptible to.

Old suppressed symptoms: Kent directed us towards another valuable class of symptoms: *old symptoms which disappeared long ago,* especially from suppression. As an example Kent mentions the case of a man who had long suffered from neuritis of the limbs, whose present symptoms did not point decisively to any of four competing remedies. But Kent discovered that in infancy he had suffered from eczema capitis, similar to the picture of Mezereum, one of the competing remedies, and on examination of the pains in the limbs it was found that they closely resembled the pains of Mezereum. This remedy proved to be curative and reproduced the original eruption.

Mute cases: A *"mute"* case (also called one with a *paucity of symptoms*) is one in which the patient has few symptoms yet feels sick all over. Why are there few symptoms? When the Vital Force is weak it may fail to throw symptoms to the surface. Very sick patients, even dying ones, often have a lack of symptoms. We have different ways to resolve mute cases.

- The prescription will probably be only a *simile* at best (because we don't have enough information to find the simillimum), but it will stimulate the Vital Force to manifest additional symptoms, leading to the correct prescription. Although the patient may feel he is getting worse because more symptoms are coming up, in reality the case is opening up and becoming more clear, and the Vital Force is becoming stronger.
- A second possibility is to use one of the *reactive* remedies of which Kent gives us 84 (K1397, "Reaction, lack of"), with 16 in bold type, including Calcarea, Carbo veg., Gelsemium, Medorrhinum, Phosphoric acid, Psorinum, Sulphur, Tarentula, and Thuja. One of the strongest reactive remedies, although not mentioned in Kent, is X-ray. These remedies will strengthen the overpowered Vital Force and restore the patient mentally and physically. Give the one which most closely matches the case.
- Another possibility is to use a remedy to *clear a lot of "debris"* (i.e. side effects from allopathic drugs), making the clinical picture more obvious so that it will be easier to make the correct prescription. The most frequently-used "clear the field" remedies are Sulphur, Nux vomica, and Thuja.
- Use the *nosode* for the active miasm (see Chapters 17).
- Give the constitutional remedy to strengthen the Vital Force, which will throw up symptoms pointing to the simillimum (see the third case on p. 212).

- For a small child, consider the symptoms or remedies of the patient's *parents*. The most common path of inheritance is from the mother to the son and from the father to the daughter. So for a boy, look at the medical history of the mother; and for a girl, at that of the father.
- Important strong symptoms which occurred *during childhood* can be useful in resolving these mute cases (even if the patient is now an adult or even elderly).
- A paucity of symptoms can be a *symptom of the remedy* in itself, if the patient is withholding information for a particular reason: the patient needing Nat. mur. is afraid to get hurt, the Sepia patient is too exhausted to talk, the Lachesis patient (although more likely to be loquacious) can be too suspicious to talk, and the Ignatia patient has a secretive instinct.
- There can be paucity of symptoms because there is *paralysis of the mind*: typical for Conium (due to sexual abstinence), Causticum (due to repetitive grief), and Helleborus (due to brain infarcts). These patients have a gradual decline in their thought process, therefore they cannot relay enough information. Long-time illness can also lead to exhaustion, indifference and forgetfulness (Phosphoric acid). In these cases we must rely on family members.
- If the case is not urgent and seems to be evolving, you can give Sac. lac. and wait until more symptoms develop. This is certainly preferable to hasty prescribing, especially if none of the above options are available. But if the patient is gravely ill with few symptoms because of an exhausted Vital Force, zig zag prescribing will be necessary to palliate and possibly cure the patient.

A perfect example of a mute case, and one which we encounter fairly often, occurs when a woman presents for infertility but a complete medical workup has shown that the woman and her partner are physiologically fully capable of having a baby. Sometimes a woman comes to us in such a situation because she wants to avoid having expensive and painful fertility treatments, but in other instances she has already been through several rounds of treatment, to no avail. If the woman tells us that she really wants to have a baby and seems emotionally as well as physically healthy, what do we prescribe on? We have no Never Well Since or any other rubrics.

One approach would be to use Thuja as a reactive remedy if the infertility is related to the sycotic miasm, as it often is (the sequelae of suppressed gonorrhea or PID). If the medical workup has shown that there are no physiological obstacles like blocked tubes, another option is to see if blockage is on the mental/emotional level. I trust the patient's own innate wisdom and ask, "If your body were trying to give you a message in this situation, what do you think it would be?" Invariably she has been able to go right to the crux of the matter.

Clinical Cases: In one infertility case, the woman had recently immigrated from Russia and had suffered terrible deprivations as a child. Her husband had started a new business in the US and like a good Sulphur had all the facts and figures at his fingertips about the cash flow and income/expense projections, but it turned out that the wife had a deep-rooted, almost delusional fear of poverty, a fear that they would not be able to provide for the child. The fear pointed to Arsenicum, but I chose to give her Phosphorus, her constitutional remedy, which also has a lot of fears and would strengthen her constitution as well as avoiding aggravations. She had had three miscarriages within the previous two years, but her next attempt at pregnancy was successful.

In another case, the patient realized that she had an unconscious fear that her life would be taken over by the baby and she wouldn't have any time left for herself. (Any parents of a newborn would say that this fear is not entirely delusional!) It turned out that as the oldest child she had been forced to take over her mother's role in caring for her four younger siblings when her mother had to be hospitalized due to mental illness. Sepia was the obvious choice for a woman who feels that her life is dominated by her family's demands to the point that she is desperate for time and space to herself. It also helped to restore her FSH and estradiol levels, which had been out of balance since she had begun fertility workups two years earlier. After only three weeks on Sepia the nurse at her fertility clinic called in a state of total surprise to say that her hormones had suddenly come into balance for the first time.

Another situation in which we sometimes encounter a mute case occurs when a patient has been given a diagnosis based on a lab test but is totally asymptomatic.

Clinical Case: A 59-year-old man consulted me for Waldenstrom's macroglobulinemia, which had been detected upon routine blood work. He was healthy and energetic, played tennis for an hour nearly every day, ate mostly grains and vegetables prepared by his wife, and had no symptoms whatsover. He was alarmed, however, when he went on the Internet and found that his disease carried a prognosis of a maximum of five years to live. There was no Never Well Since in the case; when I asked what was going on in his life in the few months before the blood work, he said that he had taken early retirement from the company where he had worked for 20 years. But he said that he had been looking forward to retirement from his sales job, which had required extensive traveling. With absolutely nothing to prescribe on (remember that we do not prescribe on blood tests) I had no choice but to give him his constitutional remedy. There was no doubt he was a Sulphur; his testy attitude, his red, patchy skin, and his attempt to bargain me down on my fee gave him away. (He shouldn't have to pay full price, he argued, because he wasn't really sick.) The remedy kicked out two key symptoms of the simillimum. First, he had a very significant dream of losing his temper at the management at his old job. In telling me the dream, he admitted with embarrassment that he had not taken early retirement, he had been fired. It was not his fault; his company had been taken over by a larger company, which was downsizing. But for a Sulphur to lose his means of supporting his family was too much of a blow to his pride, so he had kept it a secret from everyone but his wife. Causticum covered his sense of injustice and also his new sense that his legs were going out from under him ("unsteady walking and easily falling," Boericke). Causticum helped resolve his injured pride and his unsteady gait, although he never had another blood test. He refused to go back to the doctor because he was so angry at the doctor's enthusiasm for his rare disease rather than concern for his emotional state.

Food cravings and aversions: Desires and aversions to certain foods must be strongly marked to be usable at all; even then, aversions are much more valuable than desires, which are not very useful except in pregnancy. A new craving or aversion during pregnancy indicates the miasmatic state brought from the father to the mother by the child. (For example, if a pregnant woman suddenly starts craving oranges, a keynote of Medorrhinum, it may indicate that she has picked up the active sycotic miasm from her husband. Often after delivery she is likely to show this sycotic miasm herself, e.g. with recurring vaginitis.) In today's world, it is hard to find anyone who does not desire chips, sweets, or fatty foods at some point. If you ask children nowadays, they all desire pizza, hamburgers, French fries and sweets. These are useless for selecting the remedy. If a child craves nothing but bacon, this can point you to a remedy (Tuberculinum). An aversion to fatty foods or milk is also helpful because it is unusual.

There is a difference between desire and cravings: the craving is much more intense. The patient has to have the food every day and will go to any extreme to get it (for example, getting up in the middle of the night and driving to a convenience store for a chocolate bar). Often you can tell by the intensity of their answer or the way their eyes are twinkling when you mention the food. "Chocolate? I *adore* it."

Don't be fooled by patients who say, "I don't crave sweets [chocolate, chips, etc.]." Ask them if they ever eat the food and they often say, "Sure, every day." It is hard to build up a craving for something when you indulge in it every day. Likewise, when the patient has been on a special diet, restricting or increasing certain foods, ask about their habits *before* they changed their diet. People have such strongly ingrained beliefs about food in our society that it can be hard to find their natural instincts. Ask a question like, "If you didn't have to think about fat or calories or anything else, what food would taste best to you?"

Breastfeeding infants: As for the treatment of babies, if the mother is well and the baby is ill, the remedy can be given directly to the baby, dissolved in water and dabbed on the baby's lips. If the mother is ill and the baby is not, the mother should take the remedy after her last breastfeeding at night, in order to allow as many hours as possible before the baby breastfeeds again. If the mother and baby both need the same remedy, common sense must prevail: keep in mind that the baby could aggravate from multiple doses of the remedy (in a *chronic* situation; however, if they both happen to need the same *acute* remedy, the baby can handle multiple doses). On the other hand, the baby may need more doses of the remedy than the mother, if the baby is a *hyposensitive* Calcarea constitution and the mother is an extremely *hypersensitive* Phosphorus. In such cases the multiple doses which the baby receives when breastfeeding should be a bonus rather than causing a problem. Again, it also depends on the remedy needed: if the mother happened to break a limb and need Calc. phos. to mend the bone, this would benefit the baby in building its bones and no harm would be done from multiple doses.

As a practical consideration, if you are giving a nursing mother Sepia for postpartum blues, indifference, and extreme exhaustion (as frequently happens) and if she breastfeeds six times a day, the baby could get six doses of Sepia a day. The baby would then aggravate on Sepia and be awake all night, which leads to a vicious cycle: the mother gets even more exhausted and needs more Sepia. I usually resolve this dilemma by telling the mother to take a very small daily dose and potency of the remedy (6c or LM with 2 succussions) after the last breastfeeding at night. The next breastfeeding is often towards morning, leaving the mother time to use up the remedy before the next feeding. (Most likely though, a mother in a Sepia state will not even want to breastfeed until she has received enough Sepia.)

Neonatal problems: Allopathic drugs and hormones given during pregnancy frequently result in skin symptoms (eczema, diaper rash) in the baby. These can often be treated by Sulphur. Another frequent complication of allopathic drug intake is colic in babies. Legally mandatory, silver nitrate (Argentum nitricum) drops are instilled in every baby's eyes at birth to avoid ophthalmia neonatorum (gonorrheal infection possibly leading to blindness). Following the Law, "Like Cures Like" homeopathic Argentum nitricum is the top remedy for colicky babies.

Life stages: There are certain periods in life when the most significant symptoms emerge: *infancy, childhood, puberty, pregnancy, menopause,* and in the sequelae of *incompletely cured acute diseases.* When taking a case, pay attention to symptoms occurring during these periods.

Resolving contradictions: When there are many contradictions in the case (this does not mean a paucity of symptoms; there might even be too *many* symptoms), give Sac. lac. and have the patient return again two weeks later to see which symptoms prevail. Take the case again to find the *consistent* symptoms that run throughout. Waiting pays off in this case. These symptoms are the ones to prescribe on.

Symptoms occurring during acute illnesses: When an acute disease appears in a patient under chronic treatment, pay attention to the *chronic symptoms that persist* during this acute illness. They are the most important ones and should be prescribed on. Not only will they resolve the acute case but also the chronic one. If so, this is because so far you have not discovered the simillimum, only the simile. So if a chronic condition has the symptoms A, B, C, D, and E, and the symptoms B and E persist during the acute phase, then B and E are the most important symptoms to base our prescription on to resolve both the acute and chronic case.

Mental disturbances: Remember that a strong physical problem can *hide* a mental disturbance. If you treat someone for MS and the indicated remedy (e.g. Conium) does not work, then try looking for a mental/emotional disturbance underneath. If you place the Never Well Since and mental/emotional factors ahead of the chief complaint, however, you should not fall into this trap in the first place.

Start with a polychrest: What is a polychrest? It is a remedy whose essence (the mental, emotional and physical picture) is very well known. A "small remedy," on the other hand, fits only a small part of a clinical condition, usually a few physical symptoms rather than mental/emotional ones. In my own experience, if we use LM potencies and address the active miasm we can resolve the great majority of our cases with a polychrest. If there are a few superficial symptoms remaining after the polychrest has done its deep and powerful work, then we can use a small remedy targeted to these specific symptoms to clear up the rest of the picture. I have no objection to searching for a smaller remedy *if* the well-indicated polychrests fail. But I have seen too many conferences where the presenter tries to impress the participants with a small remedy which matches the case in only a few specific symptoms, often just one unusual symptom. I feel that this type of teaching is not helpful. It fails to teach universal methods which the participants could start using the very next day for all their cases. It discourages the participants, who feel that they will never be able to master Materia Medica. It highlights a remedy which the participants may never meet again in the course of their practice, and in their misguided enthusiasm they may overprescribe the remedy, to the detriment of the patient. In allopathic medicine we say, "Don't look for a zebra in the middle of New York." You are more likely to find a dog or a cat. The same reasoning goes for small remedies.

Using polychrests is effective when using LM potencies, and conversely centesimal prescribers may feel the need to match the symptom picture with great exactitude using a small remedy. Having used both centesimals and LMs extensively, my experience has been that they are qualitatively different. Centesimals are like a tall tree which has been pruned of all its side branches so that it looks like a telephone pole; you would have to stand right next to it to receive any shade from it. LMs are like great old oak trees which can shelter multitudes under their spreading branches. Or, to switch metaphors in midstream, if we think of the simillimum as the remedy which hits the bull's-eye, then centesimals are like shots from a BB gun and LMs are like a blast from a water cannon which knocks over the whole target as long as it gets anywhere close. In other words, LMs are highly effective as long as they have a general resemblance to the overall picture. I hear presenters in case conferences justify their search for small remedies by saying that the obvious polychrests did not work; but they used the polychrests in centesimal potencies, not in LMs. (Occasionally I do hear a presenter mention an LM potency, but never administered following Hahnemann's method outlined in this book.) I hear objections to using LMs from my fellow practitioners on the basis that LMs are unwieldy or take too long to master. In my experience the short time invested in learning how to use LMs is more than recouped by the time saved in prescribing and managing the followup.

Small remedies are more likely to cover only part of the symptoms, like the allopathic prescribing condemned by Hahnemann in a footnote to Aphorism 7:

> From time immemorial, adherents of the old school have used medicines in an attempt to combat and, whenever possible, to suppress *a single one* of the various symptoms of a disease. This *one-sidedness,* called *symptomatic treatment,* has rightly aroused much general contempt because through it, not only is nothing won but much also is spoiled. A single symptom of disease is no more the disease itself than a single foot is the man himself.

Based on my own clinical experience, I would advise *in 99% of cases starting with a polychrest*. A polychrest has the capacity to resolve most or all of the clinical picture, and if a few superficial symptoms are left after sufficiently long treatment with the polychrest, only then should we look for a small remedy to cover them. For instance, in my early days as a homeopath I might have opened with Sabina for a patient with uterine bleeding with big clots like pieces of liver. After failure on Sabina, a closer look at the patient would typically show the picture of Calcarea. Now I open with Calcarea to boost the patient's Vital Force. Most of the time it takes care of the Chief Complaint and several other symptoms which the patient "forgot" to mention, plus giving the patient more energy, a sense of well-being, etc. If Calcarea has completed its work and the patient still has occasional acute incidents of uterine bleeding, this would be the appropriate time to give a small remedy like Sabina. Dr. Pierre Schmidt and Dr. Jost Künzli from Switzerland, two great homeopaths, both said that unusual remedies never produce lasting constitutional cures. They may produce initial improvements which do not last or are not complete; or if the symptoms return, these remedies will not act again. When the well-indicated deep acting polychrest is given, it will work each time symptoms arise, gradually clearing all of them and increasing the resistance of the person in general.

Starting with a small remedy: There are exceptions to this rule, of course, such as the following scenarios:

- In *one-sided cases* as we discussed before: a small remedy fitting the advanced one-sided disease (e.g., advanced cancer) is necessary to increase the Vital Force first before administering a deep-working remedy. In deep-seated diseases such as TB with open cavernas, deep acting remedies such as Phosphorus and Silica would only hasten the patient to his death. Smaller lesional remedies such as Sanguinaria are required in order to boost the Vital Force.
- If the small remedy fits a *delusion or a peculiar symptom*. For example, Sabadilla has the delusion "body, erroneous ideas as to the state of his" (K22). Again, following the hierarchy of symptoms will lead to this choice by itself. Also, the remedy must be confirmed: Thuja has so many delusions about his body that it might be just a variation on a Thuja delusion. You would need other Sabadilla symptoms like a Sabadilla-type of hayfever to give Sabadilla, while in a case with a strong sycotic component this delusion would only serve to confirm Thuja.
- If the patient is basically healthy (mentally, emotionally and physically), with an intact Vital Force, but suffers from a *localized complaint* and no polychrest fits but a small remedy does. For example, right-sided carpal tunnel syndrome with a craving for sour, green apples will lead to Guaiacum.
- If *one symptom dominates* everything else (often in acute cases) to the point of threatening the patient's life, then you can provide symptomatic relief with a small remedy, as long as you follow up with the appropriate deep-working polychrest. For example, a patient may need Sambucus for his asthma attack which makes him wake up from sleep and jump out of bed between 1 and 3 a.m.. This will be followed by a deep antisycotic remedy in between attacks to prevent recurrence and provide total cure.

Prescribe by symptoms, not symbolism: Sometimes remedies are prescribed based on *symbolism* rather than on their proving symptoms, e.g. Lac leoninum, Lac dolphinum, Monkey's blood, or Salmon eggs. I even read one published case in which a prescriber chose Lac leoninum (lion's milk) because a cat came to her door while she was puzzling over the case. Not only that, she could not find the remedy in an alphabetical list and so she chose the one ahead of it in alphabetical order! Perhaps she may claim that this second remedy cured the case, but surely there must have been a more scientific method to find it. And at a time when we are trying to legitimize homeopathy in the eyes of the scientific community, I shudder to think what the average allopath would think of this prescription. In Aphorism 6 Hahnemann warned against "supersensible speculations which are not borne out in experience."

Polarity of the remedies: When remedies have a *very* typical modality, even the point of it being a keynote, they can sometimes have the *exact opposite* quality, even to the third degree (black type). For example, Lachesis has slow speech as well as hasty speech, Sulphur can have tidiness as well as its famous untidiness, and Nat. mur. can both aggravate and ameliorate at the seashore. So finding the exact opposite of a remedy keynote, *strongly expressed,* can also confirm the remedy.

Common modalities: Common symptoms can often be individualized by taking all the modalities and finding the remedy that runs through them. For instance, if there is a general aggravation from milk, fruit, fats, and acids, Sepia runs through all of these. Or in the case of a desire for oranges, sour unripe fruit, as well as salt, think Medorrhinum. Cravings for ice water, sour drinks, juicy fruits and salt will indicate Veratrum album.

Chilliness: The rubrics in the section *Chill* in Kent's repertory (K1259-1277) refer to chill *during fevers,* the single exception being the main rubric *chilliness* which refers to the patient who generally feels cold (as does the rubric "Generalities, heat, vital, want of").

Simile: After a simile prescription, the Vital Force often produces one or more *new* symptoms showing the true simillimum. Prescribe on the old picture *plus* the new symptoms.

Impatience of the patient: The patient often becomes impatient with his care because he is in the habit of focusing on the Chief Complaint. The Chief Complaint might only disappear after the mental/emotional symptoms have been resolved. What to do? Try to keep the patient preoccupied with measures that will not block the Vital Force while the correct remedy continues to work. Give Sac. lac., change the diet a little, maybe add an innocent nutritional supplement.

Skin problems: In order to avoid severe aggravations, use low potencies in skin disorders (6c, LM). The low potencies will be sufficient because the lesion is located on the most superficial area of the body and only needs a little push to be removed. On the other hand, a delusion, the deepest aberration on the mental plane, needs a bigger push: use a high potency (200c, 1M) or LM.

Isopathic Never Well Since: If there is a clear Never Well Since Penicillin in the case, we might resort as a last choice to Penicillin 6c. (I had such a case where nothing helped in which a woman lost all her hair after six months of Penicillin. Thuja and Nux vomica did not help. Penicillin 6c for a month did.)

Alternating remedies: Alternation of remedies is based on the argument that each *remedy* has its own specific sphere and manner of action upon a particular organ or tissue; and likewise each *disease* acts on a certain organ, leaving the rest of the body unaffected. By this line of reasoning, according to these prescribers, chronic heart deficiency and chronic rheumatoid arthritis can occur *simultaneously* and *independently* in the same patient, needing two different remedies which could be given in alternation. Practitioners of this method even state that each remedy will go to its designated place like members of a well-trained platoon.

But how does this argument hold up in view of our Laws and Principles?

First, we would never prescribe for the pathology (name of the disease), only for the patient with the disease. Second, the combination of the two remedies has never been proven as such, certainly never proven to create the two different independent diseases at once. Third, Hahnemann never recommended basing our choice of remedy on only a *part* of the patient's condition, e.g. first treat the heart disease and then if this is restored, treat the rheumatoid arthritis. He always insists on "the totality of the symptoms," which would include both conditions. One has only to study Traditional Chinese Medicine (see Appendix 5) to realize the interaction between the different organs, to the extent that a disease cannot affect one organ without affecting the whole person. We can honestly conclude that two or more remedies cannot act together on the Vital Force without so modifying each other that neither shall produce the effect it would if it were acting alone.

Some homeopaths might claim that Hahnemann approved of alternation. And indeed (in Aphorism 145 of the First Edition) he approved of it in some cases of old chronic diseases which have certain fixed symptoms. His main reason then was that at that time he did not have enough remedies to find the simillimum in all of his cases. But later (Aphorism 272, 5th Edition), he admonishes us that "in no case, is it a requisite to administer more than one single, simple medicine at one time." And in von Boenninghausen's *Lesser Writings* we find:

> Hahnemann never prescribed two different remedies, to be used in alternation one after the other, he always wanted to see first the effect of the one remedy, before he gave another, and this even with patients whom he treated at a distance of two or three hundred miles.[2]

Many of us may have alternated remedies in the beginning of our career, based on inexperience. But with broader knowledge, we should do this less in spite of some "successes" from alternation. There is now a worrisome trend among some homeopaths to advocate prescribing as many as five remedies at one time, believing that "this is the minimum dose that the patient needs." This "eclectic homeopathy" is becoming very popular because it seems easier than classical homeopathy, based on Hahnemann's laws and principles.

Suppression: Once the symptoms, through suppression or in the natural course of the disease, enter the deeper planes (emotional, mental), many of the physical symptoms will disappear. For example, in a Nitric acid case, as the pathology progresses, physical expressions such as cravings for fats and salty fish, offensive sweat and urine, cracks, fissures and ulcers on the skin might disappear, only to be replaced by a pessimistic outlook about health (the patient basically gives up on life), fears about death, etc. Physical symptoms disappear in proportion to the increase of mental/emotional factors. Keep in mind that giving Nitric acid will bring back the physical symptoms as part of the healing process.

CHAPTER ELEVEN

Delusions

What Precisely Are Delusions?

Since I placed delusions at the top of the hierarchy in the previous chapter on Prescribing, I feel compelled to explain some of the "mysterious" delusions in the *Repertory*. When I saw this section in the *Repertory* as a student I thought, "I probably won't be using these rubrics unless I practice on a psychiatric ward. Otherwise I don't think many people with delusions are going to walk into my office." But nothing is further from the truth. We can expand on the meaning of these rubrics, as Rajan Sankaran explains in *The Spirit of Homeopathy,* and find that they apply to many patients. If you take the delusion rubrics too literally, you will miss many opportunities for your perfect prescription. In fact your first thought should be, "Do I see any delusions [in the expanded meaning] in this patient?"

However, we must be more careful than Sankaran in how we expand these rubrics, since we give delusions top priority in our hierarchy of rubrics (unlike Sankaran, who does not prioritize his rubrics). Sankaran says a delusion can simply be a more intensely expressed version of a feeling found in the rest of the Mind section: to use his example, "Mind, unfortunate, feels" (K91) and "Delusions, unfortunate, that he is" (K34) list the same remedies. But if the remedies were different, we would have to be certain that the patient is actually experiencing a warp in her sense of reality in order to put the delusion at the top of the hierarchy. *Webster's* defines a delusion as "a misleading of the mind, a false belief or opinion, a false persistent belief not substantiated by sensory evidence," and we must be sure this kind of skew in perception is present to give this rubric top priority.

For example, if a patient says, "I feel like I am alone in the world," is it a delusion? Not if she is an elderly widow whose friends have all passed away and whose children visit rarely. But what if one of her children is a patient of ours who begs us to see his mother because, he says, no matter how many times her children call and visit it is never enough to reassure her? If she is surrounded by family and friends who care and check on her regularly, we could use

"Delusions, feels forsaken" or "Delusions, alone, that she is always" (K20), "that she is alone in the world, in a wilderness" (K20), "deserted, forsaken" (K23), "that he is friendless" (K26), etc.

When a patient expresses what sounds like a delusion, we must check his sense of reality very carefully. For example, I had a patient who told me his "Never Well Since" was that the Mafia was after him; he could hardly walk down the street without looking behind him to see if he was being followed. While this may sound like a classic paranoid delusion, in his case it was true. I was able to determine this partly by the calm, factual and detailed manner in which he told me; by the fact that he did not seem to have any other delusions; and by the plausibility of his story. He was in the restaurant business and his partner became involved with the Mafia, unbeknownst to him. His partner cheated on the Mafia and a price was put on both partners' heads. For four years my patient lived with tremendous fear and even went to prison since he did not dare testify against the mob as the government requested. I did not repertorize his expression as a delusion, but I certainly did use his fear of death to prescribe Aconite, which cured him.

Like Sankaran, we can use "delusion" to mean a feeling which becomes dominant, exaggerated and fixed, as long as we do not necessarily place it at the top of the hierarchy. When we see the patient in front of us, it is helpful to ask ourselves, "What is the essence of what is going on for this person? What is driving this person? What is her central passion in life? *Why* is she saying this?" and look for the answer among the delusion rubrics. If we expand the meaning of the delusion rubrics in this way, we will use the section on delusions almost every day.

We may even understand ourselves better by looking for our own "core delusion." Who has not felt, "Everyone in this world is against me," or "No one cares about me," or "I think they are always talking behind my back!" Unless you live in isolation, meditating as a monk in Tibet, you have experienced betrayal, grief, disappointment, frights, and monetary loss. If you have a strong Vital Force, you will experience these events as "feelings" which eventually subside. But if you have a weak Vital Force, they can become stuck and turn into "delusions," profoundly affecting your behavior and perception.

Basically I see several uses for the delusion section. If the patient has a true delusion, in the sense of a warped perception of reality which affects her behavior, then we can place it at the top of our hierarchy, and I will explain in this section how to find the delusion more easily by expanding the meaning of the rubrics in the delusion section. If a patient has a perception which can be found in the delusion section but not in the rest of the Mind section, we can use the delusion rubric and prioritize it depending on how skewed the patient's sense of reality is. If the patient's emotional expression is found both in the Delusion section and the Mind section, perhaps the delusion rubric has fewer remedies and can help us narrow our choice. (For example, "Fear, observed, of her condition being" (K46) has three remedies, while only Calcarea appears under the corresponding delusion, which is so typical of the self-conscious Calcarea: "confusion, imagines others will observe her," K22). Finally, by reading the delusion section we can look for patterns of the remedies and learn more about our Materia Medica.

Learning Materia Medica

As an exercise in learning Materia Medica, I suggested to my students that they read through the delusion section and do a differential diagnosis on the remedies listed for each rubric, or try to explain why a particular remedy is the only one listed for a delusion. For example, why does Sepia have the delusion "alone in the graveyard" (K20)? It could be because she is so exhausted that she feels dead—or because she wants so desperately to get away from everyone that she would rather be in such a solitary place!

Why do Bryonia and Phosphorus share the delusion "fancies he is doing business" (K22)? We can understand Bryonia, with his well-known preoccupation with thoughts of business even in acute ailments, and his fear of poverty ("delusions, unfortunate, that he is," K34). But why Phosphorus? I have seen this in a Phosphorus patient whose husband was wealthy, and to amuse herself she ran a little craft shop with beautiful beads and baskets where she could entertain herself all day talking to her employees and customers (mostly other Phosphoruses!) In her case the delusion was that the business was so busy that she needed four employees, and so important that she always had to carry baskets of beads around with her to impress people with how hard she was working!

I also suggested to my students that they look through the delusion section for all the rubrics for a particular remedy: they may form a pattern which indicates the central core of the mental-emotional portrait of the remedy. Here are several of the remedies we see in recurring patterns in the delusion section, with their expanded meanings.

Argentum nitricum: Argentum nitricum is well-known as the worry wart of the Materia Medica, the "What if?" remedy, always thinking of everything that could possibly go wrong. This is reflected in the many delusions of Argentum nitricum, including "appreciated, that she is not" (K21), "neglected, that he is" (K30), "repudiated by relatives, thinks is" (K31), "right, does nothing" (K31), "succeed, that he cannot, does everything wrong" (K33), "despised, that she is" (K23), and "fail, everything will" (K25). Some of Argentum nitricum's delusions are paired with corresponding "fear" rubrics: "delusions, corners of houses seem to project so that he fears he will run against them while walking in the street" (K23) with "fear, corners, to walk past certain" (K43); "delusions, houses on each side would approach and crush him" (K27), "falling, walls" (K25); "room, that the walls will crush him" (K31) with "fear, fall upon him, high walls and buildings" (K45). Argentum nitricum is a frequently-used remedy for people who refuse even to leave home because they have agoraphobia or any other phobia. And they have a great excuse for not leaving home: they get diarrhea. They always think of the worst possible things that can happen, but the fears that rule their lives are mainly unsubstantiated. Imagining all these bad things that can happen to them while walking on the streets, they feel compelled to start walking faster and faster: "delusions, die, thought he was about to, while walking thinks he will have a fit or die, which makes him walk faster" (K24).

Further, Argentum nitricum has the delusion "place, he cannot pass a certain" (K30) with the corresponding fear, "corners, to walk past certain" (K43). These would be good rubrics for superstitious people. In their expanded meaning, they show how Argentum nitricum holds himself back from doing anything, out of worry, apprehension, or fear of making a mistake. "I am willing to go only this far in these plans [or this relationship], because 'what if' something happens?" These rubrics can also reflect worry about deadlines and obligations that have to be met. Argentum nitricum patients are sensitive, cautious people, who have had bad experiences and are now unable to take any risks: they are frozen in the phobia state (even confined to one room of their house).

Arsenicum: Every practitioner has at least one Arsenicum patient: the one who is convinced he has an incurable disease but the doctors have not found it yet, so he goes from doctor to doctor, carrying his six-inch-thick medical record and suitcase full of pills. And if he doesn't have this fatal disease yet, he is sure he is about to get it: "delusions, injury, is about to receive" (K28). If the physician does not order a whole series of lab tests and spend at least two hours in consultation with him, he is convinced that the physician is not interested in curing him and then he can have the delusion "murdered, conspiring to murder him, are" (K29). This rubric can also refer to a business person who thinks that the man next door set up business to "kill him."

If you want to find 101 ways to contract a disease, then the Arsenicum patient is your walking reference library. He thinks he is surrounded by germs and is definitely the ultimate target himself, but he is also convinced that he will hurt others with his germs: "delusions, contaminates everything she touches" (K23). I had a classic case, a patient who cared for her mother while she was dying from cancer. She was instructed to be very careful not to infect her mother, who was immunosuppressed from chemotherapy and radiation. After her mother died, my patient had compulsive hand washing, and Arsenicum and Syphilinum were needed to resolve it. I have also used Arsenicum successfully for a patient who thought that she brought disease and death to everyone she came in contact with (after two of her close friends died from cancer). Of course Arsenicum also has a great fear of disease, especially cancer, and it is one of the major guilt remedies along with Aurum, Nat. mur., and Staphysagria.

The delusions of seeing insects (K28), rats (K31) and vermin (K34) reflect Arsenicum's anxiety about the future: will there be enough food, enough money? (More likely, Arsenicum is a remedy for the DT's in which the alcoholic sees rats in his delirium.) He also has the "delusions, starve, family will" (K33). He is very protective of what he has and always prepares for the worst. Arsenicum is one of the few remedies that has "eating to satiety ameliorates" (K1357) and the only one under "Desires, more than she needs" (K35), because she is afraid there won't be food at the next meal! Family members who are living off the Arsenicum can be like rats and insects eating away at his savings. Remember the saying, "I smell a rat!" He becomes mistrustful of everyone and may say, "They are all out to steal from me": "Delusions, thieves, sees" and "thieves, in the house" (K33); "thieves, that house and space under the bed are full of" (K33).

Aurum: Aurum always strives to be the best, the most successful, and risks everything to reach that goal. He wants to be the number one in school but if he thinks he has not studied enough to score 100%, he will refuse to take a test. His self-worth is based on his top performance, and this type of person will lose his self-worth when he retires, becoming deeply depressed. Aurum is a great remedy for retired people, all the more so if they have also lost their lifelong spouse. Aurum is likely to feel worthless and not needed anymore, even by his friends. He is apt to think that his longtime fellow workers don't trust him anymore and are ready to put him out to pasture. He projects his own lack of self-confidence onto others, believing that no one needs his opinion anymore. He feels that he belongs to the past and that the future is bleak. The perfectionist, guilt-ridden and dutiful nature of Aurum is reflected in the delusions "appreciated, that she is not" (K21), "right, does nothing" (K31), "succeed, that he cannot, does everything wrong" (K33), "confidence in him, his friends have lost all" (K22), and "fail, everything will" (K25). Aurum is the only black-type remedy for "delusions, neglected his duty" (K30) because of his impossible-to-achieve perfectionism: "I got one B on my report card, I utterly failed my parents," "I don't want to live anymore, I did not provide enough for my family," "My son is a nobody, it is all my fault; I was working too hard and not paying enough attention, I am not a good father or mother," or "My wife left me because I was insensitive to her, I should have listened more to her complaints, now it's too late!" This self-criticism and self-reproach bring us to the delusions "wrong, fancies he has done," (K35) and "right, does nothing" (K31). Of course he has that feeling of always having neglected someone: friends, family, job, all related to *duty*. This neglect of duty extends to his friendships: "delusions, friend, has lost the affection of" (K26).

Cannabis indica: Cannabis has more delusions than any other remedy in the Materia Medica, with thoughts whirling around in his head. We see this in patients who have used too much marijuana. Just a few of the many delusions include "absurd, ludicrous figures are present" (K20), "that he is sitting on a ball" (K21), "thinks he is bewitched" (K21), "body covered the whole earth" (K22), "of butterflies" (K22), "Christ, thinks himself to be" (K22), "clothes would fly away and become wandering stars, on becoming undressed" (K22), "of dancing satyres and nodding mandarins." Other typical delusions reflect the auditory hallucinations: "voices, hears" (K34), "bells, hearing of" (K21), "music, fancies he hears" (K29), "calls, someone" (K22). Cannabis is the top remedy for these rubrics, some of which it shares with Stramonium and Medorrhinum. A typical rubric for Cannabis is "delusions, argument, making an eloquent" (K21). This reminds me of a story of someone proving the herb in non-homeopathic doses who felt he understood the meaning of life while under its influence, so he decided to capture this insight by writing it down the next time he indulged. When he came back to reality he looked with eagerness at the paper which said, "Wow, this is great!"

Coffea: Coffee stimulates a false sense of well-being and vitality. The patient needing Coffea becomes impressionable, especially to pleasurable impressions. He thinks he is momentarily enjoying the best of all possible worlds, a veritable paradise, leading to the delusion "paradise, thought he saw" (K30). The hypersensory stimulation also leads to "ideas, abundance of" (K53) and "sleeplessness, from excessive joy" (K1253). And then he crashes, which is why Coffea is also black-type under "despair, with the pains" (K35) and why it has "sensitiveness to pain," as Kent says in his *Lectures on Materia Medica*.[1]

Fluoric acid: We can call Fluoric acid the Don Juan of the Materia Medica, even more so than Lycopodium or Medorrhinum (and we can wonder what will happen to the sacrament of marriage in the next generation which has grown up on fluoridated water). He does not want to stay married; he will say, "Look, marriage is just a piece of paper," and he certainly acts like it. "He is interested and converses pleasantly with strangers. Stands in the street ogling women as they pass by, so great is his lust." (Phatak) He can't stand being confined by wife or children, even his servants, because Don Juan needs the freedom to pursue the opposite sex. This is expressed in the delusions that "betrothal must be broken" (K21, Fl-ac. only remedy), "marriage must dissolve" (K29), "children, thinks he must drive out of the house" (K22), and "servants, thinks he must get rid of" (K31). He is completely indifferent towards those who love and serve him ("indifference, loved ones, to," and "relations, to," K55), even to any friendships, business partnerships, or commitments to other people. These can all be broken because Fluoric acid is driven to gain money and luxurious possessions. He will justify his actions, of course, as "these people are standing in my way," but in reality he is showing his inability to accept responsibility.

Kali bromatum: Poor Kali bromatum with his exaggerated sense of guilt, often instilled from an early age, in a strictly moral family where the slightest infraction is a big crime. As children Kali bromatums get nightmares; as adults they have great fear of appearing in court and of the police (looking over their shoulders when they hear a siren, certain that they must have done something wrong). As patients they tremble and wring their hands. I remember the poor schizophrenic patients I saw in the psychiatric ward, who would come to me with tears in their eyes to confess a recent murder which was just reported in that day's newspaper. This sense of guilt and persecution shows up in the delusions "that he is persecuted" (K30), "pursued, thought he was" (K31), "policeman, come into house, thought he saw" (K31), "crime, about to commit" and "as if he has committed" (K23), "arrested, is about to be" (K21), "pursued, police by" (K31) and even "brother fell overboard in her sight" (K22, Kali-br. only remedy). This latter rubric means she was watching and she let it happen, so she feels guilty of a crime. Grief and anxiety can lead to this delusion. I have seen it in a child who was walking with her younger brother. Suddenly the youngster pulled away and to the horror of the older child, he was killed. The child's guilt was so great that she refused to leave the house, thinking the police were going to arrest her. Nightmares about the event plagued her until Kali bromatum relieved her suffering.

I had a patient with cancer on one eyelid who fell in love with her ophthalmologist, although she was married. When I saw her, she had restless wringing of the hands, was silent and rather cautious in answering and looking around as if she had something to hide. Kali bromatum helped her guilty conscience, although it was too late to help the cancer. This hiding, guilty aspect is also found in "Delusions, money, sewed up in clothing" (K29) and "murder, that she is about to murder, her husband and child" (K29).

Another patient owned a successful business but sold it under pressure from his wife, who wanted more time with him. After that he became morose, depressed and told me that God punished him and made him sick for selling his business. This corresponds to yet another delusion of Kali bromatum, "delusions, vengeance, he is singled out for divine," (K34, Kali-br. only remedy). Often they have sleeplessness from grief, too, like Nat. mur. (K1253). So besides Aurum, which is the top remedy for people with depression since retirement, people can also react by going into a Kali bromatum state. It is interesting that for the different Kali's there is one theme that is important. For the Kali bich. the family is the most important, for the Kali carb. it is the fulfillment of all his duties (work and home) while for the Kali bromatum it is only business or work.

Platina: The Platina state may come from grief, from abandonment, from sexual abuse, or—like Palladium—from being overshadowed by a more attractive and outgoing sibling. Platina reacts by being very haughty and thinking that no one is good enough for her anyway; others have not seen her superior qualities or are too boorish to appreciate them. She feels she is throwing pearls before swine. Platina is the Cleopatra of the Materia Medica, too good for this world. Platina's haughtiness is expressed in the delusions "does not belong to her own family" (K21, K25), "proud" (K31), etc. The Platina patient will tell you, "My family is not good enough for me; I am ashamed of them; they are an embarrassment to me; I have nothing in common with them; no one in my family has ever amounted to anything." She wants you to believe that she has achieved a much higher status than her family and should not be tainted by association with them. Platina's religious sensibilities and feelings of superiority to the rest of the human race can be expressed as the "Delusions, devils, that all persons are" (K23). Platina's delusion rubrics could be used for patients who admit that as little girls they fantasized that they had been adopted and that at any moment a limousine would arrive to take them back to their true parents, who are wealthy and famous! Platina, like Hyoscyamus, can have many sexual delusions, possibly stemming from childhood sexual abuse. Her high sex drive makes her worry about what will happen if her husband is not there to satisfy her, leading to Platina's typical fear "husband, that he would never return, that something would happen to him" (K45). I had a patient with the typical Platina complaint of facial numbness; her symptoms resolved on Platina, then they suddenly came back. When she called to report this, my first question was, "Where is your husband?" He had just left on a business trip and she needed another dose of Platina!

Using the Delusion Rubrics in Practice

When a particular trait is outspoken and isolated: The rubric and subrubrics "Sensitive, oversensitive to the slightest noise" (K79) list 18 remedies, of which six are black type. Some may be there as part of a general irritability, like Nux vomica, or a general hyperexcitability of the nerves, like Coffea or China. But what do we do with the patient who cancels her appointment every time it rains because she can't stand the sound of windshield wipers but who is not sensitive to *anything* except certain types of sounds? I had such a patient, who came in wearing huge ear protectors like airplane mechanics use. This extreme hypersensitivity to slight sounds is expressed in the delusion "thought someone was scratching on linen or similar substance" (K31), with Asarum the only remedy (and in fact Asarum cured my patient).

Sometimes we see women with the false belief they are pregnant, in a situation of abandonment or jealousy of another woman who is pregnant. They may produce a swollen belly and even imaginary labor pains. Veratrum is the top remedy for this situation, as found in the delusions "pregnant, thought herself" (K31) and "labor, pretends to be in," (K28) as well as the rubric "feigning pregnancy" (K48).

Following are typical statements by patients and where we can find them in the delusion rubrics:

"Nobody loves me any more. I am all alone in the world." When the patient expresses a feeling of being abandoned, we might use the delusions "alone, that she is always" (K20), Pulsatilla; also "alone in the wilderness," Stramonium, or "she is alone in the world," Camphor, Hura, Platina and Pulsatilla. Pulsatilla and Stramonium are the outstanding remedies, and interestingly both are acute remedies of Calcarea, which makes sense because Calcarea is most attached to home and family and most vulnerable when the family unit is broken. Girls and little boys are more likely to become Pulsatillas in this situation, with older boys possibly going into a Stramonium state. Pulsatilla with her great need for affection and constant neediness for attention will always feel that people don't pay enough attention to her. Hence the sense of isolation because any amount of reassurance is never enough for a Pulsatilla, and any heartbreak will accentuate the feeling of being "alone in this world" no matter how many people are still fussing over her.

Stramonium has a different expression. I have seen it many times in Calcarea boys who feel abandoned by their mother whether by divorce or when she goes back to work. They react with anger and violence, smashing holes in the wall with their fists, and with lewd talk and behavior, cursing and tearing their clothes. These violent acts are actually a scream for attention. Often by the time the parents are divorced there have been years of turmoil between them during which the child feels neglected and then abandoned. One way to get attention is to misbehave, but unfortunately his violent and often sexually loaded behavior is misunderstood and condemned by the parent who then pushes the child away. I had a 15-year-old patient of a divorced mother, a big Calcarea youth who frightened his mother with his violence and his habit of exposing himself to her when he came out of the shower. His "Never Well Since" was his parents' divorce; he said, "I didn't want to have to choose between them." Stramonium and Hyoscyamus helped to bring out the youth's gentle, mild Calcarea temperament.

Two other delusions further point up the difference between Pulsatilla and Stramonium: the needy Pulsatilla can have the delusion "bed, as if someone was in, with him (K21), e.g. when sick and wanting consolation, or feeling insecure and wanting to take their mother along, even on their honeymoon! This expresses the neediness of the Pulsatilla, as we will see in the next delusion. The violent Stramonium has appropriate delusions of being attacked such as "animals jump out of the ground" (K21), reflecting his fear of bodily harm.

"You don't pay enough attention to me!" When a patient says this to us, where do we look it up? Under "Delusions, appreciated, that she is not" (K21) or "neglected, that he is" (K30). Palladium is the only remedy in both rubrics, although her "twin sister" Platina can also have this

delusion, as can Pulsatilla, the ever-needy! Palladium has "Longing, for good opinion of others" (K63) and "Flattery, desires" (K48, only remedy!). Palladium's feeling of not being appreciated can be instilled from a young age: for instance, a teenage girl can have a younger sister who is more favored by family and friends because she is more outgoing, beautiful and intelligent. Palladium's hurt feelings can easily turn into, "I feel no one appreciates me for what I am doing." A Palladium will react with wounded pride, a bad mood, and even strong language if she does not get the approval she seeks. Palladiums always need a pat on the shoulder; you constantly have to tell them: "You are great, you are doing well!" When the Palladium patient says, "You are not paying enough attention to me" she means "I want you to focus just on me, tell me how special this case is, tell me how brave I am going through this, no one is suffering like me. Please tell me."

An Arsenicum also wants your attention but tries to get it by always giving you more details of her case; she does not demand your attention in so many words, as Palladium does. Nor does Pulsatilla, who instead tries to get your attention by sweetness and pats on the arm.

"No one appreciates me!" This can also be Palladium or Platina, as just discussed. It can be the overly worried Argentum nitricum, or the depressed Aurum who has lost all self-worth and self-confidence (see discussion under Materia Medica, above). Finally, when a patient (especially a woman) tells us she is underappreciated at home or at work, it could be true; she could be an overworked Sepia trying to juggle children and a career and a husband who doesn't do housework. In this case, of course, it is not a delusion!

"Someone makes me do these bad things, I can't stop myself." If an adult says this, we will recognize it as a delusion of control, but in my practice I hear it much more often from children. We find it under the delusions "double, of being" (K24) and "mind and body separated" (K29), both Anacardium, which has the well-known keynote, "that a devil sits on his shoulder telling him what to do, while on the other shoulder sits a little angel, telling him not to do these bad things." I had an eight-year-old patient who was very rebellious, hard and cruel to her mother. Her father had been an alcoholic for many years, resulting in constant fighting between the parents. The child was deadly afraid of the father, never daring to voice her opinion. So she was caught between two opposite feelings, the fear of punishment telling her to be good; on the other hand, her suppressed anger telling her to do bad. In order to gain control of her life, and to create an outlet for her anger, her cruelty turned against her mother, the gentler parent. Although she was diagnosed as yet another ADHD case, Anacardium made remarkable changes in this girl until she agreed with her mother more easily and viewed her not as her enemy but as the friend she truly was.

"I can't help it, I keep calling my ex-girlfriend to see who answers the phone." Hyoscyamus, the most jealous of the grief remedies, will "stalk" the woman who jilted them, whether over the phone or in person. Hyoscyamus is the only remedy under "Delusions, calls for absent persons" (K22). While in a relationship, they may call their partner again and again out of jealousy, not out of sympathetic concern like Phosphorus or worried concern like Arsenicum. And if the relationship ends, they may call the former partner over and over, whether to hear her voice on the answering machine or to channel their jealousy at the new partner. O.J. Simpson was probably in a Hyoscyamus state, wild with grief, rage and jealousy. Hyoscyamus' jealousy is so intense, their actions (running around naked, stalking, lewd talk, cursing, killing) so extreme and strange that they feel they must be possessed by a devil ("Delusions, devil, possessed of a," K23). Think about the school shootings in which the killers claim to be possessed by devils. Their behavior is often triggered by a breakup with a girlfriend, a classic Hyoscyamus etiology.

"Can you help my 86-year-old mother, doctor? She doesn't recognize us any more and she doesn't even seem to know who she is." Fortunately, homeopathy can often help in this typical Alzheimer's condition. Aluminum is found in the typical Alzheimer's rubrics, "Delusions, consciousness, belongs to another" (K22); "Delusions, identity, error, of personal" (K27); and "Confusion, identity, as to his" (K15). Aluminum affects the cerebrospinal axis and so is useful when the judgement and sense of reality are disturbed, as in many Alzheimer's patients. Everything that is felt or experienced seems to be through another person's body. They have lost touch with their own physical bodies. The mind-body link appears very weak, which colors all their perceptions with an aura of unreality. In a deeper state of Aluminum they even believe that their thought process use someone else's brain ("Delusions, head belongs to another," K26, "Delusions, consciousness belongs to another," K22, "Delusions, sees, thinks someone else sees for him," K31). This situation can also been seen in teenagers suffering from heartbreak. Depressed and alienated, they walk around in a daze, not knowing who they are.

"I feel like everyone at work is on my case." If we think of Baryta carb. only for shy, bashful patients with developmental delays, with growth or mental retardation, then we will miss the opportunity to use it for people of normal or even superior intelligence who come into a Baryta carb. state by overstudying or overworking in mental work. The "carb." part of Baryta carb. is self-conscious about how others see them and is sensitive to comments, which they take as criticism, as Calcarea does. The Baryta part feels delayed, small or inadequate as will be seen in the next delusion. Baryta carb.'s feeling of being criticized at work is expressed in the delusion, "Delusions, criticized, that she is" (K23). A Calcarea is most likely to become a Baryta carb., whether at school where the Calcarea may be a good student but takes longer to

complete assignments than others; or in a business, in which the Calcarea is likely to be expert with finances but can too easily take on worries and responsibilities.

"I feel like everyone looks down on me and laughs at me. I don't dare to say anything in a conversation because I am afraid they are going to laugh at me. I never participate in sports because I might do something awkward." Some patients who were born with a Baryta carb. constitution may express themselves like this because they tend to be physically smaller as well as timid and bashful except around young children. Other patients may say this type of thing when in a Baryta carb. state. These sentiments can be found under the many delusions of Baryta carb.: "Delusions, legs, are cut off" (K28); "walk, that he walks on his knees" (K35); "laughed at" (K28); "criticized" (K23); "watched, that she is being" (K35); and "everyone is looking at her" (K29), to which Baryta carb. should be added. The first two delusions refer to the patient's (real or imagined) *smallness*, which make him feel incapable. The Baryta carb. will also say, "In comparison with other people, I feel I can't do anything properly" or "I feel like a cripple."

The Baryta carb. patient may also say, "I would rather stay at home, I feel secure at home, no one challenges me at home." This reminds us of the classic posture of the Baryta carb. child: hiding behind the sofa or her mother's skirt.

"I feel totally lost without my friend's [relative's] support." Baryta carb. can also be used for the person who suddenly feels bereft, as expressed in the delusions that he is crippled, noted above, or that "a beloved friend is sick and dying" (K32). I have seen this situation in immigrants who have just come to this country and don't speak English, and suddenly the relative who sponsored them passes away. These sentiments can also apply to the practitioner ("If you move, Doctor, I will be completely lost, I will not be able to function.") It may then be combined with Baryta carb.'s childlike shyness and fear of strangers: "I don't want to go to any other doctor, he will not be like you." Or an adult may express himself in a childlike way: "I can't do this. You have to help me."

"I don't have any contact with my family, I am ashamed to present them to my business friends. They don't amount to anything, I can't even believe they are related to me." This is probably a Platina, with her distorted view of herself (tall) versus the world (small) who tends to distance herself from her family. One of my patients in Santa Monica was one of the most famous actresses in Hollywood, but I heard from a friend of hers that she had to declare bankruptcy. She still kept driving her BMW, probably the only thing that kept her from feeling disgraced in a world where she liked to feel all-important. I saw many Platina starlets in Santa Monica, with their big flashy jewelry, surgically enhanced bodies, designer clothing and fancy cars, all designed to create the impression that they were too important to speak to ordinary mortals. They had all taken a stage name, which of course had the effect of denying their ordinary human

connection with their family.

The Platina's sense that her family would disgrace her by their ordinariness is reflected in rubric "Delusions, disgraced, that she is" (K24), a rubric which Platina shares with Sulphur. Normally we don't think of Sulphur, with his high opinion of himself, feeling disgraced. But it can happen when he loses his job or when his children don't live up to his high expectations. He may think they are lazy (as everyone else is, in a Sulphur's eye) or they don't measure up to him.

"I feel like I have a black cloud over my head" or *"Everything is black around me."* I have often heard patients say this when they need Cimicifuga, primarily women in labor or menopause. It can be found in Kent under the delusion "clouds, heavy black enveloped her" (K22), with Cimicifuga the only remedy. Women in labor need Cimicifuga when they feel depressed because their ordeal seems endless. Cimicifuga women in menopause tend to be indifferent, sitting around the house and moping, bursting into tears when you ask them something. The menopausal women who need it are so talkative that we might otherwise think of that great and loquacious menopausal remedy, Lachesis. But Cimicifuga can be distinguished from Lachesis in this situation by the typical alternation of mental/emotional with physical symptoms and by the "gloom and doom" sensation expressed in this rubric.

"I am afraid I will end up as a street person." Coming from a well-to-do adult, you know this has to be a delusion, and it can be found under "Delusions, fortune, that he was going to lose his" (K26), with Psorinum one of only two remedies. Like Bryonia, Psorinum has fear of poverty, but in Psorinum it can be related to the actual experience of extreme deprivation, such as we find in older people who lived through the Depression. No matter how financially successful they may be, they have often been indelibly stamped by the poverty of their childhood. Interestingly, Psorinum is often the best remedy for street people as well as for anyone who has suffered extreme deprivation of the basic necessities of life (food, shelter and hygiene), such as concentration camp survivors. The Psorinum person's past experience of suffering may also affect his perception of his own health, as expressed in the rubric, "Despair, recovery, of" (K36).

"My boss criticizes me in front of everyone else, but it is beneath my dignity to defend myself. I will not stoop to his level." When a patient says this, yet we see her suffering from symptoms caused by the suppression of her anger, we must think of Staphysagria. Remember that Staphysagria is one of the proud remedies, along with Platina, Palladium, and Nat. mur. The delusion "humility and lowness of others, while he is great" (K27) lists only Platina, already discussed, and Staphysagria. Staphysagria is also black-type for suffering from wounded pride, as found under "Mortification, ailments after" (K68). The proud Staphysagria tries to maintain her

dignity in a situation in which she cannot fight back, whether against a domineering parent, an abusive lover, or an unfair boss. She will repress her anger as a survival mechanism, then suffer from tics, styes, stammering, etc. Phatak's *Materia Medica* says of Staphysagria: "Great indignation about things … grieves about the consequences." She consoles herself by reminding herself that it takes an exceptional person to have so much self-control. A Nux vomica would lash out verbally in such a situation, and even a gentle Calcarea could go into a violent Stramonium state, but the Staphysagria is very sensitive to what others say about her, like Palladium. Staphysagria and Causticum share similar etiologies, but Causticum reacts actively out of a sense of injustice, whether organizing boycotts, leaping to the barricades, or planting bombs like the highly Causticum Unabomber. Staphysagrias, on the other hand, fight passively, by advocating non-violence to gain their enemies' respect through their nobility and uncompromising dignity.

"I am totally devoted to my boss. I only want the best for him. I want him to make a good impression, so I tell him how to dress for meetings, when to get his hair cut, and when to send cards to his associates." I have seen this situation in an unmarried secretary who pours all her emotional energy into pleasing her boss, in other words getting so involved with him that she almost feels she is married to him. An Ignatia will do this, and Ignatia is the only remedy under the delusion "married, that he is" (K29). The idealistic, romantic Ignatia tends to invest her entire emotional bank account in one person, often a distant or unavailable person. In this case she expects her boss to return the emotional intensity and sense of intimacy. When he does not, she sets herself up for heartbreak (for which Ignatia, of course, is one of the top remedies).

"My parents want to get rid of me." The jealousy of Hyoscyamus is based on the feeling of abandonment. It can happen to a child when another sibling is born and is found under the delusion "sold, as if he would be" (K32), with Hyoscyamus the only remedy. He feels "sold out" by the attention these parents dote on the newborn, he feels he does not belong to the family anymore. This extreme sense of abandonment leads to violent behavior with cursing, erotic behavior towards the parents (mother usually) and a strong desire to kill the sibling with a knife. Obviously such behavior does not endear him to the parents, and so the cycle of abandonment and rejection becomes a vicious one.

"I feel like a numbskull, like my head is filled with empty space. I can't remember anything. I always have to go back and check whether I turned off the iron or locked the door." This is a typical Causticum state, in which repetitive grief has brought paralysis on all three planes: mentally (forgetful), emotionally (flat affect) and physically (paralysis, torticollis, etc.). After a series of horrible events, it is as if their brain has shrunken, expressed by the delusion "space, that there is empty, between brain and skull" (K32), with Causticum the only remedy. A peculiar sensation of a

Causticum headache is "as if there were a vacuum between the frontal bone and the brain." Checking and rechecking tasks compulsively is a keynote of Causticum. I had a sad example in my practice: a grandmother babysitting for her grandchild had the traumatic experience of seeing the baby die unexpectedly in her arms. Her grief was immense, but to make matters worse, a week later the daughter-in-law accused her of being responsible for the infant's death. From then on, she suddenly lost her memory for words and familiar tasks. She was diagnosed with "early Alzheimer's" but Causticum brought her back from the twilight zone of Alzheimer's.

"I just need to make enough money to be comfortable and then I can relax," and in response to the question how much is enough, *"fifty million dollars,"* as one of my patients said! This can be found under "delusions, poor, thinks he is" (K31) or "want, fancied that he would come to" (K35). The latter rubric has Calc. fluor. and Sulph.; the former has Calc. fluor, while Sulph. is found under "delusions, thin, getting" (K33) which says the same thing on a metaphorical level. Sulphur is the collector who loves to count his money. So if he loses money (e.g. in the stock market) he feels he is getting poor. It is easy for a Sulphur to feel poor (thin) even with plenty of money in the bank. The Sulphur's life revolves around providing well for his family, so he can have tremendous anxiety about his finances.

"I have my speech memorized just fine but the moment I open my mouth to speak I can't remember a thing." This refers to the anticipation anxiety of the Lycopodium, the only remedy under the delusion "vanish, seems as if everything would" (K34). I have had Lycopodium patients who were lawyers who forgot their courtroom speeches no matter how well rehearsed, others who were students whose minds would go blank as soon as their exams started, and even a priest who would forget his sermon as soon as he mounted the pulpit. Of course this delusion implies also that he is afraid he is going to be alone (Lycopodium is a 3), or that his power will vanish. At the same time, Lycopodium can be a coward (3), hiding his true nature from the outside world while tyrannizing his family at home. He dreads being exposed, so he avoids responsibility and commitment, another well-known characteristic of Lycopodium.

"It amazes me how the least little thing can set me off whenever I get one of my headaches." Of course there can be many reasons why someone could be "at the end of their rope" (the total burnout and exhaustion of Sepia, the irritability and noise-sensitivity of Nux vomica) but we must not forget Chamomilla, as in the delusion of "vexations and offenses" (K34). Chamomilla is characterized by an unsurpassed hypersensitivity to pain (Coffea) followed by an angry accusatory response. Often the patient seems to complain of more discomfort than would be expected from the existing condition. They are ugly, cross, uncivil, and quarrelsome, irritated at every trifle. Ordinarily courteous, in pain they become impolite and angry, even cursing.

(The wife reported that their 3 year old son cried after falling around the same time her husband had one of his headaches. The husband screamed at the son and threatened him with a good whack across the face so that the child would have something to really cry about. Chamomilla was used for the husband with good results, averting a child abuse case such as we read about so often in the newspapers.)

"I'm sure my wife is cheating on me," yet she is your patient too, and you are sure she is not! This can be found under "Delusions, wife is faithless" (K35), with the violent remedies Hyoscyamus and Stramonium. One of my Hyoscyamus patients was in the habit of slapping his wife when he came home every night, saying "You know why" (meaning because she had been unfaithful, but she hadn't, so she was totally puzzled as well as hurt and humiliated). This rubric too can be expanded. "Wife" can be anyone the person trusted and counted on: a business partner, you the physician when you move to another state, or a mother who starts working when the child is three years old (and then the child becomes wild and violent).

"Ever since I took your remedy I am much worse" or *"Since I took your remedy my health is totally gone."* You may suspect your patient of being delusional if she says this after one dose of LM1, 2 succussions. If she says it after taking Sac. lac., you can be sure of it. I remember one case vividly: I gave one of my patients Nat. mur. LM1 for a heartbreak situation, but she was impatient and took a 10M on her own. While this high potency might have caused some aggravation, it certainly could not have caused her reactions for the next six months: she kept calling me to claim that she had been "poisoned by the salt, I can still taste the salt in my body." When she wanted to take the bottle to be tested with applied kinesiology, she had to have a friend carry it because she was afraid to touch it. She returned the remedy to me because she claimed the salt was coming out of it and affecting all the food in her cabinets and could even be detected in the air throughout her apartment. I realized she really needed another heartbreak remedy, Lachesis, with its suspicion and fear of being poisoned. In fact Lachesis and the other snake venoms are among the main remedies in the delusions "injury, is being injured" (K28), "injured by his surroundings" (K28), and "wrong, has suffered" (K35). The other remedies are violent remedies, Hyoscyamus, Stramonium and Lyssin: the patient usually reacts in a violent, suspicious way. When these types feel wronged, they will "bite" like a dog or snake.

Lyssin, made from the saliva of a rabid dog, is a particularly interesting remedy appearing in these rubrics. The dog depends on its master for everything—food, housing and affection—but if the master torments the dog, it arouses the dog to rage, growling and biting. This cruel, malicious behavior is often seen in child abuse and in alcoholic families.

Delusions and Their Place in Pathology

The patient's delusion, if you can find it, is of top priority in finding the simillimum. It represents the most interior level, the deepest aberration on the mental plane, as illustrated in Figure 11-1. (A more complete illustration of the same concept may be found in Figure 13-2).

We know from Hering's Laws that the Vital Force constantly tries to protect the person by pushing symptoms from the inside to the outside. This law holds true of mental and emotional symptoms as well as physical ones. For example, if our mind is overburdened with worry, we can exteriorize it by talking about it and so relieve our mental state. By the same token, when we suppress mental and emotional symptoms to the deepest level, we can produce delusions.

Once a delusion is created, the Vital Force still tries to push it to the outside through the person's relationship, profession or even his recreation. If that outlet becomes blocked, the delusion is more likely to create an imbalance in the person's life. For example, Aurums are known for being conscientious, religious, dutiful, perfectionist and guilt-ridden, to the extent that they may have the delusion that they have neglected their duty. Throughout their childhood they may pour their energy into being the top student in the class, then in young and middle adulthood they find an outlet through their work, where they may rise to be CEO of the company. The problem starts when such a person retires and this outlet becomes blocked.

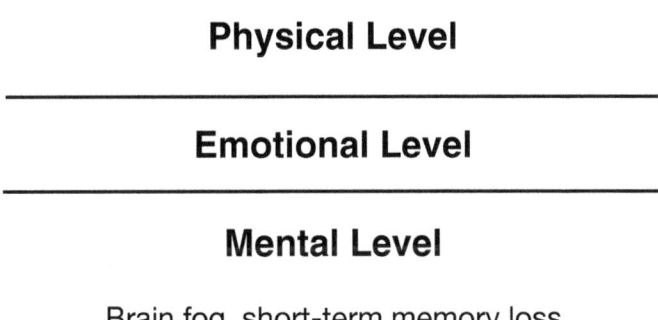

Figure 11-1, Delusions at the Deepest Level of Suppression

No wonder Aurum is the top remedy for those who become depressed when they retire. In this situation the Aurum person will typically develop heart problems (severe physical pathology) and may even commit suicide. To keep his mental, emotional and physical health, the retiree needs to find another outlet for his industriousness, competitiveness and perfectionism (or needs to take Aurum).

People typically look for an outlet for their delusion in their choice of profession: the Lycopodium with his love of power may become a politician, bureaucrat, lawyer or teacher; the Aurum with his great sense of responsibility may become a stockbroker, investing other people's hard-earned money; Sulphur with his delusions of grandeur may become a CEO or a general. Nat. mur. with her delusion of abandonment may become a psychotherapist to recreate a sense of intimacy through her profession, while Causticum may channel her sense of being wronged into battling for justice. As long as people can "live out" their inner delusion through their profession, no pathology develops. But when the outlet is blocked through retirement, a stock market crash or other reversal, pathology starts. In fact the patient will tell us, "If I only had my previous position [money, profession, etc.] back, I would be well."

If we cannot find an outlet in our profession, we may seek it in our recreation. People who enjoy facing danger and taking risks may become successful in the stock market, then become so financially well off that they need to find another outlet for their risktaking like parasailing, ballooning, or climbing Mount Everest. The current popularity of trash talk shows and of violent, sexual films may reflect a socially-acceptable outlet for the audience's inner delusions. I have seen children needing Anacardium who are fascinated with horror movies that involve cruelty, while those who need Mancinella crave supernatural horror movies such as *Poltergeist* and *The Exorcist*.

> *Clinical Case:* As an example of how a patient finds an appropriate outlet for her delusion, then develops pathology when the outlet is blocked, I think of a Platina patient I had. A bright, competitive person, she consulted me for a typical Platina complaint: numbness in the face alternating with mental/emotional symptoms of depression. A spoiled only child, she had been brought up to feel like a princess by her doting parents. Then she was treated like a queen by her husband, a high-powered executive in New York who relied heavily on her social contacts so that she was the center of attention at all their social events. The result was the typical Platina delusion of grandeur. Her numbness started when this outlet became blocked, when their first child was born. Remember that when the patient gives us a Never Well Since, we always have to ask "Why? How did it make you feel?" In her case, it meant she had to stay home instead of socializing with her husband. She said, "My whole world changed,

I was nobody special any more, I became one of the common people." She found another situation in which she could recreate this "queen" image for herself: she learned to play tennis and quickly became an extremely competitive tennis player. Although she had only been playing for two years when I met her, she would not deign to play with other newcomers to the sport and insisted on playing mixed doubles with twenty-year veterans. She was able to hold her numbness at bay as long as she was at the top of the tennis ladder, but it returned when she became pregnant again and had to give up competitive tennis.

Chapter Twelve

Aggravations, Healing Crises, and Accessory Symptoms

Similar Aggravations

A similar aggravation occurs when the patient's original symptoms become more intense. This situation, caused by the primary action of the remedy repressing the secondary action of the Vital Force, is a sign that the remedy is correct, but given in too high a dose, repeated too frequently, or re-administered too soon when it was not needed. In other words, it is a sign of the *wrong administration* of the *correct remedy*. It is hard for the patient (or the professional if he has no knowledge of homeopathy) to understand this concept. They ask: "How is it possible to cure a disease with a medicine capable of making it worse?" It bears repeating here: in the potentized remedy the material quantity of the medicine is so insignificant (no molecule of the remedy substance remains) that the crude action is almost zero. Only the dynamic (energetic) action of the remedy remains, and only for a limited amount of time.

As explained before, a similar aggravation is not at all necessary to bring about a cure. With LM potencies or 6c, there might be some aggravation *internally* (the remedy effects a subtle internal "shake-up") but this aggravation is so negligible that a cure is usually effected *before any external manifestation* of the aggravation takes place. Sometimes we will see a slight aggravation of physical symptoms lasting for a few hours or as long as a day (even with LMs). But this situation is so easily controlled that we almost welcome it, because from the first dose on it tells us we have selected the right remedy. In other words, we have the same response, for the same reason, as the Kentian prescriber who rejoices at an initial aggravation—but in the case of an LM aggravation it is so mild and transient as to be barely noticeable. And with LM potencies we can adjust the daily dose immediately to avoid further similar aggravations, even as minimal as they were. If the chief complaint was physical, even as the physical symptom persists or worsens for a few hours, the patient improves on the mental, emotional and energetic plane. He will say: "I still have my headache [original complaint] but I slept better and I have a sense of well-being. I am more peaceful, I am more optimistic." This is because the remedy acts first on the deeper spheres, the mental/emotional, shifting symptoms from this deeper level to the more superficial level, the physical.

It can happen, though, that the patient *does not feel well in spite of a mild similar homeopathic aggravation*. That would be the case in a severe mental/emotional disease where the seat of the illness is on a deeper plane. The administration of the simillimum most likely could aggravate slightly the mental/emotional symptoms while for instance *the patient's appetite and sleep improve*. This means the remedy is correct, and the practitioner has to consider with caution when to repeat the remedy (again, this is easier to control with low potencies). Imagine if someone is in an anxious, restless Arsenicum state and the practitioner repeats Arsenicum too often. What else can you expect but an aggravated state of anxiety and restlessness? Again, do not make the mistake of changing the remedy, which was well-selected.

What to do in the case of a similar aggravation? Some homeopaths claim that if a remedy produces a strong similar aggravation it is better to use allopathic medication to counteract the aggravation, rather than a homeopathic remedy, so as not to disturb the dynamic homeopathic action. Is this what Hahnemann suggested? Not at all. He stated that cases produced by a combination of chronic miasms and allopathic drug suppression are the hardest to cure.

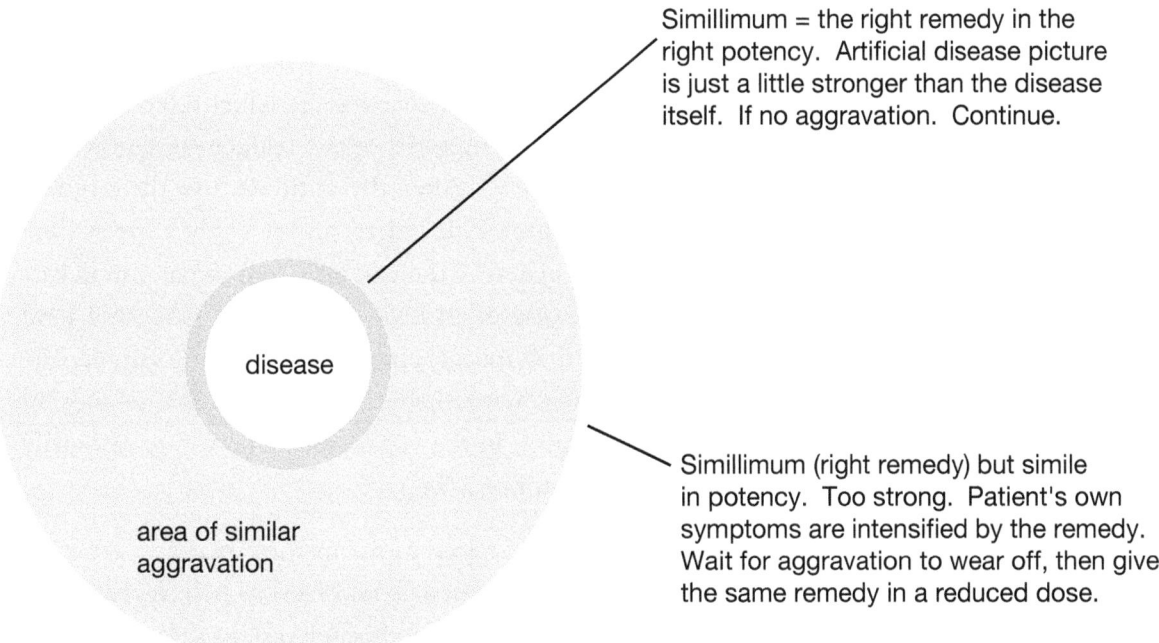

Fig. 12-1: The Similar Aggravation: Right Remedy, Too Strong

Such an approach will only confuse the case by suppression and lead the patient into a deeper state of illness.

I would not object to intervention if the situation is life-threatening because of the strong similar aggravation, as in the case of an asthma patient evolving to a status asthmaticus. Palliation is needed even if the medicine given to the patient was absolutely correct. But remember that the true definition of the simillimum is that we have chosen not only the right remedy but also the right potency and dosage. For instance, Arsenicum 30c may be the simile while 6c might be the simillimum; or Sepia LM1 8 succussions might be the simile, while Sepia LM1 2 succussions is the simillimum. Each patient resonates with one potency of a remedy, like a radio tuned to a particular frequency.

There are three ways to handle similar aggravations severe enough to require intervention, depending on the intensity of the symptoms:

- Use lower potencies of the same remedy in chronic diseases. (If you started with 6c or LM you will not run into this problem in the first place).

- If the aggravations take the form of a new active layer (created with the remedy), retake the case and use the symptoms of this new active layer to find a new remedy, which you give in a lower potency than the first one, to avoid another similar aggravation. (You would also reduce the potency of all future remedies for this patient, based on your experience with the first one.)

- Use a remedy that is a known antidote to the medicine that was used. Pick a remedy from the list of antidotes that is most similar to the symptoms of the dangerous aggravation (based on the list at the end of Kent's *Repertory*). After the antidote, use the original remedy in a lower potency (LM or 6c for chronic disorders) and possibly a lower dose (e.g. less frequent administration; and fewer pellets in the case of a centesimal potency or fewer succussions/smaller spoonfuls in the case of an LM). In my own practice I have never had to antidote a remedy except in a few unusual circumstances. (For example, one of my patients, a professional singer, gave her own remedy, Phosphorus 10M, to another singer who then developed a burning sensation in the vocal cords. She was temporarily unable to sing and had to antidote with Camphor 200c.)

Some homeopaths claim they have never seen aggravations in their practice, whether similar or dissimilar. This would be nothing short of a miracle and hard to believe. Even the most experienced old homeopaths like Kent and Hahnemann himself discuss them at length. Perhaps these homeopaths are mistaking aggravations for healing crises, discussed later in this chapter.

Sometimes if a dose is similar but too high in potency and/or dosage, the artificial disease thus created will be even greater than the original and more troublesome because it also brings up new symptoms (unhomeopathic to the case, i.e. not part of the original patient-remedy match). The Vital Force is overwhelmed and the remedy picture is no longer similar to the disease picture (because of all the added symptoms of the remedy). As Hahnemann puts it, "This is caused by the fact that the medicine used in so large a dose unfolds its other symptoms which nullify the similarity and thus establishes another dissimilar disease."[2] Thus it can establish another dissimilar disease, also chronic, in place of the former.

We may wonder how a remedy can create a chronic disease, when we are accustomed to thinking of aggravations as transient even though they may last for many months. But if the remedy punches the Vital Force down hard enough, the Vital Force may never recover. I have never seen this happen in my practice using LM potencies, however, because the aggravations created by LMs are so mild and transient; and it is rare in my experience even with centesimal potencies.

Dissimilar Aggravation

A *dissimilar* aggravation needs immediate correction because it indicates a wrong remedy. An incorrect remedy produces *new* symptoms, i.e.:
- the patient has never experienced them before,
- they are not due to the reappearance of old suppressed symptoms according to Hering's Laws,
- they are not due to the aggravation of the existing disease, and
- they are clearly produced by the remedy, rather than by a new trauma or circumstance in the patient's life adding a new symptom picture onto the existing disease picture.

These are symptoms of a troubling nature, pathogenic symptoms of the remedy that was administered, while the patient's old complaints are no better. At the same time, the general health and mental state has worsened, and the patient definitely has no sense of well-being, but rather may have a sense of malaise. The patient feels worse on all three planes, physically, emotionally and mentally.

This is true when new physical symptoms of the remedy appear alongside the patient's existing physical symptoms, in a classic dissimilar aggravation. It is also true when the patient's physical symptoms disappear and are replaced by mental/emotional symptoms. In this case we know we have the wrong remedy, as the direction of the cure is wrong (see the next chapter, Suppression). The more that new symptoms appear, the more certain we can be of a wrong prescription. What does the practitioner do in such circumstances? There are three possible scenarios:

Non-dangerous situation: The symptoms, though strong, begin to leave rapidly, thus posing no danger. The lower the potency you used, the more likely this will be the case. Wait them out and the case should return to its original state. Then retake the case and select the simillimum.

Dangerous situation: Antidote right away if the symptoms are dangerous and/or unbearable for the patient, like cluster headaches or strong palpitations in a chronic heart failure patient. The antidote will often return the case to its natural previous "status quo" state before the dissimilar remedy was given. Then take your case again fresh and select a better remedy. Waiting out numerous annoying and/or dangerous symptoms is a mistake since the remedy can graft its symptoms on the Vital Force, producing an iatrogenic or medicinal disease state more complex than the original one.

Non-dangerous but bothersome: If the symptoms are not dangerous but are persistent and disruptive, a corrective remedy should be chosen based on the combination of the *new medicinal* symptoms and the *natural* symptoms. This grand totality will correct the problem by regularizing the Vital Force and move the case towards a cure. The wrong remedy has *changed* the picture and produced a *new* state of the Vital Force. The original state of the Vital Force does

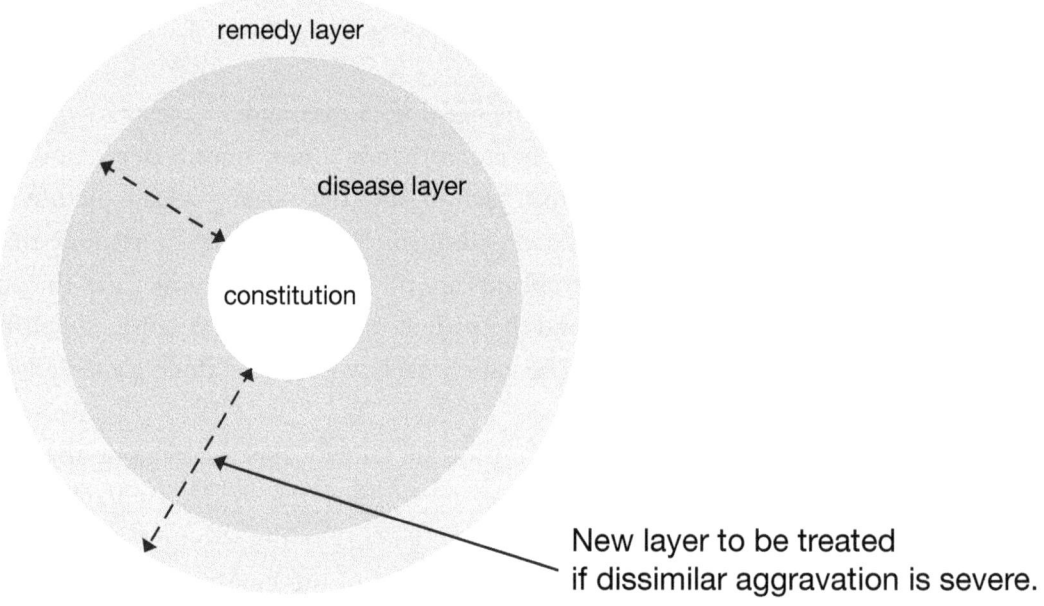

Fig. 12-2: The Dissimilar Aggravation Requiring Treatment

not exist anymore, so the original simillimum is not indicated anymore. The Vital Force has been changed by a remedy that had a negative resonance with the constitution. One always has to include the most active layer which includes the most recent symptoms (even when they are created by your mistake) when taking a case. These are the *real* indications of the patient at this moment.

A more difficult situation of dissimilar aggravation for the practitioner to manage occurs when the patient tells him at follow-up that *she is feeling well but the existing symptoms are aggravated while new ones appear.* This situation represents a *disease* aggravation because the illness is incurable despite the best efforts of the simillimum (see Chapter 16, Palliation and Incurable Diseases). In other words, the remedy has successfully brought about a sense of well-being, although temporarily aggravating the symptoms which match it and for which it was prescribed, while the underlying disease state is nevertheless worsening and creating new symptoms. This is not a dissimilar aggravation in the strictest sense of the word, because the patient has a sense of well-being. The symptoms which are not part of the patient's original symptom picture do not represent a dissimilar aggravation but rather the disease process continuing to worsen. In other words, it *may present at first as a dissimilar aggravation,* because of the new dissimilar symptoms, but once the practitioner understands what is going on, he will correctly view the situation as a *disease* aggravation.

It is easy to confuse a disease aggravation with a similar aggravation. One way to differentiate them is that the former will persist while the latter has to disappear. Another way is to assess the nature of the disease: some disease states, like TB for instance, are well-known for allowing the patient to remain fairly well mentally/emotionally up to the end, while the pathology develops silently underneath, ultimately creating fatal symptoms. I cannot stress enough that we can respond more quickly to this scenario with LMs, as the aggravation will be of *minimal duration.*

Another misleading situation of an *apparent* dissimilar aggravation—and one more frequently encountered in the practice—occurs when the patient is so focused on his disease state (typically an Arsenicum, Psorinum, or Nitric acid state) that he will *deny* the feeling of well-being *although it is present.* "I am no better, in fact I am worse," these patients will say, because for them "better" means *all* the symptoms have vanished—and short of this miracle, they will not admit to any improvement. It is understandable in this case for the practitioner to confuse a homeopathic aggravation with a disease aggravation or a dissimilar aggravation (since these patients, in their great state of anxiety, are easily influenced to find—or perhaps imagine!—new symptoms). Be aware if you have such patients. The only way to discover the truth is to cross-examine them like a lawyer, but with love. Systematically review each of the symptoms they had on their first visit, asking the exact percentage of improvement of each.

(You will be surprised at how many have improved or even disappeared on close examination.) This re-emphasizes the importance of a thorough first inquiry. The only acceptable new symptoms are rashes and discharges (and joint pains as long as the Chief Complaint was not a skin or other surface pathology). These symptoms are not a dissimilar aggravation but rather signs of a healing crisis.

Natural Healing Crisis

There is a difference between a homeopathic aggravation and a natural healing crisis. A healing crisis occurs as the disease heals from the inside to the outside, in accordance with Hering's Law: the body can express a deeper disease in the more surface manifestations of rashes, discharges, and joint pains. (Of course if the patient's Chief Complaint was a skin problem in the first place, then joint pains would not be an exterior manifestation but rather a sign of suppression.) These three types of symptoms should never be considered a dissimilar aggravation, even if the patient has never had them before, but rather a positive expression of the Vital Force reacting to the remedy and throwing off the disease. (They may also represent the return of old symptoms, because in fact many deeper diseases come from the suppression of rashes or discharges, such as the treatment of eczema with cortisone, which can lead to asthma; see the next chapter on Suppression).

These symptoms of a healing crisis should be left alone if at all possible. They should *never* be treated by changing the remedy, palliation with an acute remedy, or (of course) suppressive allopathic treatment. If the patient is uncomfortable, encourage her to slow down on the remedy and soothe the symptoms, if necessary, with non-suppressive natural treatments such as an oatmeal bath, aloe vera gel, calendula cream, or Rescue Remedy cream for skin conditions; if a rash interferes with sleep, the patient can use *herbal* (not homeopathic) valerian or passiflora.

Remember that not *every manifestation* after the intake of a homeopathic remedy is a healing crisis. Be careful of homeopaths who try to explain away every dissimilar or strong similar aggravation as a "natural healing crisis." A homeopathic aggravation is created by the *primary* action of the *remedy* while a natural healing crisis is created by the *secondary* action of the *Vital Force*.

Accessory Symptoms

Aphorisms 161-163 of the *Organon* explain accessory symptoms. Aphorism 161 addresses what we commonly think of as accessory symptoms: those typically appearing at the end of treatment, which belong to the remedy, are not part of the diminished and minimal disease picture of the patient and are thus unhomeopathic to the patient:

When medicines of longer duration of action have to combat an old or very old wasting sickness *[in other words chronic disease]* ... such heightenings of the original symptoms of the disease can then only come to light at the end of such treatments when the cure is almost or entirely completed.

While some of the symptoms that appear at the end of treatment are part of the original symptom picture, as Hahnemann states here, the majority are actually unhomeopathic to it. This latter type of accessory symptom indicates that the patient is nearing the end of the course of treatment because she has been requiring very few doses of the remedy and each one gives her an aggravation with symptoms belonging to the remedy. As her disease layer becomes smaller and smaller, the potency repeated was either the same or greater (centesimal scale) or the remedy had more succussions (LM scale). It is easy to see that as the natural disease picture dwindles and the remedy's artificial "disease picture" grows larger due to the higher potency, the remedy will cover less and less of the actual disease and will create more and more symptoms unhomeopathic to the patient (see Figure 12-3). This signifies that it is time to leave the patient alone, she is cured. All you might have to do to finish the case is to give her constitutional remedy (or another "layer" remedy if there is another layer present in the past medical history).

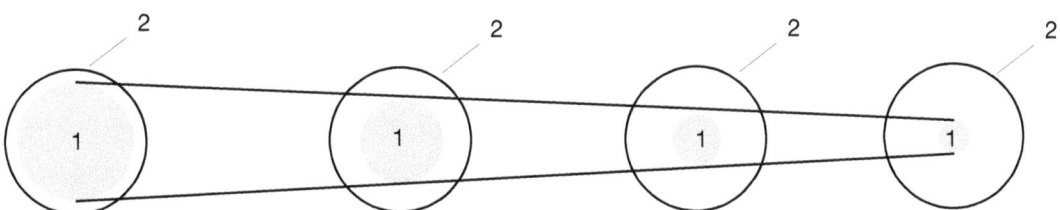

1. Disease diminishes as it is cured by the appropriate repetition of the similar remedy
2. The dissimilarity between the remedy and the patient's disease picture becomes bigger and more symptoms (un-homeopathic and accessory to the case) appear.

Fig. 12-3: Accessory Symptoms Appearing at the End of Treatment

Another kind of accessory symptom is covered by Aphorisms 162 and 163:

Because there are still only a moderate number of medicines which are exactly known as to their true, pure action, it sometimes happens that only *a portion* of the symptoms of the disease to be cured are met within the set of symptoms of the still best-fitting medicine. Consequently, this imperfect medicinal disease potency must be employed for lack of a more perfect one.

In such cases, a complete, untroublesome cure cannot be expected, because when the imperfect medicine is used, some befallments will then emerge which were not to be found earlier in the disease. These are accessory symptoms of the not-completely-fitting medicine. To be sure, this will not hamper a considerable part of the malady (i.e. the disease symptoms that are similar to the medicinal symptoms) from being expunged by this medicine, and a fair beginning of the cure arising by this means, although not without accessory ailments. With properly small medicinal doses *[i.e. LM potencies],* these accessory ailments will be moderate.

The lack of proven remedies certainly was a problem in Hahnemann's time (he had only about 200 remedies). We modern homeopaths can still struggle to find the simillimum, despite having ten times as many remedies, because the simillimum is not discovered or proven yet. The low number of modern provings (because pharmaceutical companies have no desire to test products which cannot be patented and cost only pennies) coupled to the increasing destruction of Nature and rapid extinction of species may pose a problem for finding the simillimum in some cases.

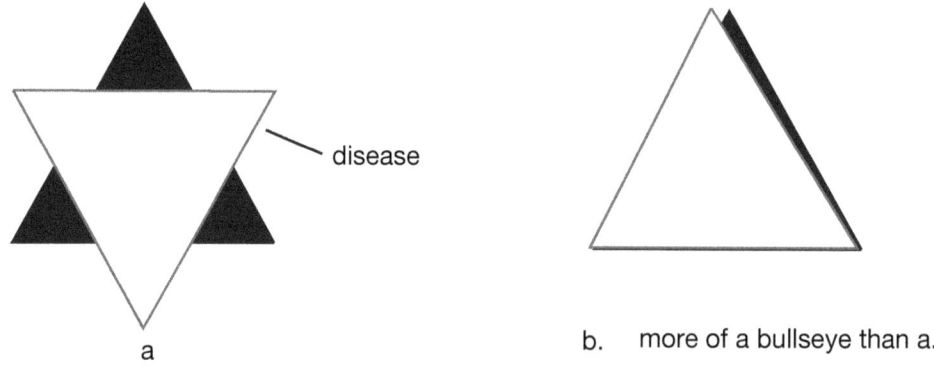

Fig. 12-4: Accessory Symptoms Appearing Due to Lack of Fit

In this case it is no wonder that a remedy will sometimes bring out "side effects" which are called accessory symptoms, unhomeopathic to the case of the patient. Hahnemann stated that it is almost impossible to find a remedy that fits the disease as perfectly as two similar triangles on top of each other. The edges that do not fit have the potential to produce accessory symptoms (see Figure 12-4). For example, in my own practice I have given Nat. mur. to a patient suffering from chronic grief, and the patient then developed Bryonia-type headaches which she had never had before. The inexperienced practitioner might consider this a dissimilar aggravation and change the remedy. But in a dissimilar aggravation the wrong remedy will manifest itself by a lack of improvement on any level while at the same time bringing out new symptoms. If it is the well-chosen remedy, however, the patient should have experienced improvement on the deeper planes, such as in processing the grief, feeling a sense of well-being, or enjoying deeper and more restful sleep. The patient often volunteers this type of information; if not, you need to ask, because one of the most common mistakes in practice is to give up too soon on the well-chosen remedy.

The same scenario may occur with a high potency acute remedy for a physical trauma: for example, I have given Rhus tox. 10M three or four times a day for an acute sprained ankle, with the result that the patient broke out in a fever blister while the ankle improved.

What to do? If the accessory symptoms are light and pass without undue suffering they are not obstacles to the cure. If they increase and persist, it is a sign that the remedy is only a partial simillimum (simile) which has done as much as it can. In this case, the case must be *retaken* and a corrective remedy given. So a partial simillimum will improve the patient only so far before one of these scenarios occurs:

- it no longer improves the case,
- the symptoms change, or
- accessory symptoms appear, increase and persist.

For all these circumstances, Hahnemann gives us guidance in Aphorism 168:

> In this way, one will more easily find an analogue, from among the known medicines, that corresponds to this new disease image. Even just a single dose of this [second] medicine, while not entirely annihilating the disease, will bring the case much closer to cure. And so one continues along (if even this medicine is not fully sufficient to restore health) examining again and again the disease state that still remains and selecting a homeopathic medicine that is as fitting as possible for it until the intention to place the patient in full possession of health is reached.

As I mentioned before, and as Hahnemann expresses in this paragraph, if the simillimum is not known yet because of our limited Materia Medica, then a successive series of similes can bring the cure in the long run (see Fig. 9-2). Each simile chips away at the symptom complex until we come to a reduced disease state for which we do have the simillimum, accomplishing our final goal: the cure of the patient.

Chapter Thirteen

Suppression

Hahnemann's Warning Two Hundred Years Ago

According to homeopathy's understanding of disease and healing, symptoms are relatively exterior manifestations of an underlying disorder; in fact, they are the expressions of the Vital Force reacting *against* a disease and not the disease itself. When the patient is treated so that some (not all) of the symptoms disappear while the underlying disorder is not addressed, the result is *suppression,* i.e. the *illusion* of cure while actually intensifying the internal disease by blocking some of its natural outlets. Hahnemann followed Nature's Laws when he warned against his colleagues' methods of driving symptoms deeper, in the false belief that a cure has been established. In Aphorism 201 he writes:

> When the human life force is burdened with a chronic disease that it cannot overwhelm with its own powers, it obviously decides (in an instinctual way) to form a local malady on a given external part … not indispensable to life … to allay the internal malady that threatens to annihilate vital organs and rob the patient of life … The local malady always remains nothing more than a part of the total disease … shifted onto a more harmless (outer) location of the body in order to allay the internal suffering.

What a wise observation—the same one made more than 5,000 years ago in Traditional Chinese Medicine, which makes "symptoms going from the interior to the exterior" part of its diagnosis of the Eight Conditions. Naturally, the body in its wisdom tries to alleviate the internal stress on the Vital Force caused by the disease or imbalance by pushing it to the exterior. Hahnemann says that although exteriorizing the symptoms does not cure the disease, at least it subdues it or makes it latent so that the individual can function. The same aphorism states:

> In this way, the presence of the external malady reduces the internal disease to silence for the present, however without being able to cure it or to essentially curtail it.

But, he says, at least it can do less harm because it is on the exterior part of the body. Hahnemann continues in Aphorism 202:

> If the local symptom is topically annihilated (by a physician ... who is of the opinion that he has thereby cured the whole disease) nature makes up for this by awakening the internal suffering and the rest of the symptoms that already existed and... *heightening the disease.*

The stronger the suppressive treatments, the more the internal symptoms will be aroused. This should be a lesson to the practitioner and patient alike not to mix allopathic and homeopathic prescriptions, mistakenly believing that this will provide "the best of both worlds." Unfortunately suppression in our era is far worse than in Hahnemann's time, when lack of hygiene and sanitation were the major factors causing disease. Today suppression is the major cause because it is so widespread and allopathic methods have become so "effective." Much stronger methods are now used, such as radiation, chemotherapy and powerful broad-spectrum antibiotics. The result is to make the homeopath's job more difficult. Most patients come to us with a history of lifelong suppression, beginning with antibiotics in infancy; the symptom picture is muddied by the lack of symptoms due to suppression; and the patient has to maintain faith in the homeopath while enduring the return of the suppressed symptoms following Hering's Law.

Natural and Artificial Suppression

Natural or Accidental Suppression: Suppression of the body's *normal* functions sometimes happens, not from medications but from the influence of an external factor. This can be a mental or emotional trauma such as fright, anger, vexation, sudden emotional shock, disappointment, grief, mental overwork, anticipation anxiety, hearing bad news, embarrassment, or humiliation; or a climate factor such as wet or excessive cold or heat. The *Repertory* is full of these rubrics like "Sleeplessness from grief" (or excitement), "Abdominal pain after vexation," "Menses suppressed, from grief" (or wet feet), "Perspiration, suppressed by chilling," and "Milk, suppressed by chilling."

We must not underestimate the power of suppression after an emotional shock in particular. As Kent used to say: "An emotional shock is equal in its suppressive powers to a thousand cups of coffee." The homeopath can resolve these conditions by prescribing for the totality, beginning with the Never Well Since. If he only addresses the symptoms, he will palliate at best, and at worst wake up a sleeping miasm. The patient will then need anti-miasmatic remedies for a full cure.

Another form of natural suppression can happen when one disease suppresses another *dissimilar* one, as Hahnemann observes in the *Organon*. An acute disease may suppress another acute one until the first one is cured; or it may suspend a chronic until the acute has run its course. For example, a chronic knee pain may be temporarily overshadowed by an acute, intense toothache.

These forms of natural suppression are fairly common and are amenable to homeopathic treatment, which will restore the suppressed natural function. They are not well treated by allopathic medicine because they do not fit its paradigm. Emotional triggers may be treated with a referral for psychotherapy (which is the next best referral besides homeopathy). But unfortunately, all too often, they are treated with neurotransmitter modulators such as Prozac and Zoloft, which only lead to further emotional suppression (as I have often heard from my patients, who complain of feeling emotionally "dead" or "flat" on these medications). As for suppression from a physical trigger, allopathic medicine does not recognize it or treat it. (The ICD-9 standard diagnostic manual does not list "suppressed menses from wet feet"!)

Artificial Suppression: Unfortunately, most doctors and patients alike look to removal of the symptoms as the goal of treatment. Recently I saw a TV ad for a herpes medication that actually boasted, "It is all about suppression!" But the most visible symptoms, the ones for which patients first request treatment, are also the Vital Force's attempts to keep the disease force on the least important external parts of the body, usually the skin. Look at the relatively innocuous initial manifestations of herpes zoster or shingles, syphilis and gonorrhea (before suppression leads to their more destructive secondary and tertiary stages).

Fifty years ago children's runny noses were treated with a quick wipe of the sleeve (efficient, cheap, and a horror for the Arsenicum mother!). Nowadays we push nasal sprays on our children and we suppress an innocuous outlet, resulting in many children suffering from asthma because their nose and cough symptoms were suppressed. Aggressive allopathic treatment tends to move the disease inward to the more important vital organs such as the lungs in this case, or the brain, heart, liver, or pelvic organs. Under homeopathic treatment correctly addressing the underlying miasm, the original suppressed manifestation should undoubtedly reappear. A homeopath with no understanding of miasms could unknowingly keep treating the surface symptoms and palliating the disease with superficial remedies rather than curing. Patients who were originally curable can thus become incurable through successive palliative treatments, whether homeopathic or allopathic. Indeed, unfortunately, the inexperienced homeopath can contribute to the phenomenon of artificial suppression by prescribing non-miasmatic remedies. If the real cause is not addressed, the disease keeps on getting worse, in spite of a few superficial symptoms being cured. This is a type of suppression since the centripetal evolution of the disease is not halted.

Some Specific Methods of Suppression

Medications of Contrary Action: We know that *all* allopathic drugs, in whatever form, assault the Vital Force, disharmonize it and add a drug picture to the disease picture (because of their primary and secondary action, as explained in Chapter Three, Laws and Principles). Different results are possible from giving an allopathic drug. If the symptoms caused by the drug (i.e. the side effects) are stronger than the natural symptoms of the disease, the symptoms of the patient will disappear (which illustrates the principle of one dissimilar disease suppressing the other). The suppression is then considered "successful" and the physician will claim to have *controlled* the disease (she never will claim to *cure* a chronic disease, as a cure is impossible without following the Law of Similars). However, if the patient's Vital Force is strong and intact, the symptoms of the patient will *reappear with the same or greater intensity* than before. The allopathic physician will call the patient *resistant to the drug*. The patient does not realize how lucky he is! Unfortunately, the physician will then resort to stronger suppressive measures.

The unfortunate soul whose Vital Force is weakened will respond to the drug with a worsened disease state which the physician will call *complications* or *side effects*. This case is different from the first scenario, which also had side effects, because in this case the original disease symptoms coexist with the new drug symptoms.

Dermatology and gynecology are responsible for more suppression than other specialties, because of their *local treatments* with creams, lotions, cauterizing and lasering. Rashes, itches, eczema and psoriasis, discharges, vaginitis, candidiasis, foot sweats and warts can all cause problems if suppressed. Western medicine recognizes genital warts in women as a risk factor for PID and infertility or cervical cancer, but it fails to recognize that *removal* of the warts *leads to* these other conditions.

The newest development in dermatology is a zinc spray for psoriasis, the most common skin ailment. I have seen many times in my own practice how skin conditions suppressed with zinc can lead to mental and emotional symptoms such as anxiety and depression. (The proof of this statement is in the cure: following the Laws of Hering, as the anxiety or depression is treated the skin condition returns temporarily, and then all the symptoms are gone for good. One of my patients suppressed his reappearing psoriasis with zinc ointment, with the inevitable result: his depression came back.) And the famous homeopath Compton Burnett, in *The Best of Burnett,* describes many cases of suppression. One was the case of an 8-month-old infant, the grandson of a physician who in spite of Burnett's protests treated the baby with zinc ointment for eczema of the scalp. Fourteen days later the suppression resulted in convulsions and death of the baby, and the grandfather shed bitter tears, realizing that his treatment had killed his grandson.[1]

Nuclear Medicine: At least Hahnemann did not have to contend with an even more severe form of suppression: radiation and radioactive isotopes. I have seen too many examples in my practice of patients who were in reasonably good health when diagnosed with cancer, whose Vital Force was irretrievably weakened by radiation and chemotherapy and whose quality of life was ruined by all the well-known side effects (hair loss, mouth sores, nausea and vomiting with resulting cachexia, etc.) It is very difficult for the homeopath to help patients whose Vital Force is so beaten down, and difficult to prove the effectiveness of homeopathy in treating cancer. The great homeopaths of the last century and the first part of this century were successful in treating many cases of cancer,[2] as homeopaths still are in India because they do not have to contend with the severe suppressive powers of radiation and chemotherapy. The homeopathic treatment of cancer is addressed in Chapter 24.

Surgery: Up until the 1880s surgery was considered a last resort. With the discovery of sterile technique and anesthesia, surgery has become the preferred mode of treatment, glamorized in the media and often expected by patients before medical options are given a chance. But surgery only removes the end-products of disease, not the imbalance in the body which created them. The human body is a work of art which should not be invaded with the surgeon's knife except as a last resort. Operations tend to be suppressive because they close an outlet for the release of a deeper internal disorder before the cause is cured (and even a plumber knows that this leads to trouble!). The surgical interventions which *are* necessary include the removal of obstructions, volvulus, embolisms, closed internal abscesses, and adhesions; repair of fractures and pyloric stenosis; and life-saving measures to re-establish vital signs. Cataract surgery is not suppressive since it involves the removal of dead tissue, although homeopathic treatment could have cured the cataracts if initiated early enough.

Surgery to remove a closed internal abscess (pyosalpinx, suppurative appendicitis with abscess formation or empyema) may or may not be necessary, depending on the indicated remedy. If Silica is indicated, it should not be given, since its well-known tendency to hasten suppuration could lead to spreading of the circumscribed area of suppuration. Here surgery should be performed instead. Calcarea carbonica could be safely given, however, because of its remarkable power to *absorb* pus.

So we cannot say that patients under competent homeopathic care never need surgery, just that they will need it less often. Why? Because most conditions requiring an operation are the last stages of disease, the structural end products rather than the functional beginnings. And homeopathy works most brilliantly in the functional stage of disease when there are many symptoms and few irreversible organic changes. Surgery may be needed for the removal of a mechanical obstruction, but first the *process* that caused it must be cured, or disease may follow in deeper, more vital regions where it cannot be cut out.

In my own practice I had a perfect example of a case in which surgery was necessary. The patient was a 45-year-old woman, who suddenly complained of strong, spastic abdominal pains. She did not respond to the well-chosen remedy, even in ever-increasing potency, and within the same day I sent her to the hospital, fearing an obstruction. After monitoring her for another day in which her condition worsened, the surgeon opened her and found one single string of an adhesion tightly wrapped around the colon. He told me it was the easiest operation he ever performed: one little snip and it was all over. So surgery saved her life—but again, the adhesion was *caused* by a previous abdominal surgery! (adhesions being a well-known unfortunate consequence of abdominal surgery). Any patient undergoing a pelvic operation should receive a single dose of Thiosinaminum 200c (3 pellets dry) followed by Graphites 6x (one teaspoon three times a day) for one month. This would greatly prevent these adhesions from occurring in the first place. And Elizabeth Wright-Hubbard used to dissolve adhesions with Kali muriaticum, even (as she admitted) prescribed on the pathology alone.

Surgical removal of polyps, hemorrhoids, fistulae, and inflamed tonsils, adenoids and appendixes should be postponed until homeopathy has been given a chance to heal them, which it often does. (Many appendix operations are not necessary; Belladonna or Bryonia can often heal an inflamed appendix. But if the inflammation does not respond quickly, a trip to the emergency room should not be delayed due to danger of peritonitis if the appendix ruptures.) In these conditions allopathic medicine seeks to remove pathology rather than cure the underlying causes, not realizing that such ultimates of disease are merely attempts at exteriorization, at protective localization. The surgeon should not operate as long as the homeopath has a hope of curing the case. Surgeons should also be well versed in medicine so that their judgment will be unbiased. Hahnemann wisely remarks that surgery, by removing external mechanical impediments, is only a means to help the Vital Force restore the injured parts of the organism.

A patient who has had many operations is dreaded by the homeopath because of the repetitive suppression; on the other hand, a patient who absolutely refuses a necessary operation is a danger to himself and the practitioner alike. Converts to homeopathy tend to become so passionate that they may refuse all allopathic treatment. Try to educate these patients to the importance of frequent supervision by a surgeon, in a situation where recommended surgery is being delayed in the hopes that homeopathic treatment will work. Ideally the surgeon should understand homeopathy, but of course this is rarely possible in the U.S. If the homeopath is not an M.D., allopathic supervision is especially important when surgery is being delayed, to protect both patient and practitioner. The first duty of a practitioner is to heal the sick, not to demonstrate a theory. We are all thoroughly convinced of homeopathic principles and of the apparent miracles possible with the right remedy; but Hahnemann himself never asked us to do anything unsafe for our patients. A homeopath must know when such a life-threatening emergency such as volvulus or intussusception can be resolved by a remedy such as Plumbum or Cuprum and when surgery is necessary. But a good homeopath rarely has to refer patients with varicose veins, hemorrhoids, or ulcers for surgery.

Palliation: Never forget that palliation of a curable case is suppression, and that it may be done quite as effectively by homeopathic remedies as by allopathic drugs. It will mask the true picture of the disease and complicate it to the point where a true cure will be hard to find. Unfortunately many homeopaths do this unknowingly. The issue of palliation will be addressed in depth in Chapter 16.

Thyroid and Adrenal Support Therapy (Glandular Suppression): The symptoms of low thyroid or adrenal function can be masked by giving glandular extracts or synthetic imitations. The result is not only suppression but also weakening of the gland as it becomes more and more dependent on the external source of the hormone. The patient will then need to take the hormone supplement for life in ever-increasing doses. This happens especially often with the common symptoms of low thyroid function (chilliness, weight gain, pallor, fatigue, etc.) These symptoms coupled to thyroid tests (TSH, T3, T4) are sufficient for physicians to prescribe thyroid for the rest of the patient's life. However, they never ask our all-important question: why is the thyroid out of balance? with the obvious corollary: how can we restore the balance so that the gland can produce its own hormones? Homeopathic treatment should be tested before resorting to replacement therapy. Thuja, Sepia, Nat. mur., and Iodum have often been used to restore function to the thyroid, although of course the simillimum can be whatever remedy is indicated. Only if the simillimum does not work will we give palliative remedies like Thyroidinum 6x (3 pellets dry to start) to prevent or limit the need for thyroid hormones.

Clinical Case: A 40-year-old woman came to me in 1996 with hypothyroidism. Her condition started in 1973 with signs of *hyper*thyroidism, treated in 1978 with radioactive Iodium, which suppressed the thyroid function to such an extent that by 1983 she became *hypo*thyroid. She did not require replacement therapy, however, as long as she was under homeopathic treatment in her native France. She stayed well until she moved to the US in 1993 and could not find a homeopathic physician at first. She was promptly put on Synthroid 0.05 mg daily. When she finally consulted with me, her time line revealed a succession of griefs including her parents' divorce, an abortion against her wishes, and her own divorce. Each of these losses was followed by a thyroid problem; but no physician had inquired as to the causality. Her case called for one of the classic grief remedies, Nat. mur. After one week on Nat. mur. LM1, 4 succussions, her old symptoms of *hyper*thyroidism came up quickly, accompanied by vivid memories of her past losses. I reduced the succussions to 2 and the Synthroid to half of her previous dose. The great sensitivity of her Phosphorus constitution brought her rapidly to an ever lower dose of Nat. mur. (only needing a dose q 14 days) and a total withdrawal of the Synthroid. Her energy stayed well and she slept well. She continued only with LM Nat. mur. prn for the next two years. She never needed another dose of Synthroid, she had no more symptoms of hypothyroidism, and her blood tests remained normal for the next two years (at which point I lost touch with her).

I have found Nat. mur. to have a profound effect on the thyroid, especially hypothyroidism (see Figure 13-1).

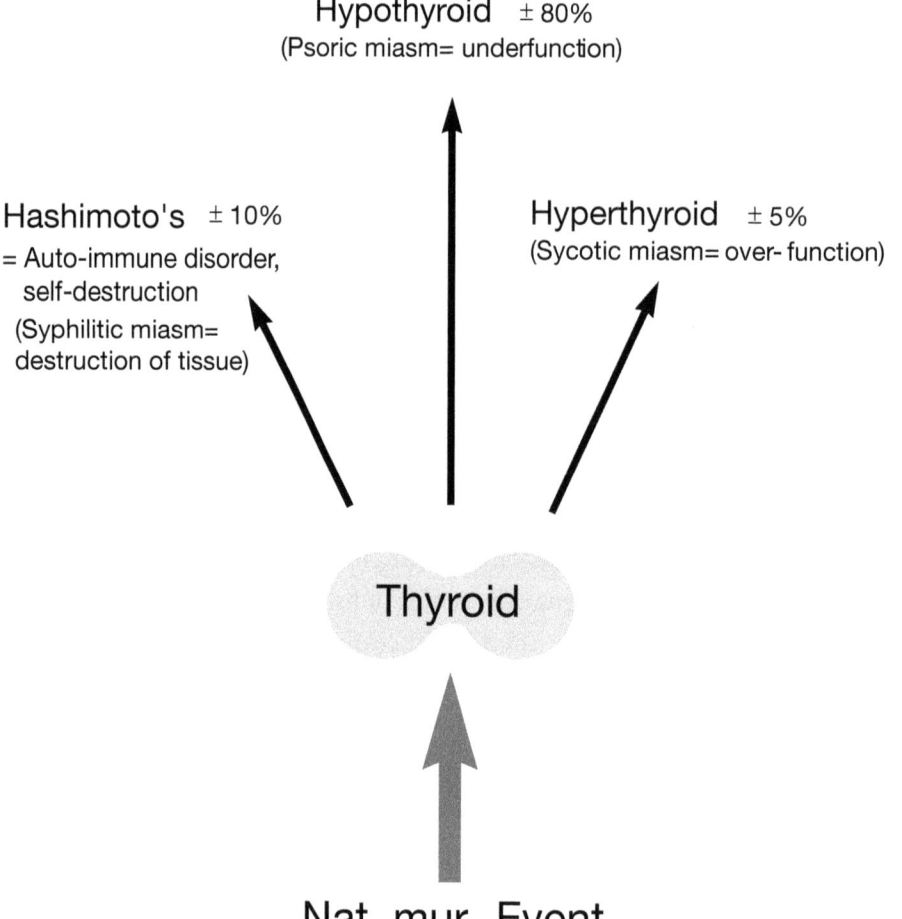

Fig. 13-1: Effect of Nat. mur. and the Miasms on the Thyroid

Treating Suppression

The sequelae of suppression are too easily accepted as sort of an evolution of the primary disease, even though allopathic treatment is actually *responsible*. In every case we must *"cherchez"* not *"la femme"* but *"la suppression,"* and when we find it many questions arise. Shall we prescribe for the symptom picture *before* the suppression took place? Shall we use the method of suppression as a symptom in our totality? Shall we prescribe primarily for the present post-suppressive syndrome? The old homeopaths had different opinions. If possible, I recommend returning to the original symptoms before the suppression took place. A perfect example is Carroll Dunham's cure of a case of deafness with Mezereum, based on the fact that Mezereum was the remedy for the eczema whose suppression led to the deafness.[3]

But there are no firm rules. The patient may have had a condition suppressed ten years ago, with the life-style, pathology and everything else changed in the meantime. In such a case you should first try prescribing on the present symptom picture, if it clearly indicates a remedy. If that does not work you will have to dig for the symptoms prior to the suppression.

As I will show in the following diagram, the suppression always drives the disease to a deeper level. An eczema case "treated" by cortisone creams, pills or injections often leads to asthma, at the second level of the physical plane (the essential organs). Five thousand years ago, the Chinese already saw this connection and placed *skin and lungs in the same element, Metal* (see Appendix 5 on Traditional Chinese Medicine). For the past hundred years, allopathic medicine has come to the conclusion that asthma and eczema are two different manifestations of the same disease. Homeopathy, on the other hand, views eczema as the disease and asthma as its suppressed form. The homeopath proves it by treating the asthma until the eczema comes back, at which point the asthma is cured for good; then he treats the eczema and cures that as well. (Unfortunately the eczema often comes back much more severely because of the suppression, to the point that the patient can hardly endure it, and it is difficult for patient and practitioner alike to let the eczema run its course—as it must if it is to be cured for good. Much will depend on the patient's confidence in the practitioner, how well he has explained the situation, and the patient's physical and mental endurance.) This is a situation in which LMs work better than centesimals because they are swifter, gentler, and easier to adjust, so that the patient will not suffer so much.

Only the strongest constitution can withstand repetitive suppressive treatments, which unfortunately usually continue until they are "successful." Figure 13-2, Levels of Suppression, shows the predictable consequences of suppression in general. (The symptoms within each layer are listed in order of deeper suppression.) It will be useful as a guideline in analyzing a case history and following the thread of how suppressive treatments (which you must always include in your inquiry) drove the illness deeper and deeper.

Outer Physical Level: the Skin
Hives, rashes
Herpes, eczema, discharges *(including from nose, ears, genitals)*
Ulceration, excoriation

Deeper Physical Levels
Joint inflammation with pains, recurrent sinusitis, fibromyalgia
Organs (heart, lungs, liver, GI tract, pelvic organs)

Deepest Physical Levels: Neurological
Vertigo, T.I.A., seizures *(no neurological damage)*
Brain infarcts, mini strokes, multiple sclerosis *(neurological damage)*

Emotional Level
Loves and hates, aversions and desires, weepiness, obsessive-compulsive behavior, recurrent dreams, apprehensions, loquacity, etc.

Indifference, lack of joie de vivre,
fears e.g. of death, darkness, misfortune, animals

Suicidal impulses and attempts, loathing of life

Mental Level
Brain fog *(occasional forgetfulness)*; loss of short-term memory

Loss of concentration, of train of thought;
forgetful of words while speaking

Mistakes in spelling, reading, calculating

Loss of long-term memory

Confusion/forgetfulness/disorientation *(does not recognize friends, well-known streets; confused as to his identity, mistakes in time—confuses present with past or future)*

Delusions *(deepest aberration)*

Fig. 13-2: Levels of Suppression

Levels of Suppression

Physical Level: There are three layers within the physical level: going from the periphery to the center, we find skin and joint symptoms, organ symptoms, and then the deepest affections on the physical plane, affections of the nervous system.

Any rashes, vesicles (as in herpes), bullae, and hives are common to the most superficial level, expressing a strong Vital Force as it tries to throw the internal disorder to a safe place, the skin. Belonging to this layer are also ulcers, excoriations, and all the discharges (from any orifice or pore). Unfortunately the patient and physician, equally misinformed, direct their most frequent forms of suppression to these conditions. The patient typically uses OTC cortisone creams and the physician treats acute "exacerbations" with high doses of oral or I.V. cortisone. This will lead to a suppression of symptoms to the next layer, that of the precious organs such as the lungs, with asthma readily accepted by allopathy as a "normal" evolution from eczema. Suppression with cortisone can also lead to ulcerative colitis, Crohn's disease, rheumatoid arthritis, and lupus. (I have seen several patients who developed lupus after taking steroids for hair transplants or alopecia areata). Traditional Chinese Medicine can explain how suppression from the skin goes mainly to the lungs and the large intestine since they are all part of the Metal group in the Five Elements. Note that the so-called auto-immune disorders are well represented in this list. Kent also cites rubrics for head congestion, head pain, eye inflammation, dim vision, ear pain, deafness, constipation, diarrhea, and chest constriction from the suppression of menses, foot sweat, and "innocent" eruptions.

If the suppressive allopathic treatment continues (especially when the patient is sensitive), neurological deficits may come up next in the form of tic douloureux, seizures, vertigo, TIA's (transient ischemic attacks, often the forerunners of strokes), brain infarcts, or multiple sclerosis. Rubrics in Kent for suppression leading to neurological symptoms include convulsions from suppressed discharges, eruptions, foot sweat, or milk; unconsciousness from suppressed menses or eruptions; and vertigo from suppressed eruptions or menses (K90, K91, K101, K1355).

Clinical Case: A 12-year-old boy came to my office with a Chief Complaint of grand-mal seizures, occurring once a month. His history was revealing and a perfect example of the above principle. He was born with eczema due to medications his mother took while pregnant (thus expressing Hering's Law: the eczema was the Vital Force's attempt to push the drugs to the exterior, the skin). The eczema was so severe that it took two years to suppress with cortisone. The moment his eczema disappeared asthma came up, and the cortisone creams were replaced with cortisone inhalers and oral steroids for the frequent acute attacks. This continued until he was eleven years old. He had his last asthma attack in December of that year and his first seizure the next month. From then on he had one seizure a month and never another asthma attack. Each time a deeper illness took the place of the previous less dangerous one, because of continued suppression. This was proved to the parents when I treated the epilepsy and the asthma returned, to be replaced by the eczema, which in turn cleared up. Five years later the boy has had no seizures, no asthma attacks and no signs of eczema.

I am only one doctor yet I have seen this scenario hundreds of times in my practice. I can only shudder at the thought of how many people are made worse every day by *well-meaning* physicians who ignore Nature's Laws and work against the Vital Force, not with it.

Emotional Level: In practice we see many emotional symptoms following suppression, the most common being depression (reflected for example in the rubric "Mind, sadness, after suppressed menses," K77). Other examples include recurrent nightmares, weepiness, obsessive-compulsive behavior and phobias such as claustrophobia, agoraphobia and fear of heights. On the deepest emotional level we find suicidal impulses. A perfect example was the patient already mentioned: he became depressed after suppressing his psoriasis with zinc ointment; the remedy relieved his depression but brought back the psoriasis; when he suppressed it again with the zinc ointment, his depression came back.

We are only one step away from the deepest level of suppression: the mental level.

Mental Level: Mental symptoms often go from an occasional forgetfulness (that dreadful brain fag) to loss of short-term memory. Concentration seems to be affected, as the patient loses her train of thoughts or even forgets simple words. (I remember a patient struggling to tell me her foot was hurting because she simply could not recall the word. In her history I found that years before, a widespread eczema was "successfully treated" with cortisone shots and ointment.) Patients make mistakes in reading, writing, calculating, balancing the checkbook and spelling at work or in school (think about all the ADD children who belong to this group). Upon further suppression, loss of long-term memory can occur and confusion as to where the patient lives or even his own identity. He may start confusing the present with the past or future. I read in the paper of one poor fellow, a university professor covered all over with an intractable case of psoriasis, who was covered with cortisone cream, wrapped in saran wrap, and placed in a sauna as a last-ditch effort at treatment. He came out of the sauna without his psoriasis—and also without his mind. He had completely lost his memory.

Finally come the deepest mental aberrations, the delusions and manias. Kent lists these mental conditions from apparently harmless suppression (rash, perspiration or menses), including insanity from suppressed eruptions or menses (K57) and mania from suppressed eruptions or menses (K64).

Remedies for Suppression

Using the diagram, the homeopath can determine how deep the suppression went and predict how the recuperation will unfold, following Hering's Laws. When we speak of the re-appearance of old symptoms we are often dealing with lifelong suppressions. In terms of remedies useful in treating suppressions, Sulphur stands first, of course. Perhaps Pulsatilla ranks second, particularly for chronic work. Apis is important for attacks on the brain following suppressions.

Dr. Knerr compiled the following list of remedies for symptoms resulting from suppression, from Hering's *Guiding Symptoms:*

Sulphur: throbbing headaches, vertigo, amblyopia and many other eye troubles; deafness from suppressed measles; asthma from suppressed itch and asthma alternating with psoriasis; convulsions and paralysis.

Apis: inflammation of the brain, hydrocephalus after suppressed eruptions in general; shortness of breath and asthma from suppressed urticaria.

Pulsatilla: asthma from suppressed rash in children, from suppressed urticaria, from suppressed eruptions in general; deafness after measles.

Arsenicum: pericarditis after suppressed measles; asthma from suppressed itch or suppressed eruptions in general.

Rhus tox.: swelling of parotid gland after scarlatina; chorea after suppressed measles.

Zincum metallicum: loss of sensation, chorea, convulsions; muscular twitching; numbness all over, better with rubbing and massage.

Ipecac: asthma from suppressed eruptions in general.

After *suppression of eruptions,* the following symptoms are helped by the noted remedies:

Convulsions	*Camphor, Stramonium, Cicuta*
Epilepsy	*Causticum, Agaricus*
Headaches	*Graphites, Nux moschata*
Paralysis	*Dulcamara*
Dyspnea with receding rash	*Bryonia*

We all know how effective *Bryonia* and *Rhus tox.* are in cases where sweat is suppressed by a sudden dash into cold water, as children love to do on hot days.

For the diarrhea of children suppressed by medications: *Opium* and *Zinc.*

For children whose mental and emotional development has been suppressed by living in a state of fear (perhaps of an alcoholic parent): *Opium*

Each of these remedies is associated with a particular form of suppression or area of expression: for instance note that *Zincum* is especially good for nervous imbalances from suppression; *Apis* has its characteristic congestion and inflammation; *Sulphur* expresses itself widely in psoric manifestations; and *Nux vomica* in older people where the suppressions are due to overuse of medications, alcohol or narcotics, or where there is much strain from business affairs. (We rarely see the indications of Nux vomica in the suppression of children's symptoms).

A clinical case of Dr. Julia Green illustrates the principle of suppression:

> During the severe influenza epidemic this boy was given up to die with double pneumonia and suspected empyema. He had been ill for 4 to 5 days. Homeopathy was tried as a last resort. After ordering an interval of several hours without drugs, I went at night to sit by the bedside and watch for symptoms. Suppression had been so violent that nothing could be observed but deep coma, irregular pulse and respiration, great pallor and entirely limp and barely alive. Finally I noticed a few fine muscular twitchings. After nearly four hours the eyelids parted and the high shrill cry came: "Rub my feet." The mother complied telling me that the child had asked for this before he went into coma and had been soothed by the rubbing. It was only one symptom but it was a peculiar one, always welcomed by the prescriber (see Kent, "Extremities, numbness, while lying," Zinc (3). A dose of Zinc 10M brought that boy to consciousness within one hour. No other medicine was needed, the dose was repeated once in the next ten days and within two weeks the boy was playing again.[4]

Another case illustrating the sequelae of suppression dates from 1854. While the medical treatment is outdated, the homeopathic treatment is still illumining. Note that the homeopath begins with polychrests, which no doubt cover the patient's overall picture as well as the suppressive treatments, before giving a specific remedy for the pathology. The homeopath's comments on how the patient was referred to him are also just as apropros now as they were 100 years ago when this case was published.

> P. B., 33 years old, called me at the end of June 1854. He had suffered from scabies, which was cured and eliminated by the ordinary dangerous method of ointments. He had been affected three times with gonorrhea and once by syphilitic ulcers. It is useless to mention the quantity of medicines which allopathy suggested for the treatment of this patient. Pills and powders, ointments, leeches, different injections, mercurial preparations, etc. We only state that by the latter treatment [the mercury] the patient suffered from excessive salivations and affection of the gums. The gonorrhea,

with all its sickly consequences, took the character of orchitis. After the prescription of leeches, ointments and purgatives of Sarsaparilla, the right testicle became swollen and hard. This manifestation took such a proportion that a prominent surgeon thought the testicle calcified and advised castration. But, as the patient objected to this, his friends advised homeopathic treatment.

This is the ordinary way by which so many patients call us. They call for help after having been ill treated by the allopaths and finally they use a medicine which they never thought would have been efficacious. Sometimes they are sent to us by the advice of the very person who ill treated them, for the getting rid of a patient whose disease could not be cured.

When I saw and examined the patient, I was extremely stuck by the large size of the testicle. It was 6.5" in length and 2.5" in breadth. It was floating in water in a state of hydrocoele. Concomitant symptoms: a feeling of weight in the scrotum with a pain during the change of the weather; arrest of gonorrheal discharge with itching in urinating; constriction of the urethra; cracking of the joints and rheumatism in the winter; tired expression of the face; skin of bad color. I administered several remedies according to symptoms: Sulphur 1M, Puls 200c, Silica 24c, Mercury 200c, Clematis 3c (I did not have a higher potency), Aurum 200c and Rhododendron 1200c. I used to give of each medicine only one dose, dissolved in a little water, which the patient took three times a day. All the above mentioned remedies produced their action more or less efficaciously, but Rhododendron acted the strongest. At last, after a treatment of four months, the patient to everyone's astonishment, completely recovered. The testicle had returned to the normal size. All other abnormalities had disappeared, and health was restored. The patient lived for another thirty years, and always enjoyed perfect health.[5]

It is my sincere hope that my allopathic colleagues will start recognizing the dangers of suppression. Otherwise the task of the homeopathic physician will continue to become more difficult, since suppression is already a major obstacle to the cure.

Chapter Fourteen

Obstacles to the Cure

When the Indicated Remedy Fails

We already mentioned that the true test of the homeopath's skill comes at the patient's second appointment. The practitioner will be confronted with many questions, one of them possibly, "I thought I had prescribed the right remedy, yet there is no reaction." It is here that the experienced homeopath will shine while the beginner will panic. What to do? What to ask? Do we admit defeat and try intuition or a good guess? This course of action may lead us to a brilliant hit but it could also lead to a hopelessly confused, mixed-up case. The better approach is to search for possible obstacles to recovery. The practicing homeopath should have a list of these obstacles in her mind which she can consult point by point like a Sherlock Holmes, leaving no stone unturned. Only then will she be able to pick up the thread that will bring her through the labyrinth of the patient's history. Let us consider step by step all the possible obstructions to the gentle, rapid and permanent cure.

The Patient Withholds Information

An incorrect prescription is not always due to the homeopath's mistake. Sometimes he does not have the essential information he needs. The patient may not feel comfortable disclosing it at first. We rely heavily on mental/emotional symptoms, but patients will not tell you that they are egotistical, secretive or unfaithful! As you get to know the patient better, he will open up to you and answer more honestly regarding his mental state. Few patients will tell you on the first visit that they are jealous or obsessive-compulsive, or that they have a sexual perversion. But as you gain their trust, you will get a more complete picture of the patient.

Sometimes the patient thinks certain events are *not worth mentioning*. Certainly the patient has been affected by the reaction of doctors who routinely discard important information as "not being pertinent" (because allopaths do not know how to use that piece of the patient's history).

Depending on the patient's *constitution* and what remedy she needs, she may not be willing to share her story with you. Where we can expect a Phosphorus person to be very open and communicative, even to smile while discussing her serious illness, a Nat. mur. patient will be on the defensive, afraid to leave her cocoon. Nat. murs. will answer the intake questionnaire on the smallest possible piece of paper, then hide it under a blank sheet of paper so no else can see it. They are upset if the receptionist calls out their name in the waiting room, as if they did not want anyone to know they were coming for an appointment. They answer verbal questions with a short "yes" or "no" and become offended by extensive questions, as if you are trying to pry open their shell. They send the silent message, "That's none of your business." Of course what they don't realize is that their behavior itself has given them away! Once a Nat. mur. warms up to her homeopath she becomes his greatest supporter, as she appreciates the one-on-one conversation and the genuine interest of the homeopath.

Clinical Case: A 23-year-old consulted me for a variety of problems including an irregular menstrual cycle, headaches, fatigue, and episodes of depression which all started (she said) since she started taking the birth control pill. I was careful to ask whether anything else happened at the onset, but she denied it. I prescribed Sepia and the only improvement was a regular menstrual cycle. It was clear that Sepia was the simile, not the simillimum, and her other symptoms pointed to Nat. mur. So I asked again about other precipitating events, specifically about any griefs or losses. She finally admitted that at the onset of her condition she had been devastated when her fiancé broke off their engagement, but she thought that "it was not important enough to mention" and "probably had nothing to do with my symptoms." The patient's misperception was the obstacle to the cure, and Nat. mur. resolved everything.

Sometimes the required information is *too painful* for the patient to divulge. I remember a Phosphorus patient suffering from rheumatoid arthritis for eight years. With each flare-up cortisone was administered, which caused an initial aggravation before her symptoms subsided. (Of course she was given the standard dosage, not adjusted for the sensitivity of a Phosphorus). I inquired about a possible trigger factor, but she denied any. When I asked, "How many children do you have?" she burst into tears and her husband had to continue the story. He revealed that their middle daughter had moved away two months before the first attack. The mother missed her and the two grandchildren terribly. But in order to cope she suppressed her grief, which the body expressed in her symptoms.

While pain and heartbreak may prevent the telltale story, *shame* can be another factor, for example if the patient has STDs in his past medical history. A professional gambler consulted me with complaints of fatigue after eating, especially worse after garlic and onions. I thought about Thuja. Since he was not willing to give me more keynotes (typical of the secretive sycotic miasm), I asked him if he ever had warts. "Genital warts twenty years ago," he said, and also that he had previously suffered from acute gonorrhea. Of course these conditions confirmed Thuja/Medorrhinum. Also his profession—gambling is a form of thrill seeking—pointed to the sycotic miasmatic remedies.

The Patient Gives a Confusing or Inadequate Report

The patient may also fail to give the necessary information about her reactions to the remedy, instead giving the misleading report that "nothing happened." Patients are not educated to note their symptoms carefully. I always ask my patients to send me reports at least every three weeks by fax or letter. (Brief weekly check-ins by phone can be even better, especially in the first month. You can suggest to your patients that they call after hours and leave a report on their progress; and if they had to adjust the remedy, to report why and what they did to adjust it. Tell them you will call back if you think they should be doing something else; otherwise you will add their message to their patient file.)

How often have I heard, when explaining what can happen after the first dose of the remedy: "You mean I have to start paying attention to my body?" As logical as this may seem to you and me, it is not always to patients who are used to allopathic drugs and expect your remedy to do wonders while they attend to more serious affairs (as if there is anything more important than health!). Many people are too distracted to pay enough attention to symptom changes.

The patient's inability or unwillingness to cooperate wholeheartedly may lessen his chances of a cure. I usually ask my patients to read one of my books (*Human Condition Critical*) which teaches them how to look for pertinent information to solve their case. Patients often submit a whole new timeline after reading the book! Keep in mind that the non-judgmental attitude of the practitioner helps to overcome shyness, shame and grief. Of course, the practitioner must re-analyze the case if the patient finally gives her the information she originally wanted.

Hypersensitive patients are a blessing and a curse: a blessing because they are so exquisitely sensitive to the remedies that they often know immediately whether the remedy is right for them; a curse because they find it so difficult to sort out their own reactions. Phosphorus patients in particular have a poor sense of boundaries between themselves and other people or other energies in the universe. When you ask them to report on their reaction when they first start taking the remedy, their response may be all over the map. One patient called to say she had stopped the remedy because she developed what felt like a sinus headache without any actual sinusitis, so she attributed it to the remedy. She called back the following day to report a false alarm. Her daughter had called from a distant city and the patient reported that her headache vanished immediately when she realized she was picking up on her daughter's sinusitis. "It happens all the time," she said matter-of-factly. "When my daughter gets a headache, I need ibuprofen."

Another Phosphorus lady reported a reaction of feeling more depressed on the remedy, then called later to say it was actually the spirit of her deceased grandmother visiting her to process some family issues. Yet another Phosphorus (a man this time) initially blamed the remedy when he felt himself growing more and more angry during an all-day meditation session, a situation which usually made him feel very peaceful. Finally, at the end of the day, he realized that he had been picking up on the energy field of the woman sitting behind him, who had been extremely upset all day. Fortunately each of these patients figured out what was really causing their reaction; most times, however, the poor homeopath is left scratching her head trying to sort out the meaning of the reactions they report! When the time comes to give them Phosphorus (which many of them need anyway) they develop a better sense of the inner core of their own being without losing their psychic sensitivities and sympathetic qualities.

The Patient Fails to Take the Remedy Correctly

If the remedy does not seem to be working, or if the patient is having a reaction quite different from what you expect, you should always make sure that the patient has actually *taken* the remedy or (in the case of LM potencies) has taken it *correctly*. Instead of repeating the instructions, ask them to explain to you *exactly* how they have taken it. From experience I can tell you that you can never be too sure of anything! Patients may drink the whole cup or succuss the cup instead of the bottle. They may assume that 4 oz. means a half cup when they are filling only a small cup, so that half the cup is barely 2 to 3 oz. Or they may use a large household spoon (closer to a tablespoon) instead of a teaspoon, which is why you should give them a standard med cup to measure their dosage with. Patients have all kinds of misconceptions about the remedies, and I am never surprised at anything any more. Some patients stop the remedy because they say it brings up suppressed sexual feelings, and one man stopped the remedy because his pain disappeared so quickly he thought I had given him morphine!

Negative Influence from Other People

>There is something harder and stronger than bronze or marble: it is prejudice.
>
>—*Horace*

The patient might be convinced that he wants your treatments, in fact he usually desires it very much. Unfortunately, negative dynamics in the family often change his mind. Family members, friends, or physicians who are opposed to your treatments (because of the unfortunate ignorance about homeopathy in this society) might tell your patient to "stop going to that quack and consult a *real* doctor." (My patients heard this all the time, even though I *am* an

M.D.!) Homeopathic treatment is often considered "substandard treatment" and homeopathic physicians have had their licenses taken away in this country precisely for that undeserved reason. (The legal situation for homeopaths in the U.S. is worse than perhaps in any other country in the world.)

Patients themselves demand and expect from their homeopaths much more than from their allopathic physicians. It is beyond imagination what the patients ask you to do: to be tactful so they don't lose their jobs, to protect them from their mother-in-law, to mediate with the schools on the vaccination issue, to get their children to eat and do their homework and their wives to enjoy sex, to change their bad habits and to give them the courage to face suffering and death. (Of course we *can* do many of these things!) They will come with a disease of 20 years' duration and say, "I am giving homeopathy one month and then if I can't see any improvement, I am going back to my real doctor."

Whenever the homeopath performs such a miracle, they consider it normal and take it in stride or even ask for the next miracle. Just to take one example among many: a couple brought their 33-year-old daughter to see me because she had been suffering from delusions, had suffered a total personality change, and was completely unable to function in life or take care of herself since a head trauma in a car accident when she was 18. They had already consulted *42 different doctors,* none of whom had been able to help in the slightest! She was completely cured and back to playing the piano after only ten doses of Nat. sulph. LM1, but her parents treated this unusual outcome as normal and never expressed any surprise or gratification. Even if some of these "miraculous" cures do not win us our patients' eternal gratitude, we must accept this as an expression of human nature and continue our beloved work. For myself, I do not need any thanks, but I would like to see homeopathy given full credit for its cures.*

Instead, unfortunately, when the homeopath performs a cure, the allopath will often claim that the diagnosis was wrong (although he himself made the diagnosis). If by chance the disease takes a turn for the worse (because it was incurable or the patient is still taking suppressive medications), the allopath will blame your remedy. Allopathy wants to have it both ways, claiming that homeopathy cannot possibly cure because the remedies have nothing in them, yet blaming the remedies for any negative outcomes. Patients will also be warned not to take these (supposedly inert and ineffective) remedies because they will interfere with

---

*Even Hahnemann complained about patients' lack of appreciation in a letter to Dr. Erhardt: "The world is ungrateful! Rich patients also should pay at each consultation immediately, otherwise they might go away without paying."[1]

medications! Often my cancer patients (who I treated mainly for the side effects of chemotherapy and radiation and to increase their quality of life) were given the misinformation that remedies could interfere with their conventional treatment. My patients often take their child to the pediatrician for a cold or ear infection. Coming home with the inevitable prescription for antibiotics, the mother would call me for a remedy, saying she didn't believe in giving her child antibiotics (of course they paid the pediatrician, but not me!). And guess what would happen if anything went wrong? Only the homeopath would get blamed.

One of my asthma patients discontinued her steroid medications in spite of explicit instructions from me (which I give to all my patients) that she must keep taking her medications until the remedy worked well enough that she didn't need them any more. She had an asthma attack that landed her in the emergency room and told her doctor that *I had instructed her* to discontinue the medication! Can you imagine the legal problems if she had died? In these dire circumstances, the homeopath often finds himself all alone and needs all his confidence, strength and courage to keep going. Yet he must, for he knows the truth of homeopathy.

Sometimes the patient will succumb to family pressure and start mixing allopathic drugs with your remedies without telling you. (While it is true we tell patients to continue any necessary medications until the remedies work, it is essential to know what medications the patient is on, when they start taking them, and what their side effects are. If patients are already on a medication, they should continue; but if they have not yet started, it would be better if they could just give homeopathy a chance and not mix the two modalities.) Since allopathic medicine and homeopathy are based on opposite laws, the homeopath's task is made more difficult (not impossible) through continued drug suppression. The homeopath has to battle constantly against heavy odds to demonstrate the superiority of homeopathy.

Excessive Use of Medications

American people are the most sensitized in the history of the world. They are severely debilitated by their effete way of life. Any pain (physical or emotional) is intolerable and even a slight discomfort must be resolved immediately. Thus the demand for fast-acting drugs has arisen, with a resulting plague of drug dependency and addiction. Sometimes the action of our remedies is hampered by drugs prescribed by the most esteemed doctor of all time—the TV commercial. Commercials induce patients to demand medications from their physicians to relieve all their ills, real or imagined. Among the four most-prescribed drugs in the U.S. are two antidepressants (Zoloft® and Prozac®) and two anti-ulcer medications (Prilosec® and Zantac®). The tremendous cost ($1,100 per patient/year) could easily be offset by homeopathic remedies at one cent a day! And now that the rules on advertising on TV are more and more relaxed, the situation will get worse.[2]

Often before the homeopath can even start the patient on the indicated remedy, she has to reverse the effects of excessive medications by prescribing Nux vomica for several weeks in an LM or 6c potency.

Clinical Case: A 30-year-old executive for a pharmaceutical company consulted me for hair loss. He led a disastrous life-style: partying, drinking, and using recreational drugs as well as medications. Nux vomica was indicated for several reasons: not only for this Sulphur person's Nux vomica life-style (competitive, ambitious, high-stress, dependent on stimulants), but also to counteract the bad effects of drugs and alcohol (Nux vomica is a great liver cleanser). As Hering's Law would predict, within five days after the first LM doses, his body was covered with itchy eruptions. I explained the cleansing effect of the remedy and encouraged him to continue it, although with fewer succussions to slow down the process. To his amazement the rash disappeared. He felt so good that he stopped taking his remedy after three weeks (you can expect that from a Nux vomica patient!). One month later when he started feeling bad again, I told him to resume the remedy. This time he broke out in an even worse rash, which prompted him to consult his physician at work. This physician claimed that if he had taken another dose of my remedy, it would have killed him because "obviously" the patient was "allergic" to my remedy. (We can forgive the doctor for not knowing that an allergic reaction is impossible because there is not even one molecule left in an LM potency. But he displayed ignorance of his own system of medicine: if the original rash were an allergic reaction, it would have gotten worse instead of disappearing under the continuing action of the remedy.) The physician had to administer three weeks of oral cortisone to "cure" the eruptions. Obviously this patient was lost to homeopathy: every time I did the right thing, a rash would have to reappear.

When the obstacle to the cure is an allopathic medication, sometimes the homeopath can resort to *tautopathy:* using a homeopathic preparation of it to counteract its side-effects. For instance, if the patient tells you that all his symptoms started since he took a round of penicillin, you can prescribe Penicillin 6c or LM. A better method would be to prescribe Thuja since it covers "Never Well Since antibiotics" and is a much broader-working remedy, covering the sycotic miasm which is so prevalent in our society. (The fact that the patient had such a reaction to an antibiotic is a good indication that the sycotic miasm was already present, because it is fueled by antibiotics). In general (as I explained in the discussion of polychrests vs. small remedies in Chapter 9), I would always open with the polychrest, Thuja in this case, and only if it failed would I resort to a specific small remedy like Penicillin. In my own practice I have only had to resort to tautopathy twice in a case like this.

Life-style Factors, Drugs and Alcohol

The patient's life-style or changes therein can influence and obstruct your treatment. If a remedy suddenly stops working, it is wise to ask your patient about any changes in life-style. I have treated patients diagnosed with Chronic Fatigue who felt so good on the remedy that they resumed their hectic night life, resulting in a disastrous downturn in their health. Common sense should have dictated that a negative life-style fueled the chronic disease, as Hahnemann expressed so wisely in Aphorism 77.

Homeopathy also has antidotes for the sins of this world. The following chart indicates which remedies can be used for immediate after-effects (like a hangover) and/or a chronic "Never Well Since" situation.

Substance	Remedy
Beer	Nux vomica, Asarum, Kali bich.
Wine	Zincum, Nux vomica
Whiskey and hard liquor	Ledum, Sulphur
Alcohol	Sulphuric acid *(the equivalent of Antabuse)*
Tea	Pulsatilla, Thuja
Coffee	Chamomilla, Nux vomica, Coffea
Fats	Pulsatilla, Nux vomica
Sugar	Argentum nitricum
Cigarettes	Caladium, Lobelia
Marijuana	Cannabis indica
Recreational drugs	Avena sativa tincture, Nux vomica
Excessive or promiscuous sex	Medorrhinum, Fluoric acid, Platina

Incurable Diseases

Obviously, the nature of the disease or the advanced state of pathology might prevent the cure. This situation is discussed at length in Chapter 16, Palliation and Incurable Diseases. We are fortunate that as homeopaths we can offer the patient great palliative treatment.

Clinical Case: A beautiful and lively 83-year-old Phosphorus lady consulted me after allopathic medicine gave up on her. After opening the abdomen and seeing how much her cancer had metastasized, her doctor simply closed her up and told to go home as she only had three months to live. Yet she lived for another two years in excellent physical and emotional condition. I will never forget her smiling face as she came on consult, always nicely dressed up and flirting (like a true Phosphorus!) and loving her "arsenic" as she called her remedy. She felt so good that she told me she planned to return for more tests, believing her cancer was gone. I knew otherwise and quietly took her daughter aside, advising her to take her mother shopping instead, which she still very much enjoyed. Repeated confirmation of her cancer could have led to a sudden downturn in her condition, as I have seen thousands of times when patients hear the "bad news" of their cancer diagnosis and their health suddenly spirals downhill. Only when there was perforation of the bladder and colon by the tumor did this patient die quickly in the hospital with only minimal suffering. But she lived those two years to the fullest extent.

Paucity of Symptoms

The Vital Force of the patient may be too weak to throw enough symptoms up to find the simillimum. Different ways of resolving such a *mute case* were described in Chapter 10, Golden Rules and Special Forms of Prescribing.

Limited Knowledge of the Materia Medica

Hahnemann writes in *Chronic Diseases:*

> As to the second* chief error in the cure of chronic diseases (the unhomeopathic choice of medicine) the homeopathic beginner (many, I am sorry to say, remain such beginners their life long) arises chiefly through inexactness, lack of earnestness, and through love of ease.[3]

While it is impossible to memorize the whole of the Materia Medica, an excellent way of learning the remedies is to study the top two or three remedies in each case. Consult several Materia Medicas, looking for symptoms which differentiate the remedies and making a list of the patient's symptoms which indicate each one. Gradually you will learn the remedies most frequently encountered in your practice.

It is a mistake of the beginner not to consult the *Repertory* and Materia Medica in front of the patient, lest he is thought not "well read" or "advanced" in his profession. My experience has been just the reverse: patients appreciate the difference from their previous experience with doctors and are favorably impressed with your care and caution. They will certainly value your hour-long intake compared to the ten-minute consult with the allopath.

---

*The first mistake was failing to give the minimum dose: "The first error I have already spoken of, and would only add that nothing is lost if the dose is given even smaller than I have prescribed. It can hardly be too small." *(ibid.)*

I suggest to my students the following *plan for systematic remedy study:*

- Considering the importance of an understanding of the miasms, start by listing the main symptoms of the remedy in several Materia Medicas and then determine which miasm each one is associated with, using the table in Appendix 3. This exercise will help you become more familiar with the symptoms of each miasm as well as with the picture of the remedy you are studying. When you are done, you can add up the symptoms appearing in each column to determine how active the remedy is against each miasm.
- Start with the mental and emotional symptoms, since the innermost being is most important. You would not give Phosphorus to one who was abnormally modest, nor Arsenicum to a slob. (This sounds like negative prescribing, but when a characteristic is so outspoken we have to find it in the patient.) Unfortunately, many of our remedies do not have a fully developed proving of mental symptoms, but where they exist they are of prime importance. For instance, take your time in studying my favorite, Margaret Tyler's beautiful portraits of the remedies in her *Homeopathic Drug Pictures.* I prefer the old masters to the modern Materia Medicas which are mainly copied from the old masters. Go to the primary source!*
- Try to find the *disease causations* associated with each remedy (its typical Never Well Since). They are of particular importance and often difficult to find in books. I have given the reader an extensive list in Appendix 2, and the reader should feel free to add to it.
- Note the *clearly marked modalities,* in other words aggravation or amelioration by such things as temperature, motion, position, touch, being jarred, etc. The marked *desires and aversions* should become etched in the student's mind.
- Next, study the *localities* of the body to which the remedy applies, and make a chart of a human figure, marking the vulnerable points of the remedy. Not only the *organs* influenced by a remedy should be noted but also the *tissues* (for example, Bryonia affects the serous membranes).
- Pick out the "strange, rare and peculiar" symptoms and the so-called keynotes of the remedy.

---

*I make an exception for Catherine Coulter's wonderful *Portraits of Homeopathic Medicines,* which are a universal favorite among my students. Coulter quotes extensively from the old masters and adds examples from her own practice as well as current literature, even cartoons, giving a modern flair and an articulate, highly literate exposition to the works of the old masters. The three volumes together only cover several dozen remedies, but they are the best place to start learning those remedies, which are among the most common polychrests.

- Learn which acute remedies are associated with each polychrest (see the chart in Chapter 10). If you know your patient consistently needs Belladonna or Rhus tox., it will help you to prescribe Calcarea for his chronic condition.
- Make a "remedy clock," a diagram showing the time of general aggravation for the remedies you are studying (because the aggravation time is often a keynote of the remedy).

Study each remedy in different Materia Medicas, as no author sees all aspects of a remedy. My favorites are Kent's *Lectures on Homeopathic Materia Medica,* Nash's *Leaders in Homeopathic Therapeutics,* Allen's *Keynotes of the Materia Medica,* Clarke's *Dictionary of Practical Materia Medica,* Hering's *Guiding Symptoms,* Tyler's *Homeopathic Drug Pictures,* Phatak's *Materia Medica of Homeopathic Medicines* and Hahnemann's *Materia Medica Pura.*

Lack of Proven Remedies

The lack of new remedy provings is an unfortunate obstacle to full knowledge of Materia Medica. The true simillimum in a case may not be known yet, since less than 1% of the possible remedy substances have been proven. We must express our appreciation, support and encouragement for those conducting modern provings so that they continue their important work. Hahnemann lamented the lack of proven remedies in his armamentarium. While we have several thousand more remedies than he did, the simillimum in a particular case may not have been discovered and proven yet. In such cases a nosode may be helpful to address the underlying miasmatic state.

Tolle Causam: Remove the Cause

Hahnemann writes in Aphorism 252 that if the well-selected remedy in the appropriate dose does not work,

> then this is a *certain* sign that the cause maintaining the disease still persists. Some circumstance is to be found in the regimen or the environment of the patient which must be gotten rid of if the cure is to permanently come to pass.

Some causalities, if continued, are stronger than any possible action of the remedy. If a chef consults you for varicose veins due to his standing in the kitchen all day long, the answer may not be a remedy, but a stool or support stockings. And freedom from the emotional suffering of a life-situation is helped mostly by escaping from it. I think of the countless children abused by an alcoholic parent or the women trapped in a loveless, even abusive marriage. Of course, I have often seen in my practice that an abused woman finds the strength through a remedy such as Staphysagria to finally leave such a relationship. How many times have I had patients on Staphysagria come back for a follow-up and say, "And by the way, I filed for divorce"! And we should not underestimate the power of Nat. mur., Anacardium, Causticum, Aurum, Carcinosin, or Mag. carb. to help a child survive an abusive parent. If the patient is really stuck in a bad situation and absolutely cannot change it (especially true in the case of a child), at least the remedy can act palliatively on an emotional level to give them the strength to endure it. However, we cannot guarantee that the chief complaint can be resolved as long as the patient is in the relationship that caused it.

The role of *diet* while using homeopathic remedies has been the topic of a long debate. Hahnemann himself warned against the use of teas, coffee, camphor and alcohol. But at that point he was mainly using single doses of a 30c (up to the fourth edition of the *Organon*), and we have seen that such antidotes are less of a concern with daily dosing. Hahnemann was afraid that his remedies would be canceled while he was struggling to convince doctors and patients alike of the efficacy of his methods, at a time when he was being viciously attacked. He continues to warn us in Aphorisms 259 and 260 of the sixth edition, although he also says: "Some of my imitators, by forbidding far more, rather indifferent things, seem to make the diet of the patient unnecessarily difficult, which is not to be sanctioned."

Unfortunately most homeopaths today, practicing according to the fourth edition, impose many unpopular restrictions on their patients. Inevitably, many patients who refuse or are unable to stop smoking, drinking coffee or alcohol, or using condiments will be lost to homeopathic treatment. And the average person's first reaction to a suggestion of homeopathic treatment is to think of all the restrictions and prohibitions he has heard about. (Oddly enough, these restrictions seem to have received more publicity than our cures!)

Coffee is the one substance most universally condemned by modern homeopaths. But the old masters did not necessarily find it an obstacle. According to Clarke:

> On account of its extensive antidotal properties, coffee has largely been condemned by homeopathic practitioners; but it should be remembered that it does not antidote all other medicines, and it is questionable if it counteracts the effect of many remedies when they are given in high potencies.[4]

And H.C. Allen remarked:

> Dr. Gallavardin published a book on the treatment of this class of patients by giving them homeopathic medicines without their knowledge or consent in tea, coffee or whatever was the ordinary drink of the patients. He brought marvelous cures in dipsomaniacs, kleptomaniacs, etc., irrespective of the habits of the patients.

The distinguished Indian homeopath S. R. Phatak writes:

I wish to bring to notice a misbelief which is very much prevalent not only among homeopaths but among lay persons also. This misbelief is that when homeopathic medicines are being given, the patient should avoid coffee, onion, garlic, etc. My own experience conclusively proves and I firmly believe that in spite of these things homeopathic remedies act, provided they are selected correctly. These substances are very convenient excuses to cover our ignorance or incapacity to select the correct remedy.

My favorite practitioner, the Swiss-born Pierre Schmidt, said, "Patients were cured even without their knowing that they are taking the remedy because the remedy was given in the wine, even in their coffee and it worked beautifully."

Wise words indeed. No doubt the same homeopaths may have advocated these restrictions elsewhere in their writings. But masters like Hahnemann and Kent recount cases in which the patient kept on drinking coffee and the remedy worked perfectly. Anyone in practice has seen the almost incomprehensible curative force of a remedy (especially in LM potencies) despite the simultaneous intake of drugs, coffee, alcohol and even the action of such suppressive measures as radiation and chemotherapy.*

In conclusion, I can say that I encourage patients to stop drinking coffee, not so much because I am afraid it will cancel the remedy, but because I consider coffee a drug acting on all the organs, tissues and vessels of the body. I encourage the reader to study Hahnemann's masterful exposé of coffee in his *Lesser Writings*.[5]

As for the homeopath prescribing dietary changes, in *acute* ailments I follow Hahnemann's rule that the patient's own inclinations should be the guide. In *chronic* illnesses, the practitioner can give the patient some advice based on her condition and the active miasm (for example, patients with an active sycotic miasm should not eat red meat). Most patients would benefit by eating less meat and fewer sweets while eating more fruits and vegetables, especially raw ones. Lifeless (cooked) food can lower the vital energy. Again, diet alone cannot cure chronic illness, whether the diet is macrobiotic, vegetarian, raw foods or any other special regimen. Since we know that true chronic diseases are caused by miasms, not diet, it stands to reason that diet alone cannot cure them. In these diseases, improving the diet can

---

*Apparently surgeons are now, out of concern for their patients' caffeine withdrawal headaches, giving them intravenous caffeine in their postop IV fluid! Aside from the obvious effects of this practice on the patients' cardiovascular systems, it is unfortunate that these physicians and patients alike don't know how Chamomilla 200c can help wean people off coffee without withdrawal headaches.[6]

remove a maintaining cause (such as sugar consumption in a diabetic) and improve the body's overall healing energy. In non-miasmatic diseases where diet does play a major role, a change of diet can be a bigger factor.

A Miasmatic Block

Sometimes the well-chosen remedy stops working because a miasm needs to be addressed. (Miasms are discussed in great depth in the third section of this book.) A miasmatic block should be suspected in the following circumstances:

- If there is TB, cancer, leukemia, genital warts, syphilis or gonorrhea in the history of the patient and/or family, usually suppressed by allopathic treatments.
- If the remedy stops working in spite of increasing the potency; we will need the relevant nosode as described in Chapter 17, Nosodes.
- When there is a paucity of symptoms.

Please refer to the different scenarios after the administration of the first dose of the well-selected remedy in the previous chapter.

The practitioner needs to clear the miasmatic block before the well-selected remedy will work again. In the course of the treatment, while working our way through the patient's layers, this may happen several times. The patient will feel as though she is "bumping against a wall" in spite of potency and dosage change.

Modern Times

It seems to me that the task of the homeopath is more and more difficult, the successes less direct and spectacular, and the failures more frequent, due to the so-called "progress" of our civilization: the chlorination and fluoridation of our water, the drugs and chemicals (and now irradiation) in our foods, air pollution, multiple vaccinations, the increasing use of X-rays, and the overuse of drugs like antibiotics and barbiturates as well as strong suppressive treatments like chemotherapy and radiation. All these factors contribute to the overwhelming suppression of natural disease manifestations, which confuses and complicates the problem in selecting our remedies.

Mistakes in Prescribing

Obviously, an incorrect prescription will become a barrier to the cure of the patient. It might be wise for the practitioner to check the following points when no progress is made in the patient's case.

Overemphasis on single symptoms: It is easy to pay too much attention to a single symptom and forget the totality. This might correctly lead you to a small remedy, but such cases are infrequent. I have too often seen practitioners basing a remedy on one single physical symptom while ignoring the patient's mental/emotional makeup. In spite of a possible favorable reaction, it will rarely lead to a cure and rather suppress the rest of the case. Remember the hierarchy of symptoms. You will minimize your labor by *starting with certain general symptoms well marked in the patient.*

Negative matching: This is probably the biggest mistake I have seen beginners make in prescribing. Frequently a patient will read about his remedy in the Materia Medica and say: "I don't have this or that aspect of this remedy, so this remedy is not for me." And unfortunately, some homeopaths reason the same way. Remember that no single prover had all the symptoms of a remedy, and neither will any patient. The symptoms of the patient must be present in the remedy selected and *not necessarily vice versa.* For instance, if you have a weepy patient with changeable moods, a recurring thick, yellow vaginal discharge, who craves fresh air and feels better moving around *but* is very thirsty, only the last symptom contraindicates Pulsatilla. It would be a grave mistake *not* to prescribe Pulsatilla in this case. I do not encourage patients to read about their remedy in the Materia Medica (because then they may start imagining every symptom listed under their remedy). But if you do, make sure to explain to them: "See what matches you positively, not negatively!"

Removing the cause: We already mentioned the importance of *tolle causam.* As Hahnemann said in Aphorism 5, "It will help the physician to bring about a cure if he can find out the data of the most probable *occasion* of an acute disease." One of the strong points of a holistic medicine such as homeopathy is that it treats the root as well as the sick branches. Don't fall into the pitfall of practicing homeopathy in an allopathic way, which can only lead to palliation but not to true cure. In fact, if the etiology is very strong, no matter what the symptoms are, the etiology will be the leader in determining your remedy. For instance, whatever the patient's symptoms (headaches, diarrhea, insomnia, vertigo, loss of memory, etc.) after a head trauma, your first choice should be Nat. sulph. (with Arnica as a backup), even if they do not appear under Nat. sulph. in the Materia Medica. The etiology, if strong and outspoken, surpasses any other element in the search for the simillimum. If there is an indignation in the history, Staphysagria should be considered. (See the Never Well Since list in Appendix 2).

A good detective looks for the onset of the disease, not the ending. Dunham cured a case of deafness with Mezereum, prescribing it because the deafness arose after the suppression of an eruption calling for Mezereum.[7] Yet Mezereum has no deafness in its provings—which disturbed Dunham very little in selecting his remedy. This demonstrates that a Chief Complaint can disappear even when the selected remedy does not cover it. So do not overemphasize the symptoms *if the etiology is clear.*

Sometimes the family history may also give a clue to the lack of response to the simillimum. If you find cancer or TB in the family history, sometimes a remarkable improvement is seen in stalled cases with a dose of Carcinosin or Tuberculinum. The *past medical history* is important as well as the family history. Repeated vaccinations, recurrent colds and other infections, suppressive treatment of warts or eruptions, or childhood illnesses might give the clue to the simillimum. Only after antidoting with remedies or nosodes covering those states (Thuja, Medorrhinum, Morbillinum, Diphtherinum, etc.) can the patient recover his health if indeed the patient was "never well since."

Following ghost etiologies: This is another frequent mistake of the beginner. A "ghost etiology" is one that does not produce symptoms or a layer. For instance, the patient had a heartbreak situation or took a high quantity of Penicillin, but the patient did *not get sick following this event*. Apparently the Vital Force was strong enough to overcome the negative impact. No prescription for this event is necessary: you would only be chasing phantoms. Symptoms occasionally appear as long as a year after a trauma or trigger but usually much more quickly (within days to weeks). An easy mistake here is to project your own feelings onto the patient. "Oh, my God, she must have been devastated when her fiancé broke off the engagement." Don't assume anything. Always ask: "How did you feel?" She might have felt relieved to escape from a bad match, and no prescription is needed. (You need to ask the patient's reaction in any case. You may be surprised at their emotional state after a triggering factor. One of my patient's emotional problems stemmed from giving birth to her only child—normally a most joyous occasion but in her case it aroused long-buried memories of her own childhood traumas.)

Ignoring the chronology and skipping layers: If the remedy for the previous layer is given, it will not be able to penetrate the current layer and it will not work effectively. You need to work your way backwards through the timeline, starting with the remedy the patient needs for her current symptoms. The current layer is determined by the current Never Well Since and the symptoms formed as a result of it. As old symptoms return, ask yourself whether they belong to the current layer (i.e., whether they stem from the same Never Well Since). If so, do not change the remedy. Symptoms returning from an earlier phase in the patient's life indicate that it is time to change the remedy (provided that they belong to a different layer, i.e. arising from a different Never Well Since). If the patient starts having dreams or powerful memories from an earlier time in her life, consider whether her current layer has been resolved (indicated by the alleviation of symptoms) and whether this earlier layer needs to be addressed.

Predetermined hierarchy: Common sense should always dictate your prescription; you do not have to rigidly follow the hierarchy of symptoms. If someone comes to you with a sprained ankle, you don't need to ask if he was abused as a child. Ask the patient, "What is the most important symptom you have today?" as it reflects the greatest leakage of energy.

Failure to underline symptoms: A general rule is to always start with certain symptoms which are *well marked in the patient*. If the patient has to think too long whether he has a certain symptom, don't use it in your prescription. At the time of the initial intake, the practitioner should indicate the intensity of the patient's symptoms with one, two or three underlines or (more practically) the numbers 1, 2 or 3 in order of increasing importance. (Of course symptoms rating a 2 or 3 are more important to record and rate than a 1.) This indication of the intensity of symptoms will be a guideline for the next prescription. The practitioner will perceive immediately what is important to the patient. And if she has to retake the case, at least she will know how the patient spontaneously expressed his complaints on the initial visit.

Overemphasis on healthy symptoms: Do not aim a remedy at healthy symptoms. If the patient is romantic, good-natured, responsible, generous and idealistic, these are healthy symptoms. Separate them from the sick symptoms which constitute the leakages of the patient's energy. Address the issues which the patient is asking for help with. This reminds me of a patient I had who became clairvoyant after a head trauma. In fact he was so good that he made a living from it. No other sequelae of the head trauma were apparent in his complaints. It would have been a mistake for me to treat the head trauma, since it could take away his psychic abilities, something the patient valued. Again, the practitioner's non-judgmental attitude is necessary. An unbalanced Sulphur practitioner might be put off by the sympathetic (or in his view, naive) outlook of the Phosphorus. It is he, not the patient who needs a remedy! As long as the symptom does not interfere with the patient's life or anyone else's, there is no treatment indicated.

Prescribing for the name of the disease: While it is good to have a certain differential in your prescribing after taking a case (knowing the top remedies for the patient's "kind" of disease), we must not forget that any remedy can cure any given disease. Often the first fatal mistake for a homeopath is to label diseases and then label drugs to match. Automatically prescribing Rhus tox. for a rheumatic case because it is called a "rheumatic remedy" is the wrong approach, similar to allopathic prescribing. It could well be that the patient needs Sulphur, not Rhus tox. Remember you are treating a *person* with rheumatism, not the rheumatism.

To say that Sepia is just a woman's remedy and therefore never given to a man is another misconception. Sepia, Pulsatilla and Graphites are more likely to be given to women, just as Lycopodium, Nux vomica and Fluoric acid are more often given to men, but there is no absolute. In this era of two-career couples and shared childrearing responsibilities, we see Nux vomica career women and Sepia single fathers.

Do not think of Sulphur and Graphites as "skin remedies." Forget the diagnosis and think of the patient. You have to say to yourself, not "this is a case of rheumatism" but "this is a Sepia patient, and whatever ails her, she needs Sepia and no other remedy." Remember what Kent told his students: to check the accuracy of your prescription, ask yourself whether you would prescribe the same remedy for the same patient if he had an entirely different diagnosis. Only if you can answer in the affirmative can you have confidence in your prescription.

Incorrect repetition of the dose: Remember the general rule for centesimals: so long as amelioration holds, *do not repeat;* and only repeat or reconsider the case, when you are sure that it is quite at an end. With LM potencies we *normally* repeat, of course, except when there is *striking* amelioration from the first dose we should not repeat so long as the amelioration holds.

Hasty prescribing and changing the remedy: You can't be too hasty with your prescription, beginner or not. A case well-thought out in the beginning will give you very little trouble later (a case well-taken is a case 90% resolved!). Conversely, if you foul the clear waters with the wrong prescription, trouble will be endless. If you are not sure, give Sac. lac. and restudy the case. A good computer program can at least speed up some aspects of the investigation. And be sure to allow sufficient time to let the remedy act. This will depend on the nature of the patient (constitutional sensitivity), the nature of the disease (acute or chronic) and the nature of the remedy, as discussed in Chapter 9 on Prescribing.

Accurate record keeping: The homeopath must keep accurate records of the patient's illnesses. Many cases result in failure from negligence in this area. It is a wise idea to keep a separate sheet recording the date and all the prescriptions for each patient (including adjustments to LMs). You need to know exactly to what remedy the patient responded, what dose and potency the patient is currently taking, etc. I staple this page inside the front cover of the patient's file, on the left, so I always have easy access to this essential information when returning calls or for follow-ups.

High potencies in advanced pathology: This point has already been emphasized in the chapter on potencies (Chapter 5). However, because of its importance, it bears repeating to state that cases of advanced pathology (cancer, diabetes, lupus, etc.) require LM or 6c potencies, *not* high potencies. Inevitably, the weakened Vital Force would not be able to sustain the blow of high potencies and the life of the patient would be in jeopardy, his downward spiral to death hastened.

Genuineness of the remedies used: It is worthwhile for the practitioner to know where her remedies are made. Imagine worrying whether your 200c is really closer in potency to a 30c! I have personally inspected the pharmacy where my remedies are made and I have full confidence in the hand successions, the sterile environment, and the meticulous procedures.

Interference from other homeopaths: It is not a good idea for a patient to see two different homeopaths simultaneously. Sometimes I have had problems when my patients consult another homeopath, whether because they are traveling or have moved far away. The other homeopath may misinterpret a report of old symptoms returning (not recognizing the Law of Hering) and change the remedy to one that suppresses the exteriorized symptoms. (See Sample Case 5 in Appendix 4 for a good example of this.) The case then goes off at a tangent, perhaps beyond recovery. We must be wary of spoiling another's work! Out of courtesy to my colleagues, I would not treat a patient who is *currently* in the care of another homeopath.

Over-reliance on computers: While computers have helped modern homeopathy in many ways, still there is one thing a computer program cannot do, which is to understand the essence of the patient. True, the computer can quickly assemble and calculate the scores of the remedies for the rubrics you put in; but the results are only as good as your rubrics. What I see when students and practitioners use computer programs is an over-emphasis on physical symptoms at the expense of the all-important mental and emotional ones, which are harder to pin down. Too many times I have seen students and participants at case conferences enter dozens of rubrics in a case, in a laudable attempt to be thorough, but the result is to skew the case too heavily towards pathological symptoms (since these are what the patient reports, whereas mental/emotional ones must be deduced.) Once the computer is turned on, the user becomes fascinated with it, drawn from one interesting thing to another, and ends up focusing on what the computer does so well: the specific modalities and concomitants of the physical particular symptoms—which is exactly what we do *not* want to base our remedies on!

I also hear students saying, after the computer calculates the 40 rubrics they have entered, "The computer says it could be Arsenicum, Mercury, Phosphorus, Silica, Sulphur, or Thuja, but I don't know which one to give." The first mistake is to think that the computer has spoken, like the Word of God, and that the remedy must be among those it has decreed. Again, the student should know the difference between these major polychrests before even beginning with the computer. There is no way you could mistake an Arsenicum patient sitting in front of you for a Phosphorus or Sulphur patient, and there is no shortcut for a thorough understanding of the polychrests. To take another example, at a recent case conference a computer-wielding participant proposed Gaertner as the solution for the case presented, obviously unaware that Gaertner is a bowel nosode and an inappropriate remedy for opening a case.

I see a fascination with computers among homeopaths, like the fascination with the Internet among many of my friends, in which the gaze becomes sucked into the screen and away from human contact. If you can understand the nature of the patient sitting in front of you, and if you can grasp the essence of how the patient was feeling when her illness began, you can solve the case better and faster than a computer, because these are exactly the things the computer will *not* tell you. Even though computers are supposed to be timesavers, my own experience with solving cases both ways is that the computer takes longer. I also feel that it reduces contact with the patient if the practitioner is looking at a computer screen while doing the intake, unlike the occasional and unobtrusive glance into the *Repertory*.

Computers have their place in homeopathy and have certainly contributed to our understanding of Materia Medica and access to the old classics, but I tell my students that they must learn case solving *without* a computer in the first two years until they have fully mastered the hierarchy of symptoms.

I would recommend using a computer *only as a last resort:* only if you have already tried one or more polychrests and they have failed to improve the patient and failed to throw up symptoms which could point to the simillimum. I would also try one of the "clear-the-case" tactics like using a nosode or a reactive remedy before resorting to the computer. With LM potencies we have the advantage that each strategy we try will show clear results within a few days or a week, so that we will not waste too much of the patient's time in trying several remedies. LM potencies also tend to highlight or clarify the patient's reaction so that it is easier to assess. The centesimal practitioner might feel more tempted to use the computer, since it can take weeks to assess the reaction to each remedy; again, I feel that this is another argument in favor of LM potencies.

For the student who (understandably) feels overwhelmed when first looking at the *Repertory*, there are excellent support materials available. *Yasgur's Homeopathic Dictionary* is indispensable for understanding the Victorian language and medical terminology of all the old masters, not just Kent. Currim's *Guide to Kent's Repertory* gives a thorough explanation of how to find things in Kent, such as the time modalities and pain rubrics. Sault's *A Modern Guide and Index to the Mental Symptoms of Kent's Repertory* provides a cross-reference for modern versions of the all-important mental/emotional rubrics. (Look up "humiliation," for example, and it will refer you to Kent's "mortification"). I encourage my students to read and re-read the Mind and Generalities sections until they come to feel, as I do, that Kent is like an old friend.

CHAPTER FIFTEEN

Management of the Case

What is more beautiful to look upon than the bud during its hourly changes to the rose in its bloom? This evolution has so often come to my mind when patiently awaiting the return of symptoms after the first prescription has exhausted its curative power. The return symptom-image unfolds the knowledge by which we know whether the first prescription was the specific or the palliative, i.e., we may know whether the remedy was deep enough to cure all the deranged vital wrong or simply a superficially acting remedy, capable of only temporary effect.

—J. T. Kent[1]

The Importance of the Second Prescription

Having learned how to select the remedy and the potency, and in how many doses to give it, the next issue is how to watch your case unfold like a bud unfurling its petals to become a rose, as in Kent's evocative image. From the patient's reports of his reaction to the remedy, the practitioner must be able to determine whether the remedy is acting at all, and if so, whether the action is favorable and what prognosis may be expected. She must know how to predict the duration of action of remedy in each individual case (much more difficult with centesimals than LMs). In short, having started the journey to cure, she must be sure she is on the right track and that she knows when and how to change remedies. Her decisions must be based on careful observation based on *seeing* the patient (no Internet or phone consultations), for what the patient reports is often misleading.

The term "the second prescription" has traditionally been used by Kentian homeopaths to mean (basically) what the practitioner does when the patient comes back for a follow-up appointment. Having given a single dose of a high centesimal potency at the first appointment, the Kentian prescriber must decide at the follow-up whether it worked as expected; if not, whether it was probably the correct remedy but there was an obstacle to the cure; or if it did, whether it was still acting or had completed its action. At that point the Kentian decides whether to re-administer the same remedy (in the same or a higher potency), to administer a new remedy, or to do nothing. The LM prescriber has received regular follow-up reports from the patient in between appointments and has made any necessary adjustments in potency and dosage along the way. The issue of whether the remedy is correct and whether it is working is usually resolved long before the first follow-up appointment. Nevertheless, the same general principles of case management apply to both Kentian and LM prescribers, so the term "the second prescription" is used here to cover basic issues of when and how to change the remedy and the potency.

The management of the patient and the question of the second prescription are crucial issues, too rarely discussed in seminars and case reports, to the detriment of students and future patients alike. Every beginning homeopath quickly learns the importance of the second prescription (while most *students* think that the *first* prescription, i.e. finding the remedy, is the Holy Grail of homeopathy). Why is it that so many patients benefit from homeopathic treatment at first but not thereafter? Most of us think the initial prescription requires all our skill and intelligence; in fact too many conferences and case reports focus on the first prescription, as if "solving the case" depended solely on this.

Yet a good clinical result depends mainly on the *second* prescription. (A prescription is only called the second one if it follows a first one that has *acted;* wrong prescriptions don't count. A bungling prescriber may have given four or five incorrect remedies and the sixth, if it really takes hold, should be considered the first prescription.) So the *accurate interpretation of the changes* occurring after the remedy has been given is, in some respects, more important than the selection of the drug and the repetition of the dose. Kent even says, "The whole future of the patient may depend upon the conclusions that the physician arrives at after the remedy has been administered."[2]

Understanding each of the following scenarios after a first prescription will keep you on the right track in chronic cases. You must have the courage and confidence to maintain a steady course no matter how much the patient wants to change a remedy because he thinks changes are not coming fast enough or thinks it is not working when old symptoms recur. How often have I seen on my telephone messages, "I am no better," yet when I talked to the patient, I found that there had been significant improvement. The patient, being used to the swift symptomatic relief of allopathic medicine, can become impatient or misunderstand the reappearance of old symptoms, increased discharges or rashes, or initial similar aggravation. Before making a second prescription the practitioner must restudy the case with the following scenarios in mind.

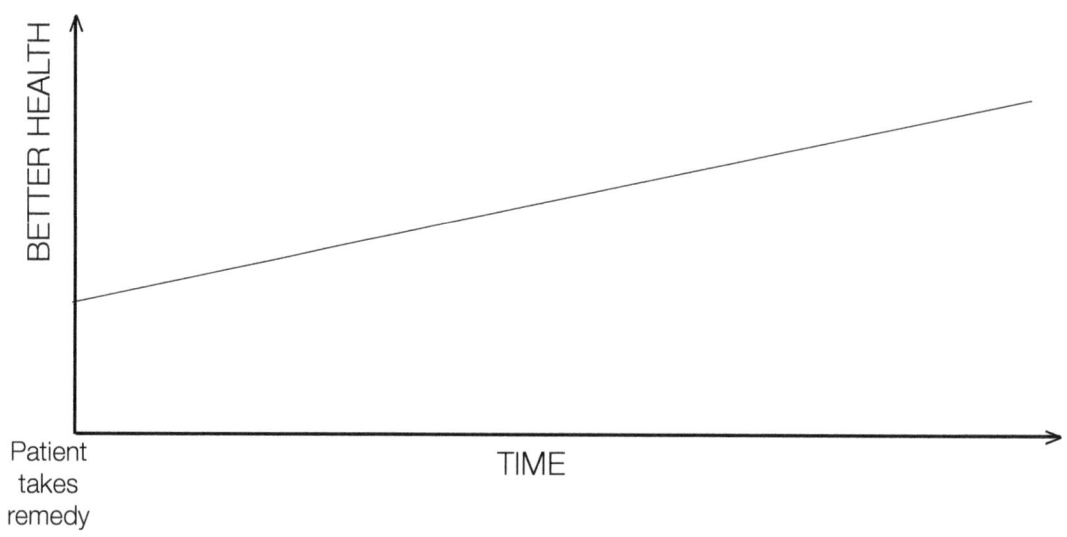

1. Immediate improvement without any aggravation

This is the ideal scenario. There is practically no observable aggravation and yet the patient recovers steadily. You have the simillimum in both remedy and potency. The patient feels a sense of well-being, his sleep pattern improves, sensitivities decrease, clarity of mind returns, symptoms disappear and calmness prevails. It is proof positive that the potency was not too high, just high enough. It also shows that there is no significant organic disease and the prognosis is very favorable.

Signs of the simillimum: Other changes that can be observed in the patient upon administering the simillimum are as follows:

- The *mental/emotional outlook* improves: since healing takes place from the inside out, the first changes are often on the mental/emotional plane. An optimistic tone replaces pessimism, and hope for full recovery replaces despair. The patient may still report that his symptoms are present to some degree (or even aggravated) but he feels the healing taking place on a deeper level and knows that he will improve.
- The patient reports feeling more *peaceful:* calm, forgiving dreams replace anguished, fighting, struggling dreams contributing to a more refreshed sleep.
- The patient needs *more sleep:* While more energy is a good sign, the need for more sleep can be an equally good or even better sign, if the sleep is deep and restful and accompanied by an underlying sense of healing. The patient often needs rest in order to repair damage on the physical level or process past traumas on the emotional level.
- There is an immediate change in the *appearance* of the patient, especially on the face. The appearance of sickness is replaced by an appearance of health. The cheeks fill up, wrinkles

seem to lessen and there is a certain brightness and cheerfulness in the face. The face takes on a healthy look so much that on the second visit, before the patient has even spoken a word, I can see that he has improved.

- *Itchiness* is a good sign, especially when the soles of the feet itch.
- *Discharges* may appear or increase: sputum, nasal or vaginal discharges, ear wax, etc. I had one patient who proudly brought in to show me the full cup of greenish discharge which emerged from his penis soon after a dose of Medorrhinum.
- Some patients even have a change in *skin color:* Caucasians and Asians become more fair-skinned, while African American skin takes on a rosy tinge, instead of the ashen tinge of illness.
- Emaciated patients often *put on weight* in the first week and continue to restore their weight steadily after that.

The simile never shows the immediate and marked improvements found above. They are clear-cut signs of the simillimum.

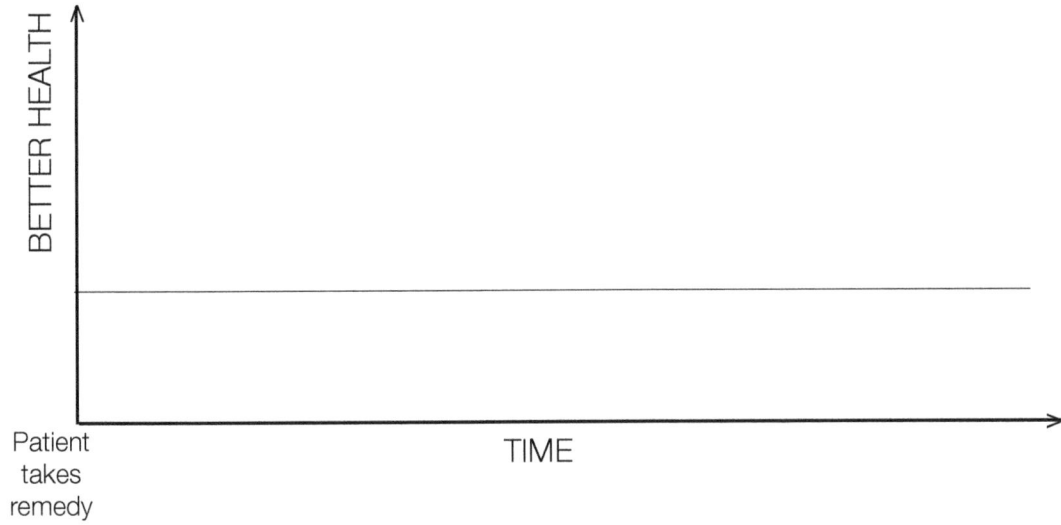

2. No reaction

There is neither aggravation nor improvement, even after three weeks (LM, 6c or 200c). Why?

- Before you change the remedy, especially when you think the prescription was well-indicated, change the potency! Go from 6c to 30c, 200c, then 1M. In case of LM potencies, increase the succussions or the amount taken from the cup or bottle. This should be your first thought after restudying the case and concluding that the remedy was indeed well-selected.

- My second thought would be that something in the patient's life-style either canceled the remedy or is a maintaining cause or an ongoing inciting cause of the disease (poor environment, continued abuse of alcohol, coffee or tea, bad eating habits, an abusive relationship, etc.). Review the history of the patient's reaction to the remedy with the patient again. Often you will hear, "I was really doing better until I started drinking every day." This roadblock must be removed, if possible, before making any change in the homeopathic remedy. You can help the patient to wean off an addictive substance with remedies; you can exhort the patient to change bad habits; but if the obstacle really cannot be removed (e.g. the patient is trapped in a bad marriage), increase the potency until you gain the desired reaction, if at all possible.
- A miasmatic block may be preventing the indicated remedy from working. You should have already noted the active miasm in the initial case-taking (see Chapter 19, Miasms). Prescribe the indicated anti-miasmatic remedy, often the corresponding nosode as an intercurrent. The tubercular miasm will reveal itself not only by the past medical history and family history but also by a specific outcome scenario: every time the patient consults you, the picture changes each time, requiring a new remedy (and reflecting the restlessness and changeability of the tubercular miasm). This scenario would indicate *Tuberculinum*.
- The patient is sluggish in reacting: he may be a hyposensitive. For example, a Calcarea type might need a higher potency, increased dose or longer time span before he will show any reaction to the remedy.

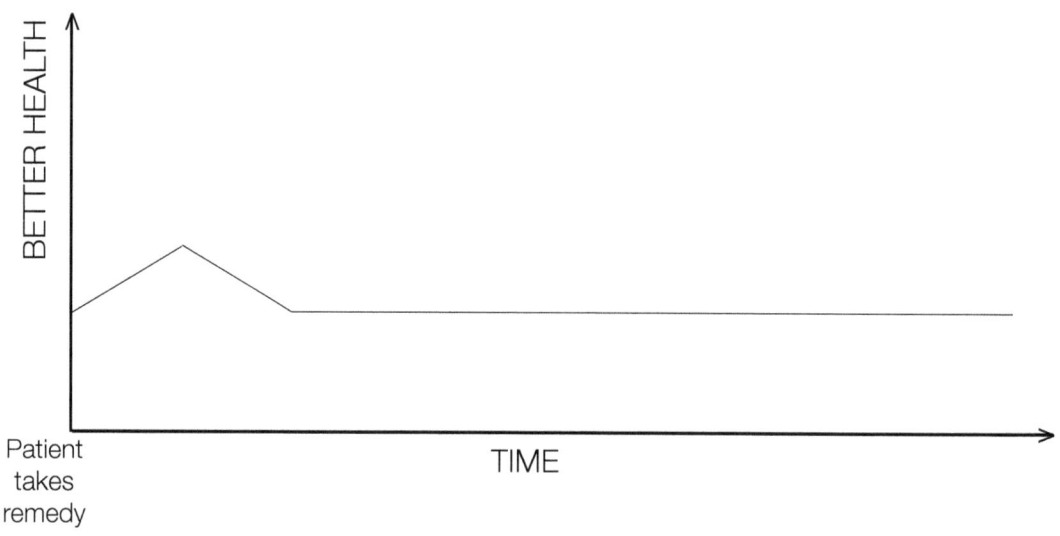

3. Initial improvement, then return of the symptoms as they were before the medicine was given.

Possible reasons include:
- First, it may be the right remedy but apparently the stimulus from the remedy was not strong enough to sustain improvement: try increasing the potency.
- A miasm may need to be removed first. After some improvement, the patient "hits a wall," the miasmatic block, and then the symptoms start to relapse. Or a deeper acting miasmatic remedy might be necessary. For example if a patient improves markedly on Silica for a week, then relapses, and Silica is repeated in a higher dose and still does not hold, *Tuberculinum* may improve the patient and sustain both its own improvement and that of further remedies. You will often return to the previous remedy after a nosode but be on the lookout for the nosode to change the symptom picture to the extent that a new remedy is indicated.
- The prescribed remedy was the simile, not the simillimum. Often you can suspect this because some superficial symptoms (like hemorrhoids) have disappeared while there is no considerable improvement for the patient as a whole. His sense of well-being, his sleep and his moods have not been affected by the remedy; none of the indications under Scenario I are present. Retake the case to find the simillimum. The patient may have withheld crucial information from you, such as the Never Well Since. The simile often stimulates the Vital Force to throw out symptoms typical of the simillimum, and you should be the lookout for them.
- Review the life-style of the patient. Often the patient has such an initial improvement that he thinks it is safe to return to old bad habits, or the patient who has suffered for years from lack of energy starts overdoing it now that she finds some of her old well-being back. The remedy is repairing, and repair takes time, patience and energy from the patient. Don't be surprised if the patient initially needs more sleep. This is an excellent reaction, telling the body to rest to save energy for the colossal repair work to be done.
- There may be organ damage beyond repair, in which case only palliation is possible. In these instances, an increase of potency would only harm. One must always be on guard for hidden pathology. Refer for an allopathic diagnostic workup if in doubt. This again accentuates the importance of pathology as explained in Chapter 4.
- Remember that the Vital Force runs in cycles or waves. Often the patient, excited about the initial progress, phones you as soon as she has a bad day. High potency prescribers should not jump to repeat the remedy. Even with LMs (if the patient has been on the same remedy for a while and is taking it prn), I would wait until I see that the patient has at least two consecutive bad days before I would allow her to repeat the dose. (If she is still taking the remedy on a daily basis, I would have her stop the remedy at that point, wait until the aggravation wears off, then repeat, even if this process took several days). Often

some incident during the day (such as an emotional upset) has temporarily interrupted the beneficial action of the remedy, and lo and behold, the remedy acts again the next day without being repeated. True curative action must not be interrupted until it is certain that the reactive force is exhausted; *watch and wait!* And if the patient is too anxious, give Sac. lac.

- The patient was improving until something interfered with the remedy: dental anesthesia or emotional trauma (hearing bad news) or the appearance of an acute illness. In this latter case, suspend the chronic remedy while giving the patient the acute indicated remedy, then resume the chronic remedy where you left off.
- This reaction is often seen in violent, rapidly progressing *acute* diseases, where the power of the remedy is used up quickly by the intensity of the disease process. Both frequent repetition *and* higher potency are necessary for a curative reaction.

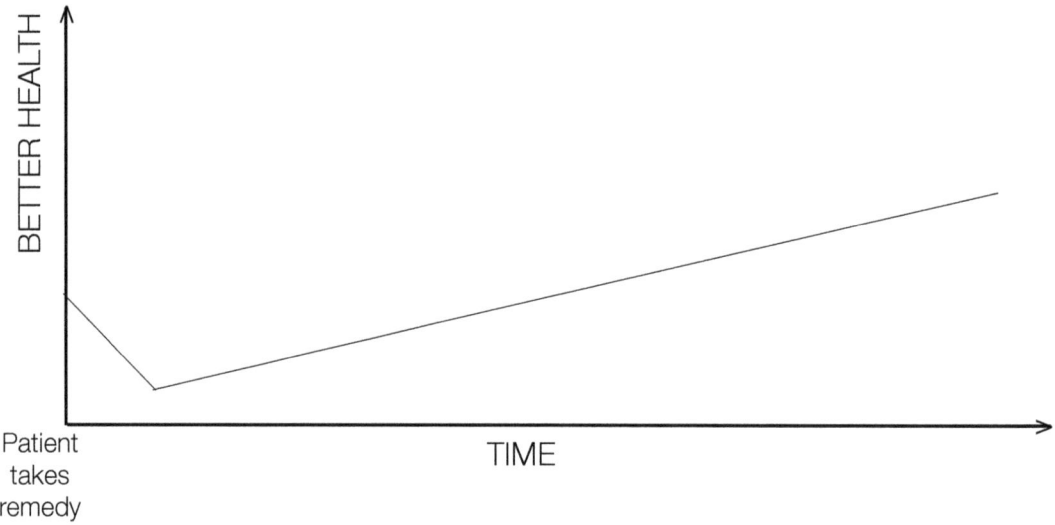

4. Quick similar aggravation followed by improvement and increase in the patient's strength

This scenario indicates an excellent prognosis: the remedy was well chosen and the improvement will be long lasting. This is the best possible reaction a high-potency prescriber can hope for (although not as good as the first scenario from the patient's point of view). The main reason for this reaction is a patient with strong vitality and good reactive power, although it can also frequently happen when the potency used was higher than necessary. A lower dilution would have avoided the aggravation. When this aggravation occurs it is usually during the first week or ten days after the remedy has been given. In LM potencies we are most likely to see this scenario with hypersensitives; with others it may occur within a week to ten days of starting a remedy, if the succussions are too high; in either case we need to reduce the succussions or amount. This scenario assures us that our remedy selection is correct and that the Vital Force's reactive power against the disease (even if complicated by allopathic medication) will give us more than a palliation. Exacerbations may arise a second or a third time after intervals of improvement. These are the waves of the reactive force, and if each succeeding one is less violent and occurs less frequently, they will gradually become ripples and then smooth waters will follow.

Some homeopaths claim that an aggravation has to be achieved or no improvement can be expected. However, every careful observer has seen cases where relief and nothing but relief has promptly followed the well-selected remedy, relief so rapid that it seemed almost like magic. A gentle reaction always leads to a more permanent cure. A slight initial aggravation and then improvement is more likely to relapse than improvement right from the start. Similar aggravations should be the exception rather than the rule if the homeopath has correctly gauged the patient's sensitivity. But when they do occur, the experienced homeopath will respect them.

In this scenario, organic changes are unlikely, and if they occur they are in non-vital organs. The prognosis is good (the case is curable). Abscesses and suppurating glands appear at times in these cases as a form of natural healing crisis and an expression of Hering's Law of exteriorization. These are good signs and should not be interfered with.

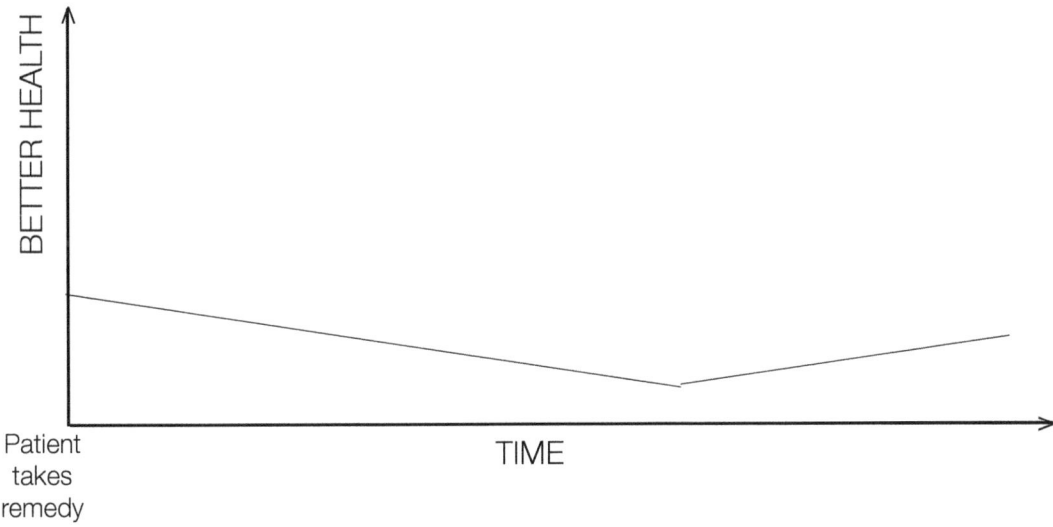

5. A long continued aggravation but eventual and slowly progressing improvement

- This reaction can occur when the potency was way too high for the reactive power of the patient, whose vitality was able to assert itself eventually, after a long struggle, and, in time, genuine curative action begins. This was a serious case and the Vital Force was barely able to start the healing process in time. Make sure that with the next dose you decrease the potency or the amount of remedy given (in cases of LM or 6c in water).
- It might indicate that the case is on the borderline of incurability, often with extensive pathology present. Make sure to refer your patient to an allopathic doctor for a diagnostic workup, if pathology has not yet been discovered. You owe it to your patient and you will have a better idea regarding the prognosis. Do not repeat too soon, but wait until the patient has sufficient strength to react to another dose and make sure this dose is in a low potency (6c or LM with 2 succussions).

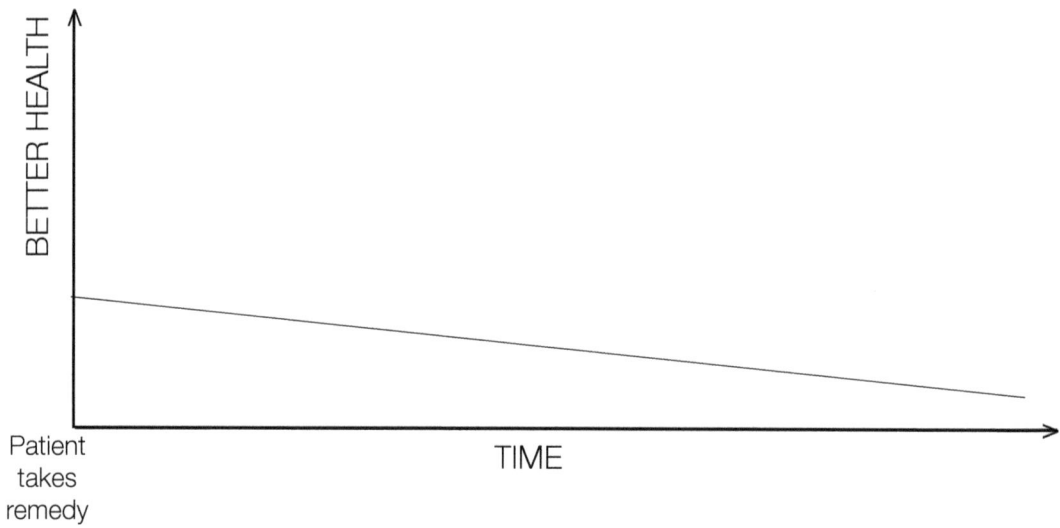

6. Prolonged aggravation and slow decline
- If the remedy was well-chosen, the case was simply incurable because of the marked irreversible organic pathology, yet the patient's vitality is still able to emit symptoms. You can only palliate with zig-zag prescribing. In other words, you will treat the *acute symptomatology*, changing the remedy as the need arises. You need to select low potency remedies (not beyond 30c) of a palliative nature in doubtful and incurable diseases.
- A second possibility, but rarer, is that the patient (usually a hypersensitive!) has been overwhelmed by the turmoil following too high a potency. In this case, if the life of the patient is threatened, the remedy must be antidoted. Then it should be repeated with greatest care and certainly in a *much* lower potency than before. One way to antidote a remedy is to give the same remedy in a lower potency, e.g. 6c.

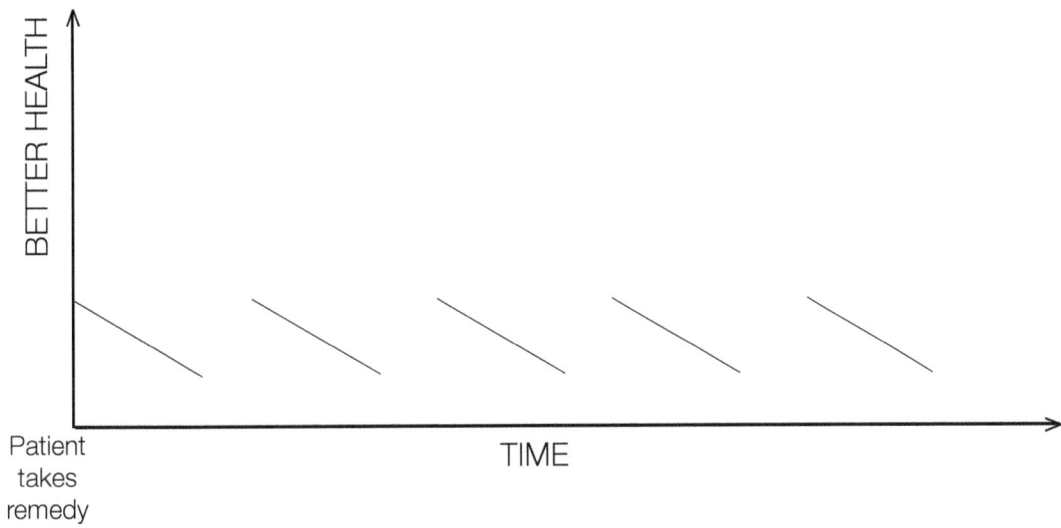

7. Aggravating reactions to every remedy

- This can happen with *extreme* hypersensitives, who react to any remedy, no matter how low the potency, with proving symptoms. Such hypersensitives are so difficult as to be almost incurable (definitely with high potencies) although they make the best provers. As mentioned before, high potencies should be avoided at all costs in these cases. Use LM with two succussions and eighth teaspoons (or even drops measured from an eyedropper), second cup, etc., 6c dry, or use the olfaction or skin method.
- Or the patient has serious unmet emotional needs (hysteria, depression, emotional abuse, etc.), or simply wants to be assured of the continued attention of the physician. Other family members should be interviewed to clarify the case. Use placebo and concentrate on the new psychological symptoms coming up.

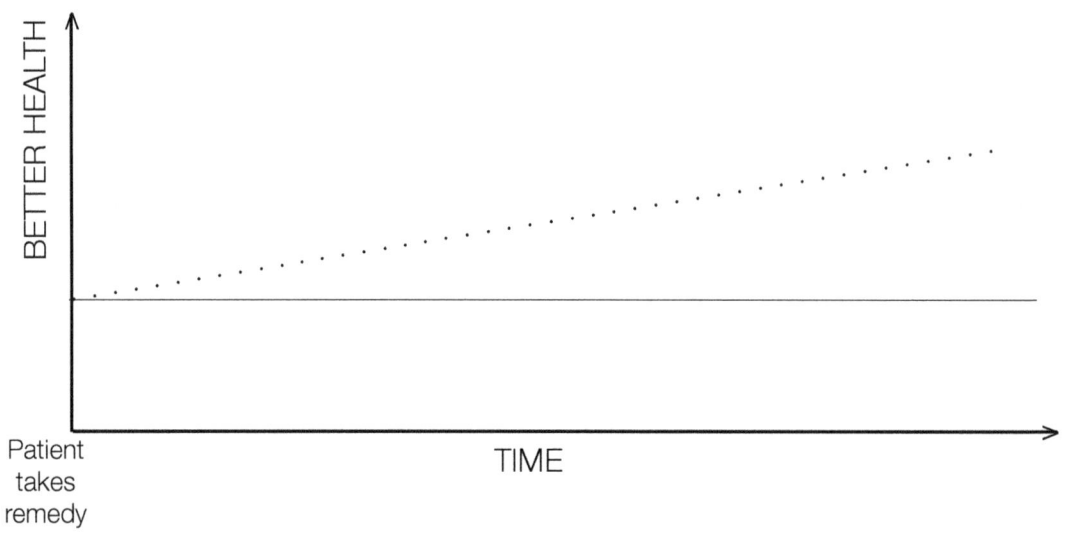

8. Symptom improvement, but no relief and no special increase in the strength or mental condition of the patient:

- Your first thought should be that you have the simile, not the simillimum: restudy the case.
- Second thought: a possible obstacle to the cure. Check the patient's life-style and home environment.
- If you are sure of the simillimum and you cannot find an obstacle to the cure, perhaps the potency was not sufficient to complete the action started; give the same remedy in a higher potency. (This would only happen in hyposensitives and normosensitives. Hypersensitives would always give you one of the signs that you have the simillimum; hyposensitives are the most likely to give you a lack of reaction.)
- This reaction is always the case when organs are scarred or partially destroyed. The remedies act favorably, but there is only so much they can do. By careful repetitions at frequent intervals, the patient may be kept comfortable for a considerable period of time, although you should not expect a cure because of the extensive pathology involved (see the next chapter, Palliation and Incurable Cases).

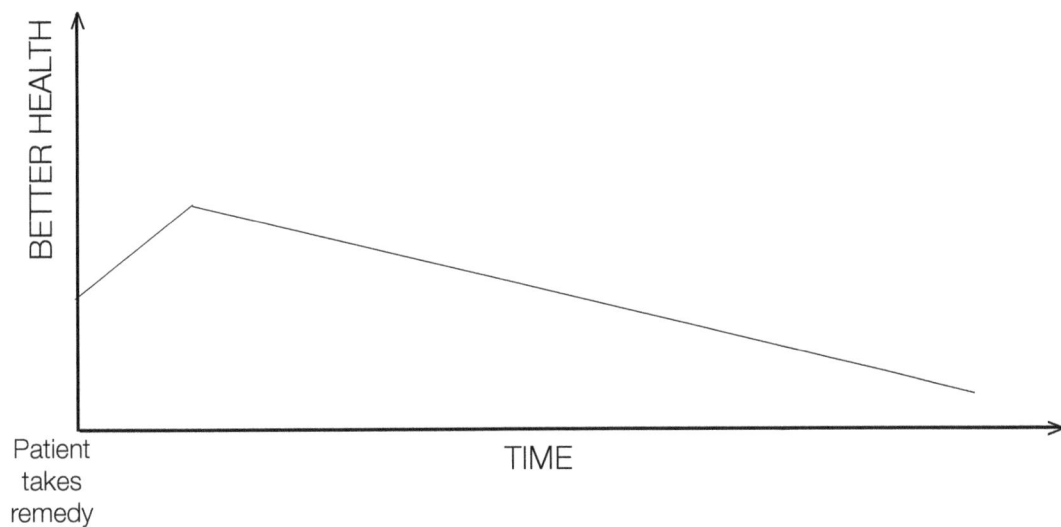

9. Rapid amelioration of the symptoms, followed in a longer or shorter period by a long aggravation

This is usually an unfavorable reaction. Possible interpretations:
- The remedy is only the simile and therefore only palliated.
- The disease is incurable.
- Don't change your remedy too hastily. Some remedies have a deferred aggravation, notably Phosphorus (up to twelve days). In other words, when Phosphorus is given as a therapeutic remedy, the patient may not react for as long as twelve days; we would expect this in a patient with a hyposensitive constitution, not a hypersensitive Phosphorus constitution.
- If the severity of the aggravation and the nature of the symptoms belong to the so-called external parts of the body—skin, mucosae, joints—while the mental and organ symptoms improve, the cure is following Hering's Law and the remedy should definitely not be changed. In chronic cases, aggravations may come and go in waves, even up to the fourth month.

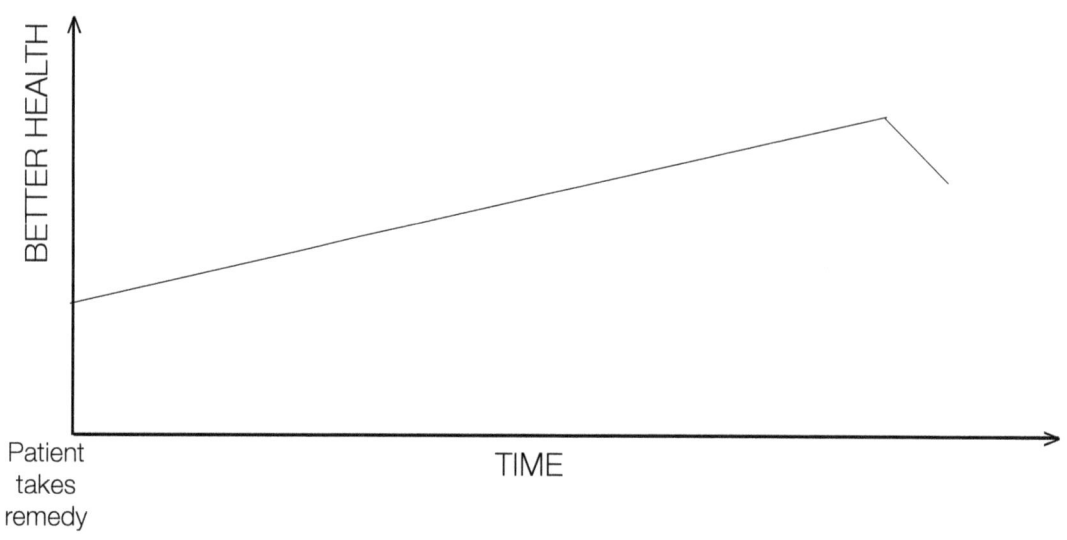

10. Longtime improvement over weeks or months, then sudden aggravation

- This scenario almost always occurs when the patient has started proving the remedy, showing accessory symptoms after taking the remedy for months with good results. It means that the patient is almost cured (or that *this* remedy has done all it can). You should stop the remedy and wait (as one always does after an aggravation). The aggravation will disappear and the patient will stay in an improved state for a long time. *Only* when symptoms start reappearing should a *single* dose of the previously indicated remedy be given (no matter what potency that was, even low), and this should be followed by immediate improvement.

- Accessory symptoms can also appear when the remedy was unnecessarily repeated. Symptoms of the remedy, unhomeopathic to the case, appear.

11. Symptoms follow Hering's Laws

This scenario is puzzling to the patient but a joy to the practitioner, who knows a *real cure* is underway. Here we should just stay with the *same* remedy, which will continue the improvement. Prognosis is good if the case is not interfered with. Old symptoms are coming back while the patient himself feels better.

Remember that the oldest ailments, among which are the constant local ailments, are the last to give way. When old symptoms come back, the *psychological* are the most important and the best guide for the selection of the remedy. For example, a patient may report that he finds himself suddenly brooding over a long-lost love or a long-deceased parent. I have had a number of patients on Nat. mur. report dreaming of deceased loved ones and of having the chance to say things in their dreams which they never had the chance to say in real life. I gave one patient Phosphoric acid for her painless diarrhea which began when her son, the last family member at home, left for college; she then re-experienced the deep grief she had felt at the deaths of her parents and her husband. (See Sample Case 5, Appendix 4).

In those rare cases in which suppressed symptoms resurface while internal symptoms aggravate, the prognosis is always doubtful. This sometimes also occurs in patients with active skin diseases.

However, if you see superficial symptoms disappear, only to be replaced by organ symptoms, stop the remedy immediately! For instance, if joint symptoms improve while asthma is aggravated, it is the wrong remedy. The disease is going in exactly the *opposite* direction of Hering's Laws. As Kent said, "To prescribe for rheumatic conditions without due regard for the other symptoms of the case is dangerous. To fit a remedy to one part or organ may jeopardize the future health or even the life of the patient." The remedy may need to be antidoted, as explained in the next scenario.

12. New symptoms appear

- The symptoms are neither old symptoms reappearing (often called "new symptoms" by the patient) nor symptoms of the remedy (similar aggravation). This is a *dissimilar* homeopathic aggravations indicating a wrong remedy. See the section on Dissimilar Aggravations in Chapter 12 for guidance. Whenever symptoms change from surface to center, the remedy should be antidoted (healing does not follow Hering's Law, as explained in the previous scenario).

- There is an exception, however: when the new symptoms indicate the remedy is working. The symptoms may be "signs of life": the moaning of a comatose patient returning to consciousness or the marked tingling in a paralyzed part when nerve function returns. In his *Lectures on Materia Medica,* Kent describes the shrieks of the Helleborus patient when sensation returns to his paralyzed extremities.* Or they may be the universal signs of

---

*Kent has wonderful advice for the homeopath treating a "stuporous" child with Helleborus:
  Just imagine these benumbed fingers and hands and limbs, this benumbed skin everywhere. What would be the most natural thing to develop? ... As he comes back to his normal nervous condition, the fingers commence to tingle, the nose and ears tingle, and the child begins to scream and toss back and forth and roll about the bed. The neighbors will come and say, "I would send that doctor away unless he gives

symptoms going from the interior to the exterior: rashes, discharges and joint pains are always good signs even if not part of the original disease picture or the remedy picture.

♦ Remember to review carefully with a patient whether a symptom is indeed new: for example, the unexpected appearance of an eruption on the skin may indicate that it had been suppressed and the patient had forgotten to mention it.

Stay With a Remedy Which Is Working

A basic rule of thumb is to *get the maximum out of each successful remedy*. A remedy which has acted well should not be changed too easily. Changing the remedy should require as much deliberation as a surgical operation! When considering a new remedy, study the totality of the present symptoms of the case, treating it like a *new* case (although as mentioned in Chapter 9, Prescribing, remedies that complement the first one or follow it well should be considered). It is said that every time a patient came to him, Hahnemann used to take the case anew. This should be a lesson to all of us. I encourage the reader to review Chapter 10, Golden Tips in Prescribing, and above all to study Kent's wonderful *Lectures on Homeopathic Philosophy*.

Repetition of the Dose

If there is an improvement of 50% the first week, the golden rule is to *slow down or stop all together!* If you don't, you will inevitably steer towards an aggravation. Do fewer succussions (in the case of LM) or start taking 6c less frequently (once a day, or every other day). In general we can say, if the *patient is better overall,* even though the local conditions may appear to be worse, the remedy is doing its work and should not be interrupted. (Of course we will decrease the dose or stop the remedy altogether temporarily, if necessary, to minimize the patient's discomfort.) The patient needs to take the remedy as infrequently as possible while still holding a gradual level of improvement. As soon as possible, start giving the remedy only as needed (prn, indicated by a slight downturn in the symptoms). If there is a striking improvement from the first dose, the patient can take the remedy on a prn basis right from the start. The rule is not to interfere when the patient expresses himself to be better.

---

something to help that child," but just as sure as you do it you will have a dead baby in twenty-four hours. You will never be able to manage one of those cases if you do not take the father… aside beforehand and tell him what is going to happen. … It is not so much the awful pains, but it is the itching, tingling and formication that cause the appearance of extreme agony.[3]

High potency prescribers will seldom have the first scenario above (immediate improvement without aggravation) because it is difficult to guess the correct potency in advance for the single dose. This first scenario is the ideal one, one every practitioner should strive for. It makes an eloquent argument for lower potencies in chronic diseases.

When the same symptoms come back *unchanged* but milder after prudent waiting (again the wait will be longer and of more uncertain duration in high centesimal potencies than in LM or 6c), the selection was correct. If the same potency fails to act, a higher one will generally do so quite promptly, as did the lower one at first.

When the picture comes back changed only by the *absence* of some symptoms, and no new symptoms appear, the remedy should never be changed until a still higher potency has been fully tested. This difficulty again is less applicable in the LM potency, since the succussions automatically raise the potency slightly higher each time the patient takes a dose.

If old symptoms arise from years ago following a remedy (Hering's Law), the remedy should not be repeated as it is clearly showing a favorable and curative action. (Even with LMs, the action of the remedy continues and might lead to an aggravation.) It is a good rule to do nothing when in doubt, but to wait until symptoms and conditions develop that point clearly to the right way. Time will be saved and danger avoided. Withholding repetition until the remedy action is fully expended requires nerve only for those who are not fully convinced of the Law of the Cure or are ignorant of its force and dependability.

Summary of Management Guidelines in Chronic Prescribing
- The ideal to be realized, as Hahnemann said, would be to treat every disease with *one single remedy and one single dose*. Unfortunately, this rarely happens because it requires a perfect correspondence of the remedy and potency to the patient. As seen in the previous chapter, Obstructions to the Cure, there are numerous difficulties preventing it.
- The repetition of the remedy requires positive and strong reasons in centesimals; in LMs the remedy is repeated unless there is striking amelioration from the first dose.
- The repetition of the remedy depends on the *nature of the remedy, the nature of the disease,* and the *potency* (Potencies, Chapter 4). The nature of the remedy refers to the *duration of its action*. Calcarea and the nosodes are well known to have a longer duration of action then such remedies as Aconite, Belladonna or Ignatia. Also, the less sensitive the patient, the more often the remedy may be repeated.
- In chronic cases, one must be careful with the repetition of centesimal potencies, and in case of doubt it is better to wait too long. More harm has been done by repeating doses than by giving a remedy too rarely.

- In acute cases, the remedy can be repeated more frequently. But we should not forget that many acute cases have been cured beautifully with a single dose of the simillimum.
- Careful observation of the patient and the disease is essential, so as to precisely ascertain which symptoms are unique to the patient and which commonly belong to the disease.

In his *Chronic Diseases*, Hahnemann teaches us:

> Nothing is more guilty than to repeat blindly and routinely a remedy, one must be guided always by the reaction of the patient and observe carefully the direction and course of the symptoms. … One must be very careful not to use prevision in the indications of homeopathic remedies and should always base his prescription on the actual totality; it is impossible to prescribe different remedies in advance, either mixed or alternated, for this is a practice absolutely aside from the principles of our doctrine. It is only empiricism, and the work of the most pitiful routine. … The homeopathic physician ought to examine the symptoms every time he prescribes; otherwise he cannot know whether the same remedy is indicated a second time, or whether a medicine is at all appropriate.[4]

We should all heed this valuable advice. And we must add, as Hahnemann says: "There are exceptions to the rule, which is, however, not the business of every beginner to discover."

Management Tips from the Old Masters

Using placebo for daily dosing: Sac. lac. (blank pellets without any remedy instilled in them) is useful if the patient is impatient; or if patients accustomed to continuing allopathic drugs even after their symptoms disappear, don't believe you when you say: "Don't take the remedy now, you are doing well." This is especially hard to understand for elderly people who are accustomed to their daily routine of taking pills. Give these patients Sac. lac. without telling them it is a placebo. Surprisingly, the patient will often say, "Doctor, this medicine is even better than the first one (the real homeopathic remedy)." Of course the patient has no clue that the first remedy is continuing to act. There is one grand rule to observe in all cases, acute or chronic, and it is this: *no symptoms, no remedy except Sac. lac.*

Do not yield to patients' demands: Patients of centesimal prescribers will become impatient and want another dose or another remedy. Patients of LM prescribers may become impatient too, if they feel their case is progressing too slowly. The practitioner needs to stand her ground. Don't forget that most patients today are accustomed to immediate effects from drugs. They will often demand immediate relief, having no tolerance for the slightest discomfort, even when these symptoms signify improvement in their health. Remedies may not produce such quick results; they may produce improvement on a deeper level, while the patient is focusing solely on the Chief Complaint; or they may even produce a healing reaction such as a discharge or rash which is encouraging to the practitioner but disconcerting to the patient. This is where a solid foundation in case management comes in. Be firm and don't let the patient dictate his treatment plan alone. It's true that we tell patients that they are the pilot and we are the co-pilot; but we definitely have to navigate! Use plenty of Sac. lac. in such cases.

Change of potency: Whenever a frequent change of potency is required, the remedy is likely to be the simile rather than the simillimum. And the further removed the remedy is from the simillimum, the more of it is needed to produce a noticeable reaction (whether more frequent repetition, higher potencies, etc.) However, there are different ways to experiment with changing the potency before changing the remedy (if the remedy is well-indicated). For example, a lower potency of the same remedy may work. Dr. Adolph Lippe advised repeating a lower potency in water every two hours until a good response is obtained, even if several days are necessary to see a reaction.

Individualize the potency to the patient: I have seen cases which did not respond to a 10M, yet they responded to the same remedy in a 200c. It is as though each patient has a certain potency which they resonate with, like tuning the dial of a radio to a particular station.

Time for the second prescription: When it is clear that the present remedy has done all it can (in increasing potencies) and/or when accessory symptoms belonging to the remedy appear), then the time is right for the next prescription (i.e., a new remedy). For guidelines in finding it, I refer you to Chapter 10, Golden Rules in Prescribing. Often the next remedy will be the complement of the first, or one of the "remedies which follow well" in the appendix to the *Repertory.* Another possibility is that a new layer has comes up, as explained in the Timeline section of Chapter 8. In this case the two remedies will not necessarily be related.

The last appearing symptom shall be the guide to the next remedy: Under the action of your first prescription, old symptoms reappear following Hering's Laws. (Remember that as long as old symptoms resurface and disappear for good, no new remedy must be considered.) Finally a *new* symptom appears, not an old symptom on its way to its final departure. It is even an error to think of a new prescription when the symptom picture is changing: you must wait for *permanency or firmness* in the symptom picture before making a prescription. Buy some time by giving Sac. lac., if you fear that the patient will resort to suppressive drugs. The first prescription may have been correct, but it is dangerous to make the second prescription in a hurry. So often I have seen beginners choose the first remedy correctly, then lose the thread of the case by changing to a new remedy because of a "new picture."

Cases with extensive suppression: After extensive surgery or long periods of allopathic medication, the system can be slow to react. The indicated remedy may need to be repeated frequently until the desired result is achieved (if using centesimal potencies). Again we see the effectiveness of LM prescribing versus centesimals, since the dose can be repeated daily, while each dose is altered through repeated succussions with an ever increasing strength. And no potency but LM's acts better and faster on suppressed cases.

Pathology may be the last to go: I have often seen the patient's symptoms improve before the pathology improves. I remember a patient with a giant bleeding stomach ulcer whose symptoms quickly disappeared under the action of the simillimum, but several months passed before X-rays revealed a significant reduction of the ulcer. In sycotic miasmatic cases with wart formation, the practitioner must be careful not to declare the patient healed until the warts have cleared up.

Signs of a complete cure: To be truly cured takes several years. When a patient is truly cured homeopathically, she is much less susceptible to acute and chronic diseases, even to epidemics. If there are occasional colds or influenza, they will be mild. Some conditions require longer treatment than others. For example, recurrent annual hay fever should gradually improve from year to year until it is cured. Many cures are slow but sure (e.g. chronic psoriasis and osteoarthritis).

Management of the Acute Case

There are several possible scenarios here:

1. Recurring acute expressions of a chronic disease

In this case, the patient may be treated acutely if coming to the practitioner for the first time during an acute attack, but thereafter the chronic condition must be addressed. For example, a child suffering from bronchitis whenever the weather changes may even grow worse if treated acutely each time. Why? Because the miasm that predisposes the child to recurrent attacks must be addressed. By not curing the root of the problem (the miasmatic state in this case), the chronic disease persists and gets worse. Addressing the underlying miasm will prevent recurrence of the acute illnesses. Acute diseases, especially if recurring, are nothing but exacerbations of a chronic miasmatic state.

2. An (unrelated) acute illness that arises during the course of chronic treatment

The chronic remedy is suspended and the acute condition is treated as in Scenario 4 below.

3. Symptoms perceived by the patient as an acute illness, but which are really part of the unfolding chronic symptom picture (aggravations, healing crises)

If you are treating a patient for asthma and he gets a runny nose, it could be an unrelated acute illness, as in the previous scenario. However, the nasal discharge could also be an expression of the body exteriorizing the lung condition, or it could be an aggravation or accessory symptom of the remedy. In none of these situations should the nasal discharge be treated with a remedy. In this case I would prefer to use a natural supplement like Vitamin C or echinacea to treat the beginnings of a cold. We call such symptoms "side shows" to the treatment of the chronic disease. Patients perceive them to be acute ailments, finding it difficult to understand that they are really part of the healing process.

4. Simple acute conditions

Obviously, management of simple acute conditions (i.e. no exacerbations of a chronic miasm) is quite different from and simpler than for chronic cases. I recommend a 200c or 1M potency of the indicated remedy, of which one pellet is dissolved by stirring briskly in 4 oz. of water. (Poppyseed pellets are preferred because they dissolve right away; larger ones may need to be crushed between two spoons or two clean pieces of paper.) The patient takes one teaspoon and 10 to 15 minutes later the case is assessed for improvement. If improvement, wait until signs of relapse to give another dose. If no improvement, stir briskly and give another teaspoon. Teaspoons may be repeated as often as every 10 to 15 minutes. As the situation improves, slow down until you are giving the remedy every 30 minutes, then every hour, then every few hours. If the patient falls asleep, it is a good sign of healing and the patient should be left alone. When he wakes he will be much improved.

If there is no improvement by the time you have finished one cup, the remedy must be incorrect (or the potency is not high enough, if you are using 30c or 200c). Depending on how sure you are of the remedy, you may give up and try another remedy before finishing the 4 oz. cup. If the remedy is the simile rather than the simillimum it may stimulate the Vital Force to throw off symptoms guiding to the simillimum; thus it is essential to observe any shift in the symptom picture. Usually if the remedy is correct you will see some improvement by the time you have given 3 doses. If a remedy works one day and the same remedy is needed the following day, make a fresh cup even if there is still liquid left from the previous day.

It is not uncommon for acute situations to require several remedies, each of which is correct at the moment it is given (like von Boenninghausen's famous croup remedies: Aconite, Hepar sulph., and Spongia).[5] Also acute situations may require several different remedies, all of which can be given within a few minutes of each other, from different cups, not from the same cup. For example, following a car accident the patient may need Aconite for the fear of almost having died and Arnica for the soft tissue trauma.

Some remedies need to be made stronger; Kali bich. for sticky, stringy mucus is a good example. I routinely give Kali bich. by the tablespoonful rather than the teaspoonful. The remedy can also be made stronger by putting it in a small spring water bottle and succussing it in between doses.

Objective criteria for assessing the reaction in acute cases:

Body temperature. The drop of temperature in an acute case is an indication that we can stop the remedy, as the remedy has taken hold of the case. Further continuation of the remedy at that point would be counterproductive. Take the temperature under the arm as the oral is far more changeable and less practical. The normal axillary temperature is about 97.5°F. Any persistent temperature rise in a chronic case, no matter how slight, always leads in time to degenerative diseases.

Pulse: The pulse remains elevated as long as the temperature is above 97.5°F. When there is high temperature with a lowered heart rate, it is an indication for Pyrogenium (sepsis, peritonitis).

Blood pressure: If a patient has a blood pressure of 90/60 and after the remedy it rises to 110/80, then the remedy was the simillimum. The simillimum always tends to normalize hypertension in adults.

CHAPTER SIXTEEN

Palliation and Incurable Diseases

A physician can only save a patient not destined to die.
—*Japanese proverb*

Where Palliation Is Not Indicated

The legitimate use of palliation, which is the temporary relief of symptoms, is in *truly incurable* cases: the root of the tree is too diseased to be cured, as it were, and the sick branches are snipped instead. In palliation, the extreme external disease manifestations—the material pathological changes—are used as the guide rather than the internal imbalance which caused them to surface. The reaction of the Vital Force is not quick or powerful enough, and the most appropriate remedy may give only temporary improvement with the patient relapsing soon after each prescription. Examples are intractable cases of cancer and the last stages of lupus (SLE), TB, diabetes, etc. Relapses in these cases indicate that the remedy can only palliate because the patient is beyond cure. As old homeopaths expressed it: "In the last stages of TB, do not give Phosphorus, Psorinum, Silica, Sulphuric acid or a metal, but give a vegetable remedy, or Tuberculinum, and hand the patient down to his grave in peace."

Unfortunately, palliation is greatly misused in modern medicine for several reasons. First, doctors routinely substitute palliation for cure in chronic diseases. Allopathic medicine accepts the impossibility of curing chronic disease to such an extent that attention is focused entirely on "controlling" the disease, i.e. suppressing the symptoms, which requires lifelong and often increasing doses of the medicine. Chronic diseases which *otherwise could be curable* are palliated over and over again until the case finally *does* become incurable because of suppression and the consequent involvement of internal organs. Another reason for overuse of palliation is the patients: not knowing the difference between palliation and cure (understandably, since medical education in this country is focused on palliation), they demand immediate relief by any means necessary. They ignore possible side-effects or the creation of worse diseases. Patients have become accustomed to "instant relief" in acute conditions and expect the same in symptoms of chronic diseases, even though allopathic palliation of acute conditions can be as harmful as in chronic conditions. When an acute condition keeps recurring, the underlying disorder needs to be treated with a chronic remedy, and treating each outbreak by palliating the symptoms distracts the sufferer from seeking a true resolution of the miasmatic background. Also it can lead to worse long-term consequences, even from the point of view of the allopathic paradigm itself. For example, the overuse of antibiotics leads to medication-resistant bacteria.

Palliation in cases which could otherwise be curable thus has destructive effects, suppressing symptoms in acute conditions and complicating the picture in chronic states.

We began by saying that palliation is appropriate in incurable cases. But what is an incurable case? Unfortunately, many cases pronounced incurable by allopathic medicine could have been cured with homeopathy, as was often demonstrated a century ago when homeopaths had more freedom to practice. Many so-called incurable cases can still be rescued, especially with LM potencies. Still others could be cured with homeopathy if we were not working in an environment dominated by allopathy. For example, the patient must be able to tolerate the discomfort or even the social stigma of any rashes, itches or discharges produced as a natural part of the healing process under Hering's Laws. Patients in our modern times can too easily resort to cortisone cream and other OTC suppressive measures which fight against the healing action of the remedy. Or patients give up too soon on homeopathy; I have often had patients say, "I will give you two weeks to cure this, otherwise I am going back to my regular doctor." They have unrealistic expectations of the time frame involved and also of what homeopathy can accomplish. It is not uncommon for the mother of an ADD child who is doing much better under homeopathic treatment to request "another remedy" because he is still protesting about having to do homework. Patients expect miracles of the homeopath—and take them for granted when they occur—which they would never ask of their "regular doctor."

In other cases, the patient is convinced of the value of homeopathy but her family is not and they pressure her to seek conventional treatment, especially when under Hering's Laws she seems to be temporarily worse. I am sure my colleagues have found, as I have, that if your remedy works they dismiss it as coincidence, saying that the remedy could not be responsible since it has nothing in it. On the other hand, if there is an aggravation or if anything goes wrong with the case for other reasons, they blame the remedy. The patient's doctor can be another obstacle: out of a sincere desire to protect her patient, but having learned nothing of homeopathy in medical school (unlike her colleagues abroad), she may try to pressure or even frighten the patient into abandoning it. Or the physician may be trained as a homeopath but pressured not to use homeopathy by the threat of government interference, the loss of license, or the loss of hospital privileges. Thus homeopaths at the turn of the millennium face a much more difficult task than the great masters of a hundred years ago who achieved dramatic cures in cancer, diabetes, TB, and so many other so-called chronic diseases.

Homeopaths can make the mistake of yielding to patients' pressure for speedy symptomatic relief. Many homeopaths practice homeopathy in an allopathic way, covering the Chief Complaint in their prescribing but neglecting the totality of the patient. This can happen when the practitioner is too busy to do a good inquiry, or when she succumbs to the patient's demands for something "for the rash on my fingers." The remedy may offer temporary relief and improve the rash, but then it reappears after three months. Or as one complaint is resolved, the internal imbalance that created it throws out new symptoms. The practitioner ends up chasing the symptoms with one remedy after another, always temporarily ameliorating some symptoms but never curing the patient. The simillimum would have removed *all* the patient's symptoms, not just the rash. Combination remedies are popular because they offer the illusion of symptomatic relief, but this shotgun approach, condemned by Hahnemann, results in palliation at best.

Thus palliation is a mistake as long as there is any hope of curing the patient. In general, the homeopath should *always treat his case as if it were curable* (with specific unusual exceptions noted below). The remedy selection process is the same, whether the patient has been declared incurable or not. Note that I said *remedy* selection, not *potency*. Low potencies *are* required in cases of advanced pathology. The homeopath knows that death is a natural part of human existence; that some cases are not curable by any means; and that the best he can do in such cases is to provide the best possible quality of life as the end approaches. This is a sphere in which homeopathy shines, as will be seen at the end of this chapter.

Palliation for the dying patient can require very *high* potencies, such as the Tuberculinum CM given by the old masters to ease the anxiety, restlessness and fear of the patient in her dying moments. This may seem a contradiction to the statement just made about low potencies when pathology is extensive. As long as there is a hope of cure, the potencies must be kept low to avoid aggravating the physical pathological symptoms. But when the case is beyond hope, the best way to help the patient in his last hours is to help him let go of life peacefully; an aggravation of suffocating mucus, for example, will not make much difference at that point. In addition, the Vital Force of the dying patient is so low, since the flame of life is about to be extinguished, that the patient has relatively few physical symptoms.

Even in these incurable cases homeopathy is superior to allopathy because the material doses of allopathic drugs have a pathogenic action. They produce new symptoms, euphemistically called side-effects, because they create a disturbance in organs where, perhaps, there was none before. They compel a defensive or eliminative reaction which exhausts the already weakened Vital Force. *The material dose is a toxic dose.* Remember from Chapter 3 that the secondary action of allopathic medicines tend to depress the Vital Force. The result in an already terminal case is to shorten the life and increase the patient's suffering. While allopathic drugs may sometimes give a temporary sense of comfort and well-being, this palliative effect is fleeting and deceptive. It is soon replaced by the weakness and irritability of the secondary action. How often have we seen in practice patients quickly succumbing to the radiation, chemotherapy and side effects of toxic drugs used to treat terminal illnesses, especially cancer. As one of my students, a hospice nurse, observed, her patients do not die of cancer but rather from the treatment, and a grim death it is. I have often seen in my practice that a patient, otherwise healthy except for an isolated tumor, declines rapidly and dies within a few months after the cancer is diagnosed and aggressive treatment initiated.

Clinical Case: I will never forget a wonderful 70-year-old man who consulted me because his wife was worried about a small lump beneath his right nipple; he was not worried because he was in perfect health, enjoying their summers in Maine. He had had this tumor for the previous two years but had refused to go to a doctor. Since I was an alternative doctor, he succumbed to his wife's insistence that he see me. My heart sank as I palpated a small mammary tumor and realized that I was legally required to refer him to a radiologist and an oncologist. As I expected, he was frightened into initiating treatment, even though he had no symptoms beyond the small localized tumor. Within two months of excision of the tumor, followed by radiation and chemotherapy, the tumor had metastasized to his brain, pressing on his ocular nerve and causing him to go blind. Six months later he was dead. I regretted that he had come to me, because otherwise he could have enjoyed several years of good health and energy. And I regretted the laws which required allopathic referral, because I know of cases in India in which homeopathic treatment has pushed a small tumor like this to the surface, causing it to burst open and discharge, then healing the skin more cleanly than any surgery.

Finally, some homeopaths yield to pressure from the patient or family in incurable cases and prescribe allopathic painkillers, believing them necessary for the patient's comfort. If such drugs were really necessary, I would be the first to urge their use. But they are not, and the true homeopath, rather than lowering his standards and compromising his principles, should simply withdraw from such a case. For homeopathy has painkillers far more effective than drugs. We have all seen Bryonia, Belladonna, Chamomilla or Hypericum instantly relieve pain which high doses of morphine could not touch. Further, as we have seen, the effects of opioids are suppressive and toxic. Remedies will not stupefy and dull the patient, cause constipation or depress the respiratory rate as opioids do.

Every good homeopath has taken cases after an allopath has said, "Nothing more can be done," and has seen those patients either recover or have their life prolonged and suffering greatly ameliorated by homeopathic treatment *alone.* Dr. Dorothy Shepard describes treating a woman with a hard tumor of the kidney causing pain so intense that massive doses of morphine could not relieve it. Shepard took her off the morphine and put her on Hekla lava 3x, which not only eased the pain, it removed all but traces of the tumor.[1] So the homeopath must have the courage of her convictions in the face of great pressure to palliate either with superficial remedies or allopathic medications.

True Indications for Palliation

When and why should a homeopath conclude that a disease such as cancer, diabetes or tuberculosis is incurable? Most incurable cases have a *paucity of symptoms.* As Hahnemann says in Aphorism 14, "All curable diseases reveal themselves to the intelligent homeopath *in signs and symptoms.*" Pathological conditions are incurable when there are no signs and symptoms on which to base a cure. *As the pathology progresses, the symptoms of the patient decrease* (i.e. symptoms of the *disease*; the patient may have many symptoms from the *treatment*). These patients rarely have the vital reaction strong enough to bring out their original symptoms, hence they are incurable. The homeopath should advise his cancer patients to stimulate their Vital Force through other means: meditation, yoga, Qi Gong, Tai Chi, Reiki, polarity therapy and other energy-based healing. These methods can increase the Vital Force, thus prolonging the patient's life and improving its quality.

The following are additional indications that a case is truly incurable:

- Cases with *irreversible and structural damage* such as advanced cases of cancer, MS, nephritis, nephrotic syndrome, etc. These cases are not the same as the "one-sided diseases" which *can* be cured with homeopathy.
- Cases where *organs are removed,* for obvious reasons. Many of these cases, however, could have been spared the operation if the root of the problem were treated homeopathically in the first place.
- Cases where the Vital Force of the patient is *too weak* and he cannot withstand the stimulus of the prescribed remedy. (This situation cannot be determined in advance; the practitioner arrives at this conclusion after repeated attempts to treat homeopathically. See further in this chapter for guidelines.)

- In cases where true chronic diseases are deeply complicated by *allopathic drug toxicity*. The case is often discouraging and at times hopeless. The patient's sufferings can be best palliated by homeopathic methods, but they often remain patients until they die. This is especially true if the suppressive medication has continued to the point of serious organic lesions. In such cases the most careful selection of remedies often disappoints us because the remedy merely palliates temporarily. We are liable to make the mistake, especially in the early years of our practice, of blaming this superficial action on the potency used. We then mistakenly repeat the remedy in a higher potency, thus increasing our patient's suffering with aggravations and adding still more medical symptoms to the picture. The real problem is that the Vital Force is too "dead"; its reactive power has been blunted or destroyed by long-continued antipathic treatment.

  Thus the reaction is weak and short, although it may be prompt because of the increasing potencies we are using. At first the remedy is strong enough to irritate (or rouse up) the Vital Force, but then it rapidly overwhelms the Vital Force. This is much more like the primary and secondary actions of an allopathic remedy. A quick favorable response to a remedy in a deeply chronic case should always be regarded with suspicion, especially if the patient is very enthusiastic over his improvement in the first few days. His cry of delight may soon be changed to one of disappointment in the following week. The effect of the remedy has been palliative and will remain so in spite of frequent repetitions or increase in potency. (Of course, this effect could also be due to incorrect selection of the remedy, based only on the most superficial symptoms—and perhaps to the patient's most annoying ones.) But in the hands of a good practitioner, it is far more often due to the Vital Force's lack of reactive power after the long-term effect of multiple medications, so retaking the case is a must. This situation is illustrated by the Figure 15-3 in the previous chapter.

Unless the case is obviously incurable following the above guidelines, the homeopath should treat it as if it were curable. But sometimes, after observing the patient's reactions to different remedies, the homeopath is forced to admit that the patient is indeed incurable. These are guidelines for the practitioner in such cases:
- After the correctly indicated remedy, the homeopathic aggravation lasts for a long time and the patient's general condition continues to deteriorate.
- After the indicated remedy, there is quick, short amelioration, followed by aggravation (this frequently happens in advanced cancer).
- The amelioration after the homeopathic aggravation does not last (i.e., the patient keeps relapsing), and there is no obstacle to the cure.
- Some of the symptoms improve but the patient does not regain a sense of well-being.

- After a well-selected remedy, the symptoms go in the opposite direction to Hering's Laws.

The management of incurable patients varies widely. No two are alike, and not infrequently the remedy works for only a few hours. The rapid change in symptoms and states demands the homeopath's constant attention. Also the closer the remedy is to the simillimum (providing the disease is terminal and incurable), the sharper and more distressing the aggravation will be, thus the need for low potencies.

Sometimes homeopathic palliation is ineffective. For example, sometimes surgery is necessary to remove late-stage pathologies which threaten the patient's comfort or even his very life, such as a large tumor blocking the trachea or GI tract.

Remedies for the Dying Patient

There is so much emphasis on preserving life in allopathic medicine that little thought has been given to accepting and easing the patient's death. Recently, however, a National Institute of Medicine panel declared that relieving suffering at the end of life should be a priority. According to the 1997 panel, "too many people suffer needlessly at the end of life." The panel viewed *optimal care* for the dying as a more significant issue than physician-assisted suicide. It also concluded that "palliative care is an invisible service now in our hospitals," strongly urging hospitals and medical schools to train doctors in end-of-life care. "Current programs do not recognize the final phases of illnesses or construct effective strategies for care and communicate sensitively with patients and those close to them," the panel concluded.

The reality of dying has been largely shunned by the news media and unrealistically romanticized by the entertainment media. The result is fear, misinformation and oversimplification that contribute to the public perception of pain and misery as inescapable. Nearly 60% of deaths in the US occur in hospitals and another 17% at nursing homes. Patients are often drugged into unconsciousness, surrounded by tubes and beeping monitors, and separated from their family and familiar home environment. In the East, death is approached as philosophically as life: death is viewed as a gate to another dimension, to be passed through consciously.

Just as we now have birthing coaches, we should have a wise and experienced coach present during the dying process to guide both patient and family. The family should be advised not to say, "Please don't die," or "We can't go on without you." When the end is inevitable, the patient should be released emotionally to die in peace. In homeopathy we have remedies to alleviate not only the patient's physical suffering but also the fear and emotional torment. This is true euthanasia, in the original sense of the word: a "good death." For example, Arsenicum or Tuberculinum in high potencies can relieve the immense anxiety, restlessness and fear of death and make the patient's final hours more comfortable.

The following are some of the top remedies indicated for the dying patient, with numbers to indicate the frequency of use. Their potency should be at least 200c and often much higher (up to CM).

Arsenicum album (3): The Arsenicum patient is known for his *fighting spirit*. Fighting illness, fighting obstacles and limitations, fighting for perfection and absolutes, and fighting the inevitable are a constant theme of his life. It stands to reason that Arsenicum would be a prime remedy for the struggles of the dying who resist death with every fiber and every cell of their being. The remedy in high potency (at least 200c) lessens the terror of the Great Unknown and eases the letting go of this life. (Boericke: "Gives quiet and ease to the last moments of life when given in high potency.") Well-known modalities of Arsenicum include thinking it is useless to take the remedy, feeling worse after midnight, desiring little sips of cold water (put Arsenicum in it), and feeling better from warmth and when the head is elevated (wanting some extra pillows).

Tarentula cubensis (3): the second-best remedy (even the favorite of some of the old masters), it soothes the final agony, especially when there is nervous restlessness, difficulty breathing, anxiety to the point of delirium, and atrocious pains with great prostration.

Lachesis (1) is another remedy for the dying (Boericke: "euthanasia") especially when, in addition to typical Lachesis indications, the patient experiences frightening spiritual struggles.

Carbo vegetalis (2) ("the corpse reviver") is a blessing to the elderly patient who spiritually is quite prepared to go but physically is gasping for air and is terrified by not being able to get enough. Guiding symptoms include complete collapse with blue, icy cold body and fear of darkness and ghosts. The patient typically is almost lifeless, but head is hot; the breath is cool, the pulse imperceptible and the respiration quickened. The patient must have air, must be fanned, and must have the windows open.

Aconite (2): for the patient who fears death, but who believes it will happen soon and even predicts the exact time. The patient typically has great anxiety, panic, and terror, with anxious restlessness and tossing about. The sufferer is rarely fully conscious, more often delirious.

Antimonium tart. (2): guiding symptoms include the death rattle; great rattling of mucus but with very little expectorated; coughing and gasping consecutively; edema and impending paralysis of the lung, in a drowsy and comatose patient.

Tuberculinum (2): also advocated in the CM potency when the death rattle is very distressing. It stops the rattling and allows the patient to go in peace.

Latrodectus mactans (3): for the anxious patient, screaming with the pain, typically in heart failure. The patient has extreme breathlessness with gasping respiration and fear of losing his breath. The skin is cold as marble.

Opium (2): for the dying person who has complete loss of consciousness, who is unable to understand or appreciate his suffering, as in a stupor. Or the patient has painlessness of all complaints, heavy, stuporous sleep, and noisy, irregular breathing (Cheyne-Stokes respiration). The patient's skin is hot and damp. She feels better from cold things and worse from heat and during and after sleep.

Rhus tox. (2): the patient suffers from extreme restlessness, with a continual change of position (very much like Arsenicum, but Arsenicum has more anxiety and prostration). There is great apprehension at night, making the patient want to get out of bed. The patient may have thoughts of suicide. He feels worse at night, during sleep, at rest, and from cold.

Veratrum album (2): The patient has attacks of pain with delirium driving her to madness, sometimes cursing and howling all night. She may have delusions that she is about to become rich. These patients are likely to suffer from collapse with extreme coldness, blueness, and weakness. Cold perspiration on the forehead is typical, and the patient feels worse at night, better from warmth.

Homeopathy truly has something to offer for humanity at every stage of life. May you enable your patient to make the great transition free from pain and with peace and dignity.

CHAPTER SEVENTEEN

The Nosodes

Definition and History

The term *nosode* refers to a remedy made from diseased tissue or discharges (from the Greek *nosos*, "disease"). Technically, a nosode is made from *pathologic material derived from vegetable, animal or human sources.* For instance, Secale cornutum and Ustilago maidis are vegetable nosodes (made from the fungi which infests rye and corn, respectively). Tuberculinum bovinum is an animal nosode (made from the sputum of a cow with bovine tuberculosis). Psorinum is a human disease product (made from the discharge from a scabies vesicle). The pathogenic discharge, fluid from an eruption, or actual diseased tissue is triturated with lactose and then potentized in the usual way. As nosodes were never used below 6c and usually in the 30th potency and upwards, there was no possibility of any disease substance remaining.

Endocrine remedies such as Adrenalinum and Thyroidinum should not be included in this group but should be studied in relation to the other glandular remedies, such as Pituitary and Folliculinum (potentized ovary tissue). These are all derived from healthy tissue, not diseased tissue, and thus are called *sarcodes* (from the Greek word *sarcos,* flesh). Continuing with the limits of our definition, Lac defloratum (skim milk) and Lac caninum (dog's milk) cannot be regarded as nosodes any more than Apis, Lachesis, or Cantharis, the latter all being normal physiological substances, although we sometimes see them listed as nosodes.

What remedies then were originally included as nosodes? The chief ones, with their disease origins, were Ambra grisea (a morbid secretion from the intestines of sperm whales), Anthracinum (anthrax), Lyssin (rabies), Malandrinum (the "grease of horses," according to Allen), Medorrhinum (gonorrhea), Psorinum (scabies), Pyrogenium (septicemia), Secale (rye ergot), Syphilinum (syphilis), Variolinum (smallpox), and Tuberculinum (tuberculosis). Of course many more were added later; two of the more popular ones are Influenzinum (influenza) and Carcinosin (cancer). When bacteriology became a flourishing branch of medicine, cultures of specific germs were used as the basis for potentized remedies, including Staphylococcin and Streptococcin (one of my favorite remedies for rheumatoid arthritis, not surprisingly since RA is a sequela of strep infections). Nosodes made from diseased tissue or discharges (particularly if the patient from whom they are taken was successfully prescribed for) have a much broader field of action and can be more safely selected than the nosodes made from individual bacterial cultures (like Staphylococcin), because the material of the nosodes is much more than the microorganisms involved. The whole environment (tissues plus microbes) has been potentized.

Long before Koch and Pasteur developed the science of bacteriology, it occurred to some homeopaths that visible disease manifestations such as skin eruptions and discharges should contain toxins which could be potentized and proven as remedies. Hahnemann was the first, doing a short proving of Psorinum. However, he would never give anything even to his most trusted followers that he had not incontrovertibly proved, and he felt that he had not proven Psorinum extensively enough to use it.

It was Hering who really promoted the use of nosodes and did many provings of nosodes. Hering was responsible for adding many categories of remedies, including the *autonosodes* made from disease substances taken directly from the patient's body. This practice made Hahnemann very protective of the laws and principles of homeopathy, as he feared that later homeopaths would change them. And indeed Wilhelm Lux, a homeopathic veterinarian, developed an offshoot of homeopathy called *isopathy* (treating a disease with potentized products of the same disease), declaring that it was based on the law "the Same Cures the Same." However, isopathic remedies have a much narrow application than homeopathic ones, since each one can only be used for one disease condition instead of having a wide range of mental, emotional and physical indications.

So are nosodes isopathy or homeopathy? Some homeopaths have long considered nosodes isopathic since they can be given in minute doses for the cure of the same disease, and it is certainly in the use of nosodes that the two schools have the most common ground. But nosodes are prescribed for a far wider range of indications than the disease from which they are derived. They are prescribed on symptoms from provings; most have a full range of mental and emotional symptoms; and they are not given for the same disease unless homeopathically indicated, any more than Rhus tox. is *always* used for poison ivy (or *only* used for poison ivy). While it is true that nosodes are not as well proven as our well-known polychrests, they are at least better and safer than vaccinations, and their indications are constantly becoming better known as they are more widely used. And nosodes have been so successful that new nosodes continued to be added. While the symptomatology for nosodes depends more on clinical experience than provings, in general, the clinical experience for most nosodes has accumulated for many years and has been checked by the experience of so many practitioners that it is considered trustworthy.

From lack of knowledge or understanding, however, nosodes have been mostly neglected or even banned. Dr. Richard Hughes, one of the first homeopaths in England, never even mentioned nosodes; but it is well known that Hughes kept out of his works everything that he thought was likely to be offensive to allopaths. Because of his influence, it was not until the next century that Margaret Tyler and Donald Foubister promoted the use of nosodes in the English-speaking world. It is unfortunate that so few homeopaths have been taught the proper uses of the nosodes, because without them it is difficult or impossible to address the miasmatic conditions underlying chronic diseases.

In spite of the negative attitude of some homeopaths, nosodes have held their place since Hahnemann's time, and the most brilliant practitioners (Hering, Swan, H. C. Allen, Foubister, Tyler, Burnett, etc.) have made the greatest use of them. H.C. Duncan of New York developed a particular type of nosodes called autogenous remedies. He prepared remedies from a patient's focal infection which could then be used for a *similar* condition in another patient (it will never be the *same*). For example, a vaginal discharge that resisted the most common indicated remedies would be treated by potentizing some of the discharge; the remedy could be used for that patient and others with similar stubborn vaginal secretions. The applications are thus broader than in isopathy but these remedies still have not been proven and thus do not have associated mental/emotional symptoms.

The nosodes have earned a bad reputation partly because some homeopaths use them isopathically. For example, if a patient has had active syphilis, they invariably prescribe Syphilinum; if gonorrhea, they automatically give Medorrhinum; and if they fail to discover either, conclude that the cause must be "tubercular" and therefore prescribe Tuberculinum. By contrast, Nash makes this comment in his *Leaders:*

> I have cured eruptions resembling itch with Psorinum, rheumatic troubles that were obstinate under usual remedies with Medorrhinum, and a long standing case of caries of the spine with Syphilinum, but in none of these cases had the patient that I could trace, itch, gonorrhea nor syphilis.[1]

In the remainder of this chapter we will examine the uses of nosodes, focusing on nosodes made from human disease products and bacteria. While the animal and vegetable nosodes are nosodes according to the technical definition, they are prescribed like other remedies in terms of indications and potency. I have had wonderful results with Ustilago, for example, for bleeding fibroids and Secale for gangrene. Massimo Mangialavori includes Ambra grisea in the family of the sea remedies, on the basis that it has taken on mental/emotional qualities from the sea creature which produces it.[2] These remedies are not used in the very specific circumstances and potencies of human nosodes. The only exceptions are Malandrinum (used by the old masters like Variolinum) and Tuberculinum (made from bovine tuberculosis).

The Use of Nosodes in Acute Cases

Based on the experience of hundreds of homeopaths, we know that nosodes are relatively ineffective in the acute conditions they were derived from. Each nosode has a far wider range of applications than its own acute disease (e.g. Influenzinum for flu, Tuberculinum or Bacillinum for TB) and for each of these acute diseases, there are many other remedies which will work better. It is probable that the acute sickness elicits such a specific reaction that other remedies are better indicated.

The great usefulness of the nosodes in acute cases lies elsewhere in two indications:

Prophylaxis in an epidemic: Generally speaking, a single dose of 30c weekly or 200c monthly will provide protection. For example, during flu epidemics the old masters gave a 30c of Influenzinum q 14 days coupled with Bacillinum (Compton Burnett's favorite) 30c once a month.

Lingering effects of disease: If a case of an acute disease *is slow in convalescence, apt to relapse,* a dose or two of its nosode will do wonders: for example, Morbillinum for a case of measles where chest catarrhal symptoms are persistent or Pertussin for a patient who only partially recovers from whooping cough. In such cases the nosode seems to give *a fresh impetus to powers of recovery.*

Certainly, we may not forget that the major polychrests Sulphur and Lycopodium are equally indicated in such circumstances and if any of them is indicated by symptoms, they should be given *before* the nosode. For example, often after flu a cough lingers which typically responds to Sulphur. But so often in these cases there is a fundamental weakness of recuperative power, which means the case has only a few vague symptoms, since characteristic symptoms are the result of the reactive power of an intact Vital Force. In this case the severe acute, lingering condition might suppress the Vital Force so that it cannot push the symptoms to the exterior on which we could prescribe the simillimum. It is precisely in these conditions—where there are no very clear indications for a remedy—that the nosode can help (as discussed in the section on Paucity of Symptoms in Chapter 10, Golden Rules and Special Forms of Prescribing).*

---

* In the history of homeopathy there has been one successful exception to the rule against treating an acute illness with the nosode made from the illness, during the pneumonia epidemic in England and Scotland after World War II. The septicemia was too severe and far too often fatal, especially for the poor patients who came into the hospital when it was far advanced, to find the simillimum by classical prescribing. For practical reasons Drs. Teale and Bach developed a *polyvalent vaccine* from several severe cases. (This was the same Dr. Bach who

The Use of Nosodes in Chronic Illness

Nosodes are a special category of remedies with special uses in chronic illness that go beyond our normal understanding of the totality of the symptoms. Following are some of their specific uses:

As a chronic remedy: Kent, H.C. Allen and other eminent homeopaths have stressed the fact that the nosodes should be prescribed on the *symptoms and not for the disease* of which the particular nosode is a product. Nosodes are no exception to the rule that remedies are prescribed on the match with the patient's symptom totality. This concept will lead the practitioner to some brilliant cures.

For example, a child with asthma attacks, better at the seashore, always better at night (worse from dawn on), who sleeps in the knee-chest position, sticking his feet out of bed because they are hot, and who is afraid of the dark and of someone behind him would clearly need Medorrhinum. In this case we would open with the nosode because according to the totality of the symptoms, no other remedy is better indicated.

The same is true if the nosode corresponds to the overall make-up of the patient. When two parents each have the same active miasm, it can become stamped on the unborn child to such an extent that it masks the innate constitution and almost becomes the constitution of the child. The Medorrhinum person, for example, loves parties, "sex, drugs and rock 'n' roll," and staying out late at night in the darkness. These people come to life at night, although they also look behind them at night all the time because of the delusion "behind him, someone is" (K30). This shows the paranoid state of sycosis (see Chapter 21, Sycosis) as it represents a subconscious fear that something is going on behind their back or that someone is about to get them. They are liars and thrill seekers, full of suspicions. This mental-emotional portrait is a clear indication of the nosode. The portraits of the nosodes of the four original chronic miasms are described later in this chapter.

As an intercurrent remedy: When a well-chosen remedy does not hold because of vital weakness and deep-seated tendencies, or if it stops working or did not act in the first place in a chronic

---

developed polyvalent vaccines from bowel nosodes, described in the next chapter, and the method of administration was similar.) The injection was given hypodermically in small isolated doses, with the effect of each dose observed before repetition was considered. After the injections the patient's body temperature would rise briefly half a degree to a degree and then fall within a couple of hours. Often no further rise of temperature would occur, and no further dose was given. Sometimes fever would return and a second dose be given. Three doses were rarely needed and never more than three to bring about a cure.

case with strong miasmatic indications, usually this indicates a *miasmatic block*. We can use a nosode to break through a miasmatic block with *intercurrent prescribing*. ("Intercurrent" means that we alternate the nosode with the top antimiasmatic remedies for the active miasm, giving a single dose of the nosode whenever the remedy stops working). This is why you need to determine the active miasm right from the first intake. And it is a good reason *not* to abandon a well-indicated remedy, because the remedy will work again after the block is removed with a nosode. For example, if Thuja has worked beautifully in a sycotic miasmatic case for several months and then it ceases to work although it is still indicated, first you should try increasing the potency and/or dose. If no further action is seen from Thuja, a single dose of Medorrhinum is administered. Allow two to three weeks for the nosode to work uninterrupted. Unless the symptom picture has then changed to the point that a different remedy is indicated (which would probably be the other top antisycotic remedy, Nat. sulph.), you would simply pick up Thuja where you left off and it will work again. (Be sure to tell an LM patient to save the partly-used bottle of Thuja which she was taking before the Medorrhinum.). For example, if the patient were halfway through a bottle of Thuja LM3, 4 successions, she would simply continue the same bottle at the same dosage level. Or if Phosphorus worked in a tubercular miasmatic case and then stopped working, give Tuberculinum.

Tuberculinum also has a particular indication which the other nosodes do not share: when symptoms are constantly changing and well-selected remedies do not help (especially in patients with low grade fevers and swollen lymph nodes who catch every cold and flu that comes around), this very changeability of symptoms would indicate Tuberculinum.

If a case is advanced by a nosode, it is best to stay with it and do nothing further as long as the action of the nosode continues. Because nosodes are such deep-working and long-acting remedies, you should wait as long as the patient continues to improve before giving another remedy. I have seen a single dose of a nosode continue to work for two months. You may also need to repeat the nosode in a 1M to make sure the terrain is completely cleared. If there is great improvement under the action of the nosode, I would prefer to repeat the nosode before returning to the remedy (or going to the next-indicated remedy). For example, if Medorrhinum is given when Thuja has stopped working, and if the patient makes great progress from the first dose of Medorrhinum, I would prefer to repeat it in a 200c or 1M before returning to Thuja (or going to the next indicated antisycotic remedy).

If the patient does not show any improvement after at least two weeks, you can introduce the previous remedy again and often it will act at that point because the nosode has removed the miasmatic block. So although the nosode might not appear to improve the case directly, it may resensitize the patient to the previous remedy. Usually it is sufficient to use the nosode in a 200c potency, one or two doses in one day (3 pellets dry, one for hypersensitives) and then wait.

Treating a Never Well Since: Using a nosode to treat a case of Never Well Since an infectious illness is similar to the acute scenario above, "Lingering Effects of a Disease," but now the disease is much more distant in the patient's past medical history. This scenario also differs in how the nosode is used: in the first case above, the nosode finishes the case, while here it can be used to open the case.

Many twentieth-century homeopaths, led by Margaret Tyler, believe that the common contagious diseases can leave lingering traces preventing full health even after the manifest symptoms have been eradicated. In other words, the patient reports being "never well since" having the flu years previously or "I never really recovered from having mono many years ago." The acquired acute miasm has become an active layer and is suppressing the patient's innate temperament. "I used to be so sharp-minded, so quick thinking, until I got mono, and now I can't remember anything, I can't follow a conversation and I feel so embarrassed."

Or the patient does not recover with the well-indicated remedies from an apparently unrelated condition, and there is a severe flu condition in the past medical history. There may be a connection even if the patient cannot remember if the current Chief Complaint and the past flu attack are related. In difficult, confused chronic illnesses, it would be wise to inquire into the past history of the patient for severe infectious diseases (shingles, measles, chickenpox, etc.). So even if an influenza was "cured," for instance with Gelsemium, it apparently "polluted" or "poisoned" the patient's economy (as the old masters called the body's functional capacity). And in order to bring the Vital Force up to par again, Influenzinum is needed to clear this residual pathology. (Give a single dose of 200c 3 pellets dry, wait several weeks and observe; if there is a strong positive response but an additional dose is needed, follow with 1M.)

This is also the case with other contagious diseases (especially childhood diseases) for which we will use the corresponding nosode, such as Morbillinum after measles, Influenzinum after the flu, or Scarlatinum after scarlet fever. Although Carcinosin is the nosode for cancer, it is used for Never Well Since mono, based on clinical experience. (It is one of the most frequently used remedies for mono, along with Arsenicum and Gelsemium.)

In such cases it is remarkable how a few doses of the corresponding nosode starts the road to recovery or at least results in a marked improvement. This nosode usually *will not finish* the case, but because of its action, the indications for the subsequent remedies become clearer and the response to them more marked. So a nosode will improve the patient significantly. In some cases it will *appear* to bring about a cure which lasts for several months to a year, but invariably, after a time, *the symptoms return, although less pronounced*. When they return, the nosode might not help but Hahnemann's antimiasmatic remedies will then complete the cure.

Of course when the Never Well Since is a vaccination, the corresponding nosode will be very useful, although we have also remedies for this situation such as Thuja, Sulphur, Malandrinum, and Silica. I would tend to try the polychrest first, but other homeopaths use DPT 200c routinely, for example, after a bad reaction to a DPT shot. Since vaccinations are known to have harmful longterm sequelae, "Never Well Since vaccination" should be suspected when the onset of the disease coincides with a vaccination, even when the patient does not make the association. While a patient is more likely to be "Never Well Since vaccination" if there was an immediate response such as a seizure or prolonged screaming, such a response does not have to be present. (Of course there is often no record or memory of the patient's response.)

Finally, when we do the patient's timeline, *any history of severe acute infection* would warrant an experimental use of the corresponding nosode in a case not responding to apparently well-selected remedies. The picture often clears with one dose of the suitable nosode and an easy prescription inevitably follows.

While the above are examples stemming from *acute* miasms, the same is true for *chronic* miasms, e.g. the patient's gonorrhea is suppressed by antibiotics, causing a sycotic state. Or a patient acquires the sycotic miasm from a sex partner. We so often see female patients with chronic vaginitis or yeast infections, dating back to the day they got married and had increased sexual activity (Never Well Since marriage!). They were innocent victims of the husband's latent or dormant sycotic miasmatic state (see Chapter 21 on the Sycotic Miasm). Even if the husband showed no symptoms (because his previous illness was strongly suppressed with Western drugs), he transmitted this miasmatic state to his spouse. Medorrhinum will be needed to clear the case. Depending on the symptoms, you may even need to open with Medorrhinum when there is a past history of gonorrhea.

To counteract a vaccination: A nosode can be used to counteract the bad effects (acute or chronic) from a vaccination for the corresponding disease. For example, Pertussin can be used for complications from DPT (because when there are problems with the DPT, it is usually linked to the Pertussis part of the vaccine). Whenever we see a child react to DPT (as is very common), we should immediately administer a dose of Pertussin or a DPT 200c. (Some parents who are committed to homeopathy have successfully used a medical or religious exemption not to have their children vaccinated; for others I would give the parents the appropriate remedy to keep on hand in case the child has a bad reaction to the vaccination.) I have successfully used Variolinum, even years later, for the long-term effects of smallpox vaccinations. I have seen patients suffering from the after-effects of this vaccination which was repeated *three times* "because it did not take the first time"! You can imagine how much "poison" is brought into the system when this vaccination is repeated. It arouses the sycotic miasm like a dormant volcano bursting into eruption, adding the speed of the sycotic miasm to the obstinacy of psora and creating cysts, tumors, boils, abscesses, and many other symptoms. Or it is added to the destructive qualities of syphilis, creating ulcerating tumors.

As a homeopathic immunization: Homeoprophylaxis can be achieved in three different ways:
- by giving the patient's *constitutional remedy*, which tends to strengthen the patient overall,
- by giving the remedy for a specific *epidemic,* which will prevent the patient from succumbing to that particular epidemic disease,
- by using the *nosode* of the acute miasm itself.

Clinical trials have demonstrated the success of using nosodes in epidemics. For example, during a meningitis epidemic in Brazil in 1974, Meningococcinum 10c was given to 18,640 children, while 6,340 children did not receive this unproven nosode. Only 4 cases of meningitis developed among the children "immunized" with the nosode, while 34 cases developed among the unprotected children. In other words, over 100 cases would have developed in this group if an equal number of children had been unprotected: they were *25 times as likely* to contract meningitis!

Von Boenninghausen was the first to suggest that nosodes could be used to prevent epidemic diseases. He suggested that Variolinum 200c is far superior to crude vaccination for smallpox and absolutely safe.

Other famous homeopaths like Margaret Tyler had good results using nosodes preventively in epidemics in the past, when they were much more common and thus it was easier to test the results. Compton Burnett wrote: "I have for the last nine years been in the habit of using vaccine matter (Variolinum) in 30c potency whenever smallpox was about and I have thus far not seen anyone so treated get variola *[smallpox]*."[3] Dr. Dorothy Shepherd wrote in *Magic of the Minimum Dose:* "Diphtheria can be more safely prevented by the homeopathic nosode Diphtherinum, given in single doses in a high potency."[4] She did clinical trials in boarding schools were epidemics were rampant. H.C. Allen used Diphtherinum for 25 years as a prophylactic and never had a patient contract the disease. It is important to note that some of the nosodes used by these eminent homeopaths were not proven, or at least not as extensively as our usual remedies. There is no time for a proving in an epidemic (as in the meningitis outbreak in Brazil.)

However, we should never routinely give children nosodes such as Morbillinum and Pertussin to replace their vaccinations as some homeopaths do. The intention is understandable: as homeopaths we would like to avoid the havoc created by frequent vaccinations, especially those made from mixed antigens. We so often see in our practice the havoc they create. But replacing the standard vaccination schedule with the corresponding nosodes is unnecessary and a waste of remedies. A much better approach (in the case of self-limiting childhood illnesses) is to let the child contract the disease naturally, treating them with the indicated remedy. Natural lifelong immunity is achieved this way, which nosodes cannot provide. (Nor can vaccinations! It makes no sense to give a rubella vaccination to little girls when the immunity is likely to wear off before they bear children. Much better to let them catch German measles, a mild childhood illness which will give them immunity throughout their childbearing years. When would you repeat the vaccination? How often and how long does the immunity last? The only way you can tell that the effect has worn off is if the patient contracts the disease!)

Other Indications
- When the paucity of symptoms in a mute case or one-sided case results in a lack of indications for any particular remedy, the nosode based on the prevalent miasmatic condition is given to open the case. (For example if the main complaints are sycotic, give Medorrhinum.) It will strengthen the Vital Force, which will then throw up symptoms on which we can prescribe. The nosode in itself might also bring improvement.
- When symptoms repeatedly relapse, this can indicate a miasmatic block to be treated with intercurrent prescribing with nosodes. (There can be other reasons for relapsing, as discussed in Chapter 15, Management of the Case.)
- The nosode can be prescribed for the miasm indicated by the patient's past medical history and family history (see Chapter 19, Miasms). The indications can be mental as well as physical. For example, a family history riddled with depression, alcoholism, drug addiction, suicide and other self-destructive behaviors will indicate the syphilitic miasm and possible need for Syphilinum. Many instances of cancer, diabetes, leukemia or pernicious anemia in the family would indicate the necessity for Carcinosin in a stalled case. A child with alabaster skin and an angelic look, with a tendency to frequent colds, flus and coughs, might require Tuberculinum if there is any family history of lung trouble or tuberculosis. Tuberculinum is also used in those children who have violent temper tantrums with kicking and screaming on the floor and those who have no perseverance or concentration. Administer your nosode as early as possible to these children; it will save a lot of time and undue suffering. Cases properly handled should leave the child with no sequelae and in better health.
- As an *autonosode*, a "vaccine" made from the patient's own disease matter (see above)
- When several remedies seem to be indicated but none of them completely fits the case, one option is to use the nosode of the active miasm. It will move the case forward enough to make the next prescription easier. This especially holds true when the remedies are associated with a particular bowel nosode (see the next chapter).

- In conditions arising from the suppression of skin lesions in particular, Psorinum is often needed. Skin conditions are so suppressed that Psorinum is needed to clear the situation (and Psorinum is also one of Kent's "reactive remedies").
- Give the nosode closest to the remedy that worked and which covers some of the patient's symptoms. If the complementary remedy does not work, the "poison" of the miasm needs to be cleared with the nosode.

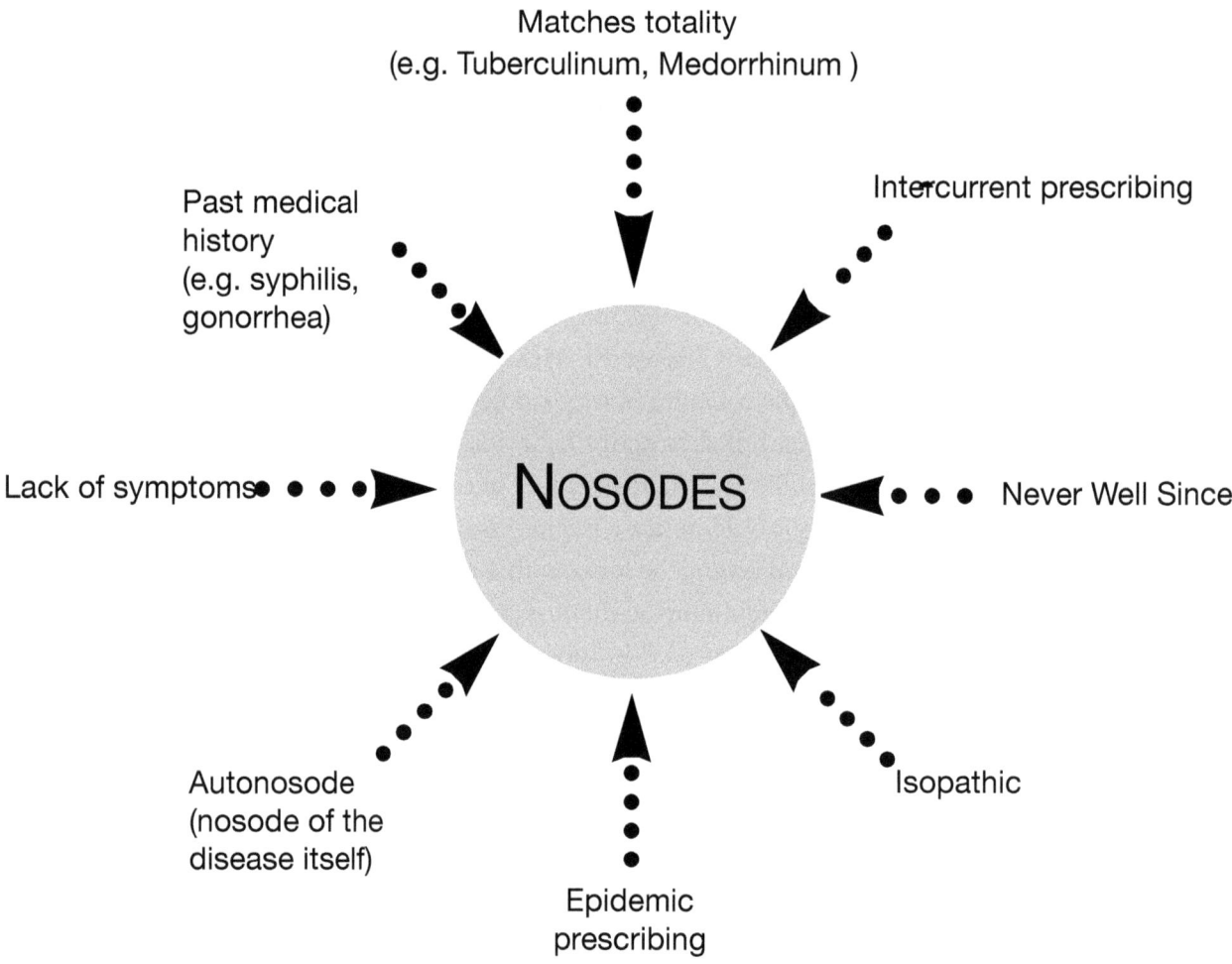

Fig. 17-1: Some Uses for Nosodes

Some Cautions about the Uses of Nosodes

Nosodes are powerful and deeply working remedies, not to be taken lightly or used too quickly. Keep them in your hand to be played like a trump card when you really need them. Do not make the mistake of prescribing a nosode if the symptoms clearly indicate a remedy. Kent says, "I have known Medorrhinum to be given and fail where Thuja would have cured promptly, because the symptoms were predominantly Thuja and not Medorrhinum."[5] Of course, if there is paucity of symptoms and a history of gonorrhea or simply a strong sycotic background, Medorrhinum will be given to clear the picture and advance the case to some extent.

Clinical case: As a reminder of how powerful nosodes are, not to be used arbitrarily, I recall a patient that came to me in desperation after being given Syphilinum by another homeopath two years before. After taking the Syphilinum, she broke out in the typical blistering, scarring rash of syphilis all over her body. The homeopath was at a loss as to how to continue the case. To make matters worse, her husband "caught" the miasm from his wife and exhibited the same rash for months after her first exposure. You can imagine the despair of the patient. She knew that allopathy could not correct her condition (would never even understand it), and her faith in homeopathy was badly shaken. (Of course, all the Syphilinum did was to stimulate the expression of a miasm present long before, but this is hard for a patient to understand). On inquiry, I discovered just how loaded her syphilitic background was: her own history and her family history included melancholy, depression, mental illness and suicide. Mercury turned out to be the simillimum, which I gave in an LM potency, 2 succussions only. After just a couple of doses, her rash came out more, which is of course a favorable reaction. But tell that to a patient who got the rash in the first place "because of homeopathy"! After only a few doses and two consultations, I did not hear from her anymore—no doubt, I thought, because she gave up on the treatment. Three years later I found out what had happened. These few LM doses of Mercury were enough to completely clear the rash for three years, when finally a little came back. But more importantly, her depression of 30 years' duration had completely lifted! Apparently in spite of so few doses and only two succussions, Mercury LM1 was powerful enough to extinguish the syphilitic miasm for a long time. I was not surprised that it was not enough to finish the job, but the homeopathic task was now easy: give her one dose of Merc. sol. LM1 at the same point where she left off. Then wait and see, giving occasional doses prn. I can only shudder at what would have happened if she had used allopathic drugs to suppress the rash. No doubt deep depression would have been a result, and homeopathy would have been wrongly blamed. But it is a lesson that nosodes must be used with great caution and only with a thorough training and good understanding.

I also shudder when I hear of homeopaths prescribing such a powerful nosode as Syphilinum indiscriminately for such vague indications as "symptoms worse at night." As we can see, Syphilinum and all nosodes are powerful drugs and not to be taken lightly.

The final section of this chapter will describe the indications for the nosodes associated with the four original chronic miasms.

Psorinum

The easiest way to remember the keynotes of Psorinum are to compare it to Sulphur, its complementary remedy. It is perhaps not surprising that Psorinum resembles Sulphur, our number one anti-psoric, when we consider that Psorinum was prepared from pus taken from mature pustules on the hands of a healthy individual who was afflicted with the itch (scabies vesicle), the origin of the psoric miasm. Psorinum resembles the "soil" from which it springs, just as there is a relationship between some plant remedies and the soil in which the plant grows (like Belladonna and Calcarea; Belladonna grows in soil rich with calcium carbonate; Pulsatilla grows in potassium-rich soil and is therefore the vegetable analog of the Kalis.)

Mental/emotional: While Sulphur can be careless (about his person and his surroundings), emotionally unstable as a ragged philosopher, full of theories and averse to physical exertion, Psorinum paints a lot more gloomy, melancholic picture. He is in a constant state of despair (Despair, of recovery K36 and Despair, religious salvation, of K36). He looks a lot like those other eternal pessimists Arsenicum and especially Nitric acid. "I am no better," these patients report to you, although they are. Psorinum has not lost all hope but he does not know what to do, as if he is caught between two walls. Everything is bleak, he sees no light breaking through the clouds above his head, all is dark about him. He takes no joy in his family, is extremely irritable and looks for solitude. Often he is driven to despair by severe itching.

While Sulphur has few fears (heights being the main one), Psorinum is full of fears. The outstanding ones are fear of poverty, insanity, disaster, fire, and failure in business (although he is prospering). Fear and despair create an inferiority complex in the Psorinum person so diametrically opposed to the self-assured, even haughty Sulphur. Psorinum's many anxieties can take the forms of guilt feelings or anxiety with oppression in the chest, great anguish in the head, driving him to pace the floor, wringing his hands and moaning. Only when he eats his meals does he cease moaning. In fact he is cross and scolds when dinner is not ready.

While the Sulphur is full of optimistic ideas and theories, grandiose as they might be, Psorinum is joyless and his ideas are sad. This great despondency makes his own life and that of others intolerable. Insufferably self-willed, he annoys those about him.

The despair of religious salvation is present because Psorinum thinks he has sinned away his last chance of divine grace: it is a fixed idea during the day and he dreams about it at night. There are horrid thoughts which he cannot get rid of at night, while he is carrying on an imaginary conversation with himself of what he would do or say in case this or that happens. Of course he gets mentally exhausted from these sleepless nights which does not help his understanding and memory during the day. He is definitely worse from emotions and mental labor. The slightest emotions cause severe trembling and wringing of the hands while the tiniest thing can give him a fright. Then there can be sudden transition from cheerfulness to sadness, or vexation without any cause.

Physical: As Margaret Tyler says in her inimitable *Homeopathic Drug Pictures,* while Sulphur is the great "unwashed" with his aversion to baths (because of aggravation of symptoms and catching cold after every bath), Psorinum is the *"great unwashable."* No matter how hard he tries he cannot get clean. His skin always looks dirty, oozes frequently and has the Psorinum sour smell or odor of rotten meat. Often there are ulcers which heal slowly. These vesicular, pustular eruptions are worse in the winter (as in Graphites). Perhaps the greatest physical modality of Psorinum is his *extreme sensitivity to cold.* He wants to be covered: the head must be covered warmly even during the summer because he is so sensitive to drafts about his head (Silica). This characteristic is so strongly marked that Psorinum usually *fails* when given to warm-blooded individuals who crave the fresh open air. Psorinum's cold sensitivity is a great mark of differentiation from the hot-blooded Sulphur. He bundles up when others like Pulsatilla, Lycopodium and Sulphur hardly feel the cold at all. Thus aggravation of Psorinum complaints in the cold or winter months is also a great characteristic of this remedy. Psorinum is also *very sensitive to atmospheric changes.* He is intensely aggravated before and during thunderstorms ("Generalities, Storm, approach of," K1403). Any change of weather affects his well-being: he is indeed a living barometer (Rhus tox.).

A striking modality of Psorinum is the *amelioration of the dyspnea on lying down* (K770, 3), contrary to orthodox medical thought. Regardless of the underlying pathological condition causing the dyspnea, whether simple pulmonary congestion, pericarditis or asthma, there is relief while recumbent. (Sulphur does not have this modality, although in Sulphur there is a relief in general from not standing, Sulphur's most dreaded position.) And Psorinum never wants the windows thrown open even though he is suffering from intense dyspnea in the heat of summer.

Periodicity is a marked feature of both Sulphur and Psorinum. Psorinum is so highly periodic that attacks (of hayfever, asthma, headaches, etc.) come on the same day, same week, same month each year. While remedies like Sanguinaria, Allium cepa, Euphrasia, Wyethia, and Sabadilla can do wonders in acute attacks of hayfever, permanently curing it requires deep-acting constitutional remedies with Psorinum being one of the most effective. Characteristic is too that Psorinum feels unusually well the day before an attack.

Both Sulphur and Psorinum are *always hungry*: Psorinum must get out of bed during the night to eat something while Sulphur is always hungry at 11 a.m. with an "all-gone" sensation. In both remedies the appetite is increased while having a headache (Psorinum 3, Sulphur 1) and eating will relieve the headache. Psorinum is one of the top remedies used to revive the Vital Force when reactions are poor (as mentioned in the section on revival remedies in Chapter 10, Golden Rules and Specific Forms of Prescribing) It is especially useful after exhaustive acute diseases when the patient despairs he will ever regain his health.

In short, the possibilities and usefulness of this interesting remedy are large indeed, when its great characteristics as described above are in evidence.

Clinical case described by H.C. Allen: A young lady came under my observation who had one of the worst cases of eczema I have ever seen. At fifteen years I remember her as attractive and brilliant, with a fine head of hair and one of the most perfect complexions of skin I ever saw. Upon questioning her I learned: family history negative [for eczema]; at fourteen years of age was vaccinated which "worked well." Six months later attended a school exhibition one very cold night in winter and face was considerably exposed. Next morning awakened with face greatly swollen, intensely red, almost unbearable itching; eyes were injected [inflamed], ears double their normal size. She called an allopathic physician who employed local and internal measures with little immediate result. Some papules formed, many of which became vesicular and not a few pustular, discharge of a thick dirty fluid which stained linen. She was of strong allopathic faith, yet after three years of local applications, she sought homeopathic treatment. She was now, at the time I saw her, taking nothing at all, had suffered for six years and was still as bad as ever, or even slightly worse. I found her in mind, though naturally bright and cheerful, very despondent, with even suicidal thoughts, complete despair of recovery. Hair dry and without luster, eyes still injected. Face, neck and much of the body was coarse, rough and of a dirty brown color with absence of perspiration. Itching intolerable, better by gentle scratching, which is continued until it bleeds. Pruritus < at night, when undressing and from warmth of the bed. Desquamation was so great that the sheet was each morning shaken and the scales swept away. I prescribed Psor. 200c, a powder each night dry on tongue for one week. Cured.[6]

This is a beautiful demonstration of how a master homeopath probes for the causality (vaccination, exposure to cold) the miasmatic background (family history negative) and captures her emotional state besides noting dutifully the modalities of the chief complaint (eczema). The result is spectacular and it is unfortunate that allopathic physicians and patients alike consider eczema incurable. Many homeopaths, myself included, have been able to repeat such successes numerous times. I just would not advise imitating Allen's dosage, every day for a week. Psorinum is a slow working nosode and one dose only of 200c would be a good start. Nevertheless, we cannot argue with success.

Medorrhinum

Medorrhinum is also known as Gonorrhinum and as Glinicum (a term coined by Compton Burnett).* It is the nosode of gonorrhea and thus of the sycotic miasm. It is indicated for someone who is reckless and immoderate, driven by his sexual desire, not even afraid of catching an STD. His motto is "sex, drugs, and rock 'n' roll." He is driven by passion, but in his passion he takes from the partner instead of giving. Woe to the women who fall for these driven passionate charmers, because the Medorrhinum thinks only about fulfilling his own sexual desires. The Medorrhinum is the hunter looking for the next intense, short-lived satisfaction. Don't expect to find him involved in a serious conversation at a party. He is cruising, showering the object of his lust with attention, but in a very sensual way. At first he might resemble a Lycopodium with his one-night stand mentality, but Lycopodium wants to make his conquests for another notch in his belt in a cold, calculating, slam-bam-thank-you-ma'am encounter. Medorrhinum is different, creating a romance of flaming passion, sweeping the woman off her feet with his eloquence, his generosity, even taking her to Paris for an impulsive romantic weekend. No wonder women fall for this charmer. And at first he plunges into the relationship heart and soul—but not for long, because he always has his eye out for the next attractive woman. As quickly as the romance flares up, it dies down, leaving the woman wondering what happened.

Medorrhinum typically swings from one extreme to the other. Don't be surprised to meet a Medorrhinum who is too timid to express his emotions (Silica) and opens up only

---

*This term confused me for a long time, especially when I read Compton Burnett singing its praises: he said it cured "more than half of my sciatica, what a record!"[7] Burnett coined his own name because he made the remedy himself and therefore, "knowing what the origin is, I want to name it myself." We certainly can grant Burnett his wish as he is one of the all-time great masters in homeopathy.

after consuming some alcohol (Nat. mur.). But usually, the erotic-aggressive instincts are heightened in the Medorrhinum, resulting in sudden brief spurts of over-activity followed by conflicts with his guilty conscience. The reaction to this conflict is *fright* conditioned by anticipation and presentiments, a mixture of fatalism and clairvoyance causing him to anticipate evils which punish him for real or imaginary sins. All this leads to his characteristic remorse, religious affections, and fear of the dark, of impending disease and of insanity (Calcarea). He is over-excited about coming events as well as bad news and the evil that he expects to overtake him. With his clairvoyance he anticipates "something will happen" and may have a delusion that "something terrible has happened." His sadness is aggravated by music and in company; he has a tendency to dwell on past unpleasant occurrences (Nat. mur.).

The second aspect of Medorrhinum is the memory deterioration. He forgets names, what he has read and the correct term for something. He is anxious if he has to meet someone at a given time. When leaving home he forgets if windows were closed or doors locked, so he must go back and repeats the procedure (Causticum). He is the procrastinator with an aversion to mental work; work seems to drive him crazy. Being forced to do mental work at school or on a job makes him irritable. In order to prevent mistakes he writes down every trivial detail. He has a strong desire to do things but he keeps putting them off. He can lose touch with reality, become tired of living and think of suicide as a solution to his torment.

He has an internal restlessness, aggravated in a closed room, ameliorated by motion and open air.

It is beyond the scope of this book to describe Medorrhinum in more detail. There are enough great Materia Medicas of the old masters which describe this intriguing remedy, and the second volume of Coulter's *Portraits of Homeopathic Medicines* features Medorrhinum and the other miasmatic nosodes.

Syphilinum (Lueticum)

As Kent so well expresses it: "Whenever the symptoms that are representative of the patient himself have been suppressed in any case of syphilis, and nothing remains but weakness and a few results of the storm that has long ago or recently passed, this nosode will cause reaction and restore order and sometimes do much curing."[8] As you can see, Kent talks about the cure of *suppressed* syphilis (which created the miasmatic state), not *acute* syphilis. (Of course this is true of nosodes in general, not only Syphilinum.)

The following well-known characteristics of Syphilinum should be compared to the syphilitic miasmatic state (Chapter 22). He has a dull mind, unable to remember names, faces, events, places. He loses the inability to remember passing occurrences, while everything that happened before the disease is remembered as distinctly as ever, almost effortlessly. There is depression, melancholy, and despair of recovery with a horrid depression. He has a terrible dread of night, anticipating the nightly aggravation of his complaints and his mental and physical exhaustion on waking. He is always washing his hands (Carc., Coca, Lac-c.) because of a delusion he is dirty. He may want to kill himself and others.

Tuberculinum

The famous homeopath Dr. Fergie Wood called Tuberculinum the "king of children's remedies" as Sulphur was the "king of adult remedies." Tuberculinum is a composite picture of Sulphur, Calcarea, Phosphorus and Silica and a deep-seated antipsoric; in fact it is a greater antipsoric than Psorinum! Its similarity to Sulphur is so great that any Sulphur case which fails to respond to Sulphur may be tentatively considered a Tuberculinum case on the strength of its Sulphur symptoms. It is especially useful when well-indicated remedies fail to work in a tubercular miasmatic case. Tuberculinum also fits cases which show a breakdown of the constitution, so that well-selected remedies don't hold because of vital weakness. And Tuberculinum has served the homeopathic physician almost better than any other remedy in the long-lasting prostration after the flu. And as Kent said: "It is an indication for Tuberculinum, when at every coming back of the case, it calls for a new remedy."

Long eyelashes, delicate appearance and hair between the shoulders are useful signs to indicate a remote tubercular history, as is suddenly getting tired. (It is the *suddenness* of onset that suggest Tuberculinum). Tuberculinum children are usually very *precocious:* they grow quickly, girls reaching puberty early and their minds growing very rapidly. They are also children who catch cold easily without knowing where and when.

Other symptoms, beginning with the mentals, include marked *irritability*; aggravation on awakening; a person who when healthy is of a lovable, even, placid disposition but becomes snappish and scrappy, positively ugly when ill. He lashes out at the slightest provocation, beside himself with rage. He has insane anger, in which he throws at you anything he can lay his hands on, followed by trembling, weakness and exhaustion. *Stubbornness* is an indication Tuberculinum shares with the psoric miasm (the tubercular miasm being a blend of psora and syphilis). I have sometimes noticed in patients who need this remedy a condition of despondency and despair of recovery, a belief that "it is no use taking a remedy, it won't help." Tuberculinum is restless, always wanting to be doing something with a *constant desire for change* of occupation, of lovers, of furniture in the house, of new toys, or for change of scene, like Calc. phos. They have *wanderlust,* as the Germans call it.

The Tuberculinum patient is anxious and melancholic, with whining and complaining. She also has *fear and apprehension,* especially of dogs (China). (Tuberculinum should probably be listed under "Fear, animals, of," K43; Tuberculinum is well-known for its fear of dogs but it has the same fear of cats, rats or horses. I have often used Tuberculinum to cure people so oversensitive to cats that they could not stay in the same room with one.) She may have loss of memory and aversion to work. Her *timidity* can be marked, due to an instinctive lack of physical power and an inability to fight for self-preservation. This may be a general attitude or take the specific form of fear of animals.

Physicals: Tuberculinum patients have a marked *air hunger* or desire for fresh air. They tend to feel chilly, yet feel as though they are suffocating in a warm room. They have an aversion to meat, which is almost impossible for them to eat (except for bacon, which they crave). They crave cold milk and are thirsty for large quantities of cold drinks. They tend to have a loss of flesh or wasting away and they are always tired. As Kent says:

> We all know what a marked feature the emaciation is in persons going into phthisis, often beginning before any other sign of TB. They are of feeble vitality, typically with a gradually increasing fatigue and weakness, and take on sicknesses easily. This is a prominent place for Tuberculinum *if the other symptoms agree.*[9]

Relaxation of the genitalia is expressed in men by nocturnal emissions and in women by prolapse of the uterus (Sepia, Lilium tig.). Women may have menstruation during lactation (Calcarea, Calc. phos., Silica, Palladium). Tuberculinum patients may have either constipation or diarrhea, which drives the patient out of bed in the morning (Sulphur). Kent tells us that this being driven out of bed in the early morning is a very common feature in cases of phthisis (pulmonary tuberculosis), or a patient going into phthisis. Their complaints aggravate from standing (Sulphur), and they can walk more easily than they can stand. They tend to have stiffness in the joints, worse on beginning to move and better from continued motion (like Rhus tox.; use Tuberculinum in these cases when Rhus tox. and Sulphur have failed).

Their sleep is troubled, and they tend to wake up worse after 3 a.m. They typically perspire during sleep, especially on the back of the neck and between the shoulder blades. Their symptoms constantly change, moving from place to place, with general aggravation from cold and damp, from change of weather and before a storm. When the symptoms imitate a different remedy at each visit think of Tuberculinum.

The *tissues* show marked symptoms: tubercular glands, adenoids and "cold abscesses." Clinically Tuberculinum cures ringworm when the other symptoms of the remedy are present (also the closely related nosode *Bacillinum,* which Compton Burnett used so successfully for ringworm). Kent let drop a hint many years ago which has been of inestimable value to us: so often a child is brought in with no symptoms other those caused by mechanical obstruction resulting from enlarged adenoids. We all know that surgical removal can bring temporary relief; but we also know the dangers of removing of the end-results of the disease without eradicating its cause. If there is no specific remedy indicated, give Tuberculinum in a series of upwards potencies (from 200c up) in intervals of approximately six to eight weeks. It will not be long before the adenoids will begin to exfoliate, the symptoms disappear and the family thinks the school doctor must have made a mistake when he said that the child needed adenoid surgery.

There are many *particulars* for Tuberculinum in the old masters' Materia Medicas (Kent, Allen, Boger, etc.). Tuberculinum may be indicated in *intermittent fevers* where the case relapses and the well-indicated remedy has failed to hold. It follows Psorinum well in hayfever. The eczema of Tuberculinum has specific characteristics: intense itching, worse at night when undressing (Rumex) and from bathing (Sulphur); immense quantities of white bran-like scales; fiery red, indurated skin with rawness and soreness.

The Tubercular Child in Your Practice

Unmistakably, the tubercular child can be classified as "difficult." These are the ones that reduce mothers to helpless tears because they are so unmanageable. You hear them screaming and everyone thinks that the mother is abusing the child—until it is time for the consultation! I have seen mothers struggling and pulling the youngster in, of whom I first saw only the legs thrown into the air, accompanied by a shrieking that went right through my bones. Before I know it, the child throws himself under the table, shrieks and kicks, while all the time claiming that he does not want to see a "stupid" doctor. Or he would not be able to be coaxed into the waiting room, let alone the consultation room, instead sitting outside on the stairs, steadfastly refusing to come in. Our Materia Medicas indeed state, "very irritable, wants to fight, no hesitancy in throwing at any one, even without a cause." It is quite a feat to pass those kicking legs to approach this child.

Try to examine this child and you will find out first-hand what stubbornness and herculean strength mean. Two or three adults are required to immobilize every part of that tiny body. But you can never stop their shrieking, which panics the rest of the children in your waiting room who think you must be torturing that poor child. Of course by this point you already know that this character needs Tuberculinum. But try popping three little pellets in his mouth. To no avail you say, "These are wonderful little sweeties" (which they are). Where other children welcome your little candies with pure joy, the Tubercular child screams, "I'm going to kill you" and manages to bite you, or clenches her teeth while you try to force the little pellets into her mouth while trying to stay out of range of those kicking legs. You think the remedy is in, but then they spit it out with great force, as if you put the vilest poison in their mouth, all the while screaming their loudest.

By then you are sure of Tuberculinum and even more determined to get it in. And hopefully you will succeed (after a struggle which leaves everyone exhausted), praying for the wonderful action of Tuberculinum. Meeting such children, I definitely understood the proving symptoms, "does not liked to be disturbed by people," and "trifles produce intense irritation," as well as "unreasonable terror in a child at a medical examination or with strangers."

Whatever you ask them, whatever you say, no matter how gently you try to coax them, the answer is "no" with a vengeance. One of these Tuberculinum characters broke the blinds in my office, while the mother, who had long ago given up, stood by helplessly. "No point in saying anything, Dr. Luc," she claimed. "She will not listen, she is argumentative and contrary with everyone."

Their excitable, difficult behavior is only matched with their restlessness and dissatisfaction. They make a mess out of your waiting room, reading a book for one second, tossing it aside the next one. They annoy other people and want to go into the drawers of your secretary's desk. Toys are kicked, broken or used to hit their mother who has to tow them into your consultation room. Have you ever seen the incredulous look on the face of those other mothers in the waiting room, who have the luck to have a nice Phosphorus or Calcarea child? They had no idea such children existed. Yet how many times my secretary or other parents would remark, months later, "That child has really changed!" And the parents and I are equally grateful for the beautiful work of Tuberculinum.

I wish some of my dentist friends could use Tuberculinum. Can you imagine trying to do dental work on a Tuberculinum child? You have a better chance of pulling teeth from a lion! But the result of a correctly applied dose of Tuberculinum is always wonderful: sudden cooperation of the child, no more fights or tears on examination, no more "killing," sitting still in the waiting room looking at pictures, plus the child gains weight (a physical correction of the characteristic tubercular wasting).

Of course you must make a distinction with equally "difficult" children: the most difficult to distinguish are the remedies related to Tuberculinum (Phosphorus, Pulsatilla, and Silica). Pulsatilla's mild, sweet and yielding disposition is well-known, but there is another side of the coin. I remember one case very well: a plump little girl, with curly hair and fair skin, but she would not answer any of my questions. If her eyes were bullets, I would have been dead long ago. And her mother told me that she shrieked so much at home when anything did not go her way that the neighbors were convinced of child abuse. Little did they know the abuse was the other way around. Tuberculinum was the top choice for this behavior, but she did not have the famous Dresden china prettiness of Tuberculinum. She was almost as broad as she was tall, she threw off her extra clothes because she was too hot, and the mother in her exasperation tried to convince me that she could be very sweet with people who she was fond of. And, the mother said, "with time she will warm up to you." I could hardly wait, but just to be sure, Pulsatilla 1M was put in her mouth which, to everyone's surprise except mine, made her the little affectionate lady we were looking for.

Indeed, a Pulsatilla can rage with the best: she has "aversion to being approached" (K9), "religious aversion to the opposite sex" (K9), and "fear of men" (K46). She is changeable, can be remarkably irritable, and can show intense dislike of people despite her neediness. And think about those earaches in your practice when the poor child is deadly afraid to be examined. Half of them are Pulsatillas!

As mentioned in Chapter 10, Golden Rules and Specific Forms of Prescribing, it is always great to follow a remedy up with its complement if you are stuck. No wonder that often Phosphorus or Silica follows after considerable improvement with Tuberculinum. Phosphorus shares with Tuberculinum the restlessness, changeability and love of travel as well as the love of beauty, art and colors. The choice of Silica is confirmed if we see its typical characteristics (such as sweaty feet, very chilly, catching cold from the slightest draft on the head or from being overheated). This is especially true if the symptoms appear after DPT or other vaccination, since Silica is one of our top remedies for Never Well Since DPT.

But it can also be that you have a constitutional Silica with a difficult nature. She hates to be touched (K89), is shy and timid (K89), and often has multiple ear infections (Silica is the chronic of Pulsatilla!). She has a big belly and puny little extremities, often with a hydrocephaloid head. She can be distinguished from a Tuberculinum child because she does not have the vehemence of a Tuberculinum, who is more stubborn and headstrong, hanging on his mother for support. Tuberculinum will be the nosode for intercurrent prescribing, though, if Silica, Phosphorus or Pulsatilla fail to work.

The poor Baryta carb. could be mistaken at first for a Tuberculinum because she is so difficult and resistant, but not for long. I had one little patient who acted like the backwards child she was. Her tongue always lolling halfway out, she was restless, stubborn and oblivious to her mother. Every time she came in, she assaulted me and my staff with her "stickering" game: stickers of every shape and color appeared on our clothes, faces, arms, and desks. Her IQ was 70, as tested by the school's psychologist. But what a difference there was from only two months of Baryta carb. LM1 and 2. The same psychologist tested her IQ at 100, she was doing her homework in the waiting room instead of "stickering" everyone, and she looked me into the eye when I asked her a question. I wish for the sake of the children that prejudice could bow to facts like these.

Chapter Eighteen
The Bowel Nosodes

Origin

Drs. Bach and Wheeler, two English physicians, presented a paper to a homeopathic medical society in 1927 entitled "The Problem of Chronic Disease." In their view, chronic disease is related to certain non-lactose fermenting bacteria. They related their experiences in treating diverse conditions with vaccines made from these organisms (injecting the nosodes, not giving them homeopathically). They contended that these bowel nosodes were a valuable addition to the homeopathic materia medica. Bach (who also developed the Bach flower remedies) concluded that psora and intestinal toxemia were identical, with chronic diseases possibly resulting from auto-intoxication of the bowels. Two Scottish physicians, John and Elizabeth Paterson, and the English physician Donald Foubister (himself a student of Elizabeth Wright-Hubbard) became great proponents of the use of bowel nosodes. The bowel nosodes are all antipsoric and cover many psoric diseases.

From the earliest records of medical history up to modern times, intestinal toxemia has been a recognized condition, treated for centuries with laxatives, colonics, cleansing diets, liver cleansers, etc. It surely is one of the marvels of nature that the intestines have been able to cope with the diversity of diet we see in different cultures. The human race was probably originally intended to live on raw foods, the fruits and foods of the tropics. Now many nations live entirely on cooked food, completely altering the intestinal content, and yet we survive. But we don't escape entirely; we suffer from a hundred and one diseases resulting from reduced strength and a loss of physical vitality. The penalty of toxemia is not immediate death but merely disease, not the extinction of the human race but rather degeneration.

When human beings live on unnatural foods, the intestinal content changes *chemically, physically and bacteriologically*. In intestinal disease, the first two components can often improve through dietary means, but the last factor can still trigger disease conditions. Changing the diet and feeding the patient lactose and acidophilus cultures change the flora only *temporarily*. The non-lactose fermenting bacteria of the same group recur again, as do the patient's symptoms. But under the influence of the curative action of the simillimum or the suitable nosode, the non-lactose bacilli begin to mutate to other groups and ultimately to disappear. This happens simultaneously with the disappearance of the symptoms, the reappearance of old symptoms, and the appearance of skin symptoms (e.g. skin rashes come back). When these symptoms finally clear, the patient has a *marked increase in vitality*. The bacilli change with the change in the patient. This has been demonstrated in before-and-after stool cultures. Of course Bach and Wheeler's presentation attracted the attention of homeopaths, since it follows the Laws of Hering.

Whether the non-lactose-fermenting bacteria are the cause or the result of the disease is still controversial. The debate about microbe versus terrain goes back to Pasteur (who, as previously quoted, said on his deathbed: "The terrain is everything, the microbe is nothing.") Virchow, the famous German naturalist, believed that microorganisms *seek* their natural habitat (diseased tissues) rather than *producing* it. By 1912 it was recognized certain non-lactose fermenting bacteria live in the intestines of both symptom-free and ill people, being especially persistent in patients with chronic diseases. These non-lactose bacilli belong to the coli typhoid group, closely related to the organisms causing typhoid, dysentery, paratyphoid, etc. In the past they had been considered unimportant and had been disregarded by bacteriologists and clinicians. But Bach and Wheeler found them in people suffering from what Hahnemann called latent psora and secondary psoric diseases.

Bach wondered why everyone is not sick if these bacilli are present in so many individuals. He discovered that first, their immediate virulence is low. A human body starting with a reasonable degree of health and a reasonably strong constitution can withstand their toxins for years without apparent inconvenience. Therefore these bacilli *cannot give rise to acute disease* or local manifestations. But the cumulative effect of their insidious and persistent poisoning over many years can give rise to chronic intestinal toxemia and thus to a great variety of chronic diseases. A breakdown often comes later in life when the body can no longer resist these organisms. It seems the nature of their toxins to affect primarily the internal secretion glands and the nervous system. Moreover, toxins from different strains of these bacilli probably attack different organs. Therefore one sufferer may show chronic arthritis, another chronic dyspepsia, another migraines or asthma, all depending on which one of these organisms is dominant. The body puts up a fight against them; improved diet and some forms of treatment can help lessen their attack. However, the most powerful weapons in this fight are the bowel nosodes potentized from these bacteria.

The clinical evidence of the bowel nosodes' curative power is well-established. Thousands of patients have been treated and 80% have seen improvement. The majority have experienced very definite relief, a good many have had brilliant results, and 10% of the results border on the miraculous.

While we now have laboratories which can analyze stool samples, these nosodes are usually prescribed on the symptoms and not based on stool cultures. The organisms which appear in the typical lab tests on stool samples in the US do not correspond to the bowel nosodes. In any case these lab tests are unnecessary. As soon as the symptomatology was worked out (as presented below) there was no more need for the type of lab testing which Bach and Wheeler did in the beginning.

Further Discoveries of Bach and Wheeler

It is important to note that *only one* of the seven types of these organisms exist at a given time in the bowels. This corresponds to Hahnemann's finding that it is impossible to have more than one disease at the same time. In spite of this principle, the type of bacteria present can certainly be *changed* by a vaccine, nosode or other remedy, which indicates that the type of organism depends on the condition of the host. In people who have not been treated homeopathically, the organism remains much more constant over a prolonged period.

It is extraordinary how rapidly the bacterial content may alter (therefore limiting the value of stool cultures). After weeks of negative culturing, within 36 hours stool samples may contain up to 100% of these abnormal bacilli. We do not know why this happens, but whatever the reason, we do know that the percentage of these bacilli bears a direct clinical relationship to the varying phases of the patient's condition.

The bowel nosodes are prepared from the pure cultures of bacteria rather than the tissues and germs together (as in Bacillinum, Psorinum, Diphtherinum, etc.). The culture used in the nosode is called a *polyvalent* preparation because the organisms from some hundreds of patients with similar symptoms are mixed together and potentized (although in their early experiments the mixtures were not potentized). The method is thus different from the *autogenous* one in which a nosode is prepared from and used for one individual patient. As discussed in the previous chapter, autogenous remedies are often not practical and will have limited usefulness. They could be useful in patients with the exact same symptoms as the patient from whom the autogenous nosode was made. Usually we prefer a polychrest to an autogenous remedy because the polychrest has been proven and has an extensive mental/emotional picture. The bowel nosodes have not been proven, but they still have a broader application than autogenous nosodes would, partly because they are taken from so many patients, and more so because they have an extensive mental/emotional picture based on clinical experience with hundreds of patients.

Originally Wheeler and Bach had excellent results in hundreds of chronic cases, resulting in demands for their injections came from all over the world. Preparing autogenous nosodes would have been impractical given the demand, so they developed seven polyvalent bowel nosodes, each covering a broad spectrum of indications. Provings in the usual sense were not done. To obtain a clinical picture, notes were kept on symptoms *associated* with the corresponding organism in the stool culture, *cured* when a particular bowel nosode was administered, or *arising* in patients who benefited from a bowel nosode (the nosode in each case being prescribed on the symptom pictures already discovered). The symptoms have been classified under each nosode. Just as with a proving record, no single patient complained of all the symptoms, nor were all of a given patient's symptoms necessarily present at the same time.

Indications

Not surprisingly, bowel nosodes have similar indications to other nosodes. One of the most frequently used methods of these nosodes is therefore *intercurrent* prescribing. Each bowel nosode is known to have a strong association with one or several polychrests. When one of these associated polychrests is well-indicated and stops working, in spite of potency increase, one possible course of action is to give the related bowel nosode (especially if there are specific indications for the bowel nosode). Either the progress of the patient continues under the action of the nosode or the indicated remedy is repeated and acts much more effectively than before. Another well-indicated use is the *paucity of symptoms* of the case. These nosodes may be looked upon as great *cleaners* or barrier removers when the polluted terrain suppresses the Vital Force. The bowel nosodes can improve the condition of the patient, in certain cases effecting a complete cure. In other cases they free the reactive power of the Vital Force so that the patient, who before gave no response, now receives marked benefit from other remedies. The bowel nosode purifies the patients, so to speak, cleaning them up until they express the symptoms of a simillimum and rendering them much more responsive to their remedy. Like any nosode, it stirs reactions so we can find the simillimum more easily. In addition, a bowel nosode brings better evacuation of the bowels and thus eases the toxic load the patient carries, therefore strengthening his Vital Force.

Like other nosodes, the bowel nosode is not necessarily the simillimum, but it helps to find it by organizing the symptom picture. If there seems to be no apparent benefit from the nosode, do not be disappointed but repeat the remedy which partially worked before, and this time you can expect a more permanent reaction. Realistically speaking, you might try to clear the field first with a remedy like Thuja, Sulphur, or Carbo veg. *before* trying the bowel nosode. Then in deciding which one to use, refer to the chart of bowel nosodes and associated remedies at the end of this chapter. For example, if Sulphur, Graphites and Calcarea were among the list of possible remedies, reference to our table would show that Morgan Pure would be indicated. Or if you are trying to decide among Phosphorus, Silica and Mercury, then Gaertner might be indicated. These were Paterson's conclusions regarding the *associated* remedies.

Administration and Repetition of the Bowel Nosodes

The general rule for any nosode is to repeat infrequently. There is no difference with the bowel nosodes—if anything, they should be repeated even *less* frequently. It must emphasized that the nosode should not be repeated for *at least three months* and indeed is often not required again for many months or years. This rule of thumb was discovered the hard way. Originally, it was thought that the higher the percentage of the non-lactose fermenting organisms, the more the nosode was indicated and unfortunately, it would be repeated too soon. The result was such an aggravation that the early experimenters learned from experience not to repeat too soon.

In the beginning these nosodes were given by injection like vaccines. The results were poor because the injections were given too frequently and at stated intervals (such as a week or ten days) regardless of the patient's response, resulting in serious overdosing and interference with the beneficial reaction. This led to giving the doses according to the response of the patient (which corresponds to the "wait and watch" method of the fourth edition of the *Organon*). When injecting nosodes to treat cases of pneumonia, Bach and Wheeler obtained better results when repeating the dose according to the patient's reaction. If the pulse rate and temperature fell after a dose, this indicated that no further treatment should be given until the pulse rate and temperature rose again. When this principle had been established for acute diseases, they realized that it might also apply to chronic cases. So they experimented and the results again were better than anticipated: the pulse and temperature would go down in subacute cases like lingering pneumonia, while other symptoms would subside in chronic cases.

Bach and Wheeler discovered that at least three months should elapse between doses because sometimes the patient did not start to improve within that time frame. If at the end of three months improvement had started, no further dose was given until every trace of improvement had stopped. The period of amelioration was found to vary from three weeks to as long as twelve months. By refusing to repeat the bowel nosode during the time of improvement, a higher percentage of good results occurred.

The bowel nosode is given either before or after a remedy, never at the same time. But if a remedy is indicated, *always* give that instead of the nosode first. Dr. Bach himself did not believe that any case was ever completely cured by these nosodes alone, however good the result. So the golden rule is always to give the indicated remedy first, only using bowel nosode to revive the case when the indicated remedy stops working. Rarely open a case with bowel nosodes (in my own experience I have *never* opened with a bowel nosode, whereas I do sometimes open with Medorrhinum or another chronic miasmatic nosode). And another remedy, often the associated one, will be needed to finish the case.

General Instructions

Some say nosodes made from the bowel organisms are most active in 12x and 30x potencies, others say 30c and 200c. We should choose the potencies for them as we do for our other remedies: with outspoken mentals we use high potencies, and where there is pathology we use 6c repeated. Furthermore, 6c is used in longstanding chronic cases which have often already been treated with numerous homeopathic remedies. If there is a combination of acute and chronic symptoms, for instance an acute bronchitis superimposed on a chronic lung condition (COPD), use 30c. Clinical observation and experience will be helpful in determining the frequency and potency of the bowel nosodes. If the nosode is showing improvement in the case, wait to readminister it until it has exhausted its action (as long as three months.) But if no improvement is seen after waiting at least three weeks, complement the action of a single dose of the nosode with repeated doses of the low potency of an associated remedy. In the chart at the end of this chapter, the associated remedy is capitalized.

Many of the excellent old homeopaths tried out these bowel nosodes, with mixed results. Some reported great results with minimal aggravations, while others cautioned about serious aggravations after bowel nosodes, even as low as 15c. Therefore, practically, in order to treat "gently," I would recommend starting with a test dose of a 6c dry.

Conclusion

We can conclude that bowel nosodes:
- are beneficially administered by mouth (instead of by injection).
- give the best results if repeated only upon cessation of improvement instead of at stated intervals (in other words, according to Hahnemann's principles).
- are capable of curing symptoms of latent psora as well as multiple so-called psoric diseases, and hence can be called antipsoric remedies; undoubtedly they are associated with chronic diseases.
- heal according to homeopathic laws or Hering's laws; they are among the deepest acting of our remedies.

- are indicated when the properly-indicated remedy fails (a standstill or plateau is reached).
- are indicated according to symptom similarity.
- are indicated when no remedy is clearly indicated (paucity of symptoms); they stir up a reaction to clear the picture.
- are indicated when the correct remedy fails to cure completely; depending on what remedies were improving partially, select the associated bowel nosode.
- are indicated when persistent symptoms don't disappear even with the right remedy.
- are indicated near the end or beginning of treatment .
- are indicated when symptoms of many remedies present themselves, but not one is clearly indicated, e.g. Mercury, Phosphorus, and Silica (all belonging to the Gaertner group) will be more clearly differentiated after giving Gaertner.

Remember, the rule is not to repeat too soon. You can easily dose too soon, you can hardly wait too long. If the improvement stops after a month, see if a new remedy is indicated (from within the associated group) rather than repeating the nosode.

Critical Views of Bowel Nosodes

Whenever our pioneers produced a new nosode, they proved it first and then used it in practice, always based on the totality of the symptoms. To prescribe a nosode on a single symptom would have been unthinkable to them. They would not have prescribed Tuberculinum because they found the bacillus of tuberculosis in the sputum. One would expect that those who developed and experimented with bowel nosodes would have followed the example of their predecessors and conducted provings. Yet in all these years none of them has been proved in the real Hahnemannian way.

Instead, Bach and Wheeler started to use them right away like allopathic vaccinations (of course, they were not homeopaths). This bacteriological prescribing was not always practical because only a few laboratory facilities were trained in such bacteriological work. Thus they had to find a method of obtaining further indications for these nosodes. This was done by setting up empirical provings, which they called "clinical provings." The stool of a patient was examined and if a species of pathogenic coli was found, the clinical symptoms of this patient were recorded. If several patients with the same pathogenic bacillus had the same clinical symptoms, then these symptoms were considered as *proved* symptoms though they were only *empirical*. They circumvented the Hahnemannian proving of the nosodes since a symptom occurring simultaneously with the pathogen may not always be related to it.

Paterson, however, really should have understood the patients' reactions to the bowel nosodes based on homeopathic principles. Instead, he was often puzzled by the unexpected phenomenon that in a patient who had previously yielded normal coli bacteria, there suddenly appeared a large number of non-lactose fermenting bacilli after the nosode was administered. (Obviously at this point he was prescribing by symptoms and not by the lab tests of fecal flora.) According to Paterson, the patient on the bowel nosode typically did not feel sick, but rather experienced some sense of well-being which he attributed to the nosode. However, after some time the case relapsed and in spite of changing the potency, he could not cure the patient. It is evident to us that the bowel nosode was a palliative (not curative) remedy which in its primary action suppressed the patient's superficial symptoms for a few weeks, but at the same time harmed his metabolism in a quiet way and caused the mutation of the bowel flora. Paterson was puzzled and could not see that the remedy was palliative rather than curative.

The danger of palliative prescribing (according to the great masters of the past, and borne out in my own experience) is that it sensitizes the patient to such an extent that when the associated remedy is given in a somewhat high potency, the patient aggravates for months without noticeable improvement afterwards. The similar aggravation is simply too much for the Vital Force to bear, causing too many symptoms unhomeopathic to the case and superimposing a remedy picture on the disease picture. Patients are not grateful when they go through all that suffering for nothing.

My conclusion? Let's not throw out the baby with the bath water: use these bowel nosodes very carefully, as a last resort, not as an opening move, and test with a 6c to avoid such complications. And as long as a bowel nosode acts, do not repeat it. Indeed bowel nosodes can produce miracles in tenacious, difficult cases. But always use the similar remedy first unless you absolutely cannot find it. In my own experience, I have used the bowel nosodes rarely and only when I am stuck, when several well-indicated remedies fail to act. Using a bowel nosode at this point has really moved these cases along. I have found them most helpful for eczema, asthma, enuresis, and anticipation anxiety, in that order.

Figure 18-1. Bowel Nosodes, Clinical Indications, and Associated Remedies

Name	Keynote	Clinical Indications	Associated Remedies
Colon Mutabile	always changing	alternating asthma and eczema	**Puls.**, Ferrum phos., Kali sulph.
Bacillus No. 7 (vitality)	mental/physical fatigue		**Kali carb., Iodum, Merc. iod.**, Arsen.iod., Bromium, Calc.iod., Ferrum iod., Kali bich., Kali brom., Kali iod., Kali nit., Nat. iod.
B. Faecalis	upset by fats/sugars		Sepia
Dysentery Co. (heart/epigastrium)	nervous tension, anticipatory, claustrophobic, shy, impressionable	chorea, duodenal ulcer, sciatica, rheumatoid endocarditis, venous circulation (varices, bruises)	**Arsenicum**, Anacardium, Argentum nit., Cadmium met., Kalmia, Veratrum alb., Veratrum vir.
Gaertner (lungs)	overactive mind or physical/emotional immaturity while mentally advanced	intractable rheumatic cases, marked emaciation, cancer, colitis celiac disease, inability to absorb fat, teething	**Merc. viv., Phos., Sil.**, Calc. fluor., Calc. sil., Kali phos., Nat. phos., Syphilinum, Phytolacca, Pulsatilla, Zinc. phos
Morgan Pure (liver-skin)	congestion	pneumonia, infantile eczema, asthma, enuresis, arthritis of the knee, hemorrhoids	**Sulph., Lyc.**, Alum., Baryta carb., Calc. carb. Calc. sulph., Digitalis, Ferrum carb., Med., Chelid., Chen., Hell., Hepar sulph., Lach., Graph., Kali–c, Mag–c, Nat-c, Petrol.
Morgan Gaertner		liver, renal colic, cholecystitis, psoriasis	Sepia, Psor., Merc. sulph., Sanguin., Tarax., Carbo sulph., Carbo veg., Tuberc.
Proteus (kidney/adrenals)	irritation of the central/peripheral nervous system (brainstorm remedy)	convulsions, epilepsy, Raynaud's, Meniere's, leg cramps, arthrosis, arthritis, numbness & tingling	**Nat. mur.**, Ammon. mur., Aurum mur., Apis, Baryta mur., Borax, Conium, Cuprum met., Calc. mur., Ferr. mur., Ignatia, Kali mur., Mag. mur., Secale
Sycotic Co. (mucous membranes, lymphoid tissues)	irritability	protracted enuresis, nasal & bronchial catarrh of children, albuminuria	**Thuja, Carc.**, Ant. tart., Calc. met., Ferrum met., Bacill., Nat. sulph., Rhus tox., Tuberc., Med.

The Dysentery Nosode

The keynote for this nosode is *nervous tension*. This is easily seen in the child needing this nosode, who is hypersensitive to the point of timidity and shyness (like the Phosphorus, who can exhibit the same shyness because of sensitivity). The face of the child expresses not so much fear as alertness. It is as if the CNS is all keyed up, in a high state of alert to react to the slightest external stimulus. For example, if you address the child or give them a compliment, they blush easily. On further observation, you might discover a slight twitching of the face or limbs (tic nerveux, chorea, facial tic); this nosode has certainly been successfully applied in these circumstances. The child is very sensitive to criticism (easily offended) and very shy in the company of strangers (Baryta carb., Calcarea).

As any other homeopathic remedy, this bowel nosode has a pathogenic predilection: it acts specifically on the duodenum. Duodenal ulcer of the adult and pyloric stenosis of the infant due to a spasm are therefore two of the indications. Another indication in children is the action on the cardiac muscle, as it will be successful in certain cases of rheumatic endocarditis.

In adults too, it has an action on the heart, and it is even called the "heart nosode" for its effectiveness in angina pectoris. The adult too, is high-strung, tense in mind and body, and very sensitive to all impressions. Above all, there is a sentiment of *nervous anticipation:* the patient has a great fear of the future and is overly conscientious. The individual is shy and lacks initiative, cannot sustain anything, and feels constantly miserable from the *fear that he cannot accomplish what he has to do*. This is the reason for his impatience and hurry, with a total inability to relax. Even in his spare time, he is bursting with feverish energy. He has a restless desire to move from place to place (like Tuberculinum). His fears are intense and multiple: of the dark, being alone, thunder and storms and narrow spaces (claustrophobia). He desires to be alone, yet has a fear of being alone.

No wonder he gets flustered and confused! Brainfag easily sets in: he forgets what he is going to say and loses his train of thought when interrupted. Depression is inevitable from the constant tension and the sense that he fails to accomplish anything. Just the thought of talking becomes too much of a strain and suicide by jumping from a roof is a possibility (Nat. sulph.).

Constant symptoms are "anxiety felt in the stomach and heart region," "nausea from excitement," and "diarrhea from excitement" (Argentum nitricum). There is a feeling of trembling, weakness, butterflies in the stomach, pain in the cardiac region with palpitations, crowding of thoughts, and muscular twitching on falling asleep with a general aggravation time of 3-6 a.m. It looks like Kali carb. and it will follow Kali carb. where this remedy only palliates. From the mental symptoms alone, it is clear that the Dysentery Co. is suitable for many people *broken down by strain and worry* (Mag carb.).

Physical symptoms: the physical symptoms of the Dysentery Co. patient are numerous. He is a chilly person, yet he has nausea and faintness in a warm room, relieved in open air (Pulsatilla). This nosode also affects the venous circulation: varicose veins, ecchymoses, Raynaud's disease with its cold white and blue fingers, etc. The nosode is also rich in gastrointestinal symptoms: poor appetite in the morning, delayed digestion, pain relieved by eating, heartburn hours after eating, thirst for cold water but which provokes pain, loose morning diarrhea (Nat. sulph., Sulphur), forcibly expelled, acrid and burning.

Angina pectoris attacks, with tightness across the chest, breathlessness and palpitations have been relieved with amazing results. However, acute remedies such as Cactus and Latrodectus mactans should be tried before the nosode. This is the only bowel nosode that can be *repeated without danger.*

Pathological conditions of the Dysentery Co.
- Angina pectoris, myocardial degeneration
- Aortic valve involvement, rheumatic endocarditis
- Chorea (specific), Tourette's, tic nerveux
- Duodenal ulcer, pyloric stenosis
- Raynaud's disease, varices, varicose veins

Clinical Case: Dysentery Co. was used with remarkable results in a little lapdog diagnosed with rheumatic endocarditis and valvular lesions after a dental cleaning, apparently while he had a strep infection. The symptoms included shortness of breath on the slightest effort, a chronic cough and complete exhaustion. The vet gave him two months to live. Naja helped minimally at first, then stopped working in spite of increased potency. Arsenicum was given with no response.

The dog was given one dose of Dys. Co. 30c. The next day, to the owner's horror, her beloved little Bichon Frisé suddenly keeled over as if dead! He got up after several hours, and the next day he was "reborn." No more exhaustion, cough or shortness of breath. He began frisking around like a puppy and stayed this way for one month, at which point some of the symptoms came back in a mild form. He was given one dose of Arsenicum 30c, the associated remedy. One year later he is still healthy with no repetition of bowel nosode or associated remedy. Note that a dose of 6c of the Dys. Co. would have avoided the frightening aggravation.

Morgan Pure

The keynote for Morgan Pure is *congestion:* an external congestion manifesting on the skin and an internal congestion, manifesting in bronchitis, asthma, bronchopneumonia, cholecystitis and jaundice. It has a selective action on the liver and skin.

It is effective in *children* with eczema starting in the face or head, then spreading over the remainder of the body, especially over the flexor surfaces of the upper and lower limbs. There is constant itching and scratching, with oozing of a bloodstained fluid (like Sulphur and Graphites). It is often indicated where Sulphur, Graphites, Psorinum and Petroleum have failed or gave only temporary relief.

In internal congestive conditions, a single dose of Morgan Pure will often turn the tide when there is a lack of response to the indicated remedy. It should also be used for Never Well Since bronchopneumonia; for pneumonia where the well-indicated Sulphur fails to relieve; and in asthma cases where Arsenicum and Nat. sulph. have failed. It works equally well in the child who has had a lot of antibiotics for recurrent bronchitis.

In the *adult,* the outstanding features of this nosode are also found on the skin: eczema with itching, oozing and scaling; intertrigo of the breast; boils, carbuncles, and acne of the shoulders, all suggesting congestion of the skin. It bears repeating: the Morgan Co. should not be given before Sulphur, Graphites, Psorinum and Petroleum have been tried and failed. It is also used in the internal congestion of congestive bronchitis, asthma, and pneumonia. It can be indicated in postzonal neuralgias (Never Well Since shingles) and in arthritis where nothing else works (worse in the morning and beginning to move (Rhus tox.), worse heat and menopause). Congestion in the liver and GI system causes heartburn, bilious attacks relieved by vomiting large quantities of bile (Nat. sulph.), cholecystitis with gall stones, and jaundice. Constipation is present in 95% of the cases. These patients desire sweets and fats and have an aversion to eggs and butter.

Mental/emotional: Patients needing Morgan Pure look like those needing Dysentery Co. with their anxiety, apprehension about health, and fear of crowds and the unknown. They are misanthropes and hypochondriacs, with feelings of doom (the world will soon come to an end), avoiding company yet worse when alone.

Morgan-Gaertner

This is a sub-group of Morgan Pure, which it resembles very much, but it is more indicated in cholecystitis and especially *renal colic.* The number one associated remedy is Lycopodium and therefore this nosode is valuable in any case which has an aggravation time of 4-8 p.m.

The patient needing Morgan-Gaertner is irritable and tense, biting his nails and fearing crowds and company.

Gaertner

Gaertner was first isolated from a food poisoning by Gaertner and was given the name *Gaertner bacillus enteritis,* the "bacillus of the intestine." It has also been called the children's nosode because in its clinical picture, we can find almost all the nutritional disorders so common in children. The keynote for Gaertner is an *undernourished body with an overactive mind*. Patients needing Gaertner look pale and thin like Silica but have the nervousness of Phosphorus. Gaertner children are physically and emotionally immature with an advanced mental ability. The nosode is applicable to many childhood diseases including celiac disease (in which the inability to absorb fats leads to failure to thrive); it is also of great value in cancer cachexia. The *causality* in general is a bad diet (junk food, canned foods), or an overly restricted healing diet such as macrobiotics. The first thing that strikes you in a Gaertner child is the malnourishment: the muscles and limbs are very poorly developed, which leads to poor coordination and clumsiness. You never use Gaertner if the patient is well-nourished.

In contrast to this poorly developed physical body, the child's central nervous system is in a hypersensitive state: the child is all brain and no brawn. The child is precocious in many ways and hypersensitive to all impressions. There are marked fears, of the dark and of being alone, with night terrors. Compare this child to the Dysentery Co. child who, although fidgety, uneasy and nervous, will not leave his chair while you are questioning him and taking notes. The Gaertner child has an inquisitive mind and must know the reason for everything you do, like why you are using the *Repertory* (Phosphorus). He prefers adult company for the mental stimulation although he has a short attention span. The child asks many questions, enjoys studying, and is often called a bookworm. He is like a mini-adult without the emotional maturity. He is wise beyond his years, an old soul, flexible, orderly, organized, and rather a follower than a leader.

The Gaertner child is *emotionally* immature, therefore needs reassurance, cuddling and company. She wants to do the right thing, to please others. They are sensitive to reprimands and cry easily but they never display temper tantrums because they simply lack the energy for it, and so they keep their problems inside.

Common indications: Besides its indication in malnutrition and wasting diseases like cancer, colitis, and celiac disease, Gaertner is the greatest teething remedy, even more than Chamomilla. In ear discharges while cutting teeth, use Gaertner 30c one time, Silica 30c one time the next day. It is indicated in digestive allergies (milk, eggs, wheat) due to the immaturity of the digestive system; in failure to thrive; and malassimilation due to antibiotics killing off the normal flora. Gaertner will rally the vitality and encourage the growth of the bowel flora. It is also effective in children with physical immaturity when Silica, Calcarea and Pulsatilla fail; in children with a history of difficult breast feeding (as well as anorexia in children and adults); and in young girls with cystitis and vaginitis (Sepia, Pulsatilla). There is a marked aggravation from milk and wheat and marked cravings for sweets, chocolate and cheese.

Proteus

In England, Proteus is called the "brainstorm remedy": nervous symptoms appear suddenly with great irritability and violent outbursts. The person can commit murder when crossed, especially before the menses. Like Tuberculinum, it is indicated in temper tantrums of children who kick and scream, especially when you say "no" to them.

The need for Proteus can result from a long nervous tense situation (like WW II, a long hostage crisis, or even a tumultuous marriage) in which the person just snaps. Aconite was of course a marvelous remedy for the British in WW II while they were bombarded, and right after the war there was a marked increase in the frequency of Proteus found in their stools. This was associated with a *long continued nerve strain*. Proteus patients can also become depressed and commit suicide. They are difficult to treat because of their rigidity and fixed ideas. They are easily startled and frightened; they tend to be confused, drawing a blank while speaking.

Further indications are Raynaud's disease (which has spasms of the capillaries of the extremities) and Meniere's disease (which has a spasm of the brain circulation). The sudden onset of the symptoms (the arousal of the storm) is evident in cases of duodenal ulcers with a tendency to perforation, where the first symptom is melena or hematemesis. Numbness and tingling of the extremities (often a first symptom of MS), epilepsy, and migraines before the menstrual cycle can all be indications for this nosode. Nat. mur. is the outstanding remedy associated with this group.

Sycotic Co.

The central idea of this remedy is *anxiety and irritability*. The mental symptoms are almost identical to Gaertner Co. with the additional factors of irritability and cross-mindedness. The general *action* is on the mucosae, well-demonstrated by diseases such as nasal and bronchial catarrh, recurrent tonsillitis of children and non-specific urethritis (NSU). The name of the remedy is based on these sycotic indications. Nocturnal enuresis and vulvovaginitis in young children often respond to this nosode. Another action of this nosode in children demands special attention: kidney involvement manifested by albuminuria, a common complaint. Sycotic Co. works equally well in asthma in which the child wakes up around 2 a.m. with a croupy cough (like Drosera). The action on the lymphoid system is seen in the overgrowth of tonsils and adenoids.

The *physical characteristics* differ greatly from those of Gaertner. To the contrary of the malnourished Gaertner, the Sycotic Co. patient is often flabby and fat, but always anemic looking. He tends to have sweating on the head at night (Calcarea), warty growths, rheumatism, premature gray hair and blinking of the eyes. There is an aversion to eggs in 50% of the cases, but cravings for butter, sweets and milk.

In adults, Sycotic Co. will often be indicated in nephritis, cystitis, pyelitis, NSU and ovarian cysts as well as PID. Asthma worse on cold days and better at the seaside (Medorrh., Carc., Nat-m.) with asthma or rheumatism that has the characteristics of Rhus tox.

Sycotic Co. is close to Thuja. If the patient has Pulsatilla and Thuja symptoms but is averse to eggs, he is likely to need Sycotic Co.

Bacillus Number 7 of Paterson

This was the seventh non-lactose fermenting bacillus observed, hence its name. The keynote is *mental and physical fatigue,* with a feeling of being unfit for mental labor, while at the same time a sense of extreme physical exhaustion. Other characteristic symptoms include a low pulse rate (often with hypotension), a tendency to syncope after sudden exertion, premature senility, and impotence.

Part Three

The Chronic Miasms

Hahnemann's Miasmatic Theory

The Psoric, Sycotic, Syphilitic, Tubercular, and Cancer Miasms

Homeopathy and Cancer

Chapter Nineteen

The Roots of Chronic Disease

History and Definitions of the Term

The term *miasm* comes from the Greek, meaning "pollution, taint." Hippocrates was the first to use it to express his concept of how infectious diseases could be carried by air, water and other sources. By the Middle Ages the term came to mean an atmospheric influence which caused illness. The doctors of Hahnemann's time used the term *miasm* to indicate the *unknown* cause of disease which pollutes the whole system so as to produce a permanent disease state. They considered syphilis the *only* existing miasm because the etiology was unknown. They did not consider sycosis, the "figwart disease," a miasm because they believed they could cure it by removing the condylomata

Hahnemann used the term *miasm* in his great theory of the origins of chronic disease. He began by separating *true* chronic diseases from diseases that were caused by mechanical or exterior conditions, which could be alleviated by modifying the environment or life-style of the patient (Aphorism 77). These conditions included traumas of all kinds, poisons, frostbite or sunstroke, and inadequate diet. Thus Hahnemann emphasized that certain diseases depended entirely on external conditions, whose removal was the first step to cure. He was a forerunner of twentieth-century proponents of prevention and treatment through a healthy life-style and natural living.

But Hahnemann also observed that the best diet, a robust constitution and healthy life-style alone could *not* help to cure a *true chronic disease*. He saw that in spite of such measures, the chronic disease unfolded into new and worse symptoms, leading inevitably to a further aggravation and death. He would caution the modern proponents of diet-based cures such as macrobiotics that if diet did not cause a disease, neither can it permanently cure it. Diet may appear to eliminate a particular expression of disease, such as a tumor in the breast, but it cannot eradicate the *tendency* to produce such a tumor, which Hahnemann attributed to the underlying miasm.

In treating his patients with chronic diseases, Hahnemann was disappointed with his results and found that the well-chosen remedy typically would work for a while but then the patient would relapse. As was characteristic of him, Hahnemann did not rest with his achievements up to that point (1816). Instead he worked tirelessly, often through the night, to study these patients' cases. In so doing he found patterns of diseases in the patients and their family histories which he felt explained the true basis of chronic disease. He called these patterns *miasms* and declared that unless the underlying miasm was extinguished, a chronic disease could not be permanently cured with homeopathy, even with the well-chosen remedy.

Hahnemann's original classic theory of miasms, expounded in *Chronic Diseases* (1828), delineated three miasms, the psoric, sycotic and syphilitic. Later homeopaths perceived the tubercular miasm, a combination of psoric and syphilitic, and the cancer miasm, based on a mixture of at least two and often three or all four of the other miasms. Some homeopaths have added others such as an AIDS miasm and vaccination miasms. The five major miasms will be addressed in this section.

Before he began prescribing antimiasmatic remedies, Hahnemann tells us frankly that he was astonished to find no progress with his remedies in treating chronic diseases. In fact, with time, patients' symptoms reappeared even stronger:

> The remedy which had been serviceable the first time would prove less useful, and when repeated again it would help still less. Then perhaps, even under the operation of the homeopathic remedy which seemed best adapted, new symptoms of disease would be added which could be removed only inadequately and imperfectly; yea, these new symptoms were at times not at all improved.[1]

Why? He did not doubt the accuracy of his law, "Like Cures Like." Could it be a lack of known remedies? Even the ever-increasing new proven remedies could not resolve the riddle of these chronic diseases. Hahnemann concluded that there must be an unknown obstacle to lasting recovery, an obstacle with its roots deep in the patient's system. He observed that when one disease disappears, it is sometimes replaced by another. Headaches disappear, colics appear. But upon closer analysis we see that these different conditions are like weeds which spring from the same root. A remedy addressing a particular weed may leave the root untouched. Until the root is taken out, it will continue to produce weeds in different parts of the patient's body. Hahnemann identified three such roots or miasms, as we have seen, and considered psora the *original* root of all diseases. This psoric theory was the result of twelve years' painstaking labor and investigation.

When Hahnemann began his research into unsolved chronic cases, he carefully recorded all the patient's current symptoms, the past medical history, and the family medical history. It was relatively easy for him to trace the venereal diseases: he could see how the residual poisons of syphilis and gonorrhea created the miasms of syphilis and sycosis, respectively. These miasms explained only one-eighth of his unsolved chronic cases, however. Setting these sycotic and syphilitic cases aside, he was still left with a large group of chronic conditions which he found difficult to classify. (In fact the list goes on for 69 pages of *Chronic Diseases*.) They included recurrent attacks of acute conditions, which, although seemingly cured at the time, would break out again upon little provocation. In analyzing thousands of such records, he always found in the patient's history *a suppression of a skin eruption*. "The obstacle to the cure of many cases seemed very often to lie in a former eruption of the itch, which was not unfrequently confessed."[2]

Hahnemann tested the psoric theory by basing his prescriptions on the original picture of the disease, going back to the suppression in the patient's past medical history or in the family history. This is why he so often opened with Sulphur: skin eruptions were usually suppressed with sulphur baths and ointments because allopathic physicians did not see the connection between skin conditions and deeper diseases. (His goal was to bring back the original skin condition; he had unsuccessfully experimented with bringing the eruption back with plasters on the skin.) His previous prescriptions were almost superficial, treating acute flare-ups of chronic diseases as though they were simple acute conditions. He based his treatment on the picture the patient presented at the time without taking the past history into account. Furthermore, in treating true acute conditions Hahnemann only used one remedy, but he realized that to eradicate the psoric root he would need a progression of antipsorics.

We can see in hindsight that his earlier method would give Hahnemann temporary success (in prescribing for acute flare-ups) but long-term failure, because the Vital Force would keep throwing out "new" diseases, which were simply new flare-ups ("weeds") of the chronic miasmatic "root." The result of this new method (treating the root) was that his unsolved cases were resolved and the patients were cured permanently. At the end of these twelve years he felt he had successfully cured enough patients with this theory that he was ready to publish it in the first edition of *Chronic Diseases* in 1828. From that time forward, Hahnemann studied and treated disease from a miasmatic perspective.

Hahnemann's theory of miasms was not well accepted among most of his followers and remains controversial among homeopaths even today. But many of the greatest homeopaths of the past, starting with Hering, Stapf, Gross, and Kent, found the miasmatic theory valuable for their practice. Kent said that treating a patient without addressing the underlying miasm is like prescribing for a "jack-in-the-box." Although many of Hahnemann's followers considered his miasmatic theory farfetched and many modern homeopaths consider it unnecessary, I believe that the proof lies in its clinical effectiveness. In my own practice I have found miasmatic prescribing to be a powerful and essential tool and I hope that my colleagues who have not yet used it will be encouraged and aided by this book to test it for themselves.

In assessing the validity of Hahnemann's miasmatic theory, we have to keep in mind that acute and chronic diseases are entirely different. We may be able to cure an isolated instance of pneumonia without addressing an underlying miasmatic state. If the patient has a tendency to recurring coughs, colds, bronchitis and pneumonia, we may even be able to cure each instance. But we will never be able to prevent recurrence without using Hahnemann's powerful tool, his miasmatic theory. (By definition, acute diseases are triggered by external factors, have a sudden onset, run a limited course and finally terminate either in recovery or death. This recovery may take place with or without the help of medicines. So we often do not even have a cure but a natural recovery. However, a spontaneous recovery of chronic cases can never occur, as we all know from the definition of chronic disease in the *Organon*. A chronic disease has the tendency to continue indefinitely.)

The Role of Miasms in Disease

A miasm, in homeopathic terms, is an invisible polluting substance which, once it gains entrance, overpowers the Vital Force and pollutes the whole system. Each miasm creates a weakness or tendency to a particular group of diseases. If not eradicated with a suitable antimiasmatic remedy, it will persist throughout the patient's life and can be transmitted to others, especially to sex partners and children. Kent called it a predisposition, a state, a dyscrasia or diathesis. This theory explains why some people develop chronic illnesses from apparently minor ailments. One acute illness can trigger the latent psora, resulting in recurring flare-ups of various acute illnesses, with the patient never completely recovering.

The acute miasms come up with such violence that they either cause imminent death or subside quickly, followed by a period of progress and recovery. As Hahnemann said in *Chronic Diseases*:

> Acute miasms have the peculiar characteristic that after they have penetrated the Vital Force the first moment of contagion, like parasites grow quickly, produce fever and then die out again and leave the living organism free. ... On the other hand chronic miasms continue to live as long as the man is seized by them is alive. They are not extinguished spontaneously like the acute miasms, but can only be annihilated by means of the potentized similar remedy, creating a stronger similar disease so that the patient is delivered from them and recovers his health.

The five major chronic miasms will be discussed in detail in the next chapters.

Miasmatic theory could be considered the true genetic theory, since miasms are transmitted to children. It also provides something analogous to genetic therapy, since the inherited miasms can be treated and the genetic transmission halted, protecting future generations. In our century we have seen the miasmatic states grow more and more powerful, partly because the miasmatic states of parents are combined and tend to concentrate in their children. An even more powerful influence, however, comes from all the triggers of miasmatic states in our modern times: physical triggers like cortisone, antibiotics, vaccinations, and birth control pills as well as mental/emotional triggers like divorce and child abuse. As each generation of children becomes weaker, we see the miasmatic expressions ranging from learning difficulties and ADHD to cancer and criminal behavior appearing earlier and earlier in childhood.

While this may seem the worst of times as the miasms become progressively more destructive, it could also be the best opportunity for homeopathy to demonstrate its effectiveness in preventing and treating these miasmatic expressions in our children. We can show how homeopathic treatment can almost immediately stop chronic tendencies from the most superficial, like recurring ear infections or vaginitis (expressions of the sycotic miasm), to the most profound, like familial tendencies to depression, bipolar disorder, alcoholism, drug addiction, and suicide (all expressions of the syphilitic miasm).

Acute Miasms

Fixed Acute Miasms: Fixed miasms are acute illnesses such as chickenpox, whooping cough and other childhood diseases which attack people only *once* in a lifetime, while the susceptibility to them all stems from a common source, the presence of active psora. Homeopathic treatment of these acute miasms strengthens the constitution and supplies the Vital Force with enhanced immunity. Margaret Tyler taught us that patients who boasted of never having had childhood diseases often fell victim to serious illnesses, including cancer, in their prime of life. Apparently something about the cancer miasm made these children non-susceptible to the childhood illnesses, a condition which in turn increased their susceptibility to cancer later in life because their Vital Force never had a chance to decrease its miasmatic burden through the outlet of the childhood diseases. Thus we now recognize this phenomenon as marker for the cancer miasm.

Recurrent Acute Miasms: Other acute infections such as cholera, yellow fever, pneumonia and diphtheria can recur repeatedly in a patient's life. These recurrent acute miasms may be so intense as to create a miasmatic block, requiring the corresponding nosode to remove it. For example, if a patient is unable to swallow after suffering from diphtheria, Causticum might be the remedy indicated by the symptoms but it might not have any effect until Diphtherinum removes the block.

Dormant, Latent, and Active Miasmatic States

Hahnemann makes a distinction between dormant, latent and active miasmatic states (although for all practical purposes we mostly see a difference between latent and active miasms). A *dormant* miasm, according to Hahnemann, is one which shows *no symptoms* of the miasm in question. It is usually discovered when the homeopath takes a complete history and investigates the time line. The situations when we see a dormant miasm are either during childhood or in an adult with a healthy life-style (mentally, emotionally and physically), giving the impression that they are healthy and free of disease. But emotions and suppressive drug actions often bring the dormant miasm to life. It is like a time bomb hidden below the stronger active layers of the case.

A *latent* miasm shows symptoms, but they are minor, transitory, and would go unnoticed except by a perceptive homeopathic observer. Hahnemann gives many examples of the latent psoric miasm, including perspiration on the head and neck, swelling of the cervical glands, epistaxis, the nose blocked with mucus, predisposition to catch colds, twitching of the limbs on going to sleep, constipation, itching of the anus, and a sour taste in the mouth. In other words, these minimal symptoms would rarely prompt a visit to the doctor and have little impact on the Vital Force. Thus miasms are generally at least latent, if not active, because their presence can usually be detected by the trained homeopathic observer. At this time the symptoms are mainly transient but as the miasm becomes *active,* it produces constant, more serious symptoms which affect the Vital Force more profoundly.

Important Principles of Miasmatic Prescribing

When not to address the miasm: In incurable diseases such as terminal diabetes or cancer, addressing the chronic miasm could weaken the Vital Force. Do not base the selection of the remedy in these cases on miasmatic symptoms, but rather palliate (with LMs or 6c). The same rule is in force for the acute exacerbations of the miasms: treat the acute symptoms with the indicated remedy (without regard to its miasmatic properties) and then when the acute condition subsides, treat the miasm to prevent recurrence.

Only one miasm is active: Two latent miasms seldom become active at the same time. Curing is relatively easy when there is a single active miasm, and much more difficult when mixed miasms are present. In this case one is usually active, holding the other one latent. If sycosis is present in any form or in any stage, it usually takes precedence. If more than one miasm is active, we are liable to have malignancy.

When more than one miasm is active: In these cases the treatment will be more complicated. First use an anti-psoric, followed by a remedy for the other dominant miasm, then follow it by an antipsoric. If the third miasm is also active, follow with a remedy for it, finishing the case with an antipsoric. In other words, psoric treatment always comes in between antisycotic and antisyphilitic remedies, and the treatment always ends with an antipsoric. More specific instructions for addressing more than one miasm will be found at the end of the chapter for each miasm.

While it sounds as though this method requires frequent zigzagging back and forth, fortunately our major remedies tend to cover more than one miasm (Lycopodium, Sulphur, and Calcarea, for example, cover all three miasms). This is another good reason to start with a polychrest which is likely to cover at least two of the miasms.

Avoid stirring up latent chronic miasms: Latent miasms can be aroused by giving a nosode incorrectly, for example solely on the basis of TB, cancer, syphilis or gonorrhea in the past medical history or family history, without any other indications for the nosode in the patient. Stirring up a latent miasm will leave the patient worse than when they began (see the description of the Syphilinum case in Chapter 17, Nosodes). The first remedy should always cover the *active* miasm. Hahnemann says in *Chronic Diseases* that in a mixed case, as one miasm is cured or disappears, *the latent one suddenly becomes active*. Wait until a latent miasm becomes active before prescribing for it. The first active miasm may need several remedies before the next miasm appears; for example, a patient with an active sycotic miasm may need Thuja, Medorrhinum and Nitric acid before psora appears.

Treating pregnant women: In *Chronic Diseases*, Hahnemann stated:

> Pregnancy offers so little obstruction to the antipsoric and hence all miasmatic treatments, that this treatment is often most necessary and useful in that condition. Most necessary because the chronic ailments are then more developed. In this state of pregnancy, the symptoms of internal miasms are often manifested more outspoken and plainly on account of the increased sensitivity of the female body.[3]

If a woman is in better health during pregnancy, as often happens because of the exteriorization just described, Hahnemann suggests treating the symptoms manifest *before the pregnancy*. He linked miscarriages, birth defects, and improper presentation of the fetus to the syphilitic miasm, which ideally should be treated before pregnancy, or at least during it. In *Chronic Diseases* Hahnemann discusses the value of giving antipsoric remedies to pregnant women:

The homeopathic treatment is indispensable in order to destroy the psora, the producer of most chronic diseases, which is given them hereditarily. Destroy it both within themselves and in the fetus, thereby protecting posterity in advance.

Of the women who had this treatment Hahnemann said, "They have given birth to children usually more healthy and stronger to the astonishment of everybody." However, pregnant women with many suppressions in their past medical history, or a habit of drug use (medical or recreational drugs), must be treated with care. A strong cleansing reaction could be stimulated which might be too hard on mother and child.

Transmission of sycosis and syphilis: Why is the sycotic or syphilitic miasm not necessarily transmitted to every sex partner? Because of the principle that two dissimilar diseases repel each other: the partner may have a stronger active miasm so wholly different from the "attacking" miasm, that it protects her from contagion. Therefore a miasm can be transmitted from father to child without the mother being affected at all. However, abnormal cravings (pica gravidarum) and aversions during pregnancy indicate the transfer of the father's miasm to the mother, carried by the child.

Treat the parents before conception: It is obvious that when the same miasm (whether sycotic or syphilitic) is strongly active in both parents, the results can be devastating for the newborn child: deformities, mental aberrations or severely emotionally disturbed children could be the outcome. This indicates the great need for antimiasmatic treatment of both parents *before* conception.

Comparative Keynotes of Hahnemann's Original Three Miasms

Psora *Hypo-,* atrophy, lack (no courage or self-confidence; weak hair, nails; lack of digestion, assimilation), weakness, timidity; inflammation, irritation and hypersensitiveness (all superficial and centripetal). Only exception: *Hyper*sensitivity.

Aggravation time: 10 a.m.–evening, worst at 12 noon

Sycosis *Hyper-,* proliferation, overgrowth, infiltration, induration, exaggeration, incoordination, restlessness, ostentation

Aggravation time: 2 a.m.–8 p.m.)

Syphilis *Dys-,* dysplasias, dystrophy, deformities, deviation, degeneration, structural destruction, ataxia, ulceration, bloody discharges; desire to kill (others and himself)

Aggravation time: 7-8 p.m. until 2-3 a.m.

CHAPTER TWENTY

Psora: the Sensitizing Miasm

History

According to Hahnemann, psora is the oldest, most universal, and most misunderstood miasm. The term comes from the Hebrew word *tsorat*, meaning "groove, defect, pollution, stigma," which was often applied to leprosy and to the great plagues. It was first used by Moses to describe leprosy several thousand years ago. The leprosy of the Israelites was one of many varieties of psora, according to Hahnemann, as were the various forms of leprosy during the Middle Ages. Another expression of psora was the malignant erysipelas in Europe during the Middle Ages called "St. Anthony's fire." Other expressions included skin eruptions of all kinds. But these external expressions of psora were changed in the course of human history by the introduction of better nutrition and hygiene, including more frequent baths and linen clothes (introduced by the crusaders). Suppressive external treatments for skin conditions were also developed (ointments of sulphur and lead, and preparations of zinc and mercury).

Hahnemann believed that psora had led to a bewildering variety of diseases because it had so many different original manifestations which had been suppressed in different individuals in the course of many centuries. Towards the end of the 15th century psora took its present form, scabies or itch. Continuous scratching stimulated the release of fluid, which led to the widespread communication of this primary manifestation of psora.

Of all the chronic miasms, psora is by far the most communicable. Syphilis and sycosis seem to require that the skin be rubbed a little but the energy of the psoric miasm can be transmitted by a mere touch, such as by shaking hands or the physician taking the pulse of an infected person. As long as psora took the form of leprosy, its spread was limited by the enforced social isolation of lepers. Although leprosy appears to be a much more dangerous condition than the almost invisible itch, psora actually became much more dangerous with this direction of suppression. The itch could be suppressed with a variety of medical treatments, leading to the formation of a legion of pervasive interior diseases. In addition to medical intervention, the rash could "spontaneously" be driven to the interior of the body. (While this involution *appeared* to be spontaneous, it was actually caused by physical and emotional traumas such as grief, fright, humiliation, and exposure to cold.)

No wonder the widespread, easily-communicable and easily-suppressed psora became the mother of all chronic diseases. Hahnemann calculated that in his time at least seven-eighths of all chronic diseases were derived from it, with sycosis and syphilis together causing the remaining eighth. Of course in Hahnemann's time (and in ours as well) doctors treated the itch locally, i.e. suppressively. Hahnemann strongly condemned this treatment, blaming it for the sufferings of humanity. He describes in *Chronic Diseases* how the physicians of his time viewed any skin condition: "Every eruption of itch is merely a local ailment of the skin, in which ailment the remaining organism takes no part at all, so that it may and must be driven away from the skin at any time and without scruple, through local applications of sulphur ointment."[1]

Hahnemann was not alone in these observations. Honest physicians of his time described numerous cases of the horrible consequences of suppressing skin rashes. In *Chronic Diseases,* Hahnemann quotes many such cases from the existing medical literature (so as not to be accused of prejudice).[2] The resulting diseases included asthma, sterility, lassitude, oppression of the chest, melancholy, swelling of the body or dropsy, anxiety, and even death. Any present homeopath still sees the results of such suppression, exacerbated by the greater effectiveness of modern treatments.

Hahnemann used the term "psora" to describe the latent susceptibility remaining in the patient from the suppression of the itch (as well as the suppression of leprosy, St. Anthony's Fire, and other skin eruptions). He considered this susceptibility in itself to be communicable (by touch or inheritance) and called it "a sort of internal itch." While Hahnemann is often considered the inventor of the miasmatic theory, he considered himself merely its careful observer, as he says in *Chronic Diseases*: "I was thus instructed by my continued observations and experiments in the last years, that the ailments and infirmities of body and soul, are but partial manifestations of the ancient miasma of leprosy and itch."[3] He also attempted to record its many manifestations in the thousands of years it has tortured humanity: his *Chronic Diseases* has 67 pages simply listing the diseases resulting from psora, which he termed "the hydra-headed monster."

Hahnemann must have moved beyond his original understanding of psora as scabies. If psora were caused by a single organism, how could it cause hundreds of diseases? And how could leprosy or St. Anthony's fire "mutate" into scabies? While the modern science of microbiology can explain the spread of these diseases (which could be considered the primary manifestations of psora), clearly Hahnemann's miasmatic theory was not limited to such microbial communication. He must have been struggling to use early-nineteenth-century language to convey an energetic transmission of disease susceptibility. In any case, a possible microbial explanation for the itch itself is not relevant for our miasmatic treatment of disease.

Using Hahnemann's powerful theory we can treat a miasmatic state before pathology emerges and we can prevent the transmission of parents' susceptibility to children. This is true preventive medicine.

Treating Psora and Its Acute Flare-ups

Hahnemann believed that acute illnesses could represent a flare-up of latent psora, as he expressed in a letter to one of his students: "This acute disease was a sudden outburst of the internal psora."[4] He envisioned latent psora like a volcano which could erupt from time to time in an acute illness of sudden onset. These sudden acute illnesses would then subside and the psora would become latent again. However, each time there was an acute flareup, the patient would be more susceptible to having another one. Hahnemann had determined that certain long-acting remedies, which he called antipsorics, were especially suited to eradicating the miasm. In provings, he found these remedies to cover the psoric miasmatic state. But he did not recommend treating the *acute* events with the antipsoric remedies, because these long-acting remedies would not work quickly enough. The antipsoric remedies were intended to remove the *tendency* to such recurring acute conditions. In other words, we do not need an antimiasmatic remedy to remove the "weeds" but we use them to eradicate the miasmatic "roots." (Of course an antipsoric remedy like Sulphur is often used acutely to treat skin conditions, but Hahnemann's point was that we choose the acute remedy simply on the indications, without taking into account its antimiasmatic properties.) Remedies are considered antipsoric if their proving symptoms match psoric indications and if they can bring back a suppressed rash.

Psora's Mechanism of Action

Hahnemann stated that the fluid in the itch vesicle contains the psoric miasm. If that fluid comes in contact with our skin, the miasm enters our organism *instantaneously*, becoming a chronic disease immediately. Hahnemann asks: "Is there in any probability any miasm in the world, which has infected from without, which does not first make the whole organism sick before the signs of it externally manifest themselves? We can only answer this question with, there is none!"[5] No eruption or itch will be seen in the first seven to fourteen days (during what is now called the incubation period). Once the whole organism is infected, a cutaneous eruption appears which is unique to psora, with voluptuous itching and a peculiar sour odor. This itching compels the patient to scratch open the vesicles, and the fluid which escapes can spread the infection to others. Hahnemann stresses the immediate transmission of this miasm, which cannot be prevented by any amount of scrubbing or douching. Hahnemann also uses this explanation for the incubation time of such acute miasmatic states such as measles, rubella, chickenpox and other childhood diseases.

It must be emphasized that the itch and/or eruption is not a local disease but the local expression of a deep internal disorder. As long as the eruption remains in its natural form, the internal psora is kept in check and the external disease can easily be cured by homeopathic remedies. But if we suppress it, the internal disease intensifies in a dangerous state called dormant or latent psora. The patient may seem to remain in good health for many years, but even a minor event can arouse this sleeping giant into one of the many chronic diseases which Hahnemann called the secondary manifestations of psora.

The primary manifestation of psora is itching, burning vesicles, which represent the Vital Force's attempt to throw the internal disorder to the surface. If they are suppressed, Hahnemann said, the internal disorder can manifest as vertigo, seizures, paralysis, insanity, and even sudden death. Hahnemann believed that everyone in the world had the psoric miasm because it was so easy to transmit (except himself because he had proved so many antipsoric remedies). He encouraged exteriorizing the psora to the skin, whether by the Vital Force's own power or by the aid of a remedy. The more it could be exteriorized, he said, the less intense would be its destructive power on a deeper plane.

Itching is the most diagnostic symptom of psora. It does not necessarily have to be present when the miasm is present; but when itching is present, psora must be, because the sycotic and syphilitic miasms do not have itching. When suppressed, it will attack the central nervous system (eczema going to stuttering or to seizures, for example). As it is transmitted from generation after generation, the susceptibility to it increases (as it does for every miasm). Since underlying psora *intensifies* whatever other miasms are present, we see the increasing activity of the other miasms in our children, resulting in cancer at an early age, learning problems like ADD, and disturbed emotional behavior (stealing without remorse and cold-blooded murders). While in Hahnemann's time psora was the dominant miasm, in my experience a great majority of patients have sycosis in some form, with catarrh or mucus as the main expression. The little children who are such mucus producers that their mothers constantly treat their runny noses are an example of this sycotic miasmatic expression. This constant suppression of the natural flow with pharmaceuticals (antibiotics, cortisone, nasal sprays, etc.) can lead to asthma (another sycotic expression).

Remedies Covering More than One Miasm

Of course not *all* the indications for psora are necessarily present in one person. In fact they are not all found in Sulphur, although Sulphur is the king of the antipsorics. Since each polychrest covers more than one miasm, we can find the indications of these miasms in the portrait of the remedy. For example, Sulphur covers sycosis and syphilis as well as psora. Sulphur's psoric indications include redness, rashes, itching, aggravation on standing, red mucous membranes, etc. But Sulphur's behavior can go to extremes, reflecting the sycotic miasm: boasting, competitiveness, studying very hard and wanting to be the best at everything. And Sulphur's syphilitic tendencies can be seen in the "ragged philosopher" described by Kent: he is not interested in anyone, he isolates himself, he does not bathe. It is as if he has given up on life, he no longer sees any way out. Calcarea is even more psoric in its proving symptoms than Sulphur, but it has abscesses and polyps (sycotic); swollen cervical glands, nosebleeds and a tendency to catch chest colds easily (tubercular miasm); syphilitic depression, melancholy, and "visions of murder and fire;"[6] and when pushed too far, Calcarea can become violent, hence we find it in the syphilitic rubric, "Desire to kill." Nitric acid, with its affinity for fissures and ulcers, is a strong syphilitic, but it has also psoric elements: chilliness, anxiety about health, despair about recovery, hypochondriasis. To know what miasms are covered by each remedy, I suggested to my students that they take all the symptoms of the remedy from a Materia Medica and classify each one according to the different miasms. In this way the proportion of the remedy associated with each miasm can be determined.

Psora's Central Idea: Lack of Strength and the Need for Support

Psora's main arenas of manifestation are the skin and nervous system. Through its neurological actions, it causes functional and subjective symptoms, never structural damage. The psoric patient is the greatest sufferer of all, not because he is in the most serious condition (he is not), but because he has so many distressing symptoms. For example, the psoric patient may have heart symptoms with great mental distress, always taking his pulse because he believes he is about to die. However, he is better off than the sycotic or syphilitic patient who dies on the spot from a heart infarct. The old masters said of the psoric patient that he is the one who lies down and prepares himself for death, then lives to be ninety.

Mental symptoms: Psoric people are hard workers in mind and body, but only for a short time, because they tire quickly. Their minds are alert and active; they have many ideas, especially worries about the future ("Ideas, abundant," K32, "Theorizing," K87, and "Thoughts intrude and crowd around each other," K87). Unfortunately they don't act on their ideas because they lack the strength. Because of their abundance of ideas and innate mental weakness, psoric people must make lists about everything: shopping lists, things to do, even lists of their lists. But then they often feel overwhelmed just by looking at their lists. They need more time than others, often being slow learners and needing to mull things over. (I asked one of my patients, a little Calcarea boy, "Who is your best friend?" His answer: "I have to mull this over." A tubercular Phosphorus would have immediately listed every child in his class.) They are deliberately slow to answer, wanting to make sure their answers are well thought out so as not to embarrass themselves. They have a fear of failure and above all, a fear of being laughed at ("Fear, observed, of her condition being," K46). While they have unusually keen and alert minds, they cannot keep to one train of thought for a very long time. While they are making a mental effort, they have a sense of bodily heat, of the heat of the room oppressing them.

The "psoric itch" expresses itself in the mental sphere as an intense mental restlessness. Psoric people are daydreamers, "sterile philosophers," building castles in the air. They may say, "If I only had a little bit more money, I could start that business." But they always feel they *lack* money and strength to do it. They find it hard to start a project (unlike the tubercular person who is a good beginner), and once started they are unlikely to finish it, since the slightest thing can interfere (the tubercular person is a bad finisher as well).

Emotional symptoms: Feeling too weak to defend themselves, psoric people tend to overcompensate to win their ongoing struggles. They feel they are too poor (even if they are millionaires) and must grasp onto whatever possessions they have, or else they won't be able to replace them. They tend to become miserly, driven by worry about the future (in contrast to the sycotic person, whose money jumps out of his pocket). Psora makes the mind intensely anxious to obtain, even by unfair means if it must, what is quite *un*necessary for his existence, like a house with 30 rooms, 25 bathrooms, and a garage for 30 cars.

These psoric people rarely will stop working; the word retirement is not in their vocabulary, even when they no longer need the money. They will work even when sick, or in the final week of pregnancy, for financial security ("Delusion, fortune, that he was going to lose his," K26, Psorinum, and "Delusion, thin, he is getting," K33, Sulphur). The psoric person does not need more possessions in reality, only in his mind: he says, "I don't want to be rich, I just want to be comfortable." But when I asked, "When would you feel comfortable financially," one psoric patient of mine answered, "When I have fifty million dollars!" The psoric person works evenings and weekends, while the tubercular person thinks, "If I had this much money, you would not catch me working." I know a couple, a psoric workaholic Sulphur husband and his free-spending tubercular Phosphorus wife. The husband, concerned about her spending, consulted a financial adviser who allocated money to each of them. When he asked his wife what she would do when she had spent her share of the money, she answered,

"Then I will just die the next day." She would never think of working to earn more!

Psoric people are chronic worriers ("itching" of the mind). They feel so weak that they think they have to constantly fight for survival, and they worry about where their next support will come from. For example, they may worry about their next paycheck (although they have plenty of money in the bank!), which reflects their "fear of failure in business" (K45, Psor.) They fear their health will fail and they will be unable to carry out what they attempt. They wake up in the middle of the night worrying about what they did the day before. "Did I offend someone? Did I find the right remedy for this patient? Did I offend my best friend by not phoning her for the last week? Did I spend too much money on my new furniture?" They worry about everything and scratch themselves because of the itch. This anxiety mainly tortures them at night, robbing them of their sleep, since they keep themselves busy during the day. Alone at night, they have time to reflect. They may feel their anxiety in the heart region, making them frequently check their pulse out of fear they are dying. Or they may feel it in the stomach ("Anxiety, in stomach," K476, Ars.).

During the 1929 crash and the Great Depression, people lived in a psoric state for a whole decade, saving all they could, and the psoric miasmatic state became deeply ingrained. Survivors of this period are definitely more cautious about spending than younger people. I had patients who always complained that they could not afford to pay me, and then later when they died, they left millions behind. I even had a patient whom I agreed to treat for free because he pleaded poverty. But then I heard from a friend of his that he had wallpapered his house with money notes. We also read in the newspaper about people who live in straitened circumstances, then leave millions to charity.

The psoric person is attached to her possessions, hoarding everything, food included. Of course she resists any change in diet, because food is enjoyment and luxury in her mind, a proof that she is successful in life. In fact she does not appreciate your good intentions in advocating a healthy diet. She loves the abundance of buffets, she likes to see food spread out on the table. If anyone in the family has more money or possessions, this might lead to a "psoric" jealousy.

A psoric person might steal out of greed, not necessity. He likes to collect things, to look at them and touch them, then put them away without doing anything with them. The house can be cluttered with ashtrays and his cupboards filled with towels taken from hotels. So the psoric person can be a kleptomaniac (although kleptomaniac could also be sycotic, if the motive is thrill-seeking, or syphilitic, if the intent is malicious, to hurt a competitor for instance).

The psoric child is apt to recognize the value of material objects at an early age. He will convince his younger sister to trade something valuable of hers for something worthless of his. He always wants to win at games, even if he has to cheat (because winning gives him a sense of strength, it bolsters his ego). Many psoric people are materialistic, not seeking higher spiritual attainment, never satisfied with what they have, never thinking they have enough to survive. (Other psoric people may be religious, spiritual, or philosophical.) As you can see, the psoric person is egotistical, his world centered around himself and his survival needs.

The timid psoric person is too shy to talk when challenged at school or in conversation. Psoric children are timid about going to school, fearing that they will fail, so they tend to be late. They don't like being the center of attention, they are easily embarrassed, and they can't stand being looked at ("Mind, looked at, cannot bear to be," K63, Ars.). Some psoric adults resort to alcohol to loosen their inhibitions enough to talk. They avoid taking initiative in school or at work. They often feel helpless, especially in school situations where they may be bullied. They easily feel overpowered by everybody and everything, even by what they see and hear ("Horrible things affect him," K52). Psoric children are very sensitive to their parents' feelings, the first to sense discord and to try to comfort their mother. This sensitiveness is carried over to "hearing bad news," to which they react with anxiety, shivering, vertigo, and fainting, as if suddenly paralyzed. (A syphilitic child will react by hitting, kicking, and breaking things.) "Never Well since fear, fright, bad news" can trigger a latent psoric miasm and require an antipsoric remedy.

Psoric children like to read history and historical novels and like to play in nature, building forts in the woods or camping on an island. They enjoy company because it means added support for their perceived "weakness." They will often say, "I can't do it, will you do it with me?" while the syphilitic gives up and says, "You do it!" When they are sick, they need constant reassurance, another form of support. And the psoric child will use any excuse to climb into bed with mummy. In the waiting room, the psoric child waits until another child approaches him; then he is glad someone has made contact with him. He feels "supported" in his play if he has company; he prefers one child to a group, where he feels lost because of his shyness. Obviously he is more a follower than a leader, and he can even show cowardice (*lack of courage*).

The psoric child constantly feels underappreciated. She is likely to be timid and bashful in the consultation room, holding onto her mother or hiding behind her, and looking at her mother when you ask her a question. She is fearful, clinging, dependent on mummy, wanting to be held, even still sucking on mummy's breast at age three. One of my dogs is very psoric: he loves to fall asleep next to me or my wife with one of his paws touching us (looking for support and love). Everyday he comes to me while I am reading at exactly the same time. I have to give him a hug, he kisses me, and then he falls asleep at my feet. It is his way of checking in: "Do you still love me?"

Because of their perceived weakness, psoric children have plenty of fears. They are afraid of bigger children and prefer to play with small children or alone with their toy soldiers or little cars. They are afraid of being late, yet always manage to be late. They are afraid to watch TV because of the scary things they see there. Psoric adults as well as children have typical psoric nightmares of things they worry about during the day. They are also afraid of being laughed at, because they know they are seen as shy, slow, or "dumb." Because of fear and insecurity, they become inflexible, hanging on to their ideas and their own ways of doing things. For example, a psoric homeopath may be dogmatic about one way of practicing, with no room for change.

The psoric person also fears high places, poverty, robbery, and losing his possessions ("Delusions, thieves, that house and space under bed are full of," K33, Ars.). He suspects anyone who does a job for him (plumber, painter, doctor, etc.) of overcharging him. He struggles continuously to have enough money, always with a nervous foreboding: today things might be going well, but tomorrow they could go downhill in a flash, or he might become ill and not have enough money to support himself. He especially fears anything that might threaten his home (darkness, storms, etc.) or his family (separation or divorce).

The little psoric boy likes to play the role of hero, carrying around a "big gun." He needs this gun to hide his fear, to give him some strength. I had this cute 3-year-old Calcarea boy who always visited me dressed as a cowboy, fireman or police officer. "I am tough, don't mess with me," his little outfits were trying to say. The psoric adult prefers a profession that shows strength, like fireman or police officer; or something related to serving others or serving food: chef or waitress, doctor or nurse. When a psoric person lies, it is not to boast (sycotic) but to appear stronger, almost out of self-protection. And with the Y2K problem around the corner, psoric people are the ones fleeing with their extended families to a big house in the country, hoarding food and supplies.

Psoric children show an early interest in religion, asking many questions about God, driven by fear as well as spirituality: "What is going to happen to me when I die?" is a frequent question, based on their fear of physical suffering. This fear of physical suffering is obvious in a psoric person who has been in a car accident: he will feel paralyzed and afraid to drive again for quite some time. He will need emotional support to overcome the shock. (This is quite different from the sycotic race car driver, who races for the thrill of it and who itches to return to it, even while recovering from his injuries in the hospital; or the syphilitic one, who considers his car a "weapon" for his aggressions, even to the point that it will kill him or someone else.) In fact, psoric people need support in fighting all their fears (like the child climbing in bed with his mother because he has nightmares). They feel paralyzed by the fears and tend to feel immobilized when angry: they don't hit back or talk back when accosted, they simmer with a red face, even feeling guilty for causing a commotion. When confronted with a frightening situation, they will run away to ask for help from a neighbor or the police.

The need for support and protection can be seen in every aspect of psoric people's life. They do not like to move away from their family. In Belgium, where I grew up, people used to go to school, marry, build a house, work, and die in the same village where they were born (the burial plot is already purchased at a young age!). This is quite different from the life-style in California, where I have also lived for many years, and where few people stay long enough to know their neighbors. (Californians are more sycotic and tubercular.) The Belgian lifestyle is solid and steady; Belgians work hard, eat well (mostly rich food), and are definitely more serious than their northern neighbors, the Dutch. Their psoric mindset is even reflected in Belgian furniture: the heavy oak furniture lasts forever and is passed down from one generation to the next. It gives a feeling of survival, of support and solidity.

The psoric teenager would join a gang because he wants to belong; he feels he needs the other boys for protection and self-confidence. If he does not find the support he so desperately needs from his family (for example, if the parents are too busy working), he may look for it in the wrong places. As a teenager he is a follower rather than a leader. If he has body piercing done, it is only to follow the others and to be part of the group. (Body piercing is usually syphilitic, since it is a form of self-mutilation, especially when done on the hidden and more sensitive, sexual parts like the nipples or penis. It can also be sycotic when the teenager flaunts it on his face to shock adults. Likewise joining a gang may be sycotic if done for adventure, to push the limits, or syphilitic if it provides the opportunity for coldblooded crime.)

You can recognize psoric people in their simple, formless, baggy clothing. They want their clothing to be protective (large, thick, and warm for the chilly psoric person) rather than the attention-getting clothing of the sycotic. Because of their stinginess, they do not like to throw out old clothes, even when they are full of holes. All hell breaks loose when the Carcinosin wife with her fastidiousness and eye for beauty throws away her psoric husband's favorite old T-shirt ("Delusion, old rags are as fine as silk," K30, Sulphur).

Physical symptoms: Because psora alone never causes structural changes, we find the psoric patient normal in size and form. (Any growths or deformations will be sycotic, syphilitic, or tubercular). Since the psoric person lacks strength, he always tries to build himself up by eating. Lacking the power to assimilate his food, he suffers constant gnawing sensations and cravings for many foods. Since pregnancy heightens psoric characteristics, the psoric woman is likely to have pica gravidarum (cravings for inedible substances). Psoric children may have the same cravings, eating sand or chalk or chewing on their pencils. Psoric people tend to crave rich, heavy foods: milk, eggs, cream, fatty foods for energy, and meat (although meat often heightens psora as well as sycosis). They are very focused on food, enjoying cooking and grocery shopping with a long list of necessities. They can't wait until mealtime, and while they may claim they "never eat," they snack constantly. Yet their system is disturbed by the slightest dietary excess, another sign of this mighty miasm. Their cravings for sweets leads to overindulgence and often to typical psoric headaches: periodic headaches which appear in the morning, growing worse as the sun rises to the zenith, and gradually ameliorating as the sun declines.

Because psoric people are too weak to maintain enough body heat, a draft or air-conditioning is unsettling, and they tend to catch cold at the slightest change of weather. Yet they can't stand the heat of the bed at night, kicking off the covers, and their symptoms are worst at noon when the sun is at its peak. They dislike wind because they feel it can push them around and knock them down. They sweat at night and tend to have excessive sweat on the forehead and scalp, hands, feet, and groin, although they may also experience a complete lack of sweat. They feel better after perspiration, as they do after all natural discharges (stool, urination, menses, etc.). Their sweat has a special sour odor, as does their breath, their stool, and all their excretions.

The psoric weakness makes it difficult for them to exercise vigorously. They have difficulty climbing stairs, so they cling to the banister out of breath. They don't like coming downstairs either, as they experience vertigo; they feel unbalanced because of their weak ankles. They don't like standing and tend to have a stoop-shouldered posture. They prefer to sit, and when sitting they slump because they don't have the strength to straighten their body. They look for support by leaning on something: a handrail, table or desk, or against a wall while standing, or as hospital patients they ask for extra pillows.

The psoric skin is pale, unhealthy, even dirty looking, with red, itching, burning rashes everywhere (no suppuration, however). The itch makes them scratch, and the more they scratch the more the rash itches and burns. This itching and burning, together with their restlessness and chronic worries, lead to insomnia and an even greater loss of energy. Of course psoric people can have perfect skin, but those who do are likely to be in the worst health on a deeper level. We tend to envy people who can live on pizza and still have perfect skin, but this means their Vital Force is not strong enough to throw their internal disorders to the surface.

Because psoric people have difficulty assimilating calcium and other minerals, they have difficulty with their hair, nails, teeth, and growth in general. Their dry, thin hair tangles and breaks easily, the ends split, and it tends to fall out after a disease. They are likely to have white streaks or prematurely grey hair. Their brittle nails break easily, and they have the tendency to bite their nails (Bar.-c.). As babies they have delayed teething (Calc-p; Calc-c.) as well as early caries (Kreos., Staph., Sil). Even if these psoric children are given calcium supplements, they can't absorb them and even get constipated from them because of the malassimilation. Their teeth are too small and lack enamel, exposing the inner part. People who grind their teeth may be psoric or tubercular. Although they need extra calcium and crave dairy products, they can't digest them and get severe diarrhea or constipation from them.

Other complications of psora include long-standing constipations, hemorrhoids, distressing headaches and a chronic tendency to boils. Although warts are mainly sycotic, we also see psoric warts: flat, soft, skin-colored, dry, and itchy. Molluscum contagiosum, with its clusters of round soft fleshy-colored balls, is also a form of psora. Ear infections develop slowly in psoric children. Over a period of several days they whine and weep about their ears aching, too weak to produce a high fever. This slow onset with low-grade fever is also found in other acute disorders (lung inflammations, gastric problems, colon problems, appendicitis with no clear picture for months, etc.).

In spite of the psoric person's weakness, the life span tends to be long. ("Creaking cars last the longest," as we say in my country.) Psoric people have disorders of sensation and function, not organic ones (at least not until old age, or not unless coupled with another miasm). For example, congestive heart failure in the elderly is typical of psora, because only the psoric patient will live long enough to develop it, while the sycotic or syphilitic patient would have already died from a heart infarct. Thus psoric people, despite their complaints and their typical "despair of recovery," are apt to survive everyone around them, including their physician.

Treatment of the Psoric Miasm

Hahnemann considered Sulphur the "king of the antipsorics" and frequently opened his cases with Sulphur in his later years to clear the effects of psora. Calcarea's proving symptoms more closely match the indications for psora, but Hahnemann was correct in opening with Sulphur rather than Calcarea, which follows Sulphur as a deeper-working antipsoric in the sequence Sulphur-Calcarea-Lycopodium. (In other words, when a patient needs both Sulphur and Calcarea, it is more effective to give Sulphur first. It also works better to give Calcarea before Lycopodium, another top antipsoric.) Other remedies frequently used in psoric conditions include Nux vomica for digestive complaints, Graphites for skin conditions, and Arsenicum for the typical psoric worries about health and finances which lead to a search for support. Surprisingly enough, Psorinum is not the most effective nosode in psoric cases: the old masters preferred Tuberculinum, finding it even more effective than Psorinum in breaking through a psoric miasmatic block. Hahnemann listed many other remedies as antipsoric in his *Chronic Diseases*, volumes 1 and 2.

What is the best time to take an antipsoric? Hahnemann tells us in *Chronic Diseases* it should be taken in the morning rather than the evening, a half an hour away from food and drinks, without going to sleep right away (sleep delays the beginning of the action of the remedy). It should not be taken just before or during the menses but about four days after the menses have begun.[7] Hahnemann also mentions that pregnancy is an ideal time to treat the mother with an antipsoric remedy, because the woman's increased sensitivity makes her internal psora manifest more plainly. Such treatment, he says, will help prevent problems of breast feeding, sore breasts, abscesses, and soreness of nipples.

Rarely will it happen in our society that only the psoric miasm is present; this only happens in a person of a strong psoric constitution who has been able to fend off the other miasms. In this case the treatment is relatively simple, although it may take years and should not be discontinued until all the signs of latent psora are eradicated. In *Chronic Diseases* Hahnemann tells us:

> When the treatment is about half completed, the diminished disease commences to return into the state of the latent psora; the symptoms grow weaker and weaker, and at the last the attentive physician will only find traces of it; but he must follow these to their complete disappearance, for the smallest remnant retains a germ for a renewal of the old ailment.[8]

He thus draws our attention to the manifold roots of the psoric miasm, which implants itself like a parasite in most of its victims. He warns us to persevere in eradicating even the slightest trace of it to avoid the recurrence of a flare-up or the formation of another psoric disease when the miasm is triggered. It is a mistake for the homeopath or patient to believe that health can be restored through a better lifestyle or improved diet, as long as traces of psora remain. While thorough antipsoric treatment may take years, the patient is encouraged to continue by his ever-increasing sense of well-being.

Cases in which psora is mixed with sycosis or syphilis will be discussed in upcoming chapters.

Chapter Twenty-One

Sycosis: The Miasm of Excess and Overgrowth

History

During Hahnemann's lifetime, the English physician John Hunter (1728-1793) was considered the sole authority on venereal disease. He believed that gonorrheal discharge and syphilitic ulcers were caused by the same venereal infection. In order to test his theory he undertook a brave but foolish (and ultimately fatal) experiment by inoculating himself with a gonorrheal discharge, using a needle that was also inoculated with syphilis. Thus he broke out with syphilis and gonorrhea, a living example of the misguided theory. Hahnemann disagreed with Hunter, as he believed that the two diseases were different and had (as he pointed out) different etiologies.* Hahnemann's observations were confirmed half a century later in 1879 by Dr. Albert Neisser (for whom the gonorrhea-causing bacteria, *Neisseria gonorrhea,* was named).

Kent's allopathic contemporaries believed, as modern physicians do, that once gonorrhea is treated and the acute symptoms subside, it is permanently cured and cannot cause systemic symptoms and cannot be transmitted. Modern medicine still has not accepted Hahnemann's viewpoint that gonorrhea which has been suppressed by medical treatment leads to latent gonorrhea, which can be inherited and which he called *sycosis*. Consistent with that position, homeopaths consider all of the tertiary manifestations of gonorrhea, as well as most if not all of the secondary ones, as solely the result of suppression by local or topical treatment of the primary discharge. Only one of Hahnemann's contemporaries, Dr. Noeggerath, had a viewpoint similar to Hahnemann's, although he was not a homeopath. Noeggerath's theory went as follows:

---

*Hahnemann agreed with Hunter about one thing: "Not one patient will escape syphilis if the chancre is destroyed by mere external applications."[1]

- That nearly all men who have had gonorrhea and have apparently been "cured" sooner or later infect their wives.
- That this infectiousness on the part of the man is usually latent, but can become perceptible in the form of an urethritis, more or less severe, following sexual intercourse. (In modern times this is often seen in the woman with recurrent vaginitis since being married to a husband with suppressed gonorrhea, although the non-specified urethritis or NSU certainly belongs to the same class.)
- That this latent gonorrhea in the man leads to a similar latent infection of the wife, which may in turn become active as the etiological factor of one or more forms of pelvic inflammation.

Noeggerath unwittingly provided support for Hahnemann's doctrine. No longer could gonorrhea be considered, as it was before, a merely local disease, as harmless as a cold in the head and as easy to cure.

Definition

Sycosis is not the same as acute gonorrhea, as some homeopaths might believe. Acute gonorrhea is acquired through sexual intercourse or transmitted from the mother to the infant during delivery through the infected birth canal. If it is treated with the right homeopathic remedy (such as Cannabis indica, Cantharis or Copaiva) and not suppressed by drugs, it is cured at once and there are no future complications. In men, the only symptom of this simple form of acute gonorrhea is the discharge from the penis. Women usually experience a mild cervical infection that remains undetected in up to 80% of cases. Since the condition remains asymptomatic, it usually remains undiagnosed and therefore, unfortunately, untreated.

The discharge in the male may last longer under homeopathic treatment than under allopathic, but when it is cured, it is never followed by stricture, enlarged prostate, or diseases of the bladder in later life. Similarly if acute gonorrhea in women were treated homeopathically, they would not suffer from pelvic inflammatory disease, infertility, ectopic pregnancies, ovarian cysts, endometriosis, or any of the other sequelae of disseminated gonorrhea, which occurs in a certain percentage of cases.

But if the acute gonorrhea is suppressed with allopathic treatment, it imposes on the patient the sycotic miasm, which will require antisycotic remedies. Sycosis was widespread in Hahnemann's time, known as the figwart disease for the shape of the typical condylomata it caused. The warts were treated with large doses of Mercury, cauterization, burning, and cutting. These growths usually were present on the genitals and usually accompanied by a thick greenish pus from the urethra. These warts often emitted a fluid smelling of fish-brine, had a cauliflower appearance, and often bled. Thus sycosis is not at all the same as acute gonorrhea; it is the appearance of condylomata (figwarts) on and around the genitalia *with or without* a greenish discharge from the urethra.

Suppression pushes the disease deeper inwards to attack the internal organs (e.g. inflammation of the genito-urinary system). If the resulting symptoms are also treated allopathically, still deeper pathology can result (such as infertility through stenosis of the fallopian tubes). This reflects the natural centripetal action of the sycotic miasm, unlike the exteriorization of psora. In other words, when psoric skin eruptions are left untreated they will naturally disappear, but the syphilitic chancre and sycotic figwart, if untreated, will naturally progress to the deeper organs. Sycosis primarily attacks the pelvic organs, but it can also affect distant organs, as in asthma and rheumatism, and the mental state, even producing insanity. Kent describes a case of asthma:

> I gave [the patient] remedies which seemed to help him for a time, but could not cure him. I knew that he had had gonorrhea but saw no correlation. Finally I gave him Nat. Sulph which cured the asthma completely, but in a short time figwarts appeared on the genitalia. I gave him Thuja, which is the complement of Nat Sulph. The figwarts disappeared and the old gonorrheal discharge appeared.[2]

This discharge may resist homeopathic treatment for years, because the miasm has become deep-seated and the discharge *should* exist as long as the miasm has not been cured. Treating the discharge as a symptom is dangerous, because this superficial prescribing will not address the miasm, and as long as the miasm remains untreated it can continue to wreak its destruction. Hahnemann warns us in Aphorism 197 of the danger of simultaneously treating such a "local malady" both internally and superficially. He explains that the external symptom, such as a discharge, serves as a guideline to how long we need to continue the systemic treatment, which we might stop too soon if we treat the local symptom superficially.

Antisycotic Remedies

Thuja, the top antisycotic remedy, is one of Hahnemann's discoveries. Practically nothing was known of its therapeutic properties until he proved it, together with Gross, Hartmann, Wagner, his son Friedrich, and a few others.

The initial enthusiasm among homeopaths about Dr. Edward Jenner's smallpox vaccination was dampened by the acute observations of von Boenninghausen. The baron discovered the effectiveness of Thuja against smallpox, however, and published his results as "Concerning the curative effects of Thuja in Smallpox."[3]

I ought to inform you of an experience of mine this winter. Since the last 6 months smallpox has appeared here and there. After giving Thuja to horses with favorable success, I used the same in the first case of smallpox that was entrusted to my treatment. It exceeded all my expectations. On the 4th day all the pustules were dried up, on the 8th day there were fallen off and no pockmarks were seen. This caused me to use Thuja in several houses where smallpox had broken out as a prophylactic, and lo and behold, no other members of the family were affected. I used in smallpox cases only a few pellets of the 200c potency.[4]

The gonorrheal discharge has been made into a homeopathic remedy (Medorrhinum, introduced by Swan). It shows in its provings such typical sycotic symptoms as rheumatism with stiffness, aching, and soreness; profuse, acrid discharges and fishy odors of the secretions; enlargement of the lymph glands; a hurried mind and a nervous, impulsive, and passionate disposition; a tendency to swing from one extreme to the other; aggravation from dampness and during the day which are typical of the sycotic miasm (such as headaches worse during the day, the opposite of the nighttime syphilitic headaches). Many severe cases of asthma, the result of suppressed gonorrhea, are speedily advanced by Medorrhinum and the symptoms of sycosis are brought out. So Medorrhinum *develops* the latent miasm, bringing up its symptoms. Medorrhinum does not *cure* the miasm or the acute gonorrhea. Medorrhinum does not work well to treat acute gonorrhea, and the miasm requires antisycotic remedies. Thus Medorrhinum acts as a *developing* remedy like Psorinum and Syphilinum. Other powerful antisycotics include Nat. sulph., Nitric acid, Lycopodium, Calcarea, Sulphur, and Arsenicum. Remedies are considered antisycotic if their proving symptoms match sycotic indications or if they can bring back a suppressed gonorrheal discharge.

Transmission of the Miasm in the Same State

Cases of gonorrhea treated with antibiotics are considered cured soon after the discharge has stopped, and the patient is told that he can safely resume sexual relations. But according to our understanding of miasms, he should wait until after the discharge has been re-established and then cleared by the appropriate antisycotic remedy. Many times we find in women's past medical history that their health broke down after marriage or after beginning a sexual relationship with a particular partner. Seeking treatment for PID, vaginal discharges, endometriosis, abdominal trouble, or yeast infections, they are often told that they are "allergic" to their partner. The partner is not likely to tell her of an infection he may have had 10 years earlier when he was 18, since he thinks it was cured at the time. His health may have also been affected with symptoms which only a homeopath would connect to the suppressed gonorrhea; or the miasm may be dormant with no symptoms present.

What is worse, the woman will catch the condition in the *same stage* it was suppressed in her sex partner. For instance, after the initial discharge has been suppressed in the man, the woman will catch the miasm in its secondary stage and will not show a discharge or other signs of acute infection. Without warning, the miasm will go directly to her deeper pelvic organs, often creating sterility. When she is treated homeopathically, she will not give off a gonorrheal discharge since it was never present in the first place. By treating this woman correctly, you cannot expect to re-establish a discharge since it was never present in the first place. (This does not preclude the possibility of a discharge produced by a healing reaction, by the simple exteriorization of an internal disorder.)

While we usually see the miasm transferred in its secondary or tertiary stage, it is actually *possible* for the acute primary disease to be transferred *years* after it was suppressed in the sex partner. Dr. E. Reininger described such a case:

> A young man of about twenty-eight years old consulted me regarding a case of rheumatism in the joints of the entire body from which he could not get relief. After examination I concluded his trouble was chronic gonorrhea. The acute infection was contracted about eight years previously. I warned the patient that in all probability there would reappear an urethral discharge (which did happen during the third week of treatment), and if it did occur not to have intercourse with his wife as in such event she would probably become infected. My warning was not heeded and the worst happened. She became infected, an acute gonorrhea developed and was treated by me for months thereafter. Here is an interval of eight years from the time of first infection, to the time of reappearance of an acute gonorrheal discharge from the urethra. This case demonstrated to me that the gonococci remained latent in his system for eight years, till reproduced as stated, and infected his wife by coition.[5]

Manifestations of Sycosis

In general, sycosis affect the soft tissues, syphilis affects the bones, and psora affects the whole system, causing a functional breakdown. Sycosis is more potent than syphilis as a cause of mental disease and moral insanity: sycosis forms a basis of much of the criminality of our own country. Like syphilis, it may remain single or mix with the other two miasms. Although sycosis and syphilis are *centripetal* while psora is centrifugal, syphilis and sycosis have an advantage over psora in that the chancre or bubo and the figwart do not disappear until they are either artificially removed or healed homeopathically from within (while the skin eruption of psora can disappear spontaneously even if not suppressed or treated). These exterior manifestations serve as a guideline for the length of therapy. The treatment is not finished until these exterior signs are gone. It is the nature of sycosis to go to the surface *only in the earlier stage,* when the constitution is still strong in the individual, producing mucus in the nose, lungs or stools. If he is too weak it will go immediately to the deeper tissues.

Sycosis was an uncommon disease in Hahnemann's time and as a rule was not taken very seriously. Unfortunately, it is now widespread and highly active, which is why cancer and malignant diseases are increasing. Sycosis gives the speed and intensity behind rapidly growing and rapidly metastasizing cancers. It is the *most venereal* of all venereal diseases, being more infectious than syphilis and only contracted through sexual intercourse (except for newborns who contract it during delivery, whereas syphilis can be spread through contact with bodily fluids or infected wounds). No wonder so many women suffer from pelvic affections (PID) and rheumatic diseases. It is a source of continual malaise, often producing sterility, chronic pelvic inflammatory disease (endometritis, endometriosis, oophoritis, etc.), anemia, rheumatism, catarrh, asthma, etc.

Like acute gonorrhea, the sycotic miasm can produce a discharge from the urethra, but in this case there is not much pain or difficulty in urination (unlike in acute gonorrhea). This condition is called *sycotic* gonorrhea (because the Neisseria gonococcus would not appear in a culture of the discharge). Recurring nonspecific urethritis (NSU), in which no particular organism can be cultured from the discharge, reflects this type of gonorrhea and an underlying sycotic miasm. While acute gonorrhea may be automatically cured over time, sycotic gonorrhea will never be cured without the proper antisycotic remedy. In other words, allopathic treatment can make a curable disease, acute gonorrhea, into an incurable one, sycosis. The following table will aid in distinguishing between acute and sycotic gonorrhea.

Sycotic Gonorrhea	**Acute Gonorrhea**
Chronic miasmatic state (root)	Acute miasm (weed which sends down the root)
Needs antisycotic remedy	Can cure spontaneously
Non-painful discharge	Painful, burning discharge
No *Neisseria g.* found (NSU)	*Neisseria gonorrhea* present
Deep disease: PID, brain	Superficial lesion: discharge

Remember that when a disease is suppressed, LM or higher potencies are necessary to sever the connection between the suppressed disease and the Vital Force. Under this treatment, symptoms subside as soon as the old discharge is re-established. Or if the genital discharge cannot be re-established, another eliminative process may appear, such as increased urination, pruritus ani or vulvae, a skin eruption, or joint symptoms. Even if these manifestations are new to the patient, the remedy is correct and should be continued.

Another primary sign of sycosis is *catarrh* or mucus. Mucus-producing infections of the eyes and especially of the nose are very common, and sycosis is responsible for the widespread sinusitis and resulting frontal headaches in our society. Sycosis gives symptoms in *joints* relieved by motion. When you can't cure joint disease with Rhus tox. although it seems to be the indicated remedy, you need an antisycotic remedy (which Rhus tox. is not). These joint symptoms are only cured when the discharge has been brought back.

Sycosis and Vaccinations

Hahnemann initially supported the smallpox vaccinations introduced by Dr. Edward Jenner in 1792 because he considered them a form of "Like Cures Like." It was von Boenninghausen who observed the negative effects of vaccinations, believing that they grafted a disease onto the patient. He used Thuja 200c at first, later Medorrhinum when it had been potentized, to protect his patients against the side effects of vaccinations which had quickly become popular.[6] Dr. Compton Burnett noticed, after many years of observation, that repeated smallpox vaccination created a condition similar to sycosis, a state he called "vaccinosis" and cured with Thuja.[7]

The connection between vaccinations and the sycotic miasm can be demonstrated by the treatment. We often see children with recurrent ear infections, colds and flu with excessive mucus production who are "Never Well Since" vaccinations. When we treat with an antisycotic remedy, not only does the Chief Complaint subside, but so do the many other sycotic manifestations in the patient. When the homeopath has finished treating the layers and still finds a sycotic influence, there is a good chance this represents the "vaccinosis" state created by multiple early vaccinations, requiring Thuja before finishing treatment with the constitutional remedy.

Having made the connection between vaccinations and sycosis, homeopaths must be alarmed at the ever-increasing number of vaccinations required for infants and small children. The first vaccination, Hepatitis B, is given when the infant is fresh from the trauma of the birth experience, followed by 20 more vaccinations by the age of two. Even within the paradigm of allopathic medicine, these early and frequent vaccinations are counterproductive because the immune system is not yet formed when the first vaccinations are given. And from a homeopathic point of view, they fuel the fire of the sycotic miasm, which is also fueled by the overuse of antibiotics and cortisone and the widespread use of birth control pills. As can be seen by the dangerous manifestations of the sycotic miasm, fueling its fire will contribute to many problems of our society, from physical problems like sterility to behavioral ones like ADHD, juvenile delinquency and violence.

Complications of Sycosis Upon Suppression

Primary Stage: *Anemia* is often the first sign of the active sycotic miasm, except for the hemolytic anemias which belong to the destructive syphilitic miasm. (The connection between sycosis and anemia has been demonstrated many times clinically. We can speculate as to the reason: the sycotic miasm attacks the kidneys along with the other pelvic organs and before detectable pathology such as cysts or nephritis appear, erythropoietin production has already been affected, reducing red blood cell production.) Also common is *prostatitis* which may continue throughout all three stages, becoming very stubborn to cure. *Rheumatism* is another frequent complication: the great majority of cases are sycotic (destructive changes in the joints are syphilitic). These are the symptoms immediately produced after suppression, demonstrating that the miasm immediately affects the entire system. Systemic symptoms do not arise if acute gonorrhea is treated homeopathically.

Secondary Stage: This stage may begin three months to two years after the primary infection, depending on the strength of the patient's constitution and how healthy her life-style is. It lasts from one to two years unless treated homeopathically. Often a single organ is affected, like the ovary or fallopian tube, as if the whole force of the disease is concentrated upon this one organ. Cyst formations are very characteristic of this secondary stage. We often see a healthy robust woman develop into a suffering invalid soon after beginning a relationship with a sycotic male, because he transmitted the miasm to her in this secondary stage.

Almost every disease in this stage is of an *inflammatory* nature, especially diseases of the pelvic and sexual organs. This miasm creates the worst forms of inflammation, infiltration of the tissues and their degeneration. In women it is most frequently found in pelvic diseases such as PID (inflammation of the fallopian tubes, cystic degeneration of ovaries and uterus). Peritonitis, endometriosis, cystitis and appendicitis are frequently caused by secondary sycosis. The discharges have a special odor: pungent, musty, or smelling of dead fish ("fish-brine" in the *Repertory*). Adhesions, abscesses, fibroid tumors, cysts, and warts are other typical manifestations of secondary sycosis, which is characterized by overgrowths of all kinds.

It is largely due to sycosis that the pelvic and abdominal cavities have become the primary arena for modern surgery. Few surgical cases in these areas are not caused by sycosis. Thus nearly all gynecology and gynecological surgery at this present time is due to the improper and unsatisfactory medical treatment of sycosis. Because it targets the fallopian tubes, sycosis in this stage often makes a woman sterile. If she is able to bear a child, the infant is frequently waxy-looking and anemic with failure to thrive. It is likely to develop purulent ophthalmia with the greenish-yellow pus typical of the sycotic miasm (versus the bland, creamy yellow of the psoric Hepar sulph. ophthalmia).

The male patient is apt to suffer from orchitis, epididymitis, prostatitis, and balanitis. Both sexes are likely to suffer from sycotic arthritis with pains and lameness across the sacrum, neuralgias in the head, and sciatic pains. Allopathic authors have even recognized and defined a disseminated gonorrheal infection in which the Neisseria bacteria enters the bloodstream, causing gonorrheal rheumatism with or without gonorrheal endocarditis and pericarditis, gonorrheal ophthalmia, conjunctivitis, gonorrheal pyemia and septicemia, PID, meningitis, and arthritis.

Tertiary Stage: This stage appears one to two years after secondary stage. The lesions are usually *skin lesions*. The first one is the warty growth, like *verruca vulgaris, filiformis* and *plana* (the common wart, thread-shaped wart, and flat wart, respectively). Psoriasis, accounting for sixty percent of all skin conditions, is often a mixture of the three miasms, with psora and sycosis dominating. *Fungal infections* like candida and all forms of ringworm are sycotic in nature, as is *Herpes zoster* (shingles).

The tertiary manifestations of all the miasms, though slower in action, always involve the *deeper* organs of the body. Lupus can often be traced to a sycosis suppressed at some point. But its full picture is created by psora, sycosis and latent syphilis, with the syphilis taking on the tubercular form. That is the reason why lupus is so difficult to cure, because the more miasms present, the more profound the disease. Another disease of sycotic origin is *gout*. Sycosis creates the susceptibility to gout, which then develops in the presence of certain foods like organ meats and wine. Gouty secretions (urate of soda) can be observed in the eyelids, rectum, mouth, nose and urethra. Another disease of sycotic origin is the *flu*.

Sycotic patients are also very sensitive to changes in *barometric pressure*. They can foretell weather changes days in advance. This means that they have *lost the power of resistance*. Before acquiring the sycotic miasm, they would not be hindered by damp weather. Now, as sycotics, their joints hurt in rain, snow or cold weather, driving them to seek relief in baths (mineral or thermal) and diet changes. Hot applications relieve their gout and rheuma, and drinking large amounts of mineral water (often alkaline) neutralizes the acid condition of their blood.

Secondary or tertiary stages of sycosis and syphilis are the result of bad treatment or suppression (according to Hahnemann, although according to modern allopathic medicine the secondary and tertiary stages will develop even if the primary stage is untreated.) After the physical inferno created by the sycotic miasm, the patient's mental/emotional breakdown starts. He becomes much more suspicious, to the point where he does not trust himself and he must go back and check or repeat what he just did. This suspicion, when turned towards others, creates one of the worst forms of jealousy. Sycotics become quarreling degenerates with a tendency to harm others and animals. They are disposed to fits of anger, and if the destructive syphilitic miasm is also present, they can harbor a smoldering rage that suddenly erupts like a volcano. We read about these unfortunate events in the newspapers: the teenager who takes a gun to school and sprays the cafeteria with bullets, or the postal worker who goes on a rampage and kills his fellow workers.

When the miasm is treated with the well-indicated antisycotic, or the Vital Force is strengthened with a healthier diet and life-style, it is likely to push out an external manifestation like a catarrh or discharge, leading to relief on the mental and emotional planes. Sycotic patients need these pathological discharges for relief and, unlike psorics, are not relieved by physiological discharges like perspiration, urination or menses. Be sure not to suppress these discharges with a remedy prescribed on the local symptoms, or the mental state can worsen again. (Usually the patient feels so much better that she will plead with you to continue the treatment despite a repugnant discharge.) Treating the sycotic miasm takes time and it is important to educate your patient that it is a systemic, not a local condition.

Sycosis in Modern Times

Reports of the sycotic mind at work appear in the newspapers every day. A recent editorial entitled "Violent kids can't be reformed" followed a crime in Los Angeles in which a group of kids kidnapped a 13-year-old, forced her into an abandoned duplex, gang raped and tortured her, and tried to set the house on fire to kill the victim. Then they killed an old neighbor who came over to investigate. The leader of the gang was 12 years old, already a hardened criminal at age 11 who had been expelled from school for fighting with knives. Another recent article described such "super predators," the young people who start out violent, stay that way, and commit much of the juvenile crimes. According to the article, each generation of these predators is more violent than the one before, and a recent study showed that 94% of these young delinquents are rearrested as adults. The article posed the question: if it is too late to save them at 12, how can we ignore them at age 6? In another article, a 6-year-old boy battered a one-month-old baby until he had a fractured skull. How could a small child do this? The article put forward several hypotheses: one blamed the mother for bad parenting, another blamed the poverty and violence the child had witnessed in his neighborhood, while another speculated that he must have been subjected to abuse himself. But many who live in these circumstances do not commit such crimes.

Only a homeopath will see these violent children as expressing the sycotic miasm, with the increase in violence a direct result of all the ways our society fuels it, whether physically through antibiotics, vaccinations, cortisone and birth control pills; emotionally through the

Fig. 21-1: The Sycotic Miasm and Suppression

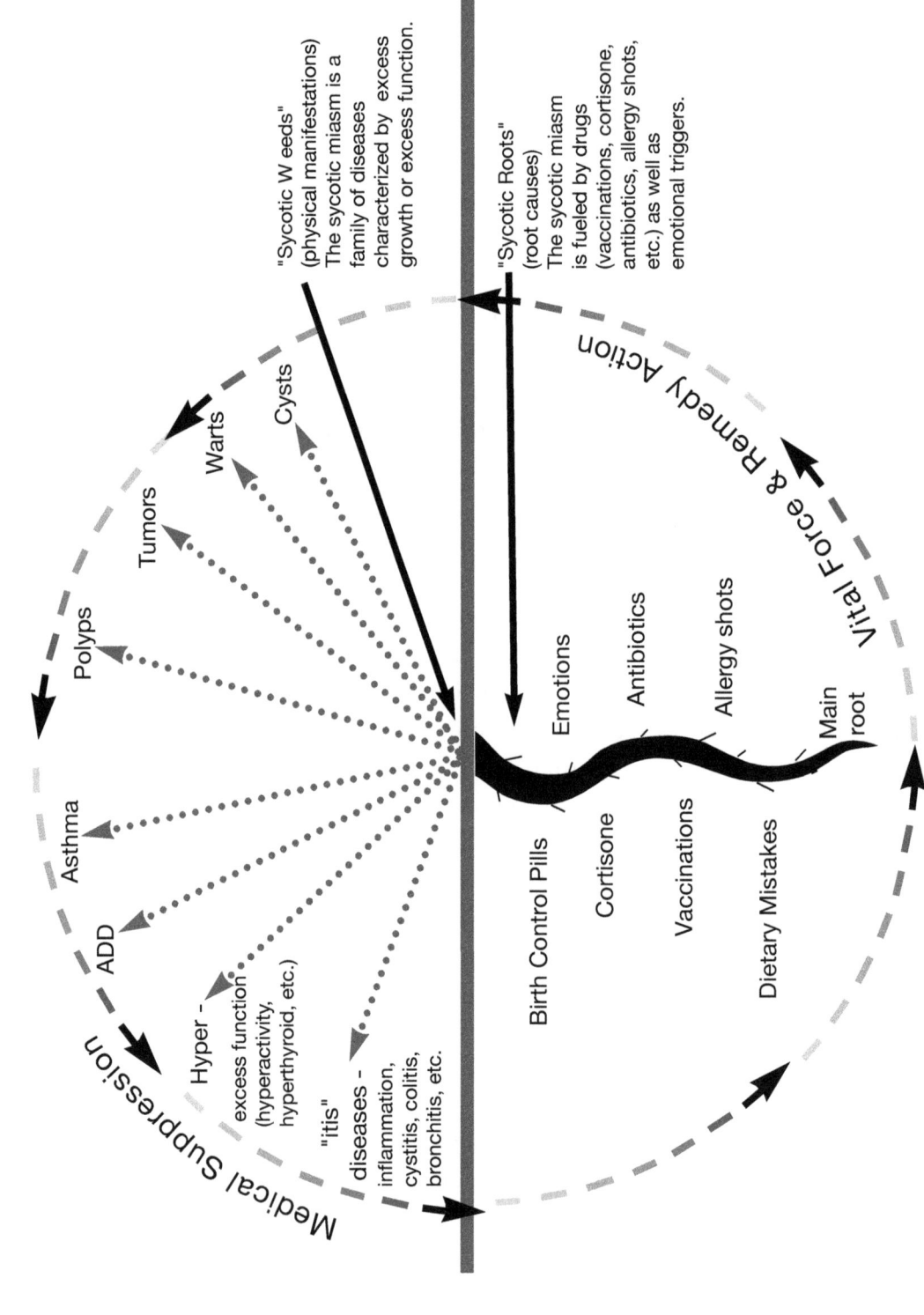

increasing traumas of separation, divorce and abuse; or mentally through video games, the Internet and the entertainment media. We can see the dominance of the sycotic miasm in our society by the illnesses our patients come with. While Hahnemann found that seven-eighths of his patients had psoric manifestations, my own experience is that most children come with their noses or ears filled with thick greenish mucus, women with vaginitis, candida and dysmenorrhea, men with prostatitis, the elderly with arthritis and rheumatism, and patients of all ages with different "-itis" diseases, all expressions of the sycotic miasm. The sycotic miasm is also constantly being created in new sufferers by the suppression of gonorrhea, which has become increasingly widespread due to the promiscuity in our society: the CDC estimates that while 600,000 new cases of gonorrhea are *reported* each year, the *actual* figure is closer to 2 to 3 million.[8]

There is another factor leading to the dominance of the sycotic miasm: it originates in promiscuous sex, the fury of its physical symptoms focuses on the reproductive system in both sexes, and it leads to ever greater sexual depravities and perversions in the sufferer, creating a vicious cycle. Each successive generation of sycotic parents concentrates the increased libido and the sexual perversions of the previous one. The old homeopaths used to say that the child born in vice has within it the germ of vicious impulse which nothing but the Grace of God, homeopathic treatment, and time can eradicate. They were fond of quoting the Gospel according to St. Luke, the physician: "For there is no good tree that bringeth forth corrupt fruit, nor again a corrupt tree that bringeth forth good fruit."[9]

Central Idea: Over-stimulation and Excessive growth

Rapid overgrowth, the central idea of the sycotic miasm, is expressed on all planes. While psora has a lack of assimilation, in sycosis the assimilation is excessive, stimulating the overgrowth. Why this overreaction? The delusions of Thuja, the greatest antisycotic, can shed some light: the delusions that the body is too thin, too brittle, delicate (K22), in other words a delusion of weakness which must be concealed in order to survive. The sycotic has discovered that he is not perfect; he has given up the continuous psoric struggle and instead he tries to survive by covering up his weaknesses. He does this by "overgrowth" on the mental and emotional plane: excessive boasting, extroverted behavior, excessive movements, all creating a smokescreen which conceals the real and imperfect person behind it. Thuja also has the delusion "building stones, appearance of" (K24): he hides his inner weakness behind a thick exterior wall. And in fact the sycotic miasm leads to overgrowth on the physical plane as well. It is as though the body is trying to create an extra protective layer behind which the person can hide, by producing warts and hyperkeratosis and a thick overgrowth of bushy hair.

Mental expressions: Mental symptoms of the miasm are not pronounced until the disease or its manifestations (discharges) are suppressed, and then they become very marked. For example, sycotics lose the train of thought in the middle of a conversation ("Thoughts, vanishing of, while speaking," K88, Thuja). There is a constant state of brainfag, so often seen in cases of chronic fatigue—the sense of being incapable of connected thought. The patient is in a state of continual doubt as to whether she has done things right. After locking the door she will go back several times to see if she did it ("Forgotten something, feels constantly as if he had," K49, Caust., Iod.). The remedies listed in this last example demonstrate beautifully how the sycotic swings from one extreme to another, from Causticum's paralysis of mind to the overstimulation or overcombustion of the Iodum. There is no middle ground in the sycotic.

There is also a partial permanent loss of memory for names of objects, streets, and people. Sycotics have absent-mindedness and forgetfulness, especially for recent happenings. They have a fear of misspelling simple words, fear of even writing a short note that might not be understood. This reflects the overgrowth or overstimulation on the mental plane: a small thought becomes a permanently exaggerated one to the point of becoming a delusion, the most extreme expression of the mental aberrations. Because of this confusion, the sycotic mind has the most fixed ideas: Thuja, the greatest antisycotic, and Cannabis indica, one of the top remedies for acute gonorrhea, have more delusions than any other remedy in the Materia Medica.

Sycotics' mental energy becomes much better at night, reflecting the daytime aggravation of sycosis: the later it becomes the more energy they have (better from 8 p.m. until 3 a.m.). These sycotic patients will work throughout the night and sleep until late in the day. They are too excited to sleep at night, even preferring mental work to sleep. Sycotic teenagers will stay up until well past midnight on school nights; then they are exhausted when they have to get up early the next day, their fatigue compounding their brainfag and short term memory loss at school.

Like all sycotic symptoms, these mental symptoms are much improved when the Vital Force can exteriorize the miasm by throwing up warts, fibrous growths, and discharges, especially from the genital tract. These sycotic warts and discharges are life-savers to the patient; where they are suppressed, malignancies often develop promptly.

Emotional expressions: The anxiety of the psoric miasm is taken to excess in the sycotic. *Anguish* is a constant symptom of sycosis, also described by sycotic patients as pain, distress, suffering, torture, torment, and agony. While the psoric person's anxiety may come and go (he constantly struggles but always thinks he can resolve it), the sycotic person's anxiety is constant. This constant state of emotional restlessness brings about a general feeling of indisposition, with a distressing sense of oppression at the epigastrium. Sycotics have an incomprehensible melancholy, with weariness. Even a short walk fatigues them so much, both mentally and physically, that they are unable to account for it. These people may appear strong and hearty to all but the trained homeopathic observer, who can see the mental strain and anxiety in the sycotics' facial expressions.

Sycotic people are not as fearful as psoric ones, but they do have a fear of the dark and of associating with strangers, avoiding anyone outside the immediate family. A peculiar symptom is the sensation that someone is behind them, that they hear whispering: they are constantly looking over their shoulders ("Fear, behind him, that someone is," K43).

As much as these negative emotions are often present, we also see the exact opposite, typical of the sycotic who always goes from one extreme to the other. They can be very expressive and spontaneous in telling you their problems. They can be the life of the waiting room, where they find a captive audience for their off-color jokes. They have an excess of sexual feelings as in everything else, their high sex drive often leading to nymphomania and masturbation. They enjoy sex because of the excitement, not out of love for their partner. They are very passionate people, but they love passion for a self-serving purpose. They are focused on themselves, not so much on the partner (who is seduced by the sycotic pretending to be romantic but hiding his real agenda, self-satisfaction). Sexual conquests are like a sport, with the sycotic "hunter" often keeping track of his "trophies" in an album or diary.

Since sycotics feel better from movement, sex becomes intensive gymnastics. The sycotic's sexual urges can be so strong that they can lead to criminality (e.g. pedophilia), but prison will not help them; homeopathy is necessary to change them. Sycotics are the ones posting and downloading pornography from the Internet, which unfortunately has helped these sexual perverts to prey on their innocent young victims. (While sexual perversions are usually ascribed to the syphilitic miasm, the sycotic miasm has them as well. Since the sycotic miasm is so much more prevalent than the syphilitic in our society, perverts are more likely to be sycotic.)

Any thrill is a stimulation to sycotic people:* climbing Mount Everest, bungee jumping (only a sycotic likes that kind of chiropractic adjustment!), white water rafting, parasailing, ballooning around the world, going to the top of a mountain by helicopter and then skiing

---

*A recent study at George Washington University in St. Louis credits a single gene with the craving for new, exciting experiences. According to Dr. Robert Cloninger, professor of genetics, researchers have not yet determined how this longer gene affects behavior. To the homeopath, of course, this thrill-seeking behavior *is* genetic, transmitted by the sycotic miasm, and unlike the geneticist, the homeopath has a way to treat it.[10]

down. The newest rage among sycotic young people is "car surfing": standing on the roof or hood of a car going 15 to 20 miles per hour and trying to stay on it when the car suddenly stops. Many of these thrill-seekers have died from head traumas. Unfortunately these stunts, glorified in the news media, attract the attention of a generation of bored sycotic youth.

Films today are geared to the predominant sycotic miasm in our society: they have action, sex and high-speed chases, plus impossible stunts, created by new techniques which provide ever more spectacular scenes of thrills and destruction. These stunts stimulate the fertile imagination of the sycotic teenager, who often pays with his life for imitating them. The warning "Do not attempt this at home" is an invitation rather than a deterrent. (Other aspects of film—the killing, violence, horror, serial murders and sadistic torture of sex victims—appeal to the syphilitic mind. The psoric prefers tearjerkers, family movies, romantic comedies, Disney films, and animal films.) The popularity of trash talk shows like the Jerry Springer show, with its focus on sex, violence, lying and cheating, plus the excitement of on-stage fights, reflects the pervasive influence of the sycotic miasm in our culture.

When sycotics kill, it is for the thrill, the excitement. They may say, "I wanted to know what it feels like to kill some one. To have that absolute sense of power over someone is the biggest thrill." They have a marked tendency to cruelty, to harm other people and even animals. The sycotic miasm produces more dishonesty, moral degeneracy, suicides, criminal insanity and mania than the other miasms. (While suicide is more *typical* of the destructive syphilitic miasm, suicide is more *frequently* caused by the sycotic miasm because it is so much more prevalent in our society. Also, the sycotic will commit suicide in a fit of passion, while the syphilitic will do it because he feels no way out of the heavy weight of depression he is experiencing.) Sycotic children will even kill small animals with their bare hands. I had a small patient with a severe sycotic case of ADD who did this, for example impaling frogs on the spikes of an iron fence. When I took the family history, his mother admitted that his father had also killed small animals as a child, and the father had obviously transmitted the sycotic miasm to the son. (This should serve as a warning to women: men who kill small animals with their bare hands may not be the best choices as marriage partners.)

On the other hand, when faced by a frightening situation sycotic people will run away as fast as they can. (Psoric people are paralyzed by fear, and syphilitics will stand and fight, even killing if necessary.) If a sycotic person is jealous she will express it in an extroverted way: she will flirt with someone else to gain her husband's attention or have sex with the first stranger she meets. She will not commit a destructive act like a syphilitic, who might throw acid on her competitor or slash her face with a razor blade. Instead, she exteriorizes her excess of emotions. Sycotics' jealousy is based on extreme suspicion: they are suspicious that they will be misunderstood, they suspect others, especially those nearest and dearest to them. Suspicion is a constant companion of the sycotic mind since they themselves are constantly trying to hide the imperfections which they no longer can deny. They know they are not what others think of them, so they think that everyone else is putting on a mask too. While the syphilitic will try to isolate and hide his entire existence, the sycotic will try to hide only one part of it, often a sexual part, such as an affair he is having.

Sycotics focus their lives on fun and thrills: sex (much of their expressions are in the sexual sphere), taking drugs, eating, earning a lot of money fast usually through gambling, playing the stock market, selling illicit drugs, even bank robbery which is an additional daredevil thrill. A sycotic wants a lot of money, not to save it, but to have fun and excitement in the present moment. If the sycotic wants to "live life to the fullest," he can't take a nine to five job. He lives life at top speed and often dies in the prime of life, but at least he "lived." He is competitive in sports, a must-win situation for him. *Carpe diem* ("seize the day") is his motto, and he never thinks about the consequences for tomorrow. Unlike the worrisome psoric, he never thinks where his next paycheck is coming from. He counts on his charm, smooth talking and often his good looks to get him what he needs.

"Short-lived" seems to be a motto of the sycotic: outbursts of anger are short, excitement is short, and they are always looking for another stimulus. A sense of urgency, impatience and hurriedness permeates their lives ("living in the fast lane"). Even the sycotic infant trembles with weak eagerness at nursing time, as if starved, until the breast or bottle is given, when it hurries so fast that it chokes or is soon exhausted. The older child at play hurries from one toy to another, eager to play but finding no joy in anything.

When a sycotic person lies, it is because he wants to boast. (The boasting of a psoric person is based on facts, on his superior knowledge, while the sycotic's boasting is not always true and serves the purpose of hiding the truth. Or it can be an exaggeration, an embroidery on the facts, another example of sycotic overgrowth.) Although the sycotic person is basically an extrovert, he will always try to conceal part of his life, the sexual or sinful part. Through his excessive outward behavior, he wants to draw your attention away from the real him, the hidden inner part. But he feels shame with great trepidation and sensitivity to being reprimanded or criticized.

Sycotic children are morbidly sensitive to correction; if chastised, they feel as if they had committed an unpardonable sin and will brood in despondency for hours and days, or lie awake half the night worrying. They may even have convulsions or contemplate suicide. Probably most of the pathetic suicides of children and teenagers are the result of inherited gonorrhea, committed as crimes of passion or as a result of using drugs and alcohol.

Sycotic behavior: Hyperstimulation on the physical plane translates into hyperactivity. It is no coincidence that the number of ADHD children has skyrocketed (their sycotic miasm fueled by mandatory vaccinations and overuse of antibiotics). While ADHD can be syphilitic or tubercular (if the child is predominantly destructive or restless, respectively), it is often sycotic. These children often have impulsivity and a thirst for excitement which makes them act as the class clown, considering the punishment worth it since they gain the admiration of their peers. They often lie to get what they want. Paying attention in school is too difficult for their wandering, brainfagged mind. Locked up in a classroom, they feel like a bird in a cage. Having to sit still is torture because they need excessive movements to feel good. They are full of mischievous behavior and often incite others to join them in their "15 minutes of fame."

Being expelled is just part of the game for sycotic teenagers and gets them "outside" where the action is. They may make a poster with their phone number and flash it to female drivers, asking for a date. Or they engage in ever more dangerous and destructive behavior, like the two teenagers recently reported in the newspaper who cruised around in their car at night, shooting at bicyclists with rubber bullets. Seeing these innocent and unsuspecting victims fall off their bikes gave them the thrill they wanted.

As sycotic teenagers become bored with the old standby stunts, they look for more and more outrageous thrills, often crossing the boundary between mischief and crime. The behavior goes from relatively innocent to mean and destructive. I had a 13-year-old patient who stole a boat late at night with his 12-year-old buddy, tried to take it to Atlantic City, drifted ashore because they could not start it, and were picked up at 3 a.m. by the police. When we hear about such antics we wonder where the parents are, but this boy announced to me defiantly that no one could tell him what to do, and in fact short of keeping him in restraints there was no way for his parents to control him.

Sycotic people are stimulated by running and dancing, and once they start dancing they will not stop for hours. The new rage among young people is the all-night "rave" in which they dance until they almost collapse and then go outside and take drugs (Ecstasy) to start all over again. The dance clubs stay open continuously from Friday night until Monday morning. No doubt these young people are excessively sycotic, easily stimulated and aroused. The musicians playing in these dance club are often sycotic themselves, leaping and jumping, throwing themselves to the floor, and undressing, which excites their sycotic audience. To make it even more colorful, their bodies are often covered by outrageous tattoos. Anything to shock, to excite, to lose control! The dancers and band members have switched their day life for a night life, which suits the most active time for the sycotic miasm (they feel better at night). Many rock stars have indulged in this life-style, eventually dying from a drug overdose (remember the Medorrhinum "theme song": "sex, drugs and rock 'n' roll").

The "pushing outward" typical of sycotic growths also shows itself in the extroverted sycotic nature: sycotic people want stimuli and fun. They are exhibitionists or do silly things to get attention. They are even attention-getters in their clothes: they wear bright colors and dye their hair fluorescent shades, or flaunt their bodies with tight jeans, miniskirts, bare midriffs and little bras. Or they wear the color of the night and dress in all black. They may wear bright red lipstick or paint their nails black. They wear rings pierced through the most visible parts of the body, to shock people. And when they stick their tongue out at you in defiance, take note of the typical very red tongue. The sycotic person is a person of extremes, never pausing in the middle ground.

Physical symptoms: Every physical manifestation of sycosis develops quickly and excessively, yet has a slow recovery. Typical acute sycotic symptoms include a high fever, ruptures, and excessive greenish-yellow pus. Sycotic appendicitis has a sudden onset, with severe pain, high fever, and a tendency to rupture, causing peritonitis. A sycotic allergic reaction will express itself as sudden epiglottitis, while the psoric reaction will develop slowly and express itself as hives. Sycotic ear infections come up quickly, producing a greenish-yellow discharge with a foul odor like fish brine or rotten cheese. A sycotic patient is usually a bad smelling one.

In sycotic dysmenorrhea, the pain is agonizing and may continue until the end of the flow. Before, during and after the menstrual period, the debility is so marked, so out of proportion to other symptoms, that it cannot be accounted for except by the sycotic miasm (which has such a devastating effect on the reproductive system). This chronic inflammation of the ovarian membranes and tubes, much aggravated during the menses, gradually subsides, only to be renewed with all its sufferings at the appearance of the next period. This shows the periodicity of the attack, another sycotic characteristic. Chronic ovarian troubles are usually sycotic.

Twitching in various parts, jerking of the head from side to side and backwards, are symptoms showing the effects of the sycotic poison on the nervous system.

While many skin conditions are psoric, sycosis can cause warty growths, some forms of acne (cystic acne and acne rosacea), and many naevi, especially those of a red, velvety appearance. Warts are typically sycotic, often brown or dark, usually growing outward with an irregular surface or cauliflower shape. Brown spots, freckles and melanomas are a sign of sycosis (because they represent an excess of pigment). Moles and papillomata may be syphilitic or sycotic. Sycotic discharges often smell like fish brine (the salt water once used to preserve fish). A British research team led by Dr. Ian R. Phillips of the University of London recently reported identifying a genetic defect that makes people smell like rotting fish. At the same time, they claim, "no cure is known for this fishy odor syndrome."[11] Homeopaths would agree that the syndrome is inherited (caused by the sycotic miasm) but would cure it with the indicated antisycotic remedy.

All forms of tinea (capitis, versicolor, etc.), herpes zoster and herpes circinatus (ringworm) are of sycotic origin. Alopecia areata or circumscripta (hair loss in patches) is sycotic, while total hair loss (alopecia totalis) is syphilitic. Other sycotic expressions include kidney stones, the majority of the parasitic diseases, and the severe forms of psoriasis (which can also be a combination of several miasms). Asthma is almost always sycotic, especially if it has the typical sycotic indications of being worse from dampness, from exercise, and in the spring; periodic and often disappearing spontaneously (the sufferer "grew out of it"). (Asthma can also be psoric if it is in the throat, while sycotic asthma is in the chest.)

All the "-itis" diseases like neuritis, vaginitis, bronchitis, cystitis, and tendinitis, are sycotic. (Appendicitis is sycotic unless it is the syphilitic type that grows silently, as if in hiding, then suddenly destroys by rupturing.) Other secondary sycotic symptoms include the inflammations and indurations of the internal organs, especially those of the reproductive system, the rectum, prostate and bladder. We already mentioned in the complications of secondary suppressed sycosis various possible conditions such as cysts, dermoid cysts, abscesses, appendicitis, PID, peritonitis, endometriosis, adhesions, strictures, stenosis, and fibroid tumors.

Severe rheumatism, either acute or chronic, must have transmitted or acquired sycosis in the background. Purulent (gonorrhea) ophthalmia is usually the first symptom in sycotic newborns, and the remedy most frequently indicated and curative is, of course, one of our best antisycotics, Argentum nitricum. Argentum nitricum (silver nitrate) has often been given to newborns in crude doses as mandatory treatment for such ophthalmia. Unfortunately, many of these babies then prove Argentum nitricum by developing colic, one of its main proving symptoms.

The sycotic infant, if born full term, may have a fleshy appearance, but instead of the natural bright flesh color, the skin has a pale yellow cast. Its movements are not vigorous, its extremities are thin and weak, and the abdomen may be enlarged. These babies have a great tendency to nasal and intestinal catarrh (colic from excessive mucus), aggravated by damp weather. The sycotic baby is "good" only when asleep. He frets and moans and cries all day and is quiet at night (the opposite of the syphilitic baby, who cries all night). He may sleep on his hands and knees, with the face buried in the pillow.

While heart defects at birth are associated with the syphilitic miasm, the sycotic miasm predisposes to later changes in the heart valves (MVP, stenosis, etc.) because of deposits and overgrowth of tissue. These are often formed after an attack of strep throat, which can cause rheumatic endocarditis when not adequately treated. Patients with these sycotic heart conditions have little of the fear or apprehension found in psoric heart patients. They may even die suddenly and without warning, with no symptoms. Anasarca is not marked in sycosis; the sufferers snuff out like candles before there is time for it to develop.

The sycotic person shows strong hair growth everywhere on the body (hirsutism); the hairs are thick and coarse. Their eyebrows and nails (thick and heavy) all express the theme of overgrowth.

Sycotic people love eating spicy, salty or sour foods, as well as enjoying meat, beer, and oranges. (I had one patient with a strong sycotic miasm who used to order oranges by the crate from California!). They eat food with extreme tastes like sour apples. Unfortunately red meat and beer arouse their latent sycosis. The sycotic patient's diet should be mainly alkaline. (For example, they should avoid nightshade plants; this is the basis for the observation that nightshade plants may aggravate arthritis, one of the "-itis" diseases associated with sycosis.)

Most sycotic symptoms are worse from dampness and from a change of weather or barometric pressure. Sycotic people don't like to live in a humid climate. Their joint problems, marked by tearing pains, are especially aggravated in wet weather as well as from rest; they are better from moving and stretching. Sycotic joint inflammations result in permanent enlargement if they ankylose. They usually attack the joints of the vertebral column, and often one knee or elbow joint. The pain appears suddenly with full intensity. There is stiffness and lameness, and the symptoms seem to indicate Rhus tox., but Rhus tox. will not help since it has little antisycotic activity. This rheumatism responds quickly to the indicated antisycotic remedy, however. While the psoric person is chilly in general, in sycosis we find *parts* of the body cold (such as the hands and feet).

When a patient seems to be making a normal recovery from an operation, then suddenly his condition takes a decided change for the worse, or perhaps sudden septic conditions appear despite the most careful sterile procedures, an underlying sycotic condition is usually responsible, roused by the shock of the operation.

Treatment of Sycosis

The strongest antisycotic is Thuja in LM potencies, followed by LM potencies of Nitric acid when the effects of Thuja are exhausted, and with Medorrhinum used as necessary for intercurrent prescribing. Of course another antisycotic remedy should be given if the symptom picture calls for it, such as Nat. sulph. which is so commonly needed for asthma in children and Arsenicum often needed for asthma in adults. Other strong antisycotics include Sulphur, Calcarea, and Lycopodium.

If sycosis is the only active miasm: When sycosis is the only active miasm and is still at the stage of the primary wart, the antisycotic treatment should be continued until the wart disappears. The external symptom, the wart, will serve as a benchmark for determining how much of the internal disease remains. If the wart is large, then the proper remedy may be administered internally *and* locally. This is the *only* instance in which Hahnemann allows local treatment (for example, a child with sycotic tendencies who develops anal warts after receiving the Hepatitis B vaccination, as I have seen a number of times in my practice). Except for *large* warts, Hahnemann said that local treatment for discharges or warts was neither necessary nor permitted. This long antisycotic treatment should be followed by antipsoric treatment, or else the latent psora may flare up at any time.

If the wart has been removed through surgery or cautery, the antisycotic treatment should continue until the scar or discolored spot at the site of removal disappears and any discharge has ceased. Parents can transmit the miasm to their offspring even if the discharge has been absent for twenty years.

If both sycosis and psora are active: First give the antipsoric remedy indicated by the totality of the symptoms. Then the sycotic miasm will come up, with symptoms indicating an antisycotic remedy. After treating the sycotic picture, resume antipsoric treatment. This process might have to be repeated several times. An antipsoric remedy will always be last.

When sycosis is active and both psora and syphilis are also present: This does not mean all three miasms are active *at the same moment* (otherwise the patient would have cancer or lupus), but the symptoms of all three miasms are present. For example, the patient's Chief Complaint may be sycotic, with years of sycotic outbreaks going back to a clear sycotic Never Well Since of vaccinations or antibiotic overuse; yet you may see the family history strongly dominated by the syphilitic miasm with indications of latent syphilis such as depression in the patient's own history. In such cases start with antisycotics, then antipsorics, then treat the syphilis, followed finally by an antipsoric again. The changing symptom picture will be your guide as to when to change remedies and which miasm is coming up. In the case of mixed miasms, only one of them will be disease-producing at one time while the other two will remain dormant (except in cases of cancer and lupus). Only treat the active miasm. Remember that whenever you resolve sycosis or syphilis you risk stirring up psora, the deepest of all miasms, so you always need to give antipsoric treatment between treating the other two and again at the end. In my experience the symptom picture always shows this: I always see psora coming up when sycosis or syphilis subsides, even if the other miasm is also present and will come up next after the psora is addressed.

CHAPTER TWENTY-TWO

Syphilis: the Destructive Miasm

History

Smallpox scars the body; syphilis, known as the "Great Pox," scars the soul as well. Traced back to 11,000 years ago in Africa, it first became pandemic in Europe in the 16th century. Like AIDS in our day, it diminished promiscuity and instituted safe sex by way of condoms called "overcoats." (Made of waxed linen, they came in only one length—an ambitious eight inches— and were held on by a ribbon threaded through the base, which could be tied in a bow for an added dash of romance.) It probably became widespread after the French soldiers of the young King Charles VIII spent many months in Naples away from their wives and entertained by prostitutes. The king himself died from syphilis at the age of 28. Its origins are unknown, however; the British called it a French disease, while the French swore it was a German disease. The Germans blamed the Spanish, who denied introducing it to the Native Americans from whom they claimed to have caught it.

Henry VIII of England was a prime example of the syphilitic miasm. Towards the end of his life his elephantine legs, swollen with edema, were covered with bloody, oozing ulcers. He never viewed his wives' disastrous pregnancies as resulting from his syphilis. His first wife bore him a stillborn daughter, a son who lived only seven weeks, and then had four miscarriages. The only surviving child had stunted growth, defective vision and a cranial deformation, and lived to be known as "Bloody Mary." He beheaded one of his wives for not providing him with an heir. The real fault, of course, lay in his syphilitic miasm, which also inspired the solution: murdering her with a sharp knife.

Physicians refused to treat syphilis victims at first, relinquishing them to barbers and charlatans, who devised the first "cure" for syphilis. They heated the victims in barrels filled with cinnabar (toxic sulfide of mercury). It cured the syphilis but killed its victims with mercury poisoning. By Hahnemann's time, physicians were treating syphilis patients but still used crude doses of mercury. It was administered until the patient began salivating excessively. The result was a "proving" of mercury, with patients suffering from mouth ulcerations, necrosis of the jaw bone, and loss of teeth. The famous violinist Paganini had already lost all his teeth to this treatment when he consulted Hahnemann in Paris for his syphilis. Hahnemann was the first physician ever to treat syphilis successfully with his minute doses of mercury, almost a hundred years ahead of Pasteur's germ theory.

Comparison with Sycosis

The difference between sycosis and syphilis is that in sycosis, the inflammation and ulceration is *in* the urethral or vaginal canal in sycosis, while in syphilis it is on the *outside* of the glans in men, on the vulva in women. As in sycosis, suppression of the chancre through drugs implants the syphilitic miasm in the organism. It goes into the same direction as sycosis: from the exterior of body to the interior (against Nature's Laws). We refer to this as the centripetal action of syphilis and sycosis as compared to the centrifugal action of psora.

The Allopathic View

Homeopathy's understanding of syphilis itself is dramatically different from that of allopathic medicine, which we will review briefly.

Primary stage: Syphilis is acquired by sexual intercourse (or contact with bodily fluids or mucous membranes) with an infected partner. The first chancre appears one to six weeks later at the point where the infection gained entrance to the body. It most often appears on the genitals but can also appear on the lips, in the mouth, on the hands or wherever the skin is broken (since it can be transmitted by direct contact with an infectious lesion). The chancre is usually hard, slightly elevated, and painless, seldom itches, and has a punched-out appearance. After removal of the chancre, buboes appear in the inguinal lymph nodes. These swollen lymph glands start on same side as the initial sore, then later extend to the other side. The inguinal glands seldom suppurate in syphilis. Although the bubo is considered part of the primary phase, it always follows the chancre: it is rarely found alone without a preceding chancre and usually the bubo only comes after the destruction of the chancre by local applications.

Secondary stage: This stage lasts several months, with some of its manifestations holding over through the tertiary stage. First maculae appear, typically on the palms and soles, then on the rest of the body. A non-itching roseolar rash appears on the back, abdomen, front of the arms and rarely on the face, followed by ulcers in the mouth and loss of hair. Iritis may also appear in this stage, usually of one eye, then of the other, with contraction of the pupil and sensitivity of the eyes to artificial and natural light. The patient often complains of a slight malaise, a draggy and achy feeling like a mild attack of flu but rarely severe enough to require bed rest.

Tertiary stage: About a third of untreated cases develop to the tertiary stage, which can begin anywhere from three to 40 years after the primary infection and can last indefinitely. Gummas (devastating, destructive lesions) may form in the skin, muscles, lungs, spleen, eyes, etc.; they may break down and form chronic abscesses. Since the gummas can affect such a wide variety of organs, the symptoms they create imitate many different diseases, which is why late stage syphilis is called "the great imitator." They are rarely seen now because of allopathic treatment. The patient complains of persistent bone pains, worse at night, and frequent, persistent or periodic unilateral, parietal and occipital headaches. The nervous system can be affected, causing deafness, blindness or insanity (neurosyphilis).

The Homeopathic View

While allopathic medicine views the secondary and tertiary phases as part of the natural course of the disease, Hahnemann's view was that they are the results of suppressive treatment. Hahnemann said that the secondary and tertiary symptoms could not break out as long as the primary chancre was left untreated. While we rarely have a chance to test this theory in the modern era, the nineteenth-century homeopaths had extensive experience with it. Kent, for example, had a patient who had a primary chancre for *45 years* without any other symptoms. Kent said, "What would be the result if the chancre was left alone? Then we could see the true nature of the disease. We could see whether it runs a certain course and recovers. But if suppressed, we get the symptoms of latent syphilis miasm" (and the unfortunate result is that the disease is considered cured).[1]

The assertion of Hahnemann and the old masters that untreated syphilis will not evolve to the secondary and tertiary stages has been contradicted by the results of the Tuskegee study (in which syphilitic patients were left untreated or treated with placebo and did in fact develop tertiary syphilis to the point of dementia.) This study has been denounced as unethical and cannot be duplicated. We have no way of turning back the clock and visiting Kent and Hahnemann as they examined their patients. But we *can* say that homeopathy can successfully treat syphilis in all three stages of its evolution, no matter what the role of suppression may be.

The old masters considered primary syphilis easy to cure with Mercury 30c. As Hahnemann said:

> The chancre remains on the same place, only increasing with the years, while the secondary symptoms of syphilis cannot break out as long as it exists. ... I have never, in my practice of more than 50 years, seen any trace of the venereal disease break out, so long as the chancre remains untouched in its place.[2]

The chancre, which immediately forms a "punched-out" ulcer, reflects the destructive nature of the miasm. Homeopathy views the secondary skin eruptions of syphilis as the Vital Force's attempts to exteriorize the infection. Under suppressive treatment, the disease is driven deeper inwards, affecting the vital organs and then the mind. When suppressed syphilis is treated homeopathically, the disease is driven outwards following Hering's Laws: the nightly bone pains and agonizing headaches are the first to heal, followed by hair loss, then throat ulcers, etc. The chancre can persist for months without affecting the patient's overall health. Under the action of the proper remedy it becomes soft and produces a copious discharge. No topical applications are necessary; the ulcer is the last to heal since it is the first to appear.

And while homeopathy views the original infection as acquired through sexual intercourse, the miasm can be acquired when this infection is suppressed, passed from parent to child, or passed to the sex partner in its dormant, latent or active state. The miasm is transmitted instantly, Hahnemann says (because it is energetic rather than material), and it has become systemic long before the chancre is formed.

If an individual with syphilis is "cured" with antibiotics, his physician will advise him that he can safely marry. But just as in sycosis, the disease can be transferred from husband to wife in the same dormant or latent stage. Then if they have a baby, it will be VDRL negative but will still manifest the *latent* symptoms of the syphilitic miasm. There will be no primary chancre, but the common symptoms of hereditary syphilis include Hutchinson's teeth, cleft palate, blindness, limb deformities, deafness, congenital heart diseases, etc. Kent describes a case in which latent syphilis was transmitted by saliva: he treated a young girl who ate with the same spoon as a friend who had mouth ulcers (a secondary form of syphilis). She broke out with the same mouth ulcers. But Kent treated her successfully and she never had a relapse.

Destruction on All Levels

The syphilitic miasm's central themes of destruction, deformity and hiding is seen on the mental, emotional and physical levels.

Mental symptoms: The mind is destroyed; these patients don't comprehend anything. They are dull, sullen, morose, stupid, and mentally heavy. You think they understand you, then you ask them something and realize that they don't remember anything. They sit expressionless, with an empty face and dead eyes. They might strike you as very reserved and silent, but it is really because they can't express themselves. (I had one patient who married a man because she thought he was the "strong, silent type" and such a good listener; she found out too late that he was silent because he had nothing to say.) The blank stare tells it all: the mind is blank, too.

In their slowness of comprehension they forget what they were about to say and then find it hard to get back their train of thought.

The same is true in reading; they must begin again and again or they lose the meaning. At least in the sycotic mind, information penetrates into the brain but is quickly forgotten. People who lose their memory after a concussion are likely to be syphilitic. They are likely to have fixed ideas developing into delusions (although less so than in sycosis). They also tend to get stuck in a thought process, as if there is a break or destruction of the train of thought.

Psychological symptoms: The syphilitic miasm shows in a family history with depression, bipolar disorder, schizophrenia or indeed any mental disease; alcoholism and other self-destructive behaviors like drug addiction; and suicides, successful or not. Syphilitic patients crave alcohol, and when this happens in a person whose psoric miasm is also active the result is to fuel the cravings and weaken the willpower, producing an alcoholism or drug addiction. Syphilitics are certainly the ones most prone to addiction.

Syphilitic people are always depressed but tend to isolate, keeping their troubles to themselves and sulking over them, the opposite of the psoric patient who seeks support by airing his troubles freely. The night oppresses the syphilitic and makes him restless and anxious. To make things worse, the syphilis person broods over his problems at night, feeling alone and hopeless about them. Despair makes his nights a continuous torture because he cannot fall asleep.

The word "hate" tends to pop up in his conversation: "I hate this life" or "I hate my job and my boss." So do expressions of his despair: "If this is life, I might as well stop it. If this is all I can expect, let's end it right now." He thinks about suicide for a long time, then all of a sudden, without warning, he jumps from a bridge or a window. Syphilitics may hate the government, society and religion and become anarchists, bombers, and destroyers. The Causticum fighter against injustice will become such a bomber if the syphilitic miasm is predominant, as it is in the Unabomber (who also demonstrates the syphilitic traits of isolation, mental illness, suspicion and distrust). Henny Heudens-Mast in a recent case conference presented the case of a nun who was a Causticum fighter against injustice, but in a psoric way: she organized support groups for disadvantaged people. She had a little trace of the syphilitic Causticum, however, and it came out at night, of course: she had a recurring dream of setting the entire city on fire.[3]

Besides hate, the syphilitic tends to be malicious. They may have violent nightmares about chasing someone to kill them, of being killed themselves, of vampires and werewolves, of killing their children or husband. Of course they are shocked by these dreams if they remember them. But the syphilitic miasm robs them of all conscience at night.

The mental-emotional symptoms of both syphilis and sycosis include marked self-condemnation and guilt feelings, because they originally were spread by promiscuous sex. The syphilitic is apt to be destructive to other people and himself. For example, he could become an alcoholic and kill himself. He also has fears that others will kill him ("Delusion, enemies, surrounded by," K23; "Delusion, enemy, everyone is," K23; "Delusion, murdered, that he would be," K29). In his mind, people follow him at night with knives and guns to kill him. Of course he has the urge to kill them too. In fact, a syphilitic person reacts to his fear by counterattacking, not with paralysis like the psoric person. Syphilitic people will always have something with them to defend and kill: a knife or a gun in extreme cases, and in more civilized cases they carry a stick, a cane, or an umbrella even if it is sunny ("Delusion, shoot, tries to, with a cane," K31). Syphilitic people have few fears, they would rather "fight than take flight" but they do have a fear of knives. When they see a knife, they have an overwhelming urge to stab somebody or themselves. Of course most will not act on it, but it does cross their mind and they must struggle to suppress the thought. They even might have a fear of killing their own children, which is sometimes seen in postpartum psychosis. Syphilitics don't trust others because they don't trust themselves. Even if they wash their hands, they will wash them again. Why? Because they want to hide something, they do not want to leave fingerprints.

Their desire to use knives and hack into something is often fulfilled in the professions they choose: a cook, or even better, a butcher, and when the syphilitic individual has greater mental capacity, a surgeon. We have seen that as long the individual can find an outlet for his delusion in his profession, recreation or relationship, he will not become sick. This is what the syphilitic individual does when he chooses such a profession. Of course, when someone becomes a butcher because he enjoys food and providing others with it, he is psoric. But the syphilitic butcher will like the feeling of hacking the flesh from the bones and of being splattered with blood. And the executioner who wielded a hatchet or guillotine in the old days was most likely syphilitic.

The syphilitic has cold-blooded cruelty, a total lack of feelings when committing a crime. They describe a murder as if they had just stepped on an insect. "You just happened to be in my way, so I will do away with you," is the underlying feeling. They express none of the excitement or thrill of the sycotic person who commits a crime of passion. They have nothing but the coldness and hardness of a professional hit man who is just doing his job.

We even see the same emotionless expression in a child. I had as a patient a ten-year-old boy with an Oedipus complex who always said to his mother, "Mom, let's get married, I will kill dad, and we'll live happily forever." He would attack his father and younger sister (who he also wanted to kill, so as to have his mother to himself) to such an extent that they had to lock him in the garage. At one point the desperate parents called me to adjust his remedy; I could hear him over the phone, bellowing from the garage that he was going to smash down the door. I will never forget his face: he never looked straight at me, because he was trying to hide, but he had cold-blooded eyes and a grimace that was absolutely chilling. He could have been a future criminal, but thank God, homeopathy saved this unfortunate child.

The syphilitic patient in the waiting room spreads the same cold feeling: "Don't talk to me," they seem to say. They are silent, have no contact with others, only spread depression to the person next to them. While a sycotic child might wave a toy gun at you out of enjoyment of the game, or a psoric little "cowboy" might swagger in pretending to be tough, a syphilitic child could come into your office with a toy gun and say, "I am going to kill you." You don't see a smile on his face, you feel the hate in the child and see the hardened look. Or he will laugh inappropriately, another syphilitic expression (like the inappropriate laughing at funerals of Nat. mur., one of its syphilitic expressions, along with its hiding and isolation). These children are the future bank robbers who hide behind black masks, who don't hesitate to kill at the slightest inconvenience without guilt or remorse. And if they get caught, they learn their trade even better in prison, such a fertile ground for the sycotic and syphilitic miasm.

While a psoric teenager might join a gang because he wants to go along with the crowd, and a sycotic teenager wants the thrill of scandalizing grown-ups, the syphilitic teenager will join a gang to satisfy his bloodthirsty feelings. They like to hurt people, to make them suffer, even to kill them. I have children as patients who have tried to hurt their younger sister, even to strangle her, or they simply play too rough with her and make her cry. Or they smile sadistically while they pull the legs off of an insect, kick the dog, or purposely break something precious to their mother. A sycotic one can do this kind of thing too, but he does it for the thrill, for amusement, or out of boredom to get a cheap thrill. The syphilitic one enjoys the absolute power he has and feels absolutely no remorse. In fact, in the world he lives in, everyone is doing it, so why not him too? These are the serial killers who abduct women and children to make sex slaves out of them and torture them while filming them.

Unfortunately war often brings such latent miasms to life, as documented in *The Rape of Nanking* about the Chino-Japanese war of 1937. Women were mutilated after being gang raped and filmed naked with their captors, who were showing off with their "trophies." Beheading captive soldiers became a national sport, with the two officers who had beheaded the most victims (106 and 105) depicted as war heroes in the Japanese newspapers.[4] (Of course the Japanese deny this version of history; if it is a fabrication, it still reflects the syphilitic mind at work.)

This cruelty can also be committed on the emotional plane. I have known an older child to relentlessly torture a younger sibling, apparently without remorse, until the victim's self-worth was absolutely zero, giving the syphilitic perpetrator the power and domination he craved. I read in the newspaper about a woman who for 21 years endured harassing phone calls from a stranger who claimed to be holding her missing daughter as a sex slave. He often called her six or seven times a night, describing "sex games" and other acts of cruelty that he claimed to be doing to her daughter. When he was caught, he showed no remorse.

Syphilitic children will also show disrespect to the physician. I had a 15-year-old patient who put his feet on my desk, right in my face, with no admonishment from his parents. Or these children simply destroy your office, not out of excitement and a sense of mischief (sycotic), but out of disrespect for authority. They damage the blinds, tear up books, and break the toys in the waiting room. Sometimes they hide their face because they don't want to get caught or they turn their chair around to avoid looking at you ("Mind, looked at, cannot be," K63, Silica). At home they lock themselves in their room, hiding from everyone and resisting the pitiful pleas of their parents.

Syphilitics like to have sex in secret because of the shame. They can have unnatural sexual feelings, preferring anal sex, harmful sex, sadomasochism, painful sex, incest, and all the other perversions you unfortunately hear about. The average person reads about these things in books and wonders, how is it possible? but the homeopath understands because he sees the seeds of the syphilitic miasm. Incest is syphilitic, for example, because it is perverse, it is kept hidden, and it is likely to lead to birth defects. No doubt the Marquis de Sade was afflicted with the syphilitic poison. Among his many malicious sexual acts, he fed "bon bons" loaded with Cantharis to his sex partners to incite their passion, knowing perfectly well that large amounts of Cantharis would cause terribly painful abdominal pains, vaginal burning in the women and priapism in the men. Even better than intercourse, he liked being flogged 700 to 800 times by his own count.[5]

Degenerates, criminals and the criminally insane invariably have a syphilitic or sycotic background. If we could only treat children showing syphilitic tendencies before they become criminals, we could empty the asylums and the prisons in one generation. We could save so much suffering for our society, not to mention expense for our state.

Syphilitics also hurt themselves. When the miasm is latent, they will do body piercing, preferably in a painful and hidden place like the penis. They will react to a heartbreak (as some of my patients have done) by burning themselves with a cigarette. Sometimes they commit suicide because their loved one has taken someone else ("Loathing of life," K62, "Suicidal disposition," K85). The psoric person will look for support after heartbreak, the sycotic for distraction, fun and excitement. If the sycotic commits suicide in this situation, it is because he is consumed by the heat of passion.

Syphilitic and sycotic teenagers will dress to shock people and dye their hair fluorescent colors. But while the sycotic does it for a thrill and to shock others, the syphilitic does it to hurt his parents' feelings. He does it out of maliciousness and meanness. He loves T-shirts and hats with skulls and cross-bones or pictures of well-known killers, like the Charles Manson T-shirt, as a show of disrespect for the rest of the world. If his parents ask him to dress up for a wedding, he will wear outrageous or offensive clothes. The protective mother might try to defend him by saying he is an independent thinker, but in reality he has contempt, pure selfishness and self-involvement.

Of course the syphilitic teenager loves to wear black, which reveals his tendency to hide. These youngsters are fascinated with Dracula, cemeteries, satanic cults and have a morbid interest in skeletons or medical books where they look up pictures of deformed people or abnormal fetuses in jars. Younger syphilitic children always play with their knights with the same theme: violence and killing. And when you ask them to draw a picture, they draw black pictures of people killing each other with drawn swords and knives while the blood flows from their severed limbs. Syphilitics often struggle with "mercurial" moods (is it not an irony that Mercury is the strongest anti-syphilitic remedy?). I had one young patient tell me in one of his more lucid moments, "I want to be less mercurial, I don't want to hide the real me!"

The syphilitic baby cries as soon as he is born, the whole night through. He does not look for his mother, does not start smiling at seven weeks, does not want to be held or touched (aversion to company, aversion to touch).

Physical symptoms: Physical symptoms can appear if the syphilitic person is mentally/emotionally strong or as an overflow from the deep-seated syphilitic mental/emotional picture. The destructive tendency of the syphilitic miasm is easily seen on the skin: cracks in the corner of the mouth, canker sores, blistering sores on the tongue and in the nose which he always picks; fissures around the anus; deep painful cracks in the heels, and rashes that ulcerate right from the onset, leaving scars. The ulcers are deep, making holes in the flesh or forming fistulas that eat away deeper and deeper into the tissues. Syphilitic ulcers are common in the throat and nose.

Warts are not only sycotic but can be syphilitic too if they are hidden under the skin, eating into the flesh. Tissues eaten away by the syphilitic miasm are stinking and offensive. The typical syphilitic ear infection is more painful at night and gives off a bloody-tinged stinking discharge. While pediatricians may caution mothers that all ear infections could possibly lead to hearing loss if untreated, in fact only syphilitic ones will cause this kind of destruction.

Destruction or ulceration does not always mean syphilis: a gastric ulcer forming after long-term gastritis can reflect the sycotic miasm. If the ulcer first shows symptoms of pain and hyperacidity, then melena, it is not syphilitic. But when the melena comes up right away, it is syphilitic, indicating the immediate destruction and bleeding of the syphilitic miasm.

Many syphilitic deformities are found in the mouth, especially the teeth, including a large split between the teeth; missing, serrated, irregularly formed, or cracked teeth; or teeth which require orthodontic work because of their incorrect position or crowding in the narrow syphilitic dental arch. The teeth erupt out of order and often decay before they are entirely through the gums (Kreos.). The child catches a cold every time a tooth appears, with the tonsils swollen and ulcerated. She may also suffer from juvenile periodontitis, a premature breakdown of the bone.

Syphilitics need to go to the dentist more than any other type, and many telltale symptoms of syphilis are found in the mouth: they may also have swollen glands in the neck and ulceration of the mucosae. The tongue can look like chopped meat, with deep cracks everywhere. (A psoric tongue looks pale with often a thick yellow coating, a sycotic one is very red, dry, often with fine cracks.) It does not help matters that in dental work, the top antisyphilitic remedy is put in the syphilitics' mouth, potentially adding a proving of Mercury to their other symptoms.

The syphilitic's hair is moist, gluey and greasy, with an offensive odor. It falls out in bunches, first from the vertex and then from the temples; the eyebrows, eyelashes, beard and genital hairs can also be affected (alopecia totalis). The eyes are another major arena of syphilitic expression, and since syphilis causes structural changes, we find its effects in astigmatism, deformities of the lens and cornea, cataracts, and ulceration in the eye. Some kinds of blindness are syphilitic (related to destruction, such as cortical blindness) as is glaucoma. It affects the meninges of the brain and the larynx and throat in general.

In the syphilis patient all the sensory senses are dulled, especially the sense of smell. Syphilis is the only miasm which causes destruction of the bones of the nose (as we can observe in leprosy, which is syphilitic as well as psoric, and leaves a hole in its victim's nose). It causes many dark-green or black scabs and crusts in the nose, which can cause an offensive odor as in ozaena. Syphilitic discharges can be greenish, like sycotic ones, or greyish, and often tinged with blood. Neither pathological discharges (from disease conditions) nor natural discharges like perspiration, urine and menses make the syphilitic patient feel better; in fact, sweating makes the syphilitic patient feel worse.

Syphilitic people's sleep is destroyed because of deep bone pains, with children waking up from "growing pains" at night (Calc-p.). All syphilitics' symptoms are worse when the sun goes down, and the farther from the sunlight, the greater the aggravation. The aggravation time is 8 p.m to 2 or 3 a.m. Syphilitic people also have a difficult time finding the right temperature. They are sensitive to heat and cold with a narrow range in comfort; Mercury, the top antisyphilitic remedy, is one of the most temperature-sensitive remedies in the Materia Medica.

The syphilitic tendency to destruction is also seen in early miscarriages, stillborn children, and the tendency to bleed during pregnancy. A recent study showed that up to 50% of young men suffer from azoospermia or lack of sperm, perhaps from the suppression of the syphilitic miasms in previous generations.

Deeper syphilitic expressions are found in birth defects affecting the most precious organs like the heart, brain and kidneys (agenesis of the brain, one kidney missing, etc.) as well as causing deformities of the bones. The miasm causes congenital heart defects like VSD, ASD, tetralogy of Fallot, single ventricle, transposition of the vessels, and location of the heart on the wrong side. Deformities include a narrow or cleft palate, harelip, missing fingers or toes (or extra ones), clubfoot, dwarfishness, a large, bulging head with soft sutures, hydrocephaloid in appearance, or a small, deformed head. It is no coincidence that allopathic medicine correlates small, lowset ears (another syphilitic expression) with birth defects and mental retardation. Intra-utero, syphilitic babies are likely to be in a malposition. Deformities of the bone also show up in exostoses, which are caused by defective nutrition of the bone.

Other syphilitic expressions are an irregular heartbeat (dysfunction of the heart), aneurysms (caused by a weakening of the arterial wall), and all blood disorders which involve the lysis of red blood cells (hemolytic anemia, purpura, ecchymoses) or platelets (idiopathic thrombocytopenic purpura, ITP). High blood pressure, being essentially a structural change in the arterial walls (arteriosclerosis), is a result of the syphilitic miasm in combination with the functional disturbances produced by psora (such as vertigo). This malignant syphilitic hypertension is different from labile or episodic hypertension without structural change as a result of grief, fright, shock or temporary stress. Diabetes is syphilitic, and gestational diabetes can be caused when the pregnancy triggers the mother's latent syphilitic miasm or the child brings the father's syphilitic miasm over to the mother.

Syphilitic headaches are frequent, intense, unilateral, parietal or occipital headaches, worse at night, worse from almost all forms of motion, from mental and physical exertion, and from warmth and heat. They feel better after cold applications and nosebleeds. Children with these manifestations will bore their head into the pillow or roll their head from side to side. Other syphilitic manifestations are locomotor ataxia or tabes dorsalis (muscular incoordination, loss of sensation, and altered deep tendon reflexes, which are first increased and later lost).

Syphilitic patients die suddenly, at a relatively young age (50-55), of a sudden stroke or a massive, first heart infarct (for example, someone who seems in good health but suddenly drops dead from shoveling snow). They are also the patients who appear healthy, who suddenly become ill, go to the doctor, are diagnosed with cancer and are dead three weeks later. A homeopath could discover and treat the syphilitic miasm before it is too late. A syphilitic case of gangrenous appendicitis or gall bladder disease is only discovered when it becomes peritonitis: there is immediate ulceration and destruction, exploding in the abdomen with infection. The end result is the same as in sycosis, but the sycotic one has immediate symptoms such as intense pain and high fever, while the syphilitic one destroys silently from within for a long time until it suddenly erupts into this violent picture.

What are some other syphilitic expressions? Multiple sclerosis (destruction of the myelin sheaths of the nerves) and Parkinson's (gradual death of the brain cells that produce dopamine) both reflect the destructive quality of syphilis. According to a recent study of 20,000 identical twins, most cases of Parkinson's disease are not caused by a defective gene but rather by exposure to as yet unknown chemicals in the environment.[6] How does the homeopath look at this? We know that defective genes are *not* good predictors of whether a particular individual will develop a certain disease. We will look for other manifestations of the syphilitic miasm in the family history. Even if both twins had the same degree of latent syphilis, one of them can be exposed to a trigger which wakes it up. While environmental factors can be a trigger, or even a dietary mistake, mental/emotional factors are the most common ones, and two twins as they grow will experience different joys and heartaches. By assessing the symptoms of latent syphilis, a good homeopath could recognize which one of two twins would be more susceptible to Parkinson's.

Van Gogh and his peculiar disease: Vincent Van Gogh (1853-1890) has recently been labeled as suffering from "Geschwind's syndrome," defined by "hypergraphia" (extensive or compulsive writing or painting), hyper-religiosity, unstable sexual behavior, intermittent aggressiveness and clingy behavior. Van Gogh showed all five traits. In addition to his prolific artwork and letters to his brother Theo, he exhibited hypersexuality, bisexuality, and homosexuality which culminated in a stormy affair with the painter Paul Gauguin. This affair resulted in the now famous self-amputation of his ear and ultimately in his suicide with a pistol. Other medical researchers believe he suffered from seizures. All miasms are present in his behavior: psora in his clinginess (looking for support), sycosis in his hypersexuality and hypergraphia (overstimulation), and syphilitic in his self-mutilation with a sharp blade and his suicide, as well as his attacking Gauguin with a razor. Other diagnoses linked to Van Gogh were depression and schizophrenia, both syphilitic expressions, and epilepsy (psoric). Without any doubt, he could have benefited from homeopathic treatment.

The Stages of Life

The three miasms can be found in the different stages of life. We have the period of youth and adolescence, where there is a struggle with growing up, a struggle with authority (parents), emotional problems, and physical exacerbations like acne around puberty. All of these reflect the continuous struggle of psora. In middle age the person has learned to accept the fact that he cannot win all his struggles and that he does not have all the answers. In order to cope and survive in the society, he has to put on his best face. Rather than always swimming upstream, like the struggling psora, he resorts to concealment and cover-up. This is the sycotic phase in life. In old age, he realizes that he is in quite a desperate and depressing situation: everyone around him is dying from cancer, infarcts, and strokes. He sees destruction everywhere and starts brooding, alone, on death. This is the syphilitic phase.

At least this is how the three ages of life were characterized until very recently. Now, through our constant suppression and fueling of the miasms, we see sycotic and syphilitic expressions from a very young age. We see cancers in small children, difficult and disobedient behavior, and cold-blooded murder, theft and sexual assault committed by schoolchildren. Suicides are now the leading cause of death among teenagers.

Treatment of the Syphilitic Miasm

Hahnemann distinguishes three different stages of treating syphilis.[7] The first phase, the uncomplicated syphilitic infection (acute syphilis) where the chancre is still intact, can be easily cured (in two weeks, according to Hahnemann) by a single dose of Merc. 30c. Hahnemann and his followers achieved this type of cure many times, with not the slightest trace of a scar remaining.

The second stage is rare in our modern world because the sycotic miasm is so widespread: the pure chronic syphilitic miasmatic state. Mercury will again bring about a cure. The difference with the previous stage is that the practitioner has now lost an indicator of the existing disease, namely the primary chancre. However, on the place where the chancre was driven inwards by local applications, there is now a discolored or reddish scar. Our cure will be effected when this scar changes to the normal healthy color of the skin.

The third and more complicated state, and the one we most often see in modern times, is the one where the syphilitic miasm has been complicated with a second or third miasm. If two or three miasms are present, often psora dominates and makes the others latent, in which case an antipsoric remedy will be first. If syphilis is strongly active and psora is latent, start with the indicated antisyphilitic. The most effective anti-syphilitics, in my experience, include Aurum, Lachesis, and Nitric acid in addition to the obvious Mercury and Syphilinum. This treatment is continued until the syphilitic miasm is subdued, at which time psoric symptoms will rear their head and an antipsoric remedy will be needed. Continue the antipsoric until most of the psoric symptoms have disappeared; then in complicated cases you may need to address the remaining syphilitic symptoms with the same antisyphilitic remedy. (If using centesimal potencies, use a higher potency than before.) Always finish with an antipsoric.

If syphilis is strongly active while sycosis and psora are both latent: Start with an antisyphilitic followed by an antipsoric, then an antisycotic and finish with an antipsoric. Although this situation was rare in Hahnemann's time, it will unfortunately become more commonplace in our practice, as indicated by the increase of cancer victims (with multiple miasms). The uncomplicated syphilitic miasm is the easiest to cure, but if it is complicated with psora or sycosis, it becomes much more difficult to cure.

If both the syphilitic and sycotic miasms are about equally active: Start with the indicated antisycotic, because the sycotic miasm is more difficult to cure. Then do an antipsoric, then treat the syphilitic miasm, and finish with an antipsoric.

Clinical Case: An ob/gyn who came to me as a patient demonstrated many of the indications for the syphilitic miasm. Despite an almost complete lack of physical symptoms, her dominant syphilitic miasm was reflected in her moods, thoughts, behavior and even her spiritual life. To begin with, her chief complaint (depression) was syphilitic, as was her family history: both sides of the family were riddled with alcoholism, depression, incest, birth defects, and even suicide. But it was the different expressions of the syphilitic miasm in her life and her personality which I found so fascinating. When I asked her what she liked most about her job, she admitted (with a guilty expression) that she actually enjoyed doing hysterectomies. She explained that she enjoyed the precise scalpel work involved in separating the internal organs. This really caught my attention, since usually women ob/gyns tend to advocate for postponing hysterectomies if at all possible. She also admitted to feeling a "spiritual high" when delivering stillborn babies with birth defects, which had become her specialty (because none of the others in her practice enjoyed doing it). The only time she would go to church would be for the funerals of these unfortunate little ones. In fact she admitted that her favorite activity as a child was to hide behind the couch with her brother and to pore over her father's medical school textbook illustrating different forms of birth defects. This tendency to hide behind the couch would make us think first of Baryta carb., but it can also be an expression of the syphilitic tendency to hide, as is the fascination with anything defective or deformed. Not only that, her father's choice of profession could also reflect the syphilitic miasm: a fascination with the most hidden, secret and pathological aspects of human nature. This doctor also mentioned that her favorite topic in medical school was studying syphilis, which she found fascinating.

I observed that when she came to my office she would sit and doodle constantly. She also mentioned that she had been praised by the nurses she worked with for washing her hands before *and* after each patient; plus changing her gloves not just between patients, as was standard, but between each separate aspect of the procedure she was doing. We might consider this an Arsenicum concern with germs and contamination, except that it was totally unconscious on her part until one of her nurses brought it to her attention by complimenting her on it. I interpreted all of these behaviors, which involved repetitive unconscious motions of the hands, as related to the compulsive handwashing of the syphilitic miasm.

It was in her relationship with her brother, however, that the syphilitic miasm was expressed most clearly. He was several years older than she, and they had slept in the same bed until they were into their teens, enjoying an emotionally intense and somewhat physically incestuous relationship. (She also thought she had probably experienced incest at the hands of one or more of her alcoholic and dysfunctional mother's "crazy" boyfriends.) She had maintained this intense relationship with her brother until he married, at which point she became irrationally jealous of his wife. In her intake she mentioned, "I don't want to kill her but I wish she didn't exist." When a patient spontaneously brings up killing someone like this, you know they are thinking about it on some unconscious level. In fact during the first interview she mentioned driving too fast and somewhat dangerously when her brother and his wife were in the car and realized it came from an unconscious desire to kill both of them. Her depression was based on her inability to form a stable long-term romantic relationship, but of course this would be impossible as long as her emotional energy was bound up in her quasi-incestuous relationship with her brother.

Clearly she needed a syphilitic remedy, and I considered opening with Syphilinum because of all the syphilitic indications. But I prefer to open with a polychrest if at all possible, and Aurum was the obvious choice for a syphilitic patient complaining of depression. Aurum did not fit in any other way, however, and Lachesis was chosen for several reasons: her precise choice of words, her "delusion" (in her own words) that she had "a god-like animal creature inside me, looking out through my eyes" and a recurring dream which, like her delusion, reflected Lachesis' religious nature, even its sense of cosmic duality. She kept dreaming of driving down a deserted road on either side of which were crucifixes, to which were nailed women who were naked from the waist up and draped in white satin from the waist down.

Her first report, after a week on Lachesis LM1, confirmed the choice. In this short time she had stopped doodling as well as excessive glove-changing and handwashing, taking on the more relaxed attitude of her colleagues. Instead she reported having a new interest in decorating her house and making it more colorful. I perceived this as her artistic interest, which had been channeled through the doodling, finding a new outlet in her interior decorating, plus a desire to replace the gloomier colors of the syphilitic miasm. She reported feeling "better than ever before in my life" and "as if a fog or funk has lifted." Her Vital Force had exteriorized her mental and emotional symptoms: she reported a little scaly patch on one lip, and the return of a white itchy spot on her tongue which she had had twenty years earlier. Only seven doses of Lachesis had "rewound" twenty years of past medical history. Less than a month later she reported stopping the remedy because she felt so much improved on all levels, including "a clearing sensation" and "clarity" about her previously unreported "destructive criticism of myself and others."

CHAPTER TWENTY-THREE:
THE TUBERCULAR AND CANCER MIASMS

The Tubercular Miasm: The Reactive/Responsive Miasm

Definition

The tubercular miasm is one of the "new miasms" like cancer and AIDS, added to the miasmatic theory after Hahnemann by Compton Burnett and later homeopaths. (Hahnemann did not consider it a separate miasm but rather a combination of miasms.) It is also called "pseudo-psora" because it primarily combines psoric and syphilitic characteristics (although the tubercular person can have some sycotic characteristics too, such as excitement, restlessness, loquacity, irritability, and a violent temper.) Tuberculosis was rampant in the nineteenth century, with many of the artists and poets of the time affected, to the point that the "tubercular" or "consumptive" artistic type became well-known: people susceptible to TB or infected by it tended to be delicate, frail, easily tired, lean and elegant, with beautiful porcelain skin, large eyes, long lashes and fine hair; they were apt to be very talented in the arts, literature or music, and tended to die an early, tragic death. (This romantic, artistic type, which appears in the literature and history of the period, corresponds very closely to the characteristics of the tubercular miasm.)

Koch discovered the tubercle bacillus, *Mycobacterium tuberculosis,* in 1882. At that time the disease was known as "phthisis" or "consumption." Hahnemann successfully treated it homeopathically long before Koch's discovery resulted in allopathic treatment. (In Kent's *Repertory* pulmonary tuberculosis is listed as "phthisis," while "tuberculosis" in the *Repertory* refers to systemic tuberculosis.) Tuberculosis most commonly infects the lungs, especially the right apex of the lung. It can also spread to serous membranes like the pleura, peritoneum, and pericardium. In children it may infect the bones (Pott's disease), joints, and lymph nodes.

The disease can be transmitted through infested cow's milk, an infected person's utensils, and spitting in public, coughing or sneezing by infected persons. The hereditary form is passed through the placenta. As is the case with the other miasms, the tubercular miasm originally results from the suppression of tuberculosis with drugs, and the miasm can then be passed to the next generation.

The traditional treatment for TB, before the modern age of antibiotics, was to send the patients to live in sanitoriums in the mountains, where they could enjoy fresh air, a restful lifestyle, and nourishing food to counteract the wasting tendency of the disease. This was a sensible treatment, as it strengthened their Vital Force. (And in fact a craving for fresh air and amelioration from it, as well as amelioration in the mountains, are all strong indications for the tubercular miasm.) The risk of spreading the infection was minimized by isolating the patients. Now instead of enjoying the fresh mountain air, TB patients are treated with hepatotoxic drugs for a year. The result is suppression, creating the tubercular miasm, and the next generation will suffer from it. The miasm is also introduced through the Mantoux test (scratch test for tuberculosis) and BCG vaccinations.

Central Ideas: Dissatisfaction (Discontentment), Restlessness and Changeability

Mental indications: Tubercular people have a great memory and are mentally keen ("Ideas, abundant, clearness of mind," K52). But their fatigue can lead to mental passivity, confusion, and aversion to mental work.

Emotional indications: Tubercular people have a cheerful, optimistic outlook and can do wonderful, artistic things. Many of our greatest artists are tubercular. They can be very good musicians, playing the violin and piano at a young age, but then they may become too impatient to continue and too restless for the disciplined practice required. I have seen the parents of these talented young tubercular patients pay a lot of money for music lessons, but to their chagrin, these children will often suddenly abandon the instrument.

Tubercular children like to have fun and to have new things. When these are not forthcoming, they throw temper tantrums. In the consulting room, they explore everything: they open your drawers, they touch everything and when you tell them to stop, they throw a temper tantrum and start breaking things. Or they break things because they are impatient and their little whims are not satisfied quickly enough. This tendency to break things is one of the syphilitic qualities of the tubercular miasm. Their restlessness makes it impossible for them to sit still and work on a puzzle like the psoric child; they are always jumping from one new thing to another. Their craving for constant newness, excitement and stimulation is a sycotic aspect of the miasm.

Constant dissatisfaction runs through their personality. "The grass is always greener in someone else's yard" for the tubercular person. No matter how good a husband a tubercular woman has, she always thinks that her real prince is yet to come like a white knight on horseback; no matter how well-provided for she is, she always longs for adventure. Anything new creates excitement for tubercular people, captures their imagination and keeps their energy level up. They are day-dreamers, changing friends and even husbands quickly. They have short but intense relationships, changing doctors all the time, changing job locations or even changing their jobs ("traveling" from job to job).

Traveling is another major theme in their lives: they love to travel everywhere but they don't stay in one place long enough to know it well. They are always moving, always looking for the next short-lived excitement. A restless inner urge drives them mercilessly from one place to the next. They may love the *sukhs* (bazaars) of the Middle East, with their bustling activities and colorful people, but they would not stay put for two hours to negotiate with a rug merchant over mint tea. And while the tubercular Phosphorus woman may say, "Let's go to the *sukhs* and get lost," driven by her thirst for adventure, the psoric Calcarea husband will worry from the moment he leaves the hotel about how to find his way back.

Tubercular travelers will buy an open-ended plane ticket because a scheduled trip is boring. They love the mountains, fresh air and open spaces (the sanitoriums of the last century were in the perfect places) but they find the ocean too boring. Extremely sensitive to all impressions, they are much more attuned than other types to the beauty of their surroundings: "Can't you see the beauty of that cloud?" they will ask indignantly of their plodding, insensitive psoric companion. (The Carcinosin will appreciate the beauty of nature as much as the tubercular, but will feel more in awe of it and will stay put longer to watch it.)

On the job or doing housework, tubercular people are like headless chickens: they look busy and run around all day from one thing to the next, but at the end not much is accomplished. Easily fatigued, they are the first to feel overwhelmed and need a little tranquilizer or glass of wine in the evening. They have the same craving for excitement as sycotic people, but sycotics have more energy and tuberculars can't keep up. Nevertheless, they never stop looking for excitement, often dancing the night away. Their enthusiasm carries them, but once they go to bed they realize they overdid it. This combination of quick physical exhaustion and discontentment leads to impatience. If they become frustrated in a project, whether making a dress or writing a letter, they quickly abandon it, tear it up, and throw it away. They are good beginners (because they are carried away by their excitement) but bad finishers (because they run out of energy and quickly become bored) so they tend to have many unfinished projects in their lives.

Physical indications: In keeping with the tubercular themes of restlessness and changeability, the physical symptoms of the tubercular miasm are ever-changing. One indication for Tuberculinum is a patient who comes back for each follow-up appointment with an entirely new set of symptoms, despite a well-prescribed remedy each time. (The Arsenicum will continue to complain at follow-ups, but will focus on her original symptoms which have not entirely cleared, as will the impossible-to-please, always pessimistic Nitric acid, who is unwilling to declare himself healed as long as 1% of his original symptoms remain. The tubercular patient will present an entirely new disease picture each time, to the frustration of the prescriber, until you recognize that this trait in itself is a keynote for Tuberculinum.)

As tuberculosis was known as "consumption" or "the wasting disease," the tubercular patient will look as though she is wasting away. Tubercular patients do not look ill, especially not in the face. Like the tuberculosis sufferers of the last century, tubercular patients will have a pale, porcelain quality to their skin and a flush on their cheeks. Tubercular children can have a delicate, angelic look, with brilliant blue eyes, long eyelashes, curly blond hair, and red lips. These are the typical slender and delicate Phosphorus or Silica children. Like the sycotic, they can have an abundance of hair growth: long, dark, downy hairs between the shoulderblades and on the arms. They tend to be feverish, always running a little temperature and sweating a lot (one of their psoric qualities), especially between the shoulder blades. They like running around, at least for a little while as long as their energy holds out. But they tend to run with headphones on, because exercise alone is not enough excitement for them.

Children born from parents with the tubercular miasm tend to have a narrow, deformed chest ("pigeon chest") and a weakness in the respiratory system, leading to frequent coughs, colds, flus, and even asthma. Being highly sensitive (another psoric quality) they also are susceptible to allergic reactions. They tend to be allergic to furry animals like dogs and cats and consequently to fear them. Their nails tend to be brittle, with white spots.

Despite their respiratory weakness, tubercular people like wind and crave fresh air ("air hunger"). Their love for travel makes them enjoy being outside. Like syphilitics, they dread artificial light more than sunlight.

Tubercular people, like sycotics, love fatty foods, milk, bacon and other smoked foods, and salt. They certainly have the greatest salt cravings of any of the miasmatic groups. They like to have bacon in the morning because they feel it stimulates them to get going. A typical tubercular trait is that they crave what they cannot assimilate: for example, they crave chocolate but it makes them sick.

Tubercular Remedies

The top tubercular remedies in my experience have been Phosphorus, Silica, Pulsatilla, and Carbo animalis, with Tuberculinum used intercurrently as the nosode.

The Cancer Miasm: The Mixed Miasm

History

When you see cancer in the family history, you can be sure that the family has at least two of the miasms active. By the same token, when you see at least two active miasms in the family history, you should be on the lookout for the cancer miasm in the patient. All four of the other miasms are necessary to develop the cancer miasm. Children who develop tumors by the age of five are likely to have family histories like this, compounded by vaccinations and suppressive treatments for childhood illnesses. When there is cancer in the family history, cancer develops at a younger age in each generation to the point that brain tumors like glioblastomas and astrocytomas are now much more common in young children than ever before. Suppression is the most important etiological factor in developing cancer: because cancer occurs when all the other miasms are active, the suppression of each of these miasms will increase the incidence of cancer in successive generations. And the younger generations are exposed to ever-increasing suppressive treatments, which are ubiquitous in the modern world. (Antibiotics, antipyretics, and in fact all the pharmaceuticals labeled "anti-" are suppressive).

Why do different cancer patients have such different outcomes? One person may seem healthy until she complains of a headache, yet one month later she has died from a brain tumor. Another may have cancer for twenty years while maintaining reasonably good health. Both were malignant cancers, yet the life span of the patient is entirely different.

The prognosis depends on the miasmatic background of the tumor. A malignant tumor that kills a patient suddenly combines the speed of the sycotic miasm with the destruction of the syphilitic. One that is slow-growing for many years is predominantly psoric. Thus the prognosis is good for a psoric cancer. Skin cancers such as squamous cell carcinoma and papillary thyroid carcinoma are slow-growing psoric tumors. A tumor can arise from any one of the miasms, or a combination of two or three of them. It does not necessarily indicate the presence of the cancer miasm, which requires an active combination of at least two of the other miasms.

Just as a patient can have the sycotic miasm without ever having had gonorrhea, or the tubercular miasm without any signs of TB in his past medical history, a patient can have the cancer miasm without necessarily having cancer, either as the Chief Complaint or in the past. If a patient presents as a Carcinosin yet has no cancer, the cure will be easier. Cancer itself can be cured homeopathically, as the old masters of the past century demonstrated many times. (Cancer does not appear in the *Repertory* under Generalities but is listed under "tumors" in the sections for the various parts of the body.) Grimmer published many cured cases of cancer in the first half of this century.[1] But these great homeopaths of the past did not have to contend with the severely suppressive treatments of our era, chemotherapy and radiation, which greatly weaken the Vital Force, and they were not threatened with legal action for providing alternative cancer treatment. In my own practice I would never hold out to a cancer patient the hope or the promise of being able to cure them. The legal situation in this country is simply too risky. Instead, I would encourage them to continue their conventional treatment and promise to offer palliation and improved quality of life, as homeopathy can easily provide for cancer patients.

The cancer miasm is the most recently identified of the five major miasms. Although we know that its nosode, Carcinosin, was used by Compton Burnett, J.H. Clarke, Kent, and others, cancer was not identified as a miasm until after the Second World War. Two homeopaths working in England at that time, Drs. Foubister and Templeton, happened to deliver two children of two different mothers, each with breast cancer during her pregnancy. These children had remarkably similar symptoms, including insomnia, crying all night, tics and blinking of the eyes, *café au lait* spots all over the body, numerous moles, and blue sclerae. Foubister deduced that these children were carrying the cancer miasm and treated them with Carcinosin, a remedy probably potentized from a breast epithelioma. The children benefited greatly from this remedy in a 30c potency. Over the years, Foubister collected several hundred such cases. If he saw children identical to the ones described, even if they were not born from a mother with cancer, he was able to treat their symptoms with Carcinosin. More importantly, he believed he was also protecting them from cancer in the future.

Since provings of Carcinosin were conducted mainly after the Second World War, Carcinosin does not appear in Kent's *Repertory*. It should be prescribed on its indications, especially its strange, rare and peculiar symptoms. It should not be given automatically because there is cancer in the family background. That is allopathic homeopathy. But you should definitely be on the lookout for indications of Carcinosin if cancer, TB, diabetes, leukemia, and/or pernicious anemia appear in the family history. Foubister found that the "Carcinosin" child often had that kind of family background rather than just cancer.

As many other homeopaths have reported, I have seen that using Carcinosin stimulates the Vital Force to throw up new indications for Psorinum, Tuberculinum, and other antipsorics. This confirms Kent's observation that cancer is the result of suppressed psora. Many of the old masters believed that the suppression of the other miasms as well leads to this state of Carcinosin, and unfortunately, often to cancer itself.

Central Idea: Suppression on All Levels and a Lack of Reactivity

Mental characteristics: The Carcinosin lack of reactivity is found in mental dullness with a lack of interest, difficulty thinking, and an aversion to conversation as well as to mental work. Carcinosins have mental inertia with a feeling of constriction. They are preoccupied but annoyed that they cannot concentrate, and they find mental work a challenge. This mental tiredness is better for sleep, even a short nap (Phos.).

Emotional characteristics: Carcinosins are very sensitive people: sensitive to people, to animals, and to beauty. They are so sensitive that they may have tears in their eyes looking at a magnificent sunset. They are astonished at beauty. Together with the tuberculars, they love travel. There is a difference, however: the tubercular travels to see the excitement in the world and will move on quickly, while the cancer personality travels to see the beauty in the world. They stay put long enough to take in the beauty wherever they go, and a camera is never far away. They love to see beautiful works of art, museums, and cathedrals. They also enjoy safaris because they love to see animals in the wild. Not only do they have no fear of thunder and lightning, they are fascinated by it. Unlike people with the other miasms, they enjoy this spectacular and beautiful display of Nature. Like the tubercular person, they love the excitement and beauty of dance.

Carcinosins are very refined, private people, keeping their thoughts to themselves, not outgoing like the tuberculars. They can be very introverted, living in their own world, and making no contact with others (the opposite of the tubercular person). In fact they hide their feelings for fear of hurting others. Even young children hide their feelings "so I don't upset mummy." When feelings are suppressed for many years to avoid hurting others, the likelihood of cancer increases.

Carcinosins are the greatest animal lovers. They are the ones who leave their estate to their pets or donate huge sums to animal shelters and save-the-whale campaigns. And when their dog dies, they bury it in the graveyard with a beautifully carved tombstone. While the tubercular person likes the mountains, the cancer person loves the sea air (and all her symptoms feel better at the seashore). Carcinosin's love for beauty leads to her fastidiousness. Unlike the Arsenicum who is fastidious out of an excessive sense of perfection, Carcinosin has fastidiousness with a purpose. The Carcinosin person loves to have the perfect house with everything matching perfectly: the paintings go with the carpets, portraits match the cabinets, and all the decorations in each room have the same theme. Their exaggerated attention to detail is focused on creating the perfect environment. They are happiest when in their beautiful home, listening to lovely, peaceful music.

Anticipation anxiety is a great indication for Carcinosin, and it should be added to the *Repertory* as a black-type remedy for "Anxiety, future, about" (K7) and "Fear, happen, something will" (K45). It takes the form of worry, sometimes amounting to anguish, for example at the late arrival of a child, husband or wife (Ars., Phos., Carc.), or the student's fear of failing an exam. What makes matters worse is that a Carcinosin feels she is powerless to control situations in her life. "I know I should get rid of this relationship," she will say, "but I feel I just can't do it." Carcinosins feel overwhelmed and can't say no to something, even when they have a premonition that it is the wrong thing to do. Part of this sense of powerlessness comes from their great lack of self-confidence, which also makes them more fastidious because they are so afraid of criticism. (Sensitivity to being reprimanded is one of their sycotic traits.) Striving for perfection is thus absolutely necessary.

Carcinosins will also stay in a relationship because they feel very responsible. This sense of duty (Sep., Aur.) can be present from a young age, as in a child who can't sleep because she hears her parents fighting and feels responsible for her parents' relationship (Mag. mur.). This sense of duty makes the Carcinosin patient always hurry in order to arrive on time (Arg-nit.).

Carcinosins have many fears, the outstanding ones being a fear of cancer (Ars., Nit-ac.), fears of narrow places and crowds (Acon., Nat-m.) and fear of heights (Sulph.). They share Sepia's marked sense of rhythm and love of dancing as well its sensitivity to music which sometimes makes them weep (Nux-v., Graph., Nat-c.). Like Phosphorus, they are sympathetic towards others. (Note that Carcinosin and Nux vomica are the only two remedies of the materia medica which have both fastidiousness and sensitivity to music.) Carcinosins make meticulous shopping lists, of course, with their favorite foods being soups and chocolate.

A patient does not necessarily become a Carcinosin because of cancer in the family history, as explained before. A Carcinosin state can develop in patients of any miasmatic background from indignation situations, especially after excessive control by a dictatorial parent (Carcinosin complements Staphysagria). This state can appear in any patient who has had a powerful experience of control, whether by fear or an excessive sense of duty; after long-lasting grief, anticipation, prolonged fear, unhappiness without any hope of improvement (like a Staphysagria state); and after vaccinations. Carcinosin is known for suicides in children and mental diseases in children. The distinguished homeopath Dr. Clarke noted that Carcinosin was useful in mental cases with a tendency to suicide and a family history of cancer.

Physical characteristics: Aside from tumors, the cancer miasm has other physical symptoms. Carcinosin children do not get the typical childhood diseases at an appropriate age; in fact anyone getting a childhood disease after puberty is likely to need Carcinosin. But Carcinosin is also needed when childhood illnesses such as pneumonia or whooping cough always attack the patient in a very severe form. And Carcinosin is needed if the child has *all* the childhood diseases, one after the other in rapid succession; if the child had the same childhood disease twice; or if there is a childhood disease with complications (such as mumps with orchitis). "Never Well Since" mononucleosis is another great indication for Carcinosin. Ulcerative colitis and Crohn's disease, which can possibly evolve into cancer, are other expressions of the cancer miasm and can respond favorably to Carcinosin (Ars., Merc.). Carcinosin can be used to treat pernicious anemia as well.

Café-au-lait spots, numerous moles, and blue sclerae were among the classic keynotes determined by Dr. Foubister. Warts on the soles and palms and molluscum contagiosum are typical for Carcinosin (also for the syphilitic miasm). Dr. Paschero of Argentina had the opportunity to administer Carcinosin pre-operatively to patients undergoing plastic surgery and found the incidence of keloid scars was greatly reduced.

Insomnia, especially in children, is one of Carcinosin's few standard symptoms. They have difficulty falling asleep and, even more, staying asleep, so they tend to catnap like Sulphur, awakened by shudders. Sometimes they lie awake most of the night with overactive ideas (Coff.) or they wake up at 4 a.m. and can't get back to sleep. They may sleep in the knee-elbow position (Med., Tub., Phos., Calc-p, Lyc., Sep.), less frequently on the back with the arms raised above the head (Puls.). Carcinosin is indicated in cases of adults and youngsters who are overworked and overtaxed because they have been subjected to undue pressure, and who complain of excessive tiredness and mental exhaustion (Sepia, Nux-v.). Dr. Templeton's provings showed this characteristic clearly.

Their food cravings can be numerous, with the outstanding ones being for chocolate (Phos.) and soups, sometimes for the fat of meat (Tub.). Dr. Templeton noted in his provings of Carcinosin the constant state of constipation with no urge to go (Morphia, Alum.), because of their lack of reactivity. Carcinosin's symptoms usually improve at the seaside (Med., even Nat-m), although they sometimes are worse at the seaside (also Nat-m.). They may have alternation of symptoms (Lac-c.) and periodicity (symptoms worse from 1-6 p.m.).

It is interesting to note that a patient's temperature is likely to rise the tenth day after taking Carcinosin. I have noticed that when patients respond at first to the indicated remedy in acute respiratory infections, including pneumonia, and then cease to respond, a dose of Carcinosin often stimulates the reaction.

Other Carcinosin expressions include bedwetting, leucorrhea in young girls (Sep., Puls.), hemophilia, aplastic anemia, hemochromatosis, leukemia, diphtheria, epilepsy, hereditary fistula, cryptorchidism, neurofibromatosis, angioma, celiac disease, and a history of twins or multiple births.

From the above picture, we can see a relationship with many different remedies (we can call them associated remedies). And indeed, many of the patients needing Carcinosin have been partially helped by remedies such as Tuberculinum, Medorrhinum, Nat. mur., and

Sepia/Nux vomica especially. When you have a patient who is not completely healing after these remedies, think Carcinosin. Staphysagria and Causticum are complementary with each other and with Carcinosin for patients suffering from a dictatorial parent. Other associated remedies are Arsenicum, Pulsatilla, Staphysagria, Phosphorus, Syphilinum, Psorinum, Lycopodium, Dysentery co. and Calc. phos. Also keep in mind that you may prescribe Carcinosin if you see symptoms in a patient belonging to more than two of the above remedies, without having a clear picture belonging to a single remedy.

Sources

The initial preparation of Carcinosin used by Dr. Foubister and Dr. Templeton was brought from the US and was probably prepared from an epithelioma of the breast. A number of different specimens are now available, prepared by A. Nelson & Co. in London. They can be prescribed by isopathic indications, in other words by the type of pathology involved:

    Carcinosin Adeno Stom.: from an epithelioma of the stomach
    Carcinosin Adeno Vesica: from an epithelioma of the bladder
    Carcinosin Scirrhinum Mammae: from scirrhous cancer of the breast
    Carcinosin Squam. Pulm.: from an epithelioma of the lung
    Carcinosin Intest. Co: from an epithelioma of the intestine.

Scenarios for Cancer Miasm Diagnosis

Understanding the difference between an active cancer miasm, a diagnosis of cancer, and the indications for Carcinosin has been a point of confusion for my students. I have found it helpful to illustrate the distinction with a series of mini-scenarios. Readers may want to check their understanding of whether the cancer miasm is involved in each case with the answers provided on the following page.

Case 1: A 50-year-old woman presents with moles which her doctors are advising her to have removed because they may be cancerous. Her past medical history reveals little besides some digestive difficulties (heartburn, flatulence) and skin problems (rashes). Her parents are both alive and active; her grandparents lived to their 90s on both sides.

Case 2: A 15-year-old girl presents with insulin-dependent diabetes mellitus. A number of relatives on her father's side have IDDM, and her mother had pernicious anemia. Her maternal great-grandmother died of TB.

Case 3: A lovely 25-year-old woman photographer with a big wide smile and bright sparkly eyes presents for dysmenorrhea and excessively heavy periods. She has no significant previous illnesses in her past medical history. In her family medical history, her father had hypertension died from a heart attack at age 64, while her mother was a smoker and suffers from COPD. In her timeline, she tells you that her father was a real tyrant who founded his own religious sect and punished the children when he caught them laughing or playing instead of studying.

Case 4: A 5-year-old boy is brought by his parents with a brain tumor (astrocytoma). He had 21 ear infections treated with antibiotics plus numerous rounds of antibiotics for colds and flus, all of which started after his 20th vaccination at age 2. Under your questioning, his parents admit that they were part of the "sex, drugs and rock 'n'roll" crowd and both had STDs. The father has had prostatitis, the mother PID.

Case 5: A young boy of 9 years old has been diagnosed with ADD. He suffers from chronic insomnia, which his parents attribute to his hyperactivity. Amazingly enough he had had no childhood diseases. In spite of his hyperactive behavior, he is a very affectionate boy and seems to have an unusual love for animals. There is no cancer or leukemia in the family, just one aunt and one uncle on the mother's side suffer from IDDM.

Case 6: A 60-year-old man went for a routine colonoscopic examination and 2 polyps were found. In the past he had suffered from recurrent tonsillitis, and at one point he was diagnosed with Reiter syndrome (iritis, urethritis, arthritis). His mother suffered all her life from RA while the father had numerous operations for nose polyps.

Answers on following page

Answer to Scenarios for Cancer Miasm Diagnosis

Case 1 miasm: psora. This woman is strongly psoric, as shown by her relative degree of good health and the types of complaints she has, as well as her family history on both sides. No matter what the allopathic diagnosis is, she does not have the cancer miasm and there is little likelihood that her moles will become cancerous. Even if they do, you will still treat them with antipsoric remedies, not with Carcinosin.

Case 2 miasm: cancer. Although her diagnosis is not cancer, nor is there any cancer in her family history, her condition indicates the cancer miasm and there are many indications in her family history.

Case 3 miasm: could be tubercular; she is probably a Phosphorus. But she may very well need Carcinosin as a result of her emotionally suppressed childhood, even though there are no indications for the cancer miasm in her or her family history.

Case 4 miasm: active sycotic miasm. The child needs to be treated with strong antisycotic remedies. This tumor does not necessarily indicate the presence of the cancer miasm.

Case 5 miasm: Cancer. The intake of Carcinosin corrected the insomnia greatly while the ADD behavior was 50% improved. The Vital Force was then able to throw new symptoms up, which showed a simillimum of Staphysagria, the complement of Carcinosin.

Case 6 miasm: active sycosis. Although polyps can be considered "tumors" in this patient, they are a relief point for his active sycotic miasm, which should have been addressed before. Medorrhinum/Thuja was greatly indicated for his Reiter syndrome and would have avoided the onset of these polyps. But the same anti-sycotic remedies will still cure these polyps, and even more, take care of the strongly present sycotic background which is present in both of his parents. Carcinosin is not indicated in this case.

CHAPTER TWENTY-FOUR

Homeopathy and Cancer

I would like to devote the final chapter of this book to the homeopathic treatment of cancer. While this may seem to contradict my cautions against allopathic prescribing (prescribing for the pathology, not the person), in fact the successful homeopathic treatment of cancer epitomizes all the techniques taught in this book. It requires an understanding of the Never Well Since, the mental/emotional state of the patient, suppression, the Laws of Hering, and the difference between palliative and curative prescribing. Above all, it requires a thorough understanding of miasmatic prescribing. Cancer indicates the presence of more than one active miasm, and different cancers reflect different miasms. Homeopathy's goal in treating cancer patients, as with all patients, is not only to cure but to prevent recurrence, and this goal is only possible with miasmatic prescribing.

Finally, cancer provides an excellent example of how homeopathy can successfully treat diseases which have eluded allopathic medicine. The allopathic claims that a cure for cancer is just around the corner remind us of the Surgeon General's announcement in 1969 that the era of infectious diseases was over. Instead of conquering infectious diseases, we see the *resurgence* of the deadly diseases of the last century (TB, cholera, etc.), the *emergence* of previously-unknown deadly infectious diseases like AIDS, and the rapid development of *antibiotic-resistant pathogens*. We see similar claims about conquering cancer, such as this one from a *Time* cover article*:* "It is a merciless disease that claims more than a half million Americans a year. But scientists are steadily unlocking its mysteries, and the fight against it may now have reached a turning point. New discoveries promise better therapies and hope against the war."[1]

What is the reality of the situation? After billions of dollars being spent in the war on cancer, not to mention the time and energy of thousands of physicians and scientists, cancer is still the second leading cause of death in this country (after cardiovascular conditions) and the second worldwide after infectious diseases (ironically enough, the other condition supposedly about to be conquered). While it used to be a disease primarily of the elderly, we see breast cancer in younger women and brain cancer in small children at a rate unheard of a generation ago. According to the American Cancer Society and the National Institutes of Health, cancer cost the U.S. over $100 billion in 1998 ($37 billion in health care expenditures,

$11 billion in productivity lost due to illness, and $59 billion in productivity lost due to untimely death).[2] The "better therapies" promised five years ago were supposed to obviate the need for harsh treatments like radiation and chemotherapy by "tricking" the cancer. Instead, the latest recommendation for all cancer patients now is to have *both* chemotherapy and radiation. Patients are suffering more than ever from the treatment, while the promised genetic therapy is nowhere in sight. Any decline in the death rate from cancer is attributable to life-style changes such as a decrease in the number of smokers, rather than better treatment. Even *The New England Journal of Medicine* and the *Journal of the National Cancer Institute* admit that many of the promising new treatments have been disappointing.[3,4]

Based on a homeopathic understanding of cancer's miasmatic roots, we can predict that this deadly plague will only become more widespread and virulent in the next century. The miasms are becoming more and more concentrated in each generation; there are many triggers for them in our modern world, as we have seen; and the suppressive treatment of cancer only serves to make it more malignant and metastatic.* Chemotherapy and radiation are so devastating to the body and the Vital Force that patients frequently die from the treatment rather than the cancer.

The National Institutes of Health and its affiliated cancer centers are currently focusing their hopes on genetic therapy; more than 100 genes have already been found which are linked to cancer and several dozen of them important in tumor formation. But where will genetics lead us? We know, for example, that only a small percentage of patients with breast cancer have the gene for it, while of those women with the gene for it, an even smaller percentage develop breast cancer. Even if we could find a way to repair the damaged gene (a quantum leap beyond identifying the gene), it would not help women who already have breast cancer. In fact, identifying the gene may backfire: it has already been used to deny insurance coverage to women with known gene markers and to frighten women in their 20s

---

*A recent unfortunate example was the case of the much-admired King Hussein of Jordan, who flew to this country for aggressive treatment of his non-Hodgkin's lymphoma. A week later he was dead of kidney and liver failure. We know that lymphoma cannot cause this kind of organ failure. Another beloved world figure provided another heart-breaking example: Jackie Onassis died only 6 months after starting a new, experimental aggressive therapy for her Hodgkin's lymphoma, during which her health rapidly declined. I have personal knowledge of another well-known case, that of Michael Landon of *Bonanza* fame: a friend of his, who was a patient of mine in California, told me that he had been doing well on alternative therapies, maintaining his health and energy and keeping the cancer at bay, but was persuaded to try a new experimental drug and died only two months later.

into having preventive mastectomies. In a recent study of the longterm effectiveness of preventive mastectomies, about 10% of high-risk women were expected to develop the disease and approximately 90% had their breasts removed unnecessarily; seven of the 614 women in the study developed breast cancer anyway, in spite of having both breasts removed.[5] Attributing cancer to a damaged chromosome does not answer homeopathy's fundamental question: Why do certain people have broken chromosomes? To answer it, we must consider the miasms and the Never Well Since.

What can we expect from homeopathic treatment for cancer? The great masters of the last century, and even of the first half of this century, were able to cure cancer rapidly and painlessly with homeopathy. Several examples of cured cases are given later in this chapter. Modern homeopaths have to content with the effects of chemotherapy and radiation, which are strongly suppressive and also weaken the patients' Vital Force to the point that it does not respond well to the remedy. When a patient comes to us with cancer, almost inevitably she has already been treated with strongly suppressive measures and usually she continues them while under homeopathic treatment. This is why we cannot hold out a hope of cure with homeopathy in the current health care environment. But we must work with consumers toward a different model in the future, in which we are free from legal restrictions and the threat of repressive legal action, and in which informed consumers may give us the opportunity to demonstrate the curative power of homeopathy.

The Causes of Cancer

The miasmatic background of cancer has been explored in the preceding chapters. Homeopathy also searches for the trauma or trigger which activated the dormant miasm. (For an excellent example of emotional and physical traumas waking up a dormant miasm, see the last case at the end of this chapter.) A study of 16 cancer patients under homeopathic treatment in England revealed emotional stressors as well as characteristic emotional traits in the etiology of their cancers.[6] These emotional stressors and traits, with a few of the top associated remedies, are as follows:

Severe emotional stress: 15 of the 16 suffered from severe emotional stress in their interpersonal relationships. They were deeply affectionate, loving and devoted to their families *(Phosphorus, Calcarea)* and 12 of the 15 were actively engaged in nursing loved ones *(Cocculus, Causticum).* If the family member's illness ended in death, then grief was added to the previous emotional strain. Other sources of grief in these patients included lost love affairs (a differential diagnosis would be needed among the many grief remedies) and lack of love from the spouse (lack of emotional nourishment) for which we think of *Nat. mur., Ignatia, Carcinosin,* and *Staphysagria.*

Personality of the patient: Whether a person reacts to stress by becoming ill depends in part on ingrained qualities of personality which belong to the innate constitution. Some of the qualities frequently found in cancer patients include the following:
- a high degree of honor, honesty, and integrity *(Nat. mur., Arsenicum)*
- conscientiousness in business, work, and study *(Aurum)*
- a deep sense of loyalty towards family, friends, and in business *(Phosphorus, Calcarea)*
- sympathy for the welfare of others and devotion to caring for others (the remedies listed in "Mind, sympathetic," K86)
- uncomplaining about their own illness (Ailments from silent grief)
- mild and gentle in nature *(Pulsatilla, Staphysagria)*
- sensitive nature and resulting fear of offending others, thus sublimating emotions and demonstrating a spirit of self-sacrifice *(Ignatia).*

Other triggers in cancer: From the teachings of the old masters and my own experience, we can identify additional triggers beyond the emotional stress noted in the British study. Among the top triggers and their associated remedies are the following:

Vaccinations: we know that any vaccination can fuel the sycotic miasm, which will put speed behind any developing tumor if combined with another active miasm (*Thuja, Silica,* the other NWS vaccination remedies). In addition, a recent study at the Baylor College of Medicine demonstrated a link between a monkey virus in pre-1963 polio vaccines and possibly hundreds of cancer deaths. The researcher, Dr. Janet Rutel, said the association between the simian virus and human cancer, "is strong enough to warrant serious concern."

Trauma: The breast and uterus are vulnerable to tumor formation following blows; *Conium* is our most valuable remedy in all cases arising from a contusion of the breast or uterus, with *Bellis perennis* also useful in breast cancer arising from a blow.

Sexual abstinence: The lack of an outlet for the normal human sexual impulse can lead to a *Conium* state, whose end pathology is an indurated cancer of the prostate, cervix, or breast. For example, a man may develop prostate cancer when his wife dies and he suddenly lacks the opportunity for sex. This situation leads to a prostate carcinoma with the following symptoms:
- a constant urge to urinate with little or not result
- urgency at night, repeatedly waking the patient, but only a few drops can be produced
- ineffectual urging with perspiration, a headache, and/or vertigo
- loss of seminal fluid by merely thinking of sex or touching a woman ("Emission, prostatic fluid, emotion, with every," and "Emission, prostatic fluid, during lascivious thoughts," both K667).
- an enlarged and hardened prostate gland.

Conium is the top remedy for cervical cancer and can still be used when the cancer has metastasized to the brain and bones.

Supporting the Family of Cancer Patients

Before we explore how homeopathy can help cancer patients themselves, we will take a look at how it can support their families in their ordeal, which often includes great anxiety, physical exhaustion, and loss of sleep when caretaking the family member throughout the night.

Nightwatching: This condition occurs in the family members of any patient whose condition requires caring for them throughout the night, when physical exhaustion is combined with emotional anguish. *Cocculus* is probably the best remedy for this situation, especially if the person becomes forgetful from exhaustion after putting out so much energy for the patient. People who need Cocculus have lost energy on all three planes: the mental plane (manifesting as forgetfulness), emotional (grief and anxiety about their family member's health), and physical (weakness, tiredness, vertigo). The Cocculus person typically manages to hold it together as long as the family member needs her, then falls apart as soon as the patient dies. *Causticum* is another useful remedy for nightwatching, but Causticum is more often indicated when the person has suffered a number of losses in a short time, resulting in a feeling of paralysis and manifesting as forgetfulness, stuttering, tics, etc. The Causticum state comes more often from the blows of repetitive griefs knocking down the Vital Force, while the Cocculus state usually comes from a lack of sleep.

Anxiety about health and fear of cancer: Family members often develop this fear when they see another family member dying from cancer. If we want to repertorize the fear of cancer, we can use "Fear, cholera, of the," K43, (because "Fear of cancer" does not appear in Kent, and cholera was the deadly disease so much dreaded in Kent's time). We can also use "Fear of death" and "Fear of impending disease," and we will see that Arsenicum is very much indicated. But Nitric acid also has anxiety about disease and fear of death, connected to a fear of the expense, dependency, and immobility resulting from a long-term degeneration. *Nitric acid* is especially indicated if the fear of cancer leads to the typical Nitric acid "4 P's" personality: pissed, pest, pessimistic, and never pleased. These people are very irritable and do not hesitate to use vulgar language. Dissatisfaction is their most prominent aspect, as well as despair about recovery to the point where they say, "nothing can be done for me" (a syphilitic expression). They are always complaining and unforgiving (syphilitic). They finally become nihilists, not believing in anything. They lose all hope and any motivation to do things. An *Arsenicum* will be less irritable and pesty, but still will keep complaining out of overriding anxiety.

Anxiety about germs (when they have to be careful about avoiding infection): Of course this is most likely *Arsenicum,* but it can also lead to obsessive handwashing, which may also indicate *Syphilinum.*

Depression: The remedy needed will depend on the particular form of depression. *Aurum* is a top remedy, especially when depression occurs in an elderly person who has lost his lifelong spouse. It could be enormously helpful in nursing homes. *Nat. mur.* is often needed after the death of a child, and *Phosphoric acid* when the quality of life is lost. Phosphoric acid stands for homesickness in its larger sense, meaning a longing for the way of life the person once had; taking care of a cancer patient requires putting one's own life on hold, which may result in a loss of career and social opportunities. Or the caretaker may feel resentment alternating with guilt, suppressed anger and irritability, indicating the need for Aurum. These emotions need to be expressed or treated, not suppressed, since otherwise they may lead to disease. Henny Heudens-Mast recently presented the case of a woman who had had to give up a career which meant everything to her in order to care for her elderly, abusive, and controlling mother. The patient's reaction, "I hope I die sooner than my mother does," just might come true, since by the time she came to Henny she already had breast cancer metastasized to the bones.[7]

Guilt that a family member has cancer: People often ask, "What did I do wrong that my child got cancer?" This leads to depression, anxiety, indecisiveness and exhaustion. *Phosphorus* and *Calcarea* personalities are especially susceptible to this kind of feeling. While *Aurum* and *Nat. mur.* are two of the top guilt remedies, look out for a delusion like "Delusion, thinks he is singled out for divine vengeance," K34, which can indicate the need for *Kali bromatum,* especially if it is confirmed by other typical Kali bromatum indications like restless hand movements or handwringing. The delusions "neglected her duty" and "wrong, fancies he has done wrong:" indicate especially Aurum first, *Ignatia* second. Aurum is strong physically and mentally, but emotionally very vulnerable.

Grief, especially when the patient dies: A differential diagnosis with our grief remedies will be necessary. No doubt *Ignatia, Nat. mur., Aurum, Phosphoric acid,* and *Cocculus* will frequently be needed in this situation. Ignatia, Nat. mur., Aurum, and Cocculus are discussed elsewhere in this chapter. Phosphoric acid appeals to those patients who derive the most comfort from close communication with and support from their loved ones (i.e. the Phosphorus and Calcarea types). The longing for the lost quality of life (metaphorically, the "homesickness" so typical of Phosphoric acid) can transform an initially bubbly personality into someone who is completely indifferent, who shuts out the world by unplugging the phone and lying in bed with her face to the wall.

Feelings of abandonment or resentment against a family member is understandable, if it occurs when one has to totally sacrifice her own time and interests to care for another, or when a child feels robbed of her childhood when it is dominated by an ill sibling. An ill grandparent or aunt may move into the household and may be resented as an intruder by children who perceive the patient as totally dominating their mother's time. Even worse, the oldest child may be forced to take on a parental role with her younger siblings, even if she is barely into her teens. Resentment may be felt against the ill person who competes for the caretaker's time, against the caretaker herself, or both. *Phosphorus, Calcarea,* and *Pulsatilla* children are especially vulnerable to feelings of abandonment. The child may react with rage (Calcarea leading into *Stramonium*) or with clinginess (Pulsatilla). Either reaction is taxing for the mother who is already mentally, emotionally, and physically exhausted. A woman may react with anger toward her dying husband ("How dare you leave me to raise the children alone?") yet feel guilty for her anger at the same time. This combination of grief, a sense of abandonment, anger, and guilt indicates that Nat. mur. can be very helpful.

Emotional Symptoms of Cancer Patients

Hearing the bad news: Any diagnosis of a potentially fatal disease is a tremendous blow to the Vital Force, and a diagnosis of cancer more so than others because of the suffering and intractable pain involved. Patients of different constitutions will react differently to this shock, however. A *Sulphur* will get as much information as possible, from books, the Internet or through a second opinion. He will not take any nonsense and his physician had better be prepared to answer some tough questions. A *Calcarea* will remain passive in his treatment plan; if given a choice, however, he will want to avoid painful procedures. A *Phosphorus* might be shocked but will keep smiling. She will be more concerned for her children and her husband than for herself, wondering, "What will they do without me?" An *Arsenicum* knew all along she would get cancer, it was just a matter of time. Fortunately, Arsenicum has a strong psoric constitution and tend to have the psoric sense of keeping up the struggle. In the Arsenicum, this will take the form of research (like the Sulphur) but with the added twist of demanding ever more lab tests just to monitor any little change in an already-diagnosed tumor. A *Pulsatilla* will start crying, reaching out to you the physician for some reassuring words. As long as you provide consolation, hope and a shoulder to lean on, a Pulsatilla will follow your treatment plan.

If the practitioner recognizes the constitution of the patient right away, a 10M dose of the constitutional remedy will be a good first prescription to support the patient's Vital Force and strengthen her on all planes. If the constitution is not immediately obvious, two remedies stand out for the acute treatment of "hearing bad news": Gelsemium and Ignatia. What is the difference?

- *Gelsemium* is helpful for the patient paralyzed by the bad news, characterized by the seven D's: dumb, dopey, dull, down, dizzy, disoriented, drowsy. These are not helpful qualities if one has to take charge of his condition and plan a possible treatment. In my practice I have found it one of the most common remedies to use when the Vital Force is knocked down by the "bad news," which is often delivered brusquely by a physician whose medical school unfortunately did not include training in this difficult and sensitive area. Upon hearing his diagnosis, all of a sudden the patient has become a "cancer victim." In order to treat a cancer patient successfully we must help bring back his Vital Force, which at this point is suffering far more from the impact of "hearing bad news" than from the cancer itself. Gelsemium will have a remarkable effect on the energy level of the patient who feels the wind knocked out of her sails, who feels exhausted yet cannot sleep (the Gelsemium keynote "sleepiness with sleeplessness").

- *Ignatia:* this patient reacts entirely differently. Her first reaction is "Why me?" and " I can't believe this is happening to me." Then there are Ignatia's three S's: sitting, sighing and sobbing. The reaction to the bad news is more hysterical and emotional: she may have difficulty swallowing, sometimes due to a globus hystericus; she sits and sighs (which means finding relief in a deep breath). She might just sit by herself, crying out loud, "God, why did you abandon me?" Sometimes she does not say a word, you just see her lips trembling, but then she can start crying hysterically. She may neglect her self-care needs, although eating the refrigerator empty when upset is a typical Ignatia sign. She may have monomania (all thoughts concentrated on one topic) or want to be carried (desiring support or continued attention). As you can see, Gelsemium reacts mainly with a lack of mental and physical energy, Ignatia mainly with emotional symptoms.

Extreme fear of death and anxiety about the disease: Because of the intensity of the impact of the bad news, the *Arsenicum* patient often takes the "symptom elevator" down to the lowest level, skipping the physical symptoms and immediately becoming submerged in the mental/emotional. The patient is tortured at night, with relentless thoughts about what to do, and with anxiety, fear and fright, especially about dying. He moves from side to side in bed, even wanting to move from one bed to another in spite of great prostration. The Arsenicum's deep-seated insecurity hinders him in this situation and his always present *dependency* on people will be even more outspoken. While an Arsenicum type tends to *want* someone constantly near him for reassurance and support, the Arsenicum cancer patient actually *needs* this. His well-known fastidiousness might well take a turn for the worse: he might become obsessive-compulsive, driving everyone around him crazy with trying to avoid the omnipresent micro-organisms. His normal anxiety about his health will become much more urgent. Death is near, in his eyes, and the practitioner will be assaulted with daily reports from the anguished Arsenicum. Thank God, his psoric nature keeps at bay the final stage in which he will view everything with suspicion (your remedy included). At that point he will lose interest in life and may even develop a suicidal disposition. Only a dose of Arsenicum can calm such a person. Other remedies for this extreme anxiety about health can be found under "Mind, fear, death, of," K44, and "Mind, fear, cholera, of the," K43.

Fear of recurrence of the cancer: We can repertorize this fear as fear of disaster *(Pulsatilla),* of impending disease *(Phosphorus, Kali carb.),* fear that her health is ruined *(Chelidonium),* fear of misfortune *(Medorrhinum, Psorinum,* and *Cimicifuga,* who feels she has a black cloud over her head), despair of recovery *(Psorinum),* and fear of suffering physical pain *(Aurum).*

Worry about the future: In addition to *Arsenicum, Argentum nitricum* is one of the top remedies for this condition, characterized by constant thoughts of "What if?" (obsessing about all the things that might go wrong).

Grief over all the losses involved in cancer: loss of health, loss of quality of life, loss of the possibility of a future (especially for a young person with a terminal condition): we will need a differential diagnosis among all our grief remedies. Two that stand out are *Pulsatilla,* when there is weepiness and clinginess with a constant desire for company, and *Nat. mur.,* when weeping is considered a childish reaction and suppressed, frequently with an aggravation of somatic complaints from suppressed grief.

Despair about the future, to the point of considering suicide: *Aurum* is one of our top suicide remedies and also covers the intractable pain associated with the later stages of cancer when it has metastasized to the bone. Aurum will relieve the pain and thus indirectly relieve the impulse to end the unbearable suffering; it will also address the suicidal impulses directly, as it has a long history of relieving depression and despair. (Hahnemann chose to experiment with Aurum as one of the early homeopathic remedies because of its use in medieval Arabic medicine for despair and suicidal depression.)

Anger at being ill: when it manifests itself as irritability, *Nux vomica* will have a calming effect. When it is accompanied by a sense of resentment and injustice, *Causticum* will be indicated.

Restlessness can have two forms, physical and mental/emotional. *Arsenicum* can cover both for cancer patients; when the restlessness comes from intractable bone pain, *Aurum* will be indicated.

Physical Symptoms of Cancer Patients Already Under Allopathic Treatment

The following remedies will be useful in treating the symptoms typical of cancer patients (as well as many other patients). The list of symptoms was gathered from patients at a prominent cancer research institution; some are produced by the tumor itself, others by the treatment. In either case the proper remedy can relieve some of their discomfort.

Shortness of breath in lung cancer patients will be helped with *Arsenicum* (which covers the terror associated with not being able to breathe) and *Carbo veg.*, which helps in any situation of hypoxia (birth trauma, drowning victims, etc.) When there are metastases to the abdomen, the dyspnea can be associated with a feeling of an elastic band across the chest or around the abdomen. This is the classic hoop or band sensation typical for *Anacardium*. Anacardium will be even more clearly indicated if the patient has a new-found tendency to swear and possibly a typical Anacardium delusion such as a separation between the mind and body or the sense of being double. Remember too the striking difference of indigestion between Anacardium and Nux vomica. The Nux vomica indigestion is worse during the digestive process, immediately after eating, and for the next two hours. But Anacardium's indigestion always *improves* with eating, only peaking two hours after eating, when the digestion is complete. Anacardium's symptoms tend to be intermittent in any case, but they always improve by eating. Anacardium also relieves distension in the abdomen.

Complications of steroids: To prevent osteoporosis, we should not hesitate to give every patient on chronic steroid use a daily dose of *Calc phos.* 6x. To prevent contagious illnesses in immune-suppressed patients, *Thuja* in a low potency (6c or LM) might be necessary. Thuja is also effective in general against the side effects of cortisone. Better than addressing the side effects, however, is to find the simillimum in the hope of obviating the need for further cortisone treatment. For the emotional upheavals associated with steroid use, *Pulsatilla* will be helpful, with its keynotes of irrational moodiness and an exaggerated need for attention.

Post-herpetic pain syndrome (the terrible burning pain which lasts for months after a shingles attack and for which allopathic medicine can provide no relief): "*Mezereum* [is] of great service in herpes zoster, both during and after for the neuralgia remaining, especially if the pains are burning."[8] *Variolinum* was Burnett's chief remedy in shingles, generally eradicating the disease, eruption and pain as well. It will also cure neuralgia left by herpes.

Post-thoracotomy pain, any post-surgical pain: *Staphysagria* is an excellent remedy in general for pain in surgical incisions, especially when it lingers months or even years after the surgery. *Calendula* 200c can be used immediately after surgery to heal the incision and prevent infection; it can be dissolved in water and taken internally as well as applied externally, as an exception to the general prohibition against applying the remedies to broken skin.

Burning pain radiating to the upper shoulders, secondary to metastatic lesions in the spine:
- Right scapula, *Bryonia* or *Chelidonium*
- In between the scapulae, *Phosphorus*
- Left scapula, *Ranunculus bulbosus*.
- Of course the other remedies for burning pains *(Rhus tox., Sulphur, Arsenicum* and *Phosphorus)* can be indicated at any time.

Intractable pain (in any condition but often seen in cancer patients): *Hypericum or Kalmia*. Both have similar pains (neuralgic, tingling, with numbness, rapidly shifting pains) but the pain of Kalmia radiates downwards. For deep bone pains arising from metastases e.g. to the spine, *Aurum* will be indicated. Aurum also covers the deep despair, even suicidal ideation, arising from relentless and unbearable pain with no relief in sight. When the pain is shooting, tearing, and stitching in the lower extremities, two remedies stand out: *Belladonna* and *Plumbum*. We all know Belladonna, but the role of Plumbum in cancer patients becomes even more apparent when we think about the atrophy, wrist drop and foot drop associated with this remedy. A great Plumbum keynote is the sense of retraction (in abdomen, cheeks, extremities, etc).

Iatrogenic consequences of radiation/chemotherapy:
- Stomatitis, so painful that the patient is unable to eat
- Dry mouth
- Persistent nausea with no relief
- Nausea that is delayed, appearing days after radiation or chemotherapy
- Gagging with vomiting
- A bitter or metallic taste in the mouth after treatment
- Sweating
- Anemia and prostration (Phosphorus is the top remedy for this condition)

Until recently, damage to the immune system was the main reason that patients had to stop chemotherapy. Now the worst part for many patients with chemotherapy or radiation is the production of mouth sores (ulcers like canker sores but much worse) on the tongue, lips, cheeks, and inside of the mouth, so painful that the patient cannot eat or talk. Cancer patients are already susceptible to wasting, and these mouth sores interfere with the absorption of much-needed nutrients. This problem has now become the number-one reason why cancer patients have to stop their therapy. Out of 1.2 million new cancer cases each year, 400,000 patients will develop oral complications from their treatment, many to the point that they will need morphine or have to stop treatment altogether. Patients who have bone marrow transplants are at even greater risk (75% to 80%) of severe oral complications. Once the lining of the mouth is damaged, patients lose a key physical barrier to infection.[9]

As for dry mouth, head and neck cancers (30,000 new cases each year) are treated with radiation which destroys salivation. Saliva is essential not only because it lubricates the mouth but also because it contains proteins that fight viruses, yeast and bacteria. Without saliva, patients have difficulty speaking, chewing, and fighting infection. But it is especially chemotherapy, more than radiation, which will damage the mouth mucosa. Tests are now underway for an experimental drug for these mouth sores, but one has to question whether this suppressive treatment will weaken the Vital Force.

Radium bromide, X-ray and Cadmium sulph. are the three remedies essential for treating the side effects of radiation/chemotherapy.

Radium bromide is used to heal radiation burns with resulting ulcerations and severe aching pains all over; and erythema, burning, and itching of the skin. Patients typically report feeling "as if my whole body is on fire." It also works well for staff members working in an X-ray department who develop dermatitis. In addition to palliating treatment-related side effects, it is a great curative remedy for many skin cancers. It also covers weakness, tiredness, and a metallic taste in the mouth.

X-ray boosts patients with low vitality, chronic fatigue, and a sick feeling after chemotherapy, radiation, or cobalt therapy. (The remedy is made by exposing water to X-ray radiation before potentizing it.) X-ray arouses the vitality, mentally and physically. It is also indicated for the mouth sores from treatment; anemia; radiation dermatitis (dry, scaly, itching eczema); and nausea with a sick feeling in the stomach. It can be used when there is paucity of symptoms because it will rouse the overpowered vitality. It is great for a deep X-ray burn (the top remedy in this condition, the second being Radium bromide).

Cadmium sulph. relieves the intense gagging and retching after chemotherapy and upper chest/abdominal radiation. It has a profound action on the stomach, especially when the patient has burning and cutting pain and even vomiting with extreme exhaustion and prostration. The patient may also have extreme chilliness. It also prevents or relieves the hair loss, anorexia, liver damage, and anemia caused by chemotherapy and radiation. It is also a great curative remedy for stomach cancer with coffee-ground vomitus.

Remedies for the Precancerous State

Allopathic medicine recognizes certain conditions as precancerous: polyps in the colon can be early signs of colon cancer, just as certain kinds of moles can be precursors of skin cancer. Even with this knowledge, allopathic medicine is unable to prevent the cancer, at least according to our homeopathic understanding of the progression of disease. Removal of the polyps or the suspicious-looking moles may lead to the illusion of preventing the cancer, but as a form of suppression it tends to accelerate the formation of cancer either at the same site or in a deeper organ. Cancer in general, even when expressed as a benign tumor, cannot be considered a local affection which initially does not affect the rest of the body. Allopathy considers a tumor as a local affliction at first, which only becomes generalized when it metastasizes (injects more of its toxins into the bloodstream). In other words, spreading is secondary. Hence the crux of the allopathic approach is to diagnose the local lesion as early as possible, and upon its discovery, to attack it and eradicate it with the strongest measures available. But in the homeopathic view, a localized tumor is like any other exterior expression of a deeper, generalized miasmatic state. A melanoma can be a point of discharge for the mighty sycotic miasm. Thus in homeopathy cancer is considered a systemic or generalized condition even *before* it expresses itself as a local exterior formation. Many moles, for instance, can lay dormant for many years, only to evolve into malignant metastasizing cancers because of the use of local suppressive techniques (surgery, laser, cauterization, radiation, etc.).

In any case, the polyp or mole represents the formation of pathology. Structural change has already taken place on the physical plane. Allopathic medicine has no effective way to predict or prevent these precancerous pathological changes. In homeopathy we turn the clock back to a previous stage, before any structural changes take place. The homeopathic view of the precancerous state is based on an understanding of the Never Well Since and the miasmatic background of the patient. We seek to cure the susceptibility to cancer before any visible or measurable change takes place (see Fig. 24-1).

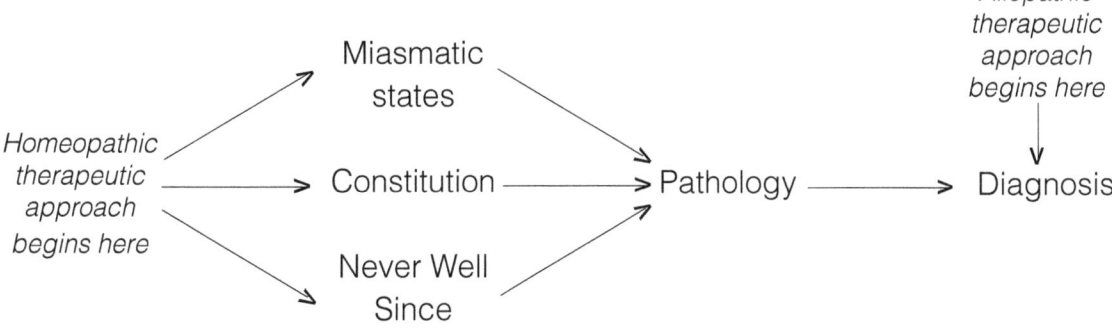

Fig. 24-1: Homeopathic and Allopathic Approaches to Treating Cancer

We have no way of proving that cancer might have developed in a particular patient, but we have the satisfaction of knowing, as the old masters found, that patients treated homeopathically have a far lower incidence of tumors than those who are not. We know that if we look at the timeline of a cancer patient, we often see an emotional trauma such as the death of a lifelong spouse just before the onset of the cancer. We also know that if we do a miasmatic analysis of the patient's past medical history and family history we will see more than one active miasm. Based on these observations, we treat patients for grief before pathology ever develops. We treat patients for the signs of an active miasm (recurrent -*itis* infections following a series of vaccinations, for example) long before the miasm can produce a tumor. This is what we consider precancerous prescribing. The top remedies useful in this situation (in a 6c or LM potency) are described below.

Keeping this in mind, homeopaths avoid tonsillectomies through careful prescribing, to avoid depriving the child of these valuable immune-system glands. Homeopaths would also rather see the child catching all the childhood diseases instead of having a multiplicity of vaccinations, in which foreign substances are injected into the bloodstream. Childhood illnesses boost the Vital Force rather than lowering it. Thus the best preventive measures for cancer involve intervention at the level of the miasms, the constitution and the Never Well Since, as expressed in Figure 24-1.

Allopathy's goal in this cycle is to establish a diagnosis of cancer, followed by a protocol treatment. Little attention is heeded to the constitution of the patient, as well as the NWS (especially the all-important mental-emotional) while the miasmatic theory in allopathy is still limited to genetic mapping without any therapeutic treatment plans linked to it. Homeopathy has already incorporated in the cancer treatment as well as the treatment of any disease, the first important three steps.

Thuja is the king of sycosis, the miasm which produces neoplasms (the proliferative or growing miasm), many of which are benign (polyps, cysts, adenomas). Remember, however, that an active sycotic miasm will put speed behind the growth of a tumor. If we see an active sycotic miasm in a patient (many -itis diseases, etc.), treating with Thuja will help to prevent the possible future formation of a sycotic tumor.

Lachesis is also one of the top remedies for precancerous and starting cancer cases, especially uterine cancer. Since it is such a great remedy for perimenopause and menopause, it is especially useful for cancer in women at this stage, especially when accompanied by vertigo, hot flashes, palpitations, and hypertension. As we would expect from Lachesis, the patient is better from menses, worse from menopause.

Lycopodium: Antipsorics like Sulphur and Lycopodium evolve towards cancer through hepatic insufficiency. Their action fortifies against the precancerous state. In confirmed cancer Lycopodium has little value, however, since it has no power over the tumoral element as do Thuja or Lachesis. The Lycopodium subject will tend to develop cancer of the liver, stomach or intestine.

Sulphur, king of the antipsorics, is reserved for the pretumoral stage (because psora gives only functional disturbances). Like Lycopodium, it has no favorable action in a confirmed cancer, even at the start. However it can help to prevent cancer of the GI tract or abdominal viscus from developing from abdominal arteriovenous hypertension, an intense portal congestion which is both arterial and venous in patients with hypertension.

Sepia, like Sulphur and Lycopodium, works better on the predisposition to cancer than on the tumor itself. It has an action similar to that just described for Sulphur, reducing abdominal congestion in the pelvis developing from portal hypertension, but in this case the condition is entirely venous and without arterial involvement (as is typical of Sepia, which is characterized by venous stasis). Unless treated with Sepia, this condition will tend to develop towards a cancer of the pelvic organs.

Petroleum is known for treating skin eruptions similar to those of Sulphur. Overexposure to petroleum (as in those working with petroleum products, like garage mechanics) can lead to skin cancer, beginning with a precancerous condition characterized by the typical Petroleum cracks in the skin < in winter and from cold.

Calcarea is indicated among the precancerous hypothyroid patients who are hypersensitive and chilly, with flaccid muscles. The subject wastes rapidly after an initial phase of false plethora and fatty invasion. (Of the other two great calcium salts, *Calc. fluor.* is only useful once cancer has already formed, while *Calc. phos.* has hardly any action either in cancer or in the precancerous state.)

Precancerous cases often require *Kali carb.* (for weakness, chills, lumbar pains, sweats, and wasting) or *Kali bich.* (for a gastric or pyloric ulcer which can develop into malignant degeneration).

Arsenicum, a very important cancer remedy, is also one of the top precancerous remedies, often indicated by the patient's prostration, agitation, burning pains, and amelioration from heat. It will bring great relief in very weak precancerous patients. There must be a nervous restlessness, a mental restlessness which is unlike the muscular restlessness of Rhus tox.

Nitric acid is effective in patients with a tendency to ulcers and fissures, debility, progressive wasting and thinning.

Cancer Remedies Proper

Of the many remedies useful in treating cancer, those prescribed purely on homeopathic indications are presented first. Next are the remedies which tend to be prescribed for their specific sphere of action in certain organs or tissues, especially when the remedies can be confirmed by mental/emotional or other homeopathic indications. At the end are certain remedies known to be specific for certain cancers, although this goes against our prohibition against allopathic prescribing. I feel they are worth including here because the old masters had the opportunity to experiment and develop a body of knowledge about remedies for cancer which we will never be able to duplicate. Kent's *Repertory* has one great rubric on page 1346 ("Cancerous affections") but many rubrics for cancer or tumors may be found throughout the repertory.

Arsenicum can be used in all forms of cancer at any stage, from the great fears and anxiety right from the time of the diagnosis, through all the stages of formation of the cancer, to relieving the fear and restlessness as the patient takes his dying breath.

Mercury is indicated when there is bleeding ulceration, aggravation at night, prostration, night sweats, oral fetor. It is especially effective digestive cancers, especially in Mercury's greatest arena of action, the mouth and throat. It is a very important remedy for metastases in the bone which eat away at the bone and cause pains worse at night. (Calcarea is the first remedy if the bone pains are as bad during the day, e.g. after breast cancer metastasizes to the bones and the bones begin to break.) Remember that Merc. corrosivus is a deeper working Merc-sol. and therefore will be greatly indicated in destructive, ulcerating, and bleeding tumors.

Nitric acid is indicated when the cancer forms ulcers, fissures or fistulas (i.e. for syphilitic cancers, like Mercury). If it cannot reverse the syphilitic destruction, at least it can relieve the pain and the wasting.

Carbo animalis is one of the best remedies for established cancer, indicated by hard tumors, indurated and swollen lymph glands, bluish discoloration, and burning pains. It has a special selective action on breast and stomach cancer and merits special mention, not only for its beneficial effects on cachexia but also for its action on the tumor itself, which may regress and become softer and less painful. It is also one of our best palliatives for cancer anywhere in the body, especially breast cancer, cervical cancer, and cancers of the glands like Hodgkin's lymphoma. Think about Carbo animalis when the case is not progressing, especially if there is ulceration. There is often weakness and depletion of vitality. The patient is chilly and susceptible to colds and infections. It has a special affinity for glands, both exocrine and endocrine. The affected organs become slowly indurated and there is great burning, especially when touched. Mentally the patient tends to be gloomy, homesick (3), and preoccupied (3) ("lost in thoughts," K64). The patient tends to feel cold, especially at night in bed, and feels worse from cold. Swollen and indurated glands can occur throughout the body (thus it is also a good AIDS remedy). The patient feels very weak (thus it is also a good chronic fatigue remedy) with burning pains. It is especially effective in cancers of the face, nose, mouth, and throat; the testes, ovaries and cervix; malignant ulcers; and breast cancer characterized by slowly progressive masses with burning sensation and lymphadenopathy.

Hydrastis (goldenseal) is known in homeopathy primarily for the treatment of cancer, especially gastric cancer, although it is equally good for breast cancer. It is especially indicated in patients with progressive debility and wasting. It improves the appetite and condition of the patient in general, including better complexion and less pain. The pus associated with Hydrastis is thick, yellow and burning, and the tongue is coated with yellow on the back and in the center (it is effective for cancers of the tongue). A long, deep and slow-acting remedy, it is also effective for many precancerous conditions such as abscesses and ulcers. It works more deeply on the liver than Carduus or Chelidonium. According to Dr. John Clarke, and later confirmed by many other great homeopaths, it has cured more cancers than any other remedy, especially of the colon, liver and stomach. Disturbances of the digestive system are always a prominent symptom.

Indications for Hydrastis in mammary cancer include:
- general exhaustion, a sensation of weakness, profound asthenia
- depression and melancholia with loss of appetite
- cancer before ulceration when pain is principal symptom
- straw-colored skin, sallow complexion
- constant pains of a burning type at the level of a mammary glands which become < at night
- hard and painful, irregular enlargement of breast with nipple retracted.

Thuja should be used, if possible, to prevent a tumor from forming in the first place when the sycotic miasm is active. However, it can also act successfully in actual cancer cases if the tumor is still localized and not too malignant. The old masters used it successfully in sarcomas, degenerated adenomas of the breast, and cutaneous epitheliomata (squamous cell carcinomas of face, lips, etc).

Iodium is indicated when the patient is weak and debilitated, wasting rapidly in spite of a good appetite (tubercular miasm). Patients who need it tend to have indurated glandular growths (breast, uterus, lymphatic glands, thyroid, etc.). It often reverses the wasting tendency and can even cause the tumor to regress, or at least it can diminish the tumor's induration and invasive tendency. (While we often think of Nat. mur. in patients with wasting, Nat. mur. is more indicated in upper-body wasting, while the cancer patient will have wasting over the whole body and thus Iodium will be indicated instead of Nat. mur.)

Silica acts especially on the connective tissues, for example in cicatricial degenerations (keloids) and in new fibrous tissue produced by sclerosis. While Thuja is mentally obsessed and Iodium is a depressed melancholic and anxious type, Silica is a hypersensitive anxious type who can also have fixed ideas like Thuja. Silica wastes very rapidly, like Iodium.

Kali iodatum, the secret ingredient in alternative cancer cures such as the Hoxsie formula, is an excellent cancer remedy. (It is known that disturbances of the potassium metabolism exist in cancers, as well as those of calcium, sodium and magnesium.) Kali iodatum is an antisyphilitic, addressing the secondary stage of the miasm. According to Grimmer, it has cured many types of tumors arising from the syphilitic or tubercular miasm, with a combination of both miasm often present in a malignancy.[10]

Calc. fluor. is the only one of the three great calcium salts which is active against cancer, especially adenocarcinomas with stony induration. It is especially effective in breast and uterine cancers with this indication. From what we know of its action on exostoses, it is not surprising that is highly effective against bony growths, although it is equally effective for fistulas and for ulcerations of the bone (syphilitic expressions). Induration (hardening) with threatening suppuration is a marked indication. Calc. phos. and Calcarea are not helpful once a tumor is formed.

A special place should be given to the cadmium salts, Cadmium sulph., Cadmium metallicum, Cadmium iodatum and Cadmium oxidatum. All these cadmiums are active against Hahnemann's three primary miasms.

Cadmium sulph. was already discussed before for the side effects of radiation and chemotherapy. One should remember the great weakness, accompanied by strong cachexia, typical for advanced cancer states. It acts mainly on the gastrointestinal tract.

Cadmium metallicum has violent vomiting and is (together with Cadmium oxidatum) the best antidote against the aluminum poisoning, so pervasive in our society.

Cadmium iodatum, like all iodatums, is warmblooded and active against cancers of all the glands (neck, tonsils, thyroid, testicles, ovaria).

Cadmium oxidatum is the most active of all the cadmium salts. It has a great reviving action in intractable cancer cases.

Conium has been used for malignant, cancerous affections of the glands; the infiltration gradually grows into a stony hardness. It is also for schirrous cancers. It has cured fibroid tumors of the uterus (Kent) and in my own experience it can change the results of a Pap smear down to a Class I from a higher class within a matter of weeks.

Bellis perennis is indicated when trauma or severe cold is the exciting factor. Give ten drops of the tincture (but not too late at night because it makes the patient restless and sleepless). It looks much like Arnica with its soreness but it has glandular involvement which is not so marked in Arnica. It also looks like Conium but can be differentiated from Conium in the large majority of cases by its painlessness.

Phytolacca is used in hard or scirrhous cancers since it can soften and diminish them. Many breast cancers as well as cancers of the uterus and rectum have been cured with Phytolacca, called the vegetable Mercury. Burning pains, soreness, restlessness and prostration are guiding symptoms.

Asteria rubens (red starfish) was used medicinally as far back as the time of Hippocrates, who used it for uterine troubles. In homeopathy it is used mainly for painful cancers of the breast, especially a hard enlarged breast cancer when the breast is more painful before the menstrual cycle as well as giving sharp pains at night. There may enlarged axillary glands and a red spot suppurating with an unusually offensive odor. This remedy, like *Carbo animalis,* can be used even when breast cancer has reached the ulcerative stage. It is especially recommended for cancer of the left breast if it feels as though it is pulled inwards (the nipple is retracted).

Sepia is useful for cancer of the pelvic organs (uterus, rectum, sigmoid colon, or prostate). Note that while Sepia is commonly used for women's reproductive disorders, it can be used for prostate cancer as well, with the typical Sepia sensation "ball, sensation of sitting on a ball" (K667).

Kreosote is effective in cancer of the cervix and vagina when characterized by bleeding ulcerations, destruction of tissues and an excoriating, fetid, burning discharge. Bleeding after intercourse can be present.

Argentum nitricum is useful for cancer of the throat, stomach or uterus. Special indications include ovarian tumors and growths that bleed easily, and of course we would expect to see the typical mental/emotional symptoms.

Cundurango is used for cancers of the eyelids, lips, esophagus, stomach, intestines, and anus. Fissures are a valuable external sign for Cundurango, especially its keynote, "a painful crack in the right corner of the mouth." It alleviates the pains in stomach cancer where there is constant burning and vomiting.

Cadmium sulphate, used for cancer of stomach, is a cross between Arsenicum and Bryonia: the patient wants to be quiet, as in Bryonia, and has burning in the stomach and vomiting, as in Arsenicum.

Cholesterinum (homeopathic cholesterol) is most often useful for cancer of the liver, especially when there is hepatomegaly. The patient is cachectic, jaundiced, and holds his hands over his liver because it hurts to walk.

Tarentula cubensis is indicated where pain and inflammation are prominent or there is a far advanced, painful cancer in the last stage. This great anti-pain, antiseptic remedy should be used especially when there is unbearable burning pain and the abscess has a dark, black, leathery appearance. For example, patients with end-stage graft-host disease following a bone marrow transplant may become totally covered with black, abscessed skin as necrosis sets in. The condition is extremely painful and high doses of pain medications are usually required.

Petroleum, one of our great remedies for skin conditions, directs itself toward surface cancers (skin and digestive mucosae) and not towards the glands.

Sedum acre and *Sedum repens* were considered powerful antitumor remedies by the old masters. I have not had the opportunity to work with them extensively so I am including them here based on the enthusiasm of the old masters, who said that in mother tincture (1x and 3x), they have an undeniable action on cancer in general, can reverse cachexia, and occasionally modify the tumor or at least retard its progress. Their principal indication is the tendency to mucosal and cutaneous fissures which are so frequent in cancer. Sedum repens acts especially on the abdominal organs.

Scrofularia nodosa acts especially on the skin, breast, uterus, and rectum, especially if there is a marked glandular invasion; it is also indicated in Hodgkin's and non-Hodgkin's lymphoma.

Sempervivum tectorum is effective in lingual, breast, rectal and other cancers, especially cancers with a tendency to aphthae or to malignant ulcers, and in scirrhous induration of the tongue.

The following remedies have been found so effective for cancers in specific areas that they can almost be prescribed by the location of the tumor:

- *Graphites* for cancer in cicatrices
- *Phosphorus* for hepatic and pancreatic cancer
- *Ornithagulum* (Star of Bethlehem) for cancer of stomach and cecum; center of action is the pylorus.

Principles for the Homeopathic Treatment of Cancer

How far advanced the pathology is will influence our method of remedy selection as well as the potency used. In the early stages, we will use our method based on the miasmatic background, the Never Well Since, the mental/emotional characteristics, and so forth. But when the pathology is full-blown it takes on a life of its own and lesional prescribing is necessary. The symptoms in the case, even the mental/emotional ones, are secondary to the tumor. For example, we usually think of emotional states as providing the ground or soil in which a disease condition develops, and therefore we use them to find the remedy. But the fear and anxiety of a patient with advanced cancer are created by the disease, not the other way around. Of course we want to address the fear, and the last clinical case in this chapter provides a good example of this approach. But this will be just one aspect of our zigzag prescribing to cover the different symptoms generated by the cancer.

Surprisingly enough, the most malignant cases do not necessarily have the poorest prognosis, as long as we use the right potency. Dr. J.H. Clarke observes that malignant tumors are more easily *acted* upon (although not necessarily cured):

> They are in a more active and, so to say, fluid state than the others. This I can amply confirm from my experience, even going further to say that they are acted upon medicinally in direct proportion to their malignancy, the most malignant of all showing infinitely stronger evidence of reaction than those which are slower in growth. For this reason I should like to sound a note of caution against acting too powerfully on far advanced malignant conditions, otherwise the sudden setting free of nature's recuperative forces may be attended with alarming consequences to the patient. Hence the vital importance of correctly judging the strength of the dose given and the frequency of its repetition.[11]

Like the other old masters, Clarke did not know about LM potencies and thus was expressing extra caution about the potency and frequency of the remedy. Even with LMs, however, we must remember that the body needs time to process and dispose of the debris produced by the breakdown of the tumor. If the blood cannot be filtered quickly enough, fatal septicemia can set in. Such a case is described by William Jackson, M.D. in an article entitled "Cancer cannot be cured, but the patient can":

> The area of the malignancy was the right testicle, which was 8 inches long and 4 inches in diameter, the prostate, the bladder, and the transverse and descending portions of the colon. The testicle had sloughed away, and was a comparatively normal organ after it was healed, about one quarter of its original size, at the time it had

completely healed, with practically no scar. The patient had urinated through the rectum for more than seven weeks, at which time he commenced to urinate from the bladder in a normal way. He recovered to such an extent that he was able to do yard chores such as mowing the lawn. After gaining to that extent, after 2 weeks he became ill again, and in about four weeks death resulted, just after his eighty-ninth anniversary *[birthday]*. Upon autopsy, I removed a full quart of pus (destroyed tissue) from the pelvic cavity before I was able to examine further. The bladder had completely healed, leaving scar tissue where the malignancy had existed before. The prostate had completely disappeared, and there were more than thirty areas on the descending and transverse colon where scar tissue existed. About half of these areas showed no evidence of malignant tissue, but the rest of them were partially healed.[12]

In approaching the patient, we must assess how much confidence she has in homeopathy, how urgent her condition is, and how much pressure she is under to pursue allopathic treatment. Legally we cannot recommend against suppressive treatment, but we can offer to support the patient no matter what choice she makes. For example, if she decides to have an operation, it is essential for her to approach it with a positive attitude. We will help her prepare for surgery with Phosphorus 200c beforehand (3 pellets dry) and afterwards if necessary (in 4 oz. of water, one teaspoon prn) to control hemorrhaging and protect against the effects of anesthesia; Calendula 200c before and after to promote wound healing and prevent infection; and Arnica 200c (before and after) to prevent swelling and extravasation. If she decides to delay an operation for several months while pursuing homeopathic treatment, we can explain this to her family and her oncologist by saying that she will gain strength for the operation. If the cancer is curable, we may see enough progress in a few months to justify postponing the suppressive treatment further. In general, it is better not to have the operation first and then begin homeopathic treatment afterwards, but sometimes surgery is urgent especially if the tumor is pressing on the vital organs.

If we are treating a patient newly diagnosed with cancer, it is usually advisable to treat the "hearing bad news" acutely with the constitutional remedy, Gelsemium or Ignatia first to strengthen the Vital Force *before* beginning the indicated remedy for the cancer.

We must remember to ask about old symptoms related to the affected organ, any traumas to the area, and any suppressive treatments. For example, in a patient with breast cancer, we would ask about symptoms during pregnancy and lactation; any blows to the breast; and any allopathic medical treatments for the cancer or any other conditions in the area (like Parlodel to stop the flow of milk, treatment for breast abscesses, or surgery for cysts).

Assessing Progress in a Cancer Case

J.G. Gilchrist gives the following benchmarks to assess the effects of a remedy in reversing tumor growth:

> We will find that the rapidity with which a remedial action is shown in a given case will depend upon the rapidity of the growth: slower in slow growths, and faster in rapid growths. It will, under the most favorable circumstances, require a long time, from days to weeks, for the effect of the remedy to be manifested. We will first note an evident gain in the patient's general condition. The pain, if any existed in the tumor, will become diminished; there will appear quite a troublesome itching or biting of the skin covering the tumor; the tumor will then remain stationary for a long time. Soon there will be a noticeable softening and increased mobility of the growth, with a change for the better in the appearance of the skin over the tumor. Should it have been discolored, it will appear more natural, should it have been adherent, it will become loosened. Of course increased mobility and softening may indicate suppuration or disintegration; but the symptoms of such an occurrence are well known and cannot be mistaken. We will now, in many cases, particularly if the tumor is a large one, notice the lymphatics in the region become somewhat enlarged, without pain or inflammation. From this point the tumor will rapidly subside and soon disappear, leaving no trace of its existence behind it.[13]

Homeopaths who treat cancer need to know this progression, both to enhance the patient's confidence and to keep a steady course with the single remedy in the face of all these changes. I have found other hints in the old masters: a severe cold with profuse coryza and much expectoration is a favorable sign, representing a natural healing crisis, because during such an attack the size of the tumor will diminish rapidly. Similarly a discharge of bloody serum from a breast indicates a tumor breaking up in the normal gland structure, while a vaginal discharge can indicate the breakdown of a cervical or uterine tumor. Itching is a positive sign of healing, in cancer as in many other conditions. The rapid growth of a tumor after administering a remedy may be terrifying to the patient, and to the practitioner if she is not expecting it; but it is often a sign of a good reaction, and the remedy should be continued until the growth stops. Another alarming development is the appearance of a tumor where none existed before; but as long as the overall condition is improving, this represents a positive evolution in the case and the remedy should not be changed.

On the other hand, sometimes we see no physical changes, no signs of a discharge or itching, yet the patient improves mentally, emotionally, and functionally with an overall increase in energy. Even if the pathology remains unchanged during this time, do not change the remedy, which is well-indicated. The potency/dosage may need to be increased before the pathology will disappear, since it is a one-sided disease.

Prompt relief of pain immediately after the remedy indicates that it is the simillimum, which will at least palliate if it is too late to cure.

In assessing the curability of patients with cancers, we must not be influenced by the size of the tumor. Instead, we will depend on the following guidelines.

- slowly or rapidly growing? (tumor doubling time)
- painful or painless?
- soft or hard?
- mobile or fixed?
- ulcerating or not?

A rapidly-growing cancer will have a poorer prognosis than a slow-growing one (at least when treated homeopathically, although this type of cancer may respond better to conventional treatment). A painful, hard, fixed, and/or ulcerating cancer is worse than when these conditions are not present. Sometimes the rapidity of growth can be predicted by the active miasms. A predominantly psoric cancer will be slow-growing while an active sycotic will create a fast-growing tumor and an active syphilitic miasm will create an ulcerating cancer. In other cases, the allopathic diagnosis can help us to determine which miasm is active, because certain cancers are known to be more rapidly growing than others. Slow growing cancers include papillary thyroid carcinoma, hemangiomas, and squamous cell carcinomas of the skin, while liver and pancreas cancers and large cell carcinomas of the lung are fast-growing, aggressive tumors.

Cancer Cases of the Old Masters

Case 1: Mrs K, 37 yrs old, married with two children by two different husbands. In 1924, patient was told that she had a tumor on the uterus, but that it would not interfere with becoming pregnant. A few months later she became pregnant and delivered a baby boy. Now she has been told by two different gynecologists that she has a big tumor on the uterus. One surgeon said she needs an operation at once, the other that she should go to the country for six weeks to get stronger and prepare for the operation.

The patient complaints of a drawing sensation deep in the lumbar region which comes on during emotional excitement and during menstruation. Menstruation has become prolonged, it lasts eight days now. The flow is red and plentiful. Whenever she douches the vagina she sees traces of blood clots in the water. There is blood on intercourse. All winter long she felt weak, unable to lift her baby. She is unrefreshed in the morning. During menses, she feels a sense of heaviness on the vertex of the head. It is like a pressure from without, > by lying and in open air, < by standing and after eating. This headache can come between periods.

She cannot stand the least bit of noise, sudden noises startle her. Music irritates her. She enjoys music, as such, but now it makes her cry. She can feel the heart beating when sitting and lying on her side, especially after the slightest emotional excitement. She does not feel her heart after walking.

She is fond of bread, but cannot eat it as it gives her a headache. Fond of salty foods. Fond of sweets but these affect her head. Is not thirsty. Sleep good but unrefreshed in the morning. She likes fresh air and enjoys being out, but for the last few years, she had desired a hot water bag at her feet in bed. She has much gas in her abdomen which makes her feel distended. This is relieved by flatus which has the smell of rotten eggs. Flatulence outspoken after milk. The stool has the same odor. There is a tendency to constipation and when not constipated, she has the feeling that the stool is insufficient. Patient has a tendency to depression and indefinite fears. Has crying spells, especially when alone, when writing or when thinking about life. She is very irritable, every little thing seems to irritate her.[14]

Treatment and followup:

Three weeks later: Patient reported that bleeding from vagina had ceased since the last menstruation which ended July 9. The period was not so painful, she did not feel weak during the period. Mentally lighter, not so depressed. Headache not so severe neither persistent during menses. Does not notice heart so much. No bad odor of stool. Better control over her mental faculties.

Analysis: The patient is reacting well so far. She is more centered and feels better mentally, emotionally and physically. If I were using centesimals, I would give Sac. lac. at this point. Using the LM potency, I would decrease the succussions and/or the dose.

The next followup was five years later. No further complaints, regular menses, q. 28 days, duration five days, profuse only two days. Patient never received another dose of the remedy. A recent gynecological examination showed complete absence of the tumor.

An analysis of this case and the remedy given is at the end of Appendix 4, Sample Cases.

Case 2: Cancer cases need a succession of remedies as the picture changes, much more so than other types of cases. A case written up by Dr. Edmund Carleton illustrates this.[15] The reader might try to find the remedies as they come up. The answers can be found at the end of Appendix 4, Sample Cases.

A business man of 55 years old was diagnosed by a specialist with cancer of the stomach and advised to have an immediate operation. The patient dreaded the operation especially since the specialist could not promise non-recurrence. His attacks of colic began in the stomach, extended to the left breast, then they were felt in the entire abdominal region and passed to the lower angle of the right shoulder blade, accompanied by a sensation of a belt pressing round the waist, with nausea and heartburn. The attacks were most severe from 11 a.m. till noon and from 4-6 p.m., when the stomach was empty and after swallowing cold substances. There existed great soreness of the stomach, made worse by the jar of stepping, > heat. Lying upon the right side caused also pain. He leaned backward to obtain relief from the excruciating pain. *Remedy A* was given in the CM potency in hot water, a tsp. every five minutes when the "colic" was on and discontinued when it abated. The remedy worked beautifully for 48 hours, and then was spent. Having giving a similar remedy [*a simile*], we were rewarded with a new picture of the disease. *[So increasing the potency will not help, we need a new remedy-Ed.].*

He now was apprehensive, restless, wanted to lie in bed a short time, next to sit in a chair, then to walk the floor, then to lie on the lounge, and so on; thirsty for little sips of water; desired external heat and was relieved by it; wanted two pillows instead of one. Of course he received *Remedy B* 200c in water q. 2 hours. This worked well for six days and then stopped. Comfort was followed by torment. He wanted one thin pillow only; his pains were paroxysmal, very marked, coming and going quickly, and characterized by throbbing, esp. at 3 p.m. and at midnight. Therefore *Remedy C* replaced remedy B. Improvement for a week was secured. Then a sudden sense of being full after eating a little, great distention from gas, and bowel rumbling from eating, all in the early evening and in last part of the day. *Remedy D, 200c* succeeded remedy C. Eight days of comfort followed then the symptoms were different. He had burning at the stomach outlet, saltish fluid rising in the mouth and offensive flatus. The medicine was changed to *Remedy E*, CM potency. It was a good prescription and helped quickly and this for 21 days.

It should be understood that during all these changes there was a real gain, each advance reaching a point a little higher than the one just before. Another remedy had to be chosen. This time the patient was thirsty for cold water, but water no colder than the room, produced nausea soon after reaching the stomach, followed by ejection of sour gas and liquid. This mighty indication of *Remedy F* reminded me of his propensity to eat salt, already mentioned. A 200c potency was given and worked for seven days. This long acting remedy in showing exhaustion so soon bore eloquent testimony to the strength and rapidity of the enemy with which we contended. I now suspected that greater results would have been gained from a single very high dose *[better, an LM dose]*. The case seemed to reverse to Remedy E. However it transpired that the flatus was hot and moist as well as offensive, < at night and after eating, flatus during diarrhea, which made the decision in favor of *Remedy G,* 200c. It worked well for twenty days.

Then an important change happened. "A faint, sinking feeling in the pit of the stomach, akin to hunger, around 11 a.m. No homeopath would miss *Remedy H*. Where was this coming from? He had been troubled in early manhood by suppurative tonsillitis. His throat was treated with powerful drugs and swabbed. His elongated uvula was amputated when he was 32. The wound bled for 4 days. Ever since then he wants to swallow and he cannot. He had bleeding piles and prolapsus of the bowel at stool, abolished by local applications. Observe a whole catalogue of suppression, followed by metastasis. What a demonstration of the truth of Hahnemann's teachings! I gave Remedy H in CM! For a number of weeks improvement followed. His complexion cleared, *the tumor disappeared,* sleep became natural and refreshing, he seemed to be well yet not strong. Then came an entirely different attack, in the guise of neuralgia which the patient informed me was an old enemy *[the Law of Hering!].* This neuralgia in the past had been suppressed by injections of morphine. Nature had taken revenge for all this abuse. How many times will it be necessary to show that no cure is ever brought by contraria? Under the influence of homeopathic remedies my patient's cancer had disappeared and his neuralgia reappeared at the original location (left occipital protuberance). He had cerebral and nervous exhaustion, sleep was impossible and he had extremely fidgety feet, especially in the evening. Without delay I gave him CM *Remedy I*. Six months later nothing wrong could be found anymore except two external piles which itched but did not bleed. A last dose of CM *Remedy J* soon cured. He remains well. *[bracketed, italicized comments added]*

Case 3: Another example of these succession of remedies is from Dr. Edmund Carleton.[16]

A middle-aged woman, the mother of one child, consulted me in April 1901 in regard to her right breast. I found a hard, irregular tumor with a retracted nipple, about the size of a goose's egg, adherent, the seat of lancinating pain. A sore lame feeling extended to the arm. The armpit glands were hard and swollen. She was a firm believer in homeopathy. My first prescription was Conium 200c, to be taken in water four times a day until improvement should be noticed. It was not sufficiently similar to the case and produced slight amelioration only. Phytolacca took its place. She had suffered pain during lactation, beginning in the nipple, radiating over the whole body when she was feeding the infant. This is characteristic of Phytolacca. (If it had been given then, would cancer have been developed later?) It held OK for ten months when improvement ceased and new symptoms appeared.

She had cherry-red lips, did not react well after a bath, and had a sinking feeling in the stomach at 11 a.m. I gave a dose of *Remedy A,* CM. It worked well for over three months, when its usefulness was ended. An irregular menstruation came on, accompanied with hot flushes, intolerance of pressure around the neck and poor sleep; all symptoms worse upon waking from sleep. *Remedy B* followed. During all these experiences the cancer became better. Two months later another dose of remedy A was needed. The medicine was effective for eleven months. In September we surveyed a vast improvement over the original case; but new indications appeared. There were more mental and physical exertion. Sharp pains in the breast were < from motion. Therefore *Remedy C,* CM was given. Improvement followed for two months. And then was rekindled by another dose of the same remedy which lasted until the beginning of next year. Jan. 7, 1902, after very close and persistent cross-questioning, I learned that the sharp pain in the breast was like a hot wire or needle thrust through the organ. I therefore prescribed with great confidence *Remedy D,* CM. It was the best prescription , helped more than any other preceded remedy and lasted over a month before repetition was needed. The second dose finished the case. She has remained well in every aspect. After a warfare which lasted three years, complete victory was ours.

Cancer Case Four: A One-Sided Disease

This is one of my own cases, presented to demonstrate miasmatic analysis of the patient's past medical history and family background. It also shows how to prescribe for advanced pathology, for the one-sided disease which has overpowered the Vital Force.

Chief Complaint: Maria is the 63-year-old divorced mother of two adult children. Her main complaint is a constant aching pain in her spine at the level of T9/T10. She was diagnosed with right-sided breast cancer in 7/97, with metastasis diagnosed 4/98 to the bone, including the cranium (9/98). She describes her back pain as "aching all over and throbbing in the mid to lower back going from left to right, and then descending to the left hip to the right hip." The pain is < 4 p.m., > 11 a.m. She also experiences a stitching and stabbing pain in the ribs and chest, making it difficult to breathe, especially on deep respiration. Pain < damp weather, movement and sitting, > lying down with several pillows behind the head. "I feel weak all the time, no energy, drained." She was tearful during the interview and expressed hope that she will beat the cancer.

Psychosocial history: Maria is now retired on disability from a career as an RN for the Veteran's Administration since her diagnosis in 19997. She weeps easily, especially when depressed or frightened. She fears being alone, fears darkness and heights. She acknowledges depression but she denies suicidal ideation. Her depression is worse upon awakening, improves as the day goes on, yet she often feels a sense of despair. Her symptoms of depression include withdrawing, crying, and withholding. She wants to be in a position of respect and authority. She admits lacking self-confidence and having poor self-esteem. She never feels she accomplished enough, feels she worked below her abilities. She does not like being alone and will even subject herself to being with others who controlling or otherwise have a negative influence on her in order to feel accepted and not to be alone. She readily admits she is jealous of others' health, money and boyfriends. She notes that others see her as caring and intelligent but also close-minded and stubborn. She describes herself as being clairvoyant since age 30.

Generalities: worse damp weather. She has been a chilly person since the onset of her illness (liked fresh air before, used to like things cold and to be outdoors). Sleeps from 11 p.m. till 11 a.m.

Timeline

Age 3-6: victim of physical and sexual abuse

Age 3: mother had psychotic depression and was hospitalized. Patient and siblings were put in different orphanages

Age 7: reacted to smallpox vaccine with high fevers and infected arm

Age 10: encephalitis

Age 11: emotionally abused and ridiculed by nun in Catholic school

Age 12: rheumatic fever for 2 months, resulted in proplapsed valve and heart murmur (wasting and cachexia for one month)

Age 19: had DPT vaccination in military

Age 19: honorable discharge from military (overdosed herself to get out of the service)

Age 20: had BCG because of not reacting to tuberculin testing

Age 21: gonorrhea (from first husband)

Age 21: warts burned off fingers, fibrocystic breasts during menses

Age 21: miscarriage at 3 months

Age 32: D&C for infertility

Age 34: cyst on left ovary

Age 36: first child born, 2 months prematurely (toxemia with bleeding)

Age 41: second child fullterm (placenta previa with bleeding)

Age 42: keratomas on face and chest removed

Age 44: traumatic divorce (due to verbal/emotional abuse); still traumatized by it.

Age 59: breast cancer: lumpectomies first right breast, then left breast. Prior to this diagnosis she had a major depression due to a "miserable" job.

Age 60: mets to bones/cranium

Has lost about 30 lbs over last two years.

Family History

Mother: "always depressed," died at age 90 from congestive heart failure. Was hospitalized for psychotic depression age 40 (?post birth of last child). Age 42: cancer of uterus (hysterectomy and radiation). Severe varicose veins, almost died from shingles; cataracts.

Father: died age 76 from CVA; age 70 Ca of larynx. Three heart attacks at a fairly young age.

Sister, age 70: depression, 3 miscarriages; hyperthyroidism; melanoma of eye (radiated); gallstones

Sister, age 67: insulin dependent diabetes, depression, pneumonia (x2)

Brother, age 60: depression

Sister, age 57: breast cancer, mets at age 45, OK for 5 years then mets to lungs and brain. Is on permanent chemotherapy.

Medications: Tamoxifen, painkillers, Compazine, Ativan.

Questions: What is the predominant miasm? What is the simillimum?

CONCLUSION

Homeopathy: Medicine for the New Millennium

> He who would gain a true knowledge of the art of healing must possess these six qualities: natural capacity; a good education and sound morals; he must have studied since youth, be in love with his work and unsparing of his time.... If an opportunity arises for helping a poor man, one should do so as best one can, for he who loves men must also love the art of healing. —*Hippocrates*

This book has been a long journey in the writing, and I want to thank my readers who have accompanied me on the long journey by reading and digesting it. Let us end the journey with some perspectives on what homeopathy has to offer medicine at this crucial juncture, at the turn of the millennium.

Some of the benefits of homeopathy are obvious. Allopathic medicine is in a devastating financial crisis, with hospitals going bankrupt all around us and nearly 50 million Americans lacking health insurance; homeopathy can offer health care which is both effective and extremely cost-effective. Many allopathic medicines and procedures cause painful or harmful side effects, to the point that allopathic practitioners come to my school in despair, declaring that they cannot in good conscience continue to practice what they know. Homeopathy, as we have seen, does not cause side effects and even enhances the quality of life as it heals.

Let us look beyond the obvious, however, and consider our role as healers, our relationship with our patients, and our purpose in healing. As homeopaths we acknowledge that we are not the healers; the patient's own healing energy effects the cure, while we lend support with the remedy. The old masters used to say that the greatest compliment that can be offered a physician is to say that he did not cure, but Nature did. In homeopathy the dynamic between practitioner and patient is more balanced, which provides greater empowerment and involvement to the patient and greater fulfillment for the practitioner. David Reilly,

M.D., who teaches homeopathy to allopathic physicians in Scotland, has found that one of the outcomes of their study is greater satisfaction and fulfillment in their work. Homeopathy challenges our minds and brings joy to our heart because with it we can truly help people who are suffering.

When we think of the goals of our homeopathic treatment, we look beyond the relief of symptoms, and even beyond the prevention of recurrence which homeopathy excels at. We seek the remedy which will help our patients live to their fullest capacity, whether mentally, emotionally, spiritually, or socially, as well as physically. We would like to see our patients use their newfound health and energy to fulfill their destined role on this earth. Hahnemann expressed this concept beautifully, defining health as the state in which "our indwelling, rational spirit can freely avail itself of this living, healthy instrument *[the body]* for the higher purpose of our existence."

When I think of the future of homeopathy in this country, I am inspired by my students, who come to homeopathy from diverse backgrounds. I envision all the students of homeopathy in this country as pioneers, taking the light of homeopathy to many different fields of medicine: from labor and delivery to nursing homes and hospice care, from chiropractic and muscular therapy to psychotherapy and pastoral counseling, from pediatrics to gynecology to geriatrics. I am inspired by my students and other homeopaths who do volunteer work, bringing the healing gift of homeopathy to the underprivileged. I see great potential for inexpensive homeopathic clinics which could offer health care to the homeless, prenatal and pediatric care to WIC families, and "barefoot doctor" homeopathic training to Third World countries. I envision homeopathy helping to alleviate some of the great unsolved social ills of our time, including juvenile delinquency, pedophilia, mental illness, and criminal behavior.

Practicing homeopathy requires mastering a massive body of information. There is no escaping the serious study required to become a master homeopath. But I believe that it requires more than knowledge. Homeopathy is based on love for our patients, love for the human condition, and compassion for all the foibles and weaknesses of humanity. Being a good homeopath requires us to understand our patients deeply. If we are to base our prescriptions on what is out of the ordinary, we must know what is ordinary in human life, which requires holding in our hearts the vast expanse of human possibilities. Homeopathy requires a powerful, disciplined mind and a loving, open heart.

I always tell my students, as they graduate from my program, "You are all lights in the darkness." May you, my dear readers, be lights in the darkness as well, as you heal and teach others to heal.

Appendices

Forms for the Practice

The Never Well Since or Ailments From

Symptoms and Their Miasms

Sample Cases and Solutions

Homeopathy and Traditional Chinese Medicine

Appendix One

Forms for the Practice:

Intake Questionnaires for Adults, Children, and Pets

Case Summary Sheet

Instructions for Patients

The following forms may used as a starting point for customized ones or may be reproduced, slightly enlarged, with the practitioner's name and address at the top.

The intake questionnaires represent only one possible set of questions. I have revised them many times over the years, discarding some questions if they tend not to yield useful information and adding others to the written questionnaire if I tend to ask it frequently in person. There are many other possible questions which I have found useful only in certain remedies. I tend to ask the patient these questions in person only if they are useful for a differential diagnosis.

The veterinary questionnaire is courtesy of one of my students, Margo Roman, D.V.M.

Adult Questionnaire

Please use a separate sheet to answer these questions.

Name:
Marital/Relationship Status:

Address:

Phone: (day)　　　　　(eve)　　　　　Referred by:

Date:　　　DOB:　　　Age:　　　Height:　　　Weight:

1 What is your chief complaint (CC)?

2 When did this problem begin? What happened in your life around that time? What do you think caused it?

3 What aggravates the CC? (certain types of foods or weather, movement, light, noise, heat/cold, or anything else that you can think of; please be specific)

4 At what time of the day or night is CC the worst? Specify an hour if you can.

5 What symptoms can you identify that accompany the CC?

General Questions

6 *Questions about the weather and environment: you only need to answer those which apply to you.*

a. In which season does the weather bother you the most?

b. How do you react to cold, hot, dry, wet or windy weather? Please mention any and all types of weather that affect you, and how.

c. How does a change of weather affect you?

d. How do you feel in bright sunlight?

e. Do you have any special reactions before, during or after a storm? Please specify.

f. How do you react to drafts of air (e.g. open window, having a fan on you) Do you like to sleep with the window open even when it's cold out?

g. How do you react to sudden changes in temperature, e.g. going from a cold environment to a hot room or vice versa?

h. What about warmth in general, warmth of the bed, of the room, of the heater or stove?

i. How do you feel at the seashore, or on high mountains?

7 What position do you dislike the most: sitting, standing, lying?

8 Do you perspire a great deal? if so, when and where on the body? (feet, head, hair, armpits, etc.)

9 What time of day tends to be a down time for you?

Mental/Emotional

10 What do you worry about? How do you deal with worries?

11 Do you tend to be neater and more fastidious than those around you, or more casual?

12 Do you cry easily? In what situations?

13 When you are upset, do you tend to tell a lot of people or keep it to yourself?

14 On what occasions do you feel despair?

15 In what circumstances do you feel jealous?

16 When and on what occasions do you feel frightened or anxious? Any fears (darkness, being alone, in crowds, altitude, flying, elevators, etc.)?

17 What are the greatest griefs that you have gone through in your life? How did you react?

18 What are the greatest joys you have had in your life?

19 In what situations do you feel the blues, depressed, sad, pessimistic?

20 What bothers you most in other people? How, if at all, do you express it?

21 Do you have a lack of self confidence and a poor sense of self worth?

22 Do you have any recurring dreams? What is the theme?

23 What would you need to feel happy?

24 What do you do for work? Ideally, what would you like to do?

25 If you had an unexpected week's vacation from work and $1000, what would you do?

26 How do other people view you?

27 What would you like to change most about yourself?

Food

28 How do you feel before, during and after meals? How do you feel if you go without a meal?

29 What would you most like to eat (if you did not have to consider calories, fat, anything you've read about the right way to eat)?

30 What foods do you dislike and refuse to eat? What foods do you react badly to, and in what way?

31 How much do you drink in a day? Include sodas, juice, coffee, tea, milk, and alcoholic beverages as well as water. How thirsty do you tend to get?

Sleep

32 What hours do you sleep? Do you tend to wake up at a particular time? Why? What makes you restless or sleepy?

33 Do you do anything during sleep? (speak, laugh, shriek, toss about, grind your teeth, snore)

34 How do you feel in the morning?

Women

35 No. of pregnancies, no. of children, no. of miscarriages, no. of abortions

36 At what age did your menses begin? If you have gone through menopause, at what age?

37 How frequently do they (or did they) come?

38 What about their duration, abundance, color, time of day when flow is greatest; any odor or clots?

39 How do you (did you) feel before, during and after menses?

Health History

40 What medications are you taking at present?

41 How frequently do you get colds and flus?

42 Have you had any childhood illnesses twice, or in a very severe form, or after puberty?

43 Have you had vaccinations since the standard childhood ones? Have you ever had an adverse or unusual reaction to a vaccination?

44 Have you had any surgery? What and when?

45 Have you had at any time (mention year): *What therapy was given?*

   a) Warts: where?   when?   how treated?

   b) Cysts: where?   when?   how treated?

   c) Polyps: where?   when?   how treated?

   d) Tumors: where?   when?   how treated?

46 Do you tend to have any discharges (nasal, vaginal, etc.)? Color, consistency:

47 *Sensitivity:*

   a) Do you tend to need a smaller dose of medications than most other people?

   b) Do you need less anesthesia than others, or have a hard time coming out of it?

   c) Do you tend to react to vitamins and herbs and/or need hypoallergenic vitamins?

   d) Are you sensitive to paint fumes, exhaust, dry cleaning fluid, fragrances, etc.?

48 *Family History:* Mention diseases, causes and ages of deaths of father, mother, sisters, brothers and grandparents on both sides

49 **Construct a time line:** Mention from birth on to the present day, all *important* events (emotional and physical traumas, heartbreaks, divorces, work-related events, diseases or traumas your mother had while being pregnant with you, family stress, death in the family or of friends, disappointments, etc.) Mention the symptoms experienced at those moments or which you can date to those traumas. Please try to write at least one page outlining major events of your life.

50 What else would you like to tell me about yourself or your condition?

Questionnaire for Children
(to be answered by the mother if possible)

Please use a separate sheet to answer these questions

Child's Name: Parents:
Address:
Phone: (day)   (eve)
Parents' marital status: Stepparents?
Date of Birth: Age: Birthweight:
Height/Length: Weight: % ile *(if known)*

1. What is the child's chief complaint (CC)?

2. When did this problem begin? What happened in the child's life around that time? What do you think caused it?

3. What aggravates the CC (certain types of foods or weather, movement, light, noise, heat/cold, being at the seashore, or anything else that you can think of)

4. At what time of the day or night is the CC the worst? Specify an hour if you can.

5. What symptoms can you identify that accompany the CC?

6. What was your predominant emotional state when pregnant with this child?

7. During the pregnancy, did you suffer any particular shocks or traumas or losses?

8. Did you take any drugs?

9. How did your food cravings and aversions change during pregnancy?

10. Were there any particular complications at birth?

11. At what age did the child reach these stages:

weaning	closing of fontanels	first milk teeth
talking	toilet training	first permanent teeth
crawling	walking	

12. How did the child react to these situations? Please try to think of mental and emotional reactions as well as any physical symptoms that may have developed.

vaccinations	birth of younger sibling	starting daycare regularly
first day at school	spending the night with a friend	
traveling with the family	going away to camp etc. without the family	

13. How many rounds of antibiotics has the child had, and for what?

14 Any skin conditions treated with cortisone cream?

15 Did the child suffer from a childhood disease with very severe symptoms? (measles, chickenpox, German measles, croup, mumps, etc.)

16 When ill or upset, does the child tend to cling to you or want to be left alone?

17 What is the child's behavior in playing with other children? Does it make a difference if the other kids are older or younger?

18 What feedback do you get from your child's teachers about behavior in class?

19 What pets do you have, and what is your child's attitude towards them?

20 a) What types of food does your child crave? Please be as specific as possible and list as many as you can.

b) What types of food does she/he refuse to eat?

c) What types of food does your child react badly to, whether physically (bloating, diarrhea, etc.) or behaviorally, and what are the reactions?

21 Any fears that are unusual for a child of your child's age (of the dark, being alone, lightning, thunder, etc.) Are there nightmares?

22 Is the child chilly? Is there excessive perspiration on the head and/or feet?

23 Is the child very affectionate when not sick?

24 Is the child unusually sympathetic (showing concern for the suffering of other children, animals, etc.)?

25 Does the child like music? What kind? Like dancing? Do symptoms (like restlessness) improve with music?

26 Is the child obstinate? How is this expressed?

27 Is the child fastidious?

28 Is the child sensitive to criticism and reprimand?

29 Can you think of any unusual or distinctive things about your child—behavior, fears, fantasies, desires, attachments, preferences in clothing, etc.?

30 Give a timeline for the child with all possible traumas, diseases, important events, deaths in the family. Describe the reaction of your child towards these events.

Questionnaire for Pets

Pet   Owner's Name

Address

Phone

Age   How long have you had your pet?   Where did you get your pet?

Vaccination history/dates: Rabies 1st   2nd   1yr/3yr   Dhllpp

Fvrcp   Leukemia   Lyme   Kennel cough   Other

Aftereffects of vaccines?

Medications

Tolerance to drugs   Diet: brand, amount

What does pet like/dislike to eat?

Water intake (amount, temp.)

Supplements or vitamins

Familial history of disease

What is pet's health problem?

When did it begin? What happened in the pet's life around this time, and what do you think caused it?

What aggravates the problem (foods, weather, noise, heat/cold, etc.)

When during the day is the problem worst?

Gvie a timeline of medical and emotional history (include surgeries, rounds of antibiotics or steroids). Please include medical records, including treatments, x-rays, lab tests, etc.

Any bowel changes (color, frequency, consistency, behavior)

Any past or present skin problems or skin lesions?

Home environment (alone, companions, restrictions, bedding)

Mental observations: reactions to fuss, consolation, scolding, noise, surrounding activity, other dogs or cats

extrovert or introvert

likes to be alone or around people

fears

Will/manner: dominant, submissive; aggressive, shy; noisy, quiet; excitable, docile; impulsive, steady; careful, clumsy; gentle, rough; obedient, disobedient, etc.

How does your animal react to a new person entering the house?

to you or a family member entering

new situations with new people

new situations with other animals

Does it show anger or hurt if you've been away for a long time? How?

Any recent personality changes?

Does your pet prefer to lie in the sun or the shade?

Where does your pet like to sleep?

In what position does it lie down?

Is there anything peculiar about your animal's behavior or symptoms?

What are your expectations about your pet being treated homeopathically?

I use the form on the opposite page as a summary sheet inside each patient's file folder. I keep this form on top, on the right hand side, and inside the left cover I staple a list of each remedy given and each time the potency (succussions, dosage) is changed.

In the space under each Chief Complaint, I list the subrubrics (sensation, location, modalities, etc.) which helps to serve as a benchmark of the patient's improvement and can be used to jog the patient's memory when assessing the reaction to the remedy at follow-up appointments.

The Never Well Since is then listed for the Chief Complaint.

If there is a second Chief Complaint, it is listed with its subrubrics and Never Well Since.

The active miasm is listed with the reasons in the patient's current or past medical history and family history.

The constitution is listed, again with reasons in this particular case.

The remedy is listed with all the indications in this particular case, as a benchmark of improvement. For example, a patient who needs Nat. mur. may notice photophobia or cravings for salty foods changing before the grief lifts.

The potency and dosage is listed, based on the constitution.

Finally, I list the different layers I see in the patient's timeline, working backwards from the current layer, with the remedy I anticipate using for each. This saves time when the patient finishes the current layer.

Chief Complaint 1:

Never Well Since:

Chief Complaint 2:

Never Well Since:

Active Miasm:

Constitution:

Remedy:

Potency/dosage:

Layers/next remedies to come up:

I give the following instruction sheet to patients along with a copy of Figure 6-3, "Driving Miss Daisy," which helps them understand the reaction we are looking for with LM potencies.

Simple Instructions for Taking Your Homeopathic Remedy

1. Succuss the bottle each time before taking a dose: that is, hit the bottle against the palm of your hand or a leather-bound book. Give it a good hard whack from a distance of two feet. This will increase the potency of the dose slightly each time so that it gradually works faster, deeper and with a more gentle effect. The number of times you succuss the bottle (typically from 2 to 8 times) will be written on the label. You may find that you need to adjust the number of successions (see **Adjusting the Dose** on the other side).

2. Take one teaspoon from the bottle and put it in a cup with 4 oz. of water (Dosage Cup). (Ideally the water should be distilled or filtered but tap water is acceptable if that is all you have.) Stir vigorously with a spoon. Use a plastic cup and spoon which you only use for this remedy, not for food or for other remedies. Label the cup for this remedy.

3. Take one teaspoon from the Dosage Cup as your daily dose. NEVER DRINK DIRECTLY FROM THE BOTTLE. This will disturb the gentle and increasingly deep-acting progression of potencies. It could cause an aggravation (temporary intensification) of your symptoms.

4. Discard the rest of the water in the cup. NEVER DRINK THE WHOLE CUP. (Hint: it's great for your plants!) Do not save it overnight. You need to make a new cup the next day after succussing the remedy bottle again. Otherwise you will not be following the methodical and systematic progression of potencies which is part of this healing system, and you may interfere with the progress of your cure.

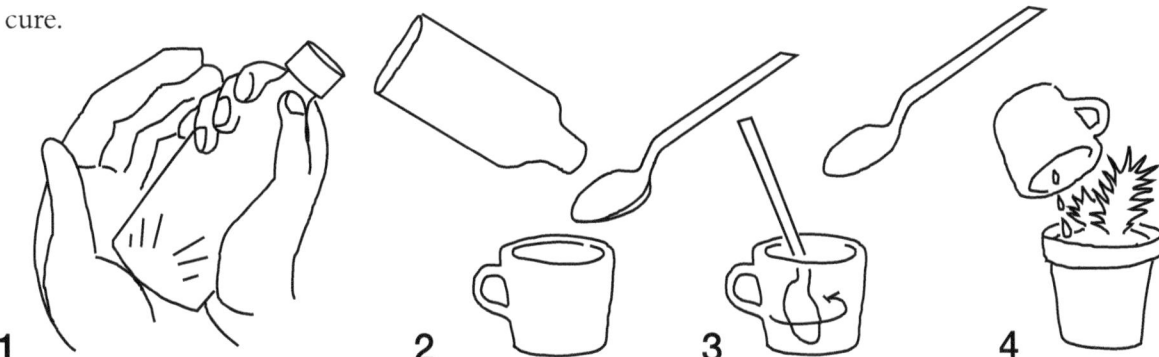

Special precautions:

- After taking your first dose, wait and don't take the remedy the next day. Observe.
- Try to keep it out of direct sunlight and away from heat (e.g. in the glove compartment of your car on a hot day). Avoid having it x-rayed when traveling.
- Do not eat anything for 15 minutes before or after taking your remedy.
- Caffeinated coffee may alter the effects of the remedy. Drinking more than one cup a day may antidote the remedy. If one cup is drunk, take the remedy at least 1 hour later. (Tea is acceptable, as are other caffeine-containing foods like cola and chocolate).
- If you have symptoms related to your menstrual cycle, don't start a new remedy (LM1) while having PMS or during your menstrual cycle, as your symptoms may aggravate.

Symptoms Which You Think Are Caused by the Remedy

If you experience a new symptom (whether mental, emotional or physical) and you think the remedy may be causing it, please ask yourself these questions:

- Is there anything in my life which could have caused this reaction? Did I just eat an unfamiliar food or hear some bad news? Was I involved in a fender-bender? If so, it was not the remedy.
- Have I ever experienced these symptoms before, at any time in my life? If so, it's a good sign, a sign that the remedy is bringing forward old symptoms to be fully healed. Usually people only experience "a shadow of their former symptoms," not a real illness and nothing to worry about. Keep going with the remedy unless the symptoms become uncomfortable, in which case stop for two days and adjust the dose (see below).
- If you have *never* experienced the symptom, and you can't explain it any other way, it *may* be caused by the remedy. Stop the remedy, call the office, and if you get the answering machine leave a detailed description of the symptoms. Wait for further instructions.

Adjusting the Dose

If your **existing** symptoms get worse (this is called an 'aggravation'), stop taking the remedy for AT LEAST TWO DAYS OR LONGER until they stop. Then start taking the same remedy again but SUCCUSS IT TWO LESS TIMES. For example, if you were succussing it 8 times, start again at 6 times.

If you once again get an aggravation, stop again as above, and start again at 2 less succussions, until you are down to 2 succussions. You can't do 0 succussions (not effective), so to adjust the remedy downward, follow these instructions for "making a second cup":

Put 1/2 tsp. from the bottle into your 4 oz. cup, pour 1/2 tsp. from this cup into *another* 4 oz cup of pure water. Stir as usual and drink 1/2 tsp. from this *second* cup. Discard the remainder of both cups.

If this is still too strong, you may need to use 1/4 or even 1/8 tsp. at each step.

Answers to Commonly Asked Questions

Does it matter if I succuss the remedy, then get interrupted and don't take it right away? No, the power of the succussions is still in there.

Does it succuss the remedy if I take it traveling with me and it gets jounced around? No, the succussion has to be a hard and direct thwack.

Should I stop taking my prescription medication? No. You should continue to take it until you have an opportunity to consult with the physician who prescribed it, who is the only person who can be responsible for your discontinuing it. Some medications are dangerous if discontinued suddenly.

What time of day should I take it? Generally in the evening, except for these remedies which should be taken in the morning so that they don't keep you awake at night: Ignatia, Phosphorus, Arsenicum, Sepia and Nat. mur. The most important thing is to take it consistently at about the same time of day.

Can I reuse the same cup? Yes, as long as you are taking the same remedy. It doesn't matter what potency (LM1, LM2, etc.) But when you start a new remedy, you need a new cup. Washing it is not enough to take out the traces of the former remedy, which may interfere with your new one.

What if I spill it? Call the office for a replacement. You'll have to make it "catch up" to the old bottle by removing as many teaspoons and succussing it as many times as the first bottle.

Appendix Two

Never Well Since or Ailments From

A number after a remedy indicates the frequency of use; when the remedies in a list are not numbered, they are approximately equal in frequency; in either case, they should always be prescribed on the other indications of the remedy.

Any remedy appearing in this list should receive a score of 3 (black-type) when scoring the 10-rubric chart.

Mental/Emotional Factors

Ambition, deceived: Nux-v. #1, Sulphur #2
Anger: Nux-v., Cham., Coloc., Plat.
    with anxiety: Ars. #1, Nux-v. #2
    with fright: Acon.
    with indignation: Staph. #1, Coloc. #2
    with grief: Cocc.
    with silent grief: Ign. #1, Staph.
    with vexation: Staph. #1, Cham., Plat.
    with wrath and vehemence: Cham., Lyc., Nux-v.
    suppressed: Staph. #1
Anticipation: Gels. #1, Ign. #2, Arg-n. #3, Carc.
Anxiety: Calc-c.
Bad news: Ign. or Gels. #1; Caust. or Calc-c. #2
Betrayal: Lyc., Nat. mur.
Broken heart: Nat. mur., Ign., Lach.
Business failure: Gels., Nux-v., Silica
Cares and worries (*especially about welfare of family members and friends*): Calc-c. #1, Phos. #2
Contradiction: Nux-v., Calc-c., Lyc.
Death of a child: Ignatia

Death of parents or friends: Ignatia #1, Caust. #2 *(repetitive grief)*

Debauchery: Nux-v.

Disappointed love: Nat. mur., Ign., Phos. acid., Puls., Lach., Plat.

Disappointment: Lyc. #1, Ignatia

Discords between chief and subordinates: Nux-v., Sulphur

Discords between parents and children, competition between children: Nux-v., Sulphur

Domination, children dominated by parents: Carc. #1, Nat. mur., Staph.

Egotism: Sulphur, Platina, Lyc., Calc-c., Silica

Embarrassment: Sulphur #1, Ignatia, Calc-c., Ambra grisea

Emotional shock: Aconite (#1), Lach., Opium

Excessive sex: Sepia, Phos. acid. *(lost excessive seminal fluid)*

Excitement, emotional *(also called "happy surprise")*: Coffea #1, Acon., Puls., Plat.

Excitement, religious: Veratrum album

Failure in business (bankruptcy): Ambra grisea (#1), Nux-v., Lyc.

Fear: Opium *(of past events)*; Aconite *(of present, just happened)*; Gelsemium *(of future)*. Also Ign. and Carc.

Financial loss: Aurum *(if suicidal)*; Ars., Kali-ar. *(if not)*

Fortune, reverse of: Aurum, Ars., Ignatia

Fright: Aconite (#1), Lach., Opium *(paralyzed, in a daze)*; Acon. for the present, Opium for the past, Gels. for the future; Carc.

    during menses: Ignatia

    with vexation: Ignatia or Aurum (#1); Plat., Phos., or Opium (#2)

Grief or death of beloved one: Nat. mur.; Aur. met. *(if suicidal, feels like life is gone)*

Grief, repetitive: Causticum, Phos. acid., Ambra grisea

Hearing bad news: Ign. or Gels. #1; Causticum or Calc-c. #2

Honor, wounded: Staph. #1, Nat. mur. #2

Hurry: Tarent., Sulph. acid., Med., Sulph., Arg. Nit., Nux-v., Iodium

Incest: Staphysagria, Sepia

Indignation, insults: Staph., Nat. mur.

Infertility (due to heartbreak): Nat. mur., Staph.

Jealousy: Lachesis, Hyosc.

Joy, excessive: Coffea

Lack of sleep while nursing loved ones: Cocculus (#1), Caust., Phos., Zincum

Lack of emotional nourishment: Nat. mur. #1 by far *(also other grief/abandonment remedies; also think of Sepia if the patient lacked emotional nourishment as a child because the mother was in a Sepia state and the patient had to take over the mother's duties)*

Laughing, excessive: Coffea

Headaches after excessive laughing: Iris, Phos.

Literary or scientific failure: Sulphur, Nux-v.

Love, disappointed, lesbian: Sepia, Platina

Loss of spouse: Aurum

Meditation: Phos.

Mental exertion: Silica, Kali phos.

Money, from losing: Ars., Aurum

Mortification, with anger: Staph. *(throws things)*, Aurum *(complete withdrawal, aversion to all around him)*

Nightwatching: Cocculus (#1), Caust., Phos., Zincum

Overambition: Nux-v.

Overresponsibility: Nux-v., Calc-c., Sepia

Overstudy: Kali phos., Nux-v., Sil., Carc., Zincum

Parental (excessive) control: Carc., Staph., Anac., Kali-br.

Postpartum depression: Sepia

Rage, fury: Nux-v.

Rape: Staph. (#1), Caust. (#2), Sepia, Anacardium *(if split personality)*

Remorse: Aurum

Reproach *(being criticized by others):* Opium #1, Ignatia, Staph.

Reputation, loss of: Sulph. #1, Nux-v. #2

Rudeness of others: Staph. #1, Lyc. #2

Sadness: Aur., Ign., Nat. mur., Phos. acid., Staph., Cocc., Calc-c.

Scorn (being scorned): Nux-v., Staph.

Sexual abstinence: Conium

Sexual abuse: Staph. (#1), Caust. (#2), Anac., Sepia

Sexual activity, increased: Medorrhinum

Sexual excesses: Phos. acid.

Sexual excitement: Plat. *(women)*; Sulph., Lyc., Calc-c. *(men)*

Shame: Staph., Ignatia, Nat. mur., Lyc., Coloc., Bell., Phos-ac.

Shock, acute sudden: Aconite, Ignatia

Stage fright: Arg. nit. (#1), Gels., Lyc., Kali phos.

Suppressed anger: Staph., Coloc., Carc., Ign.

Surprises, pleasant: Coffea #1, Acon., Opium, Puls.

Traumatic accident *(fear from accident, especially with hyperventilation/shortness of breath):* Carbo veg.

Unhappiness: Carcinosin

Work, mental *(key: T = thinking, R = reading, W = writing):* Calc-c. (T,R,W), Calc. phos. (R), Nat. mur. (T,R,W), Nux-v. (T), Sulphur (T)

Worry for future: Arg-n., Ars.

External Factors

Climate

Altitude sickness: Coca, Carbo veg., Calc. *(< ascending,)* Sil.

Dampness: Nat. sulph., Dulc.

Dry wind: Acon., Caust., Hepar sulph.

Frostbite: Agar., Ars.

Heat stroke: Verat-a. #1 (chronic), Glonoin (acute) *(headaches)*, Sol. (acute), Bell. (acute), Nat. carb. *(headaches)*

Lightning, being struck by: Phos., Nux-v.

Mountain sickness: Coca, Carbo veg., Calc. *(< ascending),* Sil.

Seashore: Nat. mur., Sepia, Med., Carc.

Storms: Phos., Rhododendron

Sun *(symptoms worse from sun):* Nat. mur., Glonoin, Nat. carb., Verat.

Trauma

Bleeding: China, Phos-ac., Ferrum met., Plat.

Cut: Calendula

Electrocution: Phos.

Excessive bleeding: China, Phos-ac.

Head, falling on: Arnica *(especially if bleeding, pressure on brain)*, Nat. sulph. *(if nerve damage, tingling, or mental changes)*, Opium, Hell.

Overlifting: Calc-c., Graph.

Spine: Nat. sulph.

Stroke: Lachesis, Crotalus, Vipera, *snake venoms in general*

Trauma: Arnica

Whiplash: Rhus tox.

Wound: Calendula

OTHER

Abortions, repetitive: Sepia, Helonias *(chronic fatigue since)*
Acute infectious disease: Carbo veg., Psor., Sulphur, Tuberc.
Anesthesia: Phos., Opium
Antibiotics, allergy shots, cortisone: Thuja
Antibiotics: Thuja, Nit-ac. *(diarrhea)*, Arsenicum
Bad hygiene: Psorinum
Birth control pill: Sepia (#1), Thuja *(#2)*, Puls. *(#2)*, Folliculinum 3x or 6x *(#2)*
Childbirth: Sepia *(exhaustion)*, Caulophyllum, China *(loss of blood)*, Ferr-m. *(loss of blood)*, Helonias dioica *(exhaustion)*, Pyrogenium *(sepsis)*, Pulsatilla *(bleeding, retentio placentae)*
Childhood disease: Sulphur, Psorinum, or the nosode of the disease
Childhood infection, severe: Carcinosin
Concentration camp: Psorinum
Cortisone, excessive: Thuja #1, Causticum
Cystoscopy: Staph.
Delivery (childbirth): Sepia
Diarrhea, loss of fluids from: China
Diphtheria: Diphtherinum
Drugs (medical, street): Nux-v., Sulphur, Thuja
DTP vaccination: Sil., DPT homeopathic
Fertility drugs, hormonal therapies: Sepia, Thuja, Nux-v.
Flu shots: Gels.
Flu: Influenzinum, Gelsemium, Chin-a., Psorinum, Sulphur, Tub. *(if prostration)*
Gall bladder removed: China
Gonorrhea: Medorrhinum
Herpes zoster *(postzonal neuralgias, migraines)*: Mezereum
Hormonal treatment: Sepia
Hysterectomy: Sepia
Lead poisoning: Plumbum, Nux-v.
Marriage *(recurring vaginal infections since)*: Med., Thuja, Staph.
Measles: Morbillinum, Drosera, Kali-c.
Mono: Gelsemium (#1), Carcinosin, Merc-sol.
Morphine addiction: Morphinum, Op., Av. Sat.
Multiple vaccinations *(especially if they don't "take" and need to be readministered)*: Thuja (#1), Pyrogenium
Nursing: Sepia

Overuse of drugs (medical or street drugs): Nux-v.
Penicillin: Penicillinum
Pneumonia: Phos. (#1), Lyc., Carbo-veg., Sulphur, Tuberculinum, Bacillinum
Polio: Lathyrus sativa
Poverty, bad living circumstances: Psorinum
Radiation/chemotherapy: Cadmium sulph.
Sepsis *(appendicitis, gangrenous gall bladder, puerperal fever, peritonitis, etc.)*: Pyrogenium (#1), Gunpowder
Spinal tap: Hypericum
Suppressed eczema: Sulphur
Suppressed sweat: Sulphur, Sil., Thuja, Calc-c., Merc.
Surgery: Staphysagria *(for painful incision)*, Hypericum
Traveler's diarrhea: Arsenicum *(polluted water)*, China *(after spoiled meat, or diarrhea with bloating)*, Zingiber
Vaccination for yellow fever: Crotalus
Vaccination: Thuja (#1), Silica, Carcinosum, Pyrogen *(multiple)*, Variolinum *(smallpox)*
Viral hepatitis: Phos.
Virus: Lathyrus sativa
Whooping cough, attack of: Tuberculinum, Carcinosin

Diet
Alcohol, overuse of: Nux-v., Ranunculus bulbosa
Beer: Nux-v.
Coffee: Cham., Coffea
Fatty foods: Puls., Sulphur, Nux-v.
Food poisoning: Ars. *(diarrhea and fever)*, Verat. *(diarrhea and vomiting)*, China *(diarrhea and bloating)*; Zingiber *(after intake of melon)*
Hangover: Nux-v.
Hepatitis *(from cirrhosis of liver due to alcoholism)*: Sulph. acid, Lyc.; *plus Carduus marianus tincture*
Milk: Nat-c., Calc-c.
Overuse of alcohol: Nux-v.
Partying, excessive: Nux-v.
Pork: Puls.
Tea: Thuja, Puls., Paris quadrifolia
Tobacco: Lobelia, Calad., Sepia *(neuralgia of face)*, Lyc. *(impotence)*, Ars. *(antidote to chewing tobacco)*

Veal *(aggravated from eating):* China, Kali nitricum, Ipecac
Wine: Zincum

Internal factors

Fever: China
Hepatitis: Phos. (#1), Nat. sulph., Mag-m. *(chronic fatigue since)*
Hormonal therapies: Sepia
Loss of fluids: China and Ferrum-m. *(blood loss, dehydration)*, Phos-ac. *(loss of semen, excessive sex/masturbation)*
Masturbation (in women): Plat., Origanum *(in young girls)*
Masturbation (in men): Phos-ac. *(loss of spermatic fluid)*, Lyc., Kali-br.
Menopause: Lachesis (#1), Sepia, Puls., Graphites
Miscarriage: Sepia, Caulophyllum
Puberty: Pulsatilla, Sepia
Sweating: China
Vomiting, loss of fluids from: China

APPENDIX THREE

Symptoms and Their Miasms

Key: P = psoric, Syc = sycotic, Syp = syphilitic, T = tubercular, C = cancer

Physical Symptoms	P	Syc	Syp	T	C
Abscess		x			
Abscess with fistula				x	
Acne, rosacea or vulgaris				x	
seborrheic, cystic, scarring		x			
Acromegaly			x		
Addison's disease				x	
Adenomas		x			
Adhesions		x			
Aggravations, dampness, from		x			
meat, from	x	x			
milk, from	x				
sea, proximity to		x			
spring, during		x			
Allergies	x	x			x
Alopecia, after acute disease	x				
Amaurosis (blindness)			x		
Amenorrhea	x				
Amyloidosis			x		
Anasarca		x			

	P	Syc	Syp	T	C
Anemia, in most cases		x			
hemolytic			x		
severe form					x
Aneurysm			x		
Angina pectoris		x	x		
Ankylosis of joints		x			
Aphthosis, chronic			x		
Apoplexy			x		
Appendicitis		x			
gangrenous			x		
Appetite, loss of	x				
during menses				x	
in morning				x	
Arteriosclerosis			x		
Arthritis		x			
Arthrosis deformans			x		
Ascites		x			
Asthma < spring, < damp weather, paroxysmal, on exertion,		x			
and/or in chest		x			
in throat	x				
Astigmatism			x	x	
Ataxia			x		
Atrophy			x		
Aversion, meat, to			x		
wind, to	x				
Azoospermia			x		
Babies, old looking			x		
Barber's itch		x			

	P	Syc	Syp	T	C
Bechterew's disease					x
Bleed, tendency to				x	
Boils, recurrent	x				
Bone pains, deep			x		
Breast swelling, before menses	x				
Café-au-lait spots					x
Calluses on soles of feet	x			x	
Cancer, sarcoma			x		
Candida albicans		x			
Caries, bones			x		
Caries, teeth			x		x
early appearing	x	x			
Carpal tunnel syndrome				x	
Cataract			x		
after suppressed eczema	x				
Catarrh, chronic		x			
Cellulitis		x			
Cheeks, flushed					x
Chickenpox		x			
Childhood diseases absent					x
after puberty					x
the same one recurs twice					x
one after another					x
Children, sickly or thin				x	
Chilly	x			x	
Chorea			x		
Club-foot			x		x
Celiac disease					x

	P	Syc	Syp	T	C
Cold, lack of vital heat	x			x	
Colds, strong tendency to catch				x	
Colic		x			
Colitis ulcerosa			x		x
Condylomata		x			
Constipation, longterm	x				
Cracks, skin			x		
Cravings, bacon				x	
chocolate				x	x
fat	x			x	
fried food	x				
hot foods	x	x			
meat	x	x			
milk	x				
oranges		x			
pica gravidarum	x				
rich foods	x				
salt	x			x	
soups					x
sour	x	x			
spicy foods	x	x			
sweets	x				
tobacco				x	
unnatural (chalk, sand)	x				
Crohn's disease				x	x
Cryptorchidism			x		
Cysts		x			
Deafness	x			x	

	P	Syc	Syp	T	C
Deformities			x		
gestational			x		
Diarrhea, bloody			x		
chronic, green		x			
in morning	x				
Digestion, easily disturbed	x				
malabsorption	x				
Diplopia			x		
Discharge, fish-brine		x			
greenish; green-yellow		x			
greenish with blood			x		
offensive		x	x		
watery, acrid		x			
Disorders, functional	x				
Down's syndrome					x
Dupuytren's disease			x		
Dwarfism			x		x
Dyslexia			x	x	
Dysmenorrhea, chronic		x			x
painful, excruciating	x	x		x	
Dysplasia, hip			x		
Ears, short			x		
sticking out			x		
low-placed			x		
Eclampsia		x			
Ecchymosis, tendency to				x	
Ectopy vesicae			x		
Eczema, itching	x				

Eczema, *continued*	P	Syc	Syp	T	C
bleeding			x		
head, crusty				x	
dry		x			
pustular			x		
scaly	x				
papulous		x			
Edema		x			
Endometriosis		x			
Enuresis nocturna			x	x	x
Epilepsy		x	x		x
Epistaxis				x	
difficult to stop				x	
during menses				x	
improves sx				x	
Erection disturbances	x				
at night			x		
Erythema nodosum				x	
Excretions, sour	x				
Exostosis			x		
Extremities, cold		x		x	
numbness	x				
Eyebrows, loss of			x		
unruly		x			
Eyelashes, long and silky				x	
loss of			x		
Eyes, black rings under				x	
Face, angelic				x	
asymmetrical			x		

Face, *continued*	P	Syc	Syp	T	C
grey			x		
porcelain complexion				x	
Fatigue, sudden				x	
Feet, flat			x		
Fertility, excessive				x	
Fever, unknown origin				x	
high		x			
low or absent while sick	x				
Fibroids		x			
Fingers, missing			x		
Fistulas and fissures			x	x	
Flatulence	x				
Flu	x				
Freckles, multiple				x	
Gallstones		x			
Gangrene			x		
Gigantism			x		
Gingiva, bleeding				x	
spongy and weak				x	
Glands, swollen	x			x	
Glaucoma			x		
Glottitis		x			
Gout		x			
Grave's disease (hyperthyroidism)		x		x	
Hair, abundant (hirsutism)		x			
abundant, along spine or in lumbar region, dark and long			x		
alopecia areata		x			
alopecia, in patches			x		

Hair, *continued*	P	Syc	Syp	T	C
alopecia totalis			x		
coarse and thick		x			
dry and thin	x				
ends split	x				
gluey, greasy			x		
grey, early	x				
late appearing			x		
loss, excessive	x				
lustreless				x	
sparse			x		
white streak	x				
Hallux valgus			x	x	
varus			x		
Hayfever, < fall		x			
light	x				
severe				x	
Headaches, < at noon	x				
< exertion, > cold, vertex			x		
after school				x	
occipital, < night, < heat			x		
periodic				x	
Healing, wounds, slow		x			
Heart, congenital malformations			x		
congestive heart failure	x				
dropsical	x				
sudden death, infarct		x	x		
valvular lesions		x		x	
Heart disease, functional (not organic)	x				

	P	Syc	Syp	T	C
Heat, < of the bed	x				
Heat, flushes of	x				
Hemangioma		x			
Hemianopsy			x		
Hemochromatosis					x
Hemophilia			x	x	x
Hemorrhoids	x	x			
Hepatitis, of newborn		x			
Hepatosplenomegaly, congenital			x		
Hernia, after birth		x			
Herpes simplex I and II		x			
Herpes zoster		x			
Hoarseness		x			
Hodgkin's disease			x		
Hordeolum		x			
Hunger, voracious	x				
at night	x				
Hydramnion			x		
Hydrocephaly			x	x	
Hydrocele		x			
Hyperemesis gravidarum	x				
Hypersensitivity to noise or smells	x				
Impetigo contagiosa		x			
Impotence	x	x			
Incontinence, stress	x				
Infantilism			x	x	
Insomnia, in infants and children					x
on falling asleep, because of worry	x				

	P	Syc	Syp	T	C
Intertrigo		x			
Intolerance to fats	x				
-itis diseases (cystitis, vaginitis, bronchitis, etc.)		x			
Kidney stones		x			
Kidneys, multip or single			x		
Legs, bowlegged (varus)			x		
Legs, knock-kneed (valgus)			x		
Leprosy			x		
Lesions, slow growing	x				
fast growing		x	x		
Leucorrhea		x			
Leukemia		x			x
Lice	x				
Lipomas		x			
Low grade fevers	x				
Lung diseases, alternating with mental diseases				x	
alternating with rectal sx					x
Lupus erythematosus		x			
Luxation, congenital hip			x		
Malposition, babies			x		
Melanoma		x			
Menarche, delayed					x
Meniere's disease			x		
Menses, exhausting, abundant				x	
Migraine, < before menses				x	
< nights			x		
before menses, strong				x	
chronic		x			

	P	Syc	Syp	T	C
Migraine, *continued*					
chronic, since childhood			x		
for several days			x		
nosebleeds amel.				x	
on weekends	x		x		
periodic				x	
Miscarriage, 2nd or 3rd month		x			
Miscarriages, repetitive			x		
Molluscum contagiosum	x				
Mononucleosis					x
Multiple births			x		
Multiple sclerosis			x		
Naevus		x			
hairy		x			
spider		x			
Nails, break easily	x			x	
ingrowing	x			x	
paper thin			x	x	
thick		x			
white spots				x	
Nasal polyposis		x			x
Nausea in pregnancy	x				
Necrosis of bone, without new bone formation			x		
with formation of new bone		x			
Neurofibromatosis					x
Night, improvement of sx		x			
worsening of sx			x		
Nightblindness (hemeralopia)			x		
Nose, redness with capillaries		x			

	P	Syc	Syp	T	C
Nose, saddle			x		
Oligospermia			x		
Onset of disease, slow	x				
sudden		x			
Ophthalmia, purulent		x			
Osteogenesis imperfecta			x	x	
Osteomalacia			x	x	
Osteomyelitis			x		
Osteoporosis			x		
Ovarian cysts		x			
Ovaries, inflammation of		x			
Overgrowth, fleshy		x			
Ozaena		x	x		
with fetid odor			x		
Paget's disease			x		
Palate, cleft			x		
narrow			x		
Papillomata		x			
Paralysis, progressive			x		
Parkinson's disease			x		
Pectus excavatus			x		
Pemphigus			x		
Peritonitis		x			
Perspiration amel.	x			x	
excessive	x				
head/neck	x				
oily	x				
sour	x				

	P	Syc	Syp	T	C
Petechiae, tendency to				x	
Peyroni's disease			x		
Phimosis		x			
Photophobia	x				
Physical symptoms, always changing				x	
Poliomyelitis			x		
Polyposis		x			
Poison oak susceptibility				x	
Pregnancy, feels better during	x				
Priapism, at night			x		
in the day	x				
Prostate enlargement		x			
inflammation		x			
Pruritis	x				
Psoriasis		x		x	
Ptosis			x		
Pulse, fast		x			
irregular			x		
slow	x				
Pupil reflex absent			x		
Purpura			x		
Pyloric stenosis		x	x		
Raynaud's disease			x		
Recovery, slow		x			
Rheumatism		x			
Salivation, extreme			x		
sticky			x		
Sarcoma			x		

	P	Syc	Syp	T	C
Scabies	x				
Scheuermann's disease				x	
Sclerae, blue				x	x
Seashore, symptoms improve at		x			x
Seminal emissions, daytime	x				
night			x		
without erections	x				
Sensory senses, dull			x		
Skin, burning	x				
cracks	x		x		
dirty looking	x				
dry	x				
fissures			x		
fistula			x		
itching	x				
pale	x				
slowly healing				x	
transparent				x	
ulcers			x		
unhealthy	x				
Smell, loss of			x		
sour	x				
stinking		x	x		
Spina bifida			x		
Stenosis		x			
Sterility (infertility)		x			
Stimulated, aroused, easily		x			
Strabismus			x		

	P	Syc	Syp	T	C
Stricture of rectum, esophagus, trachea, urethra		x			
Symptoms < at night			x		
< change of weather, barometric pressure		x			
< dampness		x			
> natural discharges, after	x				
> unnatural discharges, after		x			
Syndactyly			x		
Taste, bitter	x				
burnt	x				
loss of			x		
metallic			x		
Teeth, black			x		
calcium buildup				x	
caries			x		x
caries, early	x		x		
cracks			x		
fall out early			x		
grinding	x				
grown together			x		
Hutchinson's			x		
missing			x		
not erupting			x		
position incorrect			x		
serrated			x		
small (microdentism)			x		
spaced out (diastema)			x		
Teething, delayed	x				
early caries	x	x			

	P	Syc	Syp	T	C
Teething, continued					
small teeth	x				
Testes, undescended			x	x	
Tic nerveux			x	x	x
Tinea, all kinds (ca*pitis, co*rporis, etc.)		x			
Tires easily, mentally/physically	x			x	
Toenails, ingrowing			x		
Tongue, cracks			x		
red		x			
Tonsils, enlarged or pustular				x	
Trismus (lockjaw)		x			
Twin pregnancies			x		
Twitching, of muscles		x			
Ulceration, immediate			x		
Varicose veins, early		x			
Veins, visible				x	
Vertigo	x				
Vesicles		x			
Vitiligo	x		x	x	
Walk, late learning to			x		
Warts, digitata or filiform		x			
flat, dry and itchy	x				
penetrating, deep			x		
soles			x		x
vulgaris		x			
Wasting (chronic unintended loss of weight)				x	
Weakness, need for support	x				
Whooping cough				x	
severe					x

Mental/emotional symptoms	P	Syc	Syp	T	C
Abundance of ideas	x				
Addictive personalities			x		
Admonition, sensitive to		x			
Absentmindedness			x		
Air castles, making	x				
Alcoholism, hereditary			x		
social	x	x		x	
business-related	x				
Alert, active mind	x				
Alzheimer's			x		
Anguish		x			
Anxiety, anticipation	x				x
health, about	x				
heart region, in	x				
poverty, about	x				
Artistic				x	x
Autism			x		
Avarice	x				
Boasting		x			
Body piercing		x	x		
Breaking things			x	x	
Carried, child wants to be		x			
Cheerful		x		x	
Clinging	x				
Cognitive limitations			x		x
Cold-blooded (e.g. murderer)			x		
Company, likes	x			x	
Concealment		x			

	P	Syc	Syp	T	C
Consolation, needing	x				
Contact, breaking off, with family			x		
Courage, lack of (cowardice)	x				
Cries all day long, child		x			
all night long, child		x			
Criminal insanity		x	x		
Criminality		x	x		
Criticism, sensitive to		x			
Cruelty		x	x		
Crying, cannot speak without		x			
Dancing, love for		x		x	x
Delusion, alone, she is, in the world	x				
asylum, that she will be sent to	x				
body, brittle	x				
body is thin	x				
crime, is about to commit a			x		
criminal, that he is a			x		
enemies, surrounded by			x		
enemy, everyone is an			x		
fail, everything will	x		x		
fortune, that he was going to lose his	x				
identity, errors of personal			x		
inconsolable over fancied		x			
murdered, he would be			x		
persecuted, that he is		x			
pursued, thought he was		x	x		
sick, imagines himself	x				
someone is behind him		x			

	P	Syc	Syp	T	C
Delusions, *continued*					
thieves, sees	x				
watched, that she is being		x			
Dementia praecox			x		
Depression			x		
Despair, about recovery	x				
Destructive			x		
Details, eye for					x
Discipline, lack of, in children		x	x		
Dishonesty		x			
Dislike for children			x		
because of suffering	x				
Disrespect			x		
Dissatisfaction				x	
Dogmatic	x				
Drug addiction, including prescription medication		x	x		
Drugs, use of street		x			
Dullness of mind			x		x
Easily distracted	x				
Egotism	x				
Embarrassed, easily	x				
Excitement seekers		x		x	
Exhibitionists		x			
Expressionless			x		
Extrovert		x		x	
Fastidious, emphasis on sense of beauty					x
emphasis on efficiency	x				
emphasis on contagiousness/insecurity			x		
Fear of artificial light			x	x	

Fears, *continued*	P	Syc	Syp	T	C
being alone	x			x	
being late	x				
cats, dogs, furry animals				x	
darkness	x				
disease	x				
doom, impending	x				
dying	x				
failure in business	x				
ghosts	x				
heights	x				x
insanity	x				
knives			x		
lightning	x			x	
narrow places	x				x
night			x		
people are going to steal from him	x				
physical suffering	x				
rape	x		x		
robbers	x				
storms	x			x	
strangers		x			
thunder and lightning	x			x	
watching TV, of seeing horrible things	x				
Fearful in general	x				
Followers, need support, dependent on others	x				
Foolish, clownish behavior, in children			x		
in adults		x			
Forgetful, read, for what they have		x	x		

	P	Syc	Syp	T	C
Forgetful, say, for what they are about to			x		
Forgotten something, feels constantly he has		x			
Greed	x				
Handwashing, obsessive-compulsive			x		x
Hate			x		
Hiding			x		
Hoarding, collecting	x				
Hopelessness about recovery	x		x	x	
Horrible things affect him	x				
Hurried		x		x	x
Hyperactivity		x			
Hypersensitivity (emotional)	x			x	x
Hypochondria	x			x	
Hyposexuality	x				
Hysteria				x	
Ideas, abundant	x				
fixed		x	x		
Idiocy, children			x		
Impatient		x		x	
Impotence	x				
Inspection of genitalia, tendency to		x			
Introvert					x
Irresolution	x				
Isolation			x		
Jealousy	x	x	x		
Kill, desire to		x	x		
Kleptomania, for thrills		x			
for possessions	x				

	P	Syc	Syp	T	C
Laughing inappropriately			x		
Looked at, cannot bear to be	x				
Loquacious		x			
Love, for mountains				x	
for animals	x				x
for ocean		x			x
Lying		x			
Masturbation		x			
Materialistic	x				
Melancholy, with lassitude			x		
Memory, brainfag, constant		x			
Memory loss, beginning		x			
sudden			x		
short-term		x			
for names of persons or things		x	x		
Mental illness		x	x		
in children			x		x
Moral degeneracy		x	x		
Morose			x		
Nightmares, about killing, being killed, wolves			x		
Nymphomania		x			
Obstinacy	x				
Overwhelmed, easily				x	
Perversions		x	x		
Protection, need for	x				
Pyromania		x			
Reflective	x				
Religious	x				

	P	Syc	Syp	T	C
Remorseless		x	x		
Reprimands, sensitive to		x			
Sado-masochism			x		
Sadness			x		
Schizophrenia			x		
in adolescents					x
Secretive			x		
Self-condemnation		x	x		
Self-mutilation			x		
Sex, group		x	x		
Sex, perverse			x		
Shame		x			
Shameless			x		
Slow learner	x		x		
Spiritual	x				
Sterilization, voluntarily, at young age			x		
Stuttering			x		
Suicidal impulses		x	x		
in young people		x			
Support, needs	x				
Suspicion		x			
Tearing things			x		
Temper tantrums	x			x	
Theorizing	x				
Thoughts, lose train of		x			
Thrill seekers		x			
Thunder and lightning, fascinated with					x
fear of	x			x	

	P	Syc	Syp	T	C
Timid, bashful	x				
Tires easily, mentally/physically	x			x	
Travel, love for, cosmopolitan				x	x
Unforgiving attitude			x		
Worry, about future	x				

APPENDIX FOUR

Sample Cases

These are a few of the cases used in my school to demonstrate different principles of rubric selection and case analysis for beginning students. The first three are fictional, written to help beginning students practice and build confidence. The remaining cases are from real patients, with names and identifying details changed; all quotes are in the patients' own words. Students who want to gain the maximum benefit from this book may want to attempt solving the cases, comparing their answers with those given at the end of this appendix.

Exercise for the first four cases:

First list all possible rubrics in the case with their page number in Kent, according to the hierarchy of symptoms.

Then choose 10 of the rubrics and justify your choice of rubrics.

Make a scoring chart, choose your remedy, and justify your choice.

Sample Case 1

Miss Juliet (the other half of Romeo) is 23 years old and comes into my office weeping. As soon as she gets my attention, though, she flashes a big smile (and her quick change in temperament really *does* get my attention). When I ask what brings her to me, she says dysmenorrhea. When I ask her for details, she says the symptoms change all the time. When I ask about her period, she says she usually gets it late (40-day cycle) and it lasts for 10 days; it only flows during the day and there are clots in the flow. She has crying spells premenstrually and also during her period. While she is telling me this she starts weeping again, although I can't see any particular reason for this. She feels her Chief Complaint stems from the time when her father died when she was 12.

She tells me that she loves to talk to people when she is sad about something, because it always makes her feel better. But she feels so lonely that she says, "I feel all alone in this world!" (I know this is not true, since her parents are also my patients and they adore their two daughters.) She tells me she does not have many fears, although she confides that sometimes she feels she "is going crazy." Although she loves company, she is rather afraid of men. She feels that she has no self-confidence, and she is jealous of her younger sister who, she tells me, "gets all the attention." She dreams of black animals and sometimes has dreams of romantic situations. She likes to eat things cold, disliking warm drinks as well as high-fat and rich foods. In general she feels the worst around sunset; she always cries and feels sad around that time. She tells me she is warm-blooded and feels weak in a hot room. She hates stuffy rooms and usually opens the windows, as she craves fresh air which makes her feel better. She can't stand it when it's really windy. After I reassure her that I can help her, she smiles and says, "I knew you would make me better!"

Sample Case 2

Mr. Al seemed like a handful. When I asked what brought him to me, he said: "I'm going to be honest with you, Doctor, I don't have much good to say about doctors. I know what I am doing, people say I have a big ego and always want the last word, but I don't care. My biggest problem is this rash on my arm. It itches and burns like hell, especially at night when I am in bed and also when I take a shower. It feels better when I scratch it, but then I scratch it until it bleeds. I've had it since I was a kid. My mother told me that my father had it too, but I have a lot of my own ideas about what caused it. I think the summer has something to do with it, then the poison ivy I got when I was a child and the cream I got for it aggravated it. And you never know, maybe I think I ate too many apples as a child, I drank too little and I never took the vitamins that my mother tried to give me. Anyway, I hate this rash, it looks so ugly! Now don't try to give me any of those fancy creams like other doctors do, I know better than anyone that they don't help. I have a special position in this society, Doctor, I truly believe that few people are on the same level as me. But you know, I'm worried about money, I used to have a lot more. I can't stop thinking about it and I am afraid I will end up as a street person. *[I know from the kind of car he drives and his address that these are totally unrealistic fears.]* I'm not afraid of anything, although I have to admit I don't like to cross over high bridges because I always get dizzy. So I would never go to Egypt to climb the pyramids. I would rather go to Germany for my favorite foods: spicy sausages and their famous beers. I hate milk, I think that's one of the causes of my rash. And I can't help it that I have to sprint out of my bed around 5 a.m. because I always get diarrhea. Oh, I always sleep with my feet sticking out from under the covers and can you believe it, I often have dreams that come true a couple of days later. OK! I hope you can figure out my remedy right away with that info, because I'm in a hurry. And maybe you can give me a remedy for the headaches I always get in bed and strangely enough, mostly in the winter.

Sample Case 3

Ms. Ellie, 25 years old, 5", 118 lbs. has two chief complaints. First, pressing headaches, located on the forehead, < approaching thunderstorms, and > with cold applications. These headaches have been present as long as she can remember, even back to childhood. Her second group of complaints is more serious. She says that she has the sensation that her body is "very fragile." She always has been pretty fearful but now she constantly thinks she is "about to die" although there is no apparent reason to support this since her MD found nothing on a complete physical examination. She usually wakes up around 3 a.m., which she says is her worst time as she feels bad in general ("can't put my finger on it"). Sometimes she wakes up at 4 a.m. after which she has a hard time falling asleep because she has a feeling in her abdomen "as if something is alive in there." What increases this anxiety, especially at night after dinner, is that she does not know who she is and that while walking with her dog, she gets lost in her own neighborhood. "And I can't believe it how sensitive I have become to music lately, I hear a tune and I start crying! How weird!"

She swears to me that these weird sensations started after she got hepatitis vaccinations before her trip to Africa. Looking at her face when she tells me how much she enjoys traveling, it seems to be worth all her present suffering. "Indeed," she tells me, "I will never give up my travels, there is so much to see and I don't want to be stuck in a small town all my life." And as she is telling me all these troubles, she never loses her smile and does not seem in the least concerned.

She is very loquacious and vivacious. She loves going to fortune tellers and sitting in on seances with a medium. Even now as an adult she does not like the dark or being alone. She loves chocolate and salty potato chips but has an aversion to other sweets.

Sample Case 4

David M., age 46, 5'9", 210 lb.

CC: I feel totally inadequate and impotent in all phases of my life. I struggle every day with constant feelings of low self-esteem, inadequacy and self-pity. My colon was removed due to ulcerative colitis 14 years ago. During this time I was involved in a troubled marriage and was on the brink of divorce (my wife admitted to me she was gay).

Mental/emotional: afraid when not in control of a situation e.g. when faced with a task or confrontation. Lacks skills, confidence to complete the task. Everything is a struggle to get through. Fears failure, altitude, paralysis: not forging ahead to take on a task without worrying about mistakes or criticism.

People see him as nice guy, kind and caring. Deals with stress by "looking for something to eat." Eating gives comfort. Escapes by thinking about past hunting experiences, sexual fantasies. Sometimes a song goes around in his head and he can't get it out.

Greatest sources of stress: family-owned business and marriage (see Timeline).

Dislikes in other people: aggressive behavior, immaturity, not listening, not caring, selfish. Avoids that person. Never confronts or criticizes. Would like a profession with a defined skill/experience so he can feel secure and confident.

Jealous when he observes someone performing their job/profession with ease and confidence. Also "when I see an attractive and sexy woman with another man. I am jealous because I perceive that man as confident, self-assured and able to satisfy that woman sexually and emotionally."

To be happy: "I would like to be someone else." What bothers him: lack of self-confidence, fear of failure, fear of taking control of situations; would like not to give in so easily, to be able to fight for what is right for him.

I crave carbos, grains, sugars, dairy, chocolate. Prefers cold drinks, big gulps, likes water/juice mix, iced tea. Dislikes hot, humid weather. Hot person. Does not perspire much. Sleeps 10 p.m.–4 a.m. Sometimes rested; most times wishes he could stay in bed longer.

Timeline: Kindergarten very traumatic; first day cried hysterically for mother.

Childhood was stressful; a handful of kids on block were intimidators. Afraid of being beaten or harassed. Always felt down about himself. Discovered that right leg was shorter than left leg. Felt very inadequate when not as agile as other kids in climbing or running. Sixth grade, joined Boy Scouts after much hesitation. Never had the drive to go to Eagle Scout.

Teachers in grammar school commented that he had potential but did not apply himself. Always fearful his father would die and he would be alone. Father worked all the time in his tavern. Always told how tough his father was; war stories, good fighter. The father tried to teach patient to fight.

Frightened when entering high school. Played football, baseball. Confidence started to grow. During a school physical the doctor described him as robust; he felt great!

Parents critical, babied him, "did nothing to build my self-confidence."

Injured his knee playing football just when he was building his confidence. A few months later diagnosed with ulcerative colitis. This development changed his life forever. "Destroyed my self-confidence. I was sick, no cure, crapping in my pants. Couldn't think of anything else. I felt hopeless, self-pitying."

"High school a nightmare. Every day sitting in class, crapping in my pants, running to the bathroom. Chose a college 10 miles from home so I could return home if an accident happened, and it often did. I was going backward, depending on my parents again. I hated my life.

During high school dated a few girls but scared, afraid to act out my sexual feelings. No one to talk to, afraid to confront."

"Met my first wife before ulcerative colitis. After I became sick she stayed with me. I married her because I knew no one else would want me. I settled! Marriage was the last thing I needed but I wanted to be away from my parents, on my own. At 23 I was ill-prepared to face the complexities of love, life and career—still true at 46!"

"Went to work at small firm after many rejections. Crapping in my pants every day."

"Sex was a disaster during my teenage years and my marriage. Always afraid I was taking advantage of a girl in high school. My first wife and I were both virgins when we married; unfulfilled sex life."

"Throughout my twenties several hospital stays, constant feelings of self-pity. Always want to be someone else, jealous of other people. Quit my job, went to work for my father, felt frail and sickly, jealous of everyone else's job and sex life.

"1982-83 large intestine removed, afraid polyps might become cancerous. My wife hardly came to the hospital to visit me. Surgery brought on a complication I have agonized over every second of every day: partial impotence.

"During this time my wife told me she was gay and was filing for divorce. I was single and impotent. How could I start dating and a relationship?

"Began therapy which tried to focus my attention on the relationship, not solely on sex. I wanted sex, I still do.

"Met an attractive woman, sex was OK but never the way I wanted it to be. After several years of dating she wanted to marry and have children. I knew I couldn't be responsible for children so I broke up with her. I was devastated, still think about her every day.

"1989-90 my family sold the restaurant, I lost my job, it terrified me. Went into a state of depression, thought constantly about suicide. Finally got a job with an accounting firm. Quit to go into business with my sister and brother-in-law; made a terrible mistake."

"Several relationships during this time, but I ended all of them. Felt inadequate sexually, emotionally, physically, intellectually. Hated every moment.

"Met my present wife, Leona, in 1994. Perceived her as strong and decisive, all the qualities I lacked. Very attracted to her. She was very sexy. I hoped our love would grow.

"She had vaginal problems so there would not be any demands on me sexually.

"Bought a business, more stress. Struggled for a year to keep it going despite attempts from former owners to ruin me. Leona and I fought every day. Since we were married, terrible arguments, horrible fights. She would call me names, degrade my personality. We have never truly made love. Sex is practically non-existent. She is always pushing me away, telling me I'm annoying.

Sample Case 5, illustrating a principle of management

This is the case of a 43-year-old woman who had three acute attacks of diarrhea in bed, which were painless and did not wake her up. After each attack, totally loose bowel movements continued for about two hours after she woke up. She had no cramps, but she had an intense headache and debilitating fatigue. These three attacks were about two weeks apart. The first two attacks came when she was on a trip, the third one at home. Before the first attack, her only child (a son) went to college in another state. She had been widowed 4 years earlier and had lost both parents within the past few years. I knew that she had a hypersensitive Phosphorus constitution.

Question 1: What remedy do you give and in what potency/dosage? Without doing the scoring chart, just think about the case and what you know of the remedies.

Question 2: You are treating her over the phone and she only has 200c potencies available. What do you advise?

The result from the remedy was a deep sense of grief, which she felt for several days and which slowly lifted with time. She went to a homeopath in her area, who claimed that the remedy was incorrect; he said it was only for the acute attacks, and that by taking it in between attacks, she was proving the remedy. He immediately suggested a different remedy.

Question 3: What should the homeopath have asked before coming to this conclusion? What do you expect the patient would have answered? How should he have interpreted her reaction to the remedy?

Sample Case 6 for Miasmatic Analysis

This student case has been included because it provides an excellent example of miasmatic analysis and also provides the opportunity to review decision-making on what potency to use.

One of my students got to know one of his neighbors, Joe, a 45 year old man, on an occasional walk with their dogs. Joe's main topic of conversation was his complaining about anyone in his life: his co-workers, family, children, the drivers on the road, and especially the police. Obviously, Joe seemed troubled. He often became beet red when telling of his altercations. The latest of them was the previous week. The police driving by his house heard terrible abusive language and thought someone was abusing his wife, but Joe was just upset because he had spilled a pan of water on himself. The arrival of the police only aggravated the outburst, and he turned the verbal abuse toward them. His rage grew more intense: he got into such an argument with his brother while doing errands in another town that he had an incredible vulgar outburst and decided to hitchhike home in the pouring rain. Obviously his Chief Complaint was anger, and road rage was another expression: he could not stand "lousy" drivers and his favorite part of the car was the horn.

Joe stated that he had numerous medical conditions and had been placed on many medications. However, he was not taking them because he believed they might be harmful to him and they would not help anyway. He had hemorrhoids which bled frequently and gave him sharp, stitching pains. He felt as though his rectum was torn, and he had periods of constipation and diarrhea. He also had had warts on his hands, cauterized two years earlier. He had numerous small red itching eruptions on his thighs. He also complained he heard crackling in his ears (a symptom present since childhood) and could hear his own voice reverberating in his ears. He had a cracking sensation in his jaws and difficulty swallowing (food seemed to get lodged). Some of his complaints and his emotional behavior were definitely worse in the morning upon awaking. He suffers from severe temporal headaches, worse at night and only improving with cold applications. He states he does not trust doctors because they have never done anything to help. He seemed more relaxed after telling all this, as he had never told it to anyone. My student figured it was the best time to find out the root of his problem.

Joe related that when he was in the seventh grade his brother, who was five years older, was killed. His brother was very popular and very protective of Joe, always walking him to school. His brother was killed in a motorcycle accident just after an argument with Joe, and Joe was the one who found his body. He waited there for 20 minutes until the police came. The worst part of the whole event, he said, was that after the police arrived, they placed him in his father's van and would not let him out. He viewed this as an act of cruelty, became hysterical, and smashed the interior of the van.

His brother's death was the beginning of the family break up. The father became very abusive, physically and emotionally, and had numerous affairs. When a classmate made a derogatory remark about Joe's brother, Joe became enraged and hysterical, tipping over desks and throwing anything he could get his hands on. After several more outbursts he was put in a special class (although he had never had any problems in school before). He said he never fit in after that and only had one close friend in life. He could not hold a job because of altercations with co-workers; he has little ambition to work which causes him much distress. He feels that working for himself, by himself, may be a solution, so he works as a house painter.

A remedy was given (a 30c in 4 oz of water) and he took about 2 oz. Thirty minutes later, he moved his jaw and said that the cracking was gone and he could not remember when it had not bothered him. The next day he went on a five-mile walk and said he felt great. He also said that his wife asked him if he had been drinking (he is a non-drinker) since she could not remember ever seeing him so relaxed. The next day he walked for two miles without complaining of anything, saying, "I am just enjoying the scenery.

After three or four days his symptoms came back. The same remedy was given in an LM1 potency, 8 succussions, with instructions to take one tsp. and wait, then resume if no aggravations. About two days later, he had another outburst, this time at a police officer who was directing traffic. The succussions were adjusted down to 2. Upon the next contact three weeks later, Joe admitted he had been in a mental hospital. After another outburst of rage he had become despondent and depressed. His wife drove him to the mental hospital, where he was diagnosed with depression. He had only taken two doses of the remedy; his wife confirmed that over the years he had seen numerous doctors for numerous prescriptions but never took them.

His wife said then, "He has been this way since they brought that bike into the house." The family home had been sold recently, and Joe kept the motorcycle on which his brother was killed. He planned to get a bunch of bikers together and destroy it with a sledge hammer for a charity fundraiser.

Family History:
Mother: alcoholism, aneurysm of brain, stroke in one eye, tear in her colon
 Father: quadruple bypass operation, after 3 major heart attacks, first one age 49
Brothers: one brother died in accident; other brother had muscular dystrophy and atrophy of shoulders
Grandparents: Mother's side: grandmother had severe deforming arthritis
 Father's side: grandfather died of stomach ulcer in his early 30s.

Questions: What is the remedy? Do two separate analyses, one with the 10-rubric chart and one analyzing the symptoms for the active miasm. Discuss the top remedies in the scoring chart based on the miasmatic analysis.

Sample Case 7 for Miasmatic Analysis

Ms. C., a 21-year-old Egyptian woman, treated by one of my students when my student travels home to Egypt. Her CC is a menstrual cycle which is painful, prolonged and abundant. Her period lasts about 9 days, strong bleeding, red and clots. Medication makes it worse. Also a fibroadenoma was discovered and removed when she was 19. It was at this point that the first consult was done. The patient is tall, very slender, well proportioned, with dark complexion and features, anxious look. She is a tomboy (dressed in pants all her life).

"I worry a lot, especially at night when it gets dark. I think about my mother and sister and about my studies. I get up at night to check if they are OK in bed and sometimes I crawl in bed with my mom. I feel more responsible for my family since my father died (7 years ago). [She was not at all close to her father. However, C. has been a worrier from age 4 on, she used to panic easily about her younger sister and follow her everywhere.] My studies are not going very well. I work hard but with no results. My memory is not good. I often get colds, runny nose, fever and sore throat, I am anemic, I feel tired. I faint when I do vigorous exercise. My energy level is better at night. I prefer to stay up late and wake up late too. I am always cold in the winter, my extremities especially.

"I have one best friend. I would never think of leaving a friend. It would hurt too much. Sometimes I like to talk about my problems, sometimes not. I don't like people to know who I am. I prefer not to talk at the university because people might misunderstand me. [In her four years at the university she has not made one friend. She studies psychology. At this time, C. has one good friend, M.. However, according to C. she has started to behave very strange lately, trying to avoid her. M. got engaged recently and C. is very upset and anxious about this].

"When I cry, it is silently. I do not have violent anger. If I am upset, I will only talk about it when I feel like it. I am a neat person, I hate a mess. Everything has to be arranged well, I even will pick things up that are not mine too. It takes me a long time to get attached to someone. I cannot make friends easily. I am a trusting person, not malicious or suspicious.

"Marriage has to be an ideal love story, including living happily ever after. [She says she would like to marry someone whom she loves at first sight. He has to be perfect and have a good amount of money too!] I met someone, was not too interested at first, but I am still going out with him. I do not want to get married early, there is no need to leave my home; I feel more secure at home with my mother than with a husband. This boyfriend is exactly like me. We talk about our problems but I still feel more attached and closer to my mother than to him. I want to stay young. Getting married will make me older. I do not want to be pushed, it makes me nervous.

"I am not very happy with my life, I want to be like before [i.e. when M. was her real friend and acting normal]. My extreme happiness is to be with this best friend. I am both optimistic and pessimistic. I like attention, someone to care about me all the time. I like people to call me on the phone, but if they don't, I still call them. When I got the fibroma, I was very worried and thought of the worst. My stool is normal. I like cold drinks. I dislike fatty foods. I become quickly full after eating a little. I am not very thirsty, not even in summer. I like to drink soft drinks. I like salty foods. My appetite is changeable, either I am very hungry or not at all. I love pasta most of all and feel more energetic after eating."

Family History:

Father was depressed for a long time. Depression in cycles, 6 months on, 6 months off. He had feelings of inability to perform, was very sensitive to other people's opinion of him. Very attached to wife and children. He died at age 45 in a cab on the way to the airport, his BP rose so sharply because he was worried about leaving his family to go on a trip for two months abroad. He had HTN and kidney problems all his life. C. was not too attached to him.

Mother has had no special health problems except now is in an exhausted Sepia state.

Pulsatilla 30c was given (3 pellets, q. day for 15 days). The 16th day one dose of 200c and one month later, 1M.

First report 3 months later:

"My period is shorter, but still painful. I put on some weight. I am always hungry, especially before my period. I am more perceptive about my problems and fighting to improve. My studying is better, I feel less anxious about my mother and sister. I still think marriage is a load and I do not want it. My major problem I think is with my head, not with my feelings. My boyfriend (the same one) loves me more than I love him. I feel restless about this whole situation. My cold extremities have improved. I have bad dreams about M. I am scared for her, when I remember the dreams I become anxious. M. still calls me on the phone, she is keeping the friendship normal but at a distance. I do not want that, it has to be like it used to be. I am scared to be attached to her. I feel neglected, my thoughts are to keep away from her, because my feelings are not 100% OK. I am scared I might deviate towards girls. I am not trying to feel like this."

Second report 5 months later:

"I have ups and downs, two weeks good, two weeks bad. Before I was never good. My anxiety is better although I still feel worse at night. I like to sleep with my feet out of the covers, they feel hot. When I am anxious I do not know for what reason, because I am no longer worried about my family. I am seeing a psychiatrist now, she helps me talk of my problems. With M. it is not completely over. I go though phases. I am angry at her now, mainly because she puts me into a problem which I cannot solve. I cannot solve the fact that I feel things towards her that I should not feel towards a girl and I am angry that we are no longer friends. I do not care about my life, it is just flowing and it used to be much better. I can no longer continue with my boyfriend, I have tried hard, but really I have no feelings toward him. He knows I do not love him, I never did. I am waiting to tell him we will break up but I am scared I will upset him. How will I tell him? All my friends are boys, I have neutral feelings towards them. My dreams are insecure, if I have a bad dream it is about her. My period is long in duration, but no longer painful."

A new remedy was given, *Phosphorus* 200c, two months later another 200c. She phoned after the first dose that she had left her boyfriend.

Third report 5 months later:

"I was physically attached to M. for three years, we did things together (would not specify). Now I feel the same toward other girls. The problem is still there. All my life is around this issue, I am upset at M. but I do not feel jealous. I feel I am obsessed: girls are attractive, I look at them the way boys look at them and I am upset. I am relieved I have left my boyfriend. When a boy tells me about his girlfriend, I feel upset because I do not have that. I imagine myself in a boy's place, not a girl's. I am upset at these thoughts."

Took Phosphorus 1M.

Two weeks later:

"I no longer feel haunted and upset about my thoughts towards girls. I can control my thoughts, I think of them, but it does not bother me that I cannot be with these girls I see. Please help me more; it sometimes bothers me so much, I feel pain in my chest."

One week later:

"I feel I am about to collapse and I am helpless. I cannot control myself as much as before. How lucky are boys to be able to love girls without restrictions. I am suffocating because when I love someone, I will not be able to talk about it with anyone. This is killing me. I am really fed up, my doctor says there is no solution, I just have to cope. I cannot cope when I am stuck with something that has only one option that upsets God, thus I do not consider it an option. So I am stuck with something that has no options and I feel suffocated. I feel really sad these days, I got used to holding on, but these days I can't anymore. I need HELPPPPPPP!"

Phosphorus 6c was sent, to be taken every day.

Two weeks later:

"I am better than the past few weeks. A day after taking the medicine, I dreamt about M. The dream altered my mood a bit for the whole day as I dreamt that I was very much attached to her emotionally. When I woke up I wished the dream would come true. I am trying not to be desperate although I really wish I could have this opportunity with someone like M. again."

Questions: What is the remedy? Do two separate analyses, one with the 10-rubric chart and one by analyzing the symptoms for the active miasm. Discuss the top remedies in the scoring chart based on the miasmatic analysis. What do you think of the prescription of Pulsatilla and Phosphorus?

Sample Case 8

One of my students submitted the following case:

A 35-year-old woman presented with twitching of the face, a pronounced tic, almost as a pronounced grimacing, affecting sometimes a part of the face, sometimes her whole mouth, most of the face, and even extending to the neck especially when speaking of something emotionally charged. She looked much younger than her age and had an 8 year-old daughter.

It was a difficult interview as she seemed to be unable to focus on questions posed to her. I observed that she had a look of "Am I right in coming here? Is it okay for me to be here, or should I bolt immediately?" She often looked like she could as easily run away as stay. I felt it necessary to give her lots of reassurance.

What came up quickly were issues relating to marital difficulties. She complained with great emotion that her husband argues and fights with her in front of her daughter. "I've asked him not to, but he keeps on. He is very domineering towards me, at times abusive (not physically). Sometimes he threatens to put me in a mental hospital." From here she jumps quickly to her mother and tells me "she can be pretty domineering too." I observed a great emotional quality in what she said, a sense of outrage in some instances, often a partially expressed thought, followed by an exceedingly hopeful "do you see what I mean?"

"Even as a child I did not too well in school, I was three years behind in reading and two years ahead in speaking. I don't learn information, I absorb it like a sponge." And at one point, out of the blue, she says, "Sometimes when I talk I get stuck in the middle of a sentence. And I get really confused and lose my concentration when I have to think too much."

She says she is easily intimidated. She refers to herself several times as a victim type. She says that in high school "I had a good time. I was in performance after performance, always center stage." She was interested in art and psychology and wanted to become an art therapist. At age 22 she became pregnant and was devastated since she had a strong Catholic upbringing. At that moment, she says, "I was so lonely that I used to phone the Samaritans for someone to talk to."

Observations from my part include this patient's extreme sensitivity. The moment she enters the room, she immediately feels the unconscious motivations, particularly the disturbing ones, of everyone present. She is constantly in an acutely anxious and painful state. She seems to perceive these painful things in a childish way and to be hurt constantly. Recently she was suspended from work because "I got upset." She was standing preoccupied, absorbed in something she was doing, when her supervisor suddenly appeared next to her. She reacted in a very forceful, anxious way and explained to me that she was afraid she was going to be hit by the supervisor. "I was intimidated." Clairvoyance enters the picture too: she predicted

Princess Diana's death, the recent bombing of Sudan, an uncle's disease, a child's death, and so on. Of course her husband tells her she is crazy when she makes these predictions. She says, "I get blamed for everything, and now it's happening at work, too." She lists types of food, weather, movement, light, and noise as aggravating factors and late afternoons and evenings as aggravation times.

As she leaves, she turns hesitantly, almost hunching over, and waits for my guidance. "Should I close the door or is okay to leave it open?" She has a very anxious look on her face, which I have noted throughout the interview.

Question: Find the remedy doing an analysis according to the miasms and to the ten rubrics.

Sample Veterinary Case

Case of Ali, my Calcarea female bull mastiff. From an early age on, Ali would wake up at night between midnight and 2 a.m. with a severe attack of itching. She moaned from the pain, scratching until it bled. It was always the left ear, which would become very hot, purplish or dark red during an attack, which would last for about 30 minutes. Sometimes, but rather rarely, the attack was around 3 p.m. This was the case almost every night, and my wife (who treats the dogs like her children) begged me to find a cure. At first I considered it a psoric (itching) situation, related to the psoric miasm which is usually predominant in Calcarea. Thinking it was an acute expression of her dominant miasm, I gave her Sulphur and Psorinum intermittently when indicated. At first the attacks were diminished in frequency, which gave me hope that I was on the right track. But after a while, progress slowed and then halted completely. I reanalyzed the active miasm, based on the time of the attacks (only at night) and suspected the presence of an active syphilitic miasm. I found the simillimum when Ali got her period (these dogs get it twice a year for about 17 days). During this time the attacks almost entirely stopped. This marked modality of "better from menses" indicated Lachesis, confirmed by other indications: purplish or dark red color, left ear, sometimes going to the right, and always at night, waking the dog from sleep (sleep aggravates).

I decided to give an LM1 of Lachesis, 8 succ., thinking about her slow-reacting Calcarea constitution. The next day she had an immediate serious aggravation, which taught me that she was more sensitive than I thought. Of course no more remedy was given, and immediately amazing results began to develop. For the next two weeks, she produced a thin greenish vaginal discharge. Eureka! Hering's Law was in effect. Then a small papilloma on one of her nipples started to grow enormously to the size of a golf ball, but elongated. After two months, half of it had completely dried up. Furthermore, two cysts appeared on her left leg and a papilloma on the left side of her chest, the size of a nipple (good signs of exteriorization of the miasm). She can now go two weeks without an attack (remember it was daily!). If she does get one, it is very short and much less intense (she just shakes her ear for a minute without scratching). No other dose is given unless she has two severe attacks in a row, and then only 2 successions in the second cup. Her energy has perked up, she likes walking now and is very playful. Lachesis is the simillimum without any doubt. What do I expect? There has been no further discharge but I expect the growth on her nipple to dry up and fall off. And of course attacks should decrease even further. This case teaches us that miasms are present in animals (and I suspect they will become worse and worse with inbreeding), that homeopathic laws are followed as well as in human beings, and that homeopathic remedies can be very effective in animals.

Solutions to Sample Cases

Sample Case I: Miss Juliet, CC dysmenorrhea

A list of all possible rubrics:

Delusions	Delusions, alone, she is in the world, K20
	Delusions, insane, that she will become, K28
Never Well Since	Ailments from grief, K51
Mental/emotional	Weeping, telling of her sickness, K94
	Fear of insanity, K45
	Fear, men, of, K46
	Jealousy, K60
	Company, desire for, K12
	Confidence, want of, K13
	Mood, changeable, K68
	Consolation ameliorates, K16
	Sleep, dreams, black forms, beasts, K1236
	Sleep, dreams, amorous, K1235
Generalities	Gen., weakness, warm room, K1420
	Gen., warm room, aggr., K1413
	Gen., air, open, desire for, K1344
	Gen., evenings, twilight aggr., K1342
	Gen., wind, K1422
Food cravings/Aversions	Stomach, desires, cold food, K484
	Stomach, aversions, drinks, warm, K480
	Stomach, aversions, fats and rich foods, K480
Chief Complaint	Genitalia female, menses, painful, K727
	irregular, late K727
	clotted, K725
	daytime only, K724
	protracted, K728
	Mind, weeping, before and during, K94
	Mind, sadness, before and during, K77

Assessment:

We have many more than 10 rubrics to choose from. In such a case, choose medium-sized rubrics, avoiding those which have too many or too few remedies (of course, delusions and NWS are exceptions). Using this reasoning, here are my 10 favorite rubrics:

1. Delusion, alone, she is, in the world
2. NWS Ailments from grief
3. Mind, fear of insanity
4. Mind, fear, men, of
5. Mind, jealousy
6. Mind, confidence, want of
7. Gen., twilight aggr.
8. Gen., wind, aggr
9. Stomach, aversion, fats, rich foods
10. Menses, painful, and weeping, menses during

I chose as one of the generalities "twilight aggr." as it is an aggravation in time which is always important. The weeping with menses could have been included with the mental/emotional rubrics.

Remedies	1	2	3	4	5	6	7	8	9	10	a	Score
Camphor	1				1							
Hura		1										
Platina	2	2	1					1		2		
Puls.	2	2	3	2	2	2	3	3	3	3	2	11/27
Aurum		3		2		2						
Caust.		3			1	2	1					
Cocc.		3								2		
Ignatia		3	1	1		1						
Lachesis		3	1	1	3	1		2		3		7/14
Nat. mur.		3	2	1		1	1		2	2		7/12
Ph-ac		3			1							
Staph.		3			1		1					

Discussion: Pulsatilla is clearly the the top remedy no matter what rubrics are chosen (because it was written to dramatize the keynotes of Pulsatilla). Reading about it in the Materia Medica, we can see that it has all the characteristics from the case and is easily distinguished from Lachesis and Nat. mur., the next remedies in line.

Sample Case 2: Mr. Al, CC itchy rash

List of all possible rubrics:

Delusions	Delusion, poor, that he is, K31
	Delusion, fancies that he would come to want, K35
	Delusion, superiority, K33
	Delusion, great person, is, K33
	Delusion, fortune, that he was going to lose his, K26
	Delusion, better than others, that he is, K21
	Delusion, thinks he is divine, K24
	Delusion, humility and lowness of others, while he is great, K27
NWS	Skin, eruptions, suppressed, K1319
Mental/emotional	Mind, censorious, K10
	Mind, egotism, K39
	Mind, theorizing, K87
	Mind, disgust, K37
	Mind, haughty, K51
	Mind, fear, high places, K45
	Mind, high places aggravate, K51
	Mind, hurry, K52
	Mind, impatience, K53
	Mind, doubtful about recovery, K37
	Mind, thoughts, persistent (about his perceived "poverty")
	Mind, thoughts, persistent, K87
	Mind, thoughts, tormenting, K88
	Mind, dictatorial, K36
	Mind, discontented, K36
	Mind, haughty, K51
	Mind, quarrelsome, K70
	Mind, fear of poverty, K46
	Mind, anxiety, future, about, K7
	Sleep, dreams, prophetic, K1242

	Sleep, dreams of events not yet taken place, K1239
	Sleep, dreams clairvoyant, K1237
Generalities	Generalities, vertigo, high places, K100
	Rectum, diarrhea, morning, driven out of bed, K609
	Rectum, diarrhea, morning, waking with urging, K610
	Generalities, evening, K1342
	Generalities, night, K1342
	Generalities, winter in, K1422
	Generalities, in summer, K1404
	Generalities, lying in bed aggravates, K1374
Food	Stomach, desires, highly seasoned foods, K485
	Stomach, desires, beer, K484
	Stomach, aversion, to milk, K480
	Generalities, food, milk; aggr., K1364
Sleep	Sleep, position, limbs, uncovered, inclined to have, K1247
	Sleep, waking, 5 AM, with urging to stool, K1255
Chief Complaint	Skin, eruptions, itching and burning at night, K1327
	itching < night, K1314
	itching, > scratching, till bleeding, K1328
	itching, voluptuous, K1329
	itching < warmth of bed K1314
	itching, evening, in bed, K1327
	itching, scratching amel., K1328
	from bathing, K1345
CC2	Headaches, evening, in bed, K135
	winter headaches, K152

Before choosing among the many rubrics, I always ask my students to get a sense of the case (the essence). If you want to describe this personality in one word, it would be "fiery." He is fiery and burning in all aspects, even in his swearing; there is a great intensity about this person. He is not a yielding, changeable character like a Pulsatilla, nor a friendly, sympathethic idea of a Phosphorus, nor an overworked Sepia, not even the stubborn, yet cautious, even timid Calcarea. Of course, Mr. Al thinks the world of himself, definitely considering himself several notches higher in the hierarchy than most people, which could also indicate the haughtiness of a Platina. What stands out is his fear of losing his possessions; he also has great anxiety about health, although that could be an Arsenicum too. Let's see where these remedies are in our repertorizing. With so many rubrics available, we want to choose the ones that reflect this patient the best.

This is one possible choice of 10 rubrics for repertorizing:
1. Delusion, fancies, that he would come to want, K35
2. Delusion, great person is, K26
3. NWS, skin, eruptions, suppressed, K1319
4. Mind, egotism, K39
5. Mind, censorious, critical, K10
6. Mind, fear of high places, K45
7. Sleep, dreams of events not yet taken place, K1239
8. Rectum, diarrhea, morning, driven out of bed, K609
9. Stomach, desires, highly seasoned foods, K485
10. Skin, eruptions, rash, K1317
    a. itching, voluptuous, K1329
    b. itching, > scratching, till bleeding, K1328
    c. itching and burning at night, K1327

Rem.	1	2	3	4	5	6	7	8	9	10	a	b	c	Score
Calc-f	1													
Sulphur	1	1	3	2	3	1	2	3	3	3	3	2	3	13/30
Agaricus		2									2			
Cann-i		2												
Platina		2		3	2									3/7
Veratrum		1	1		2									
Calcarea				2	1					2				
Silica				2	1			2				2		4/7
Lachesis				2	2							2		3/6
Ars.					3									
Sepia					2				1	2	1			4/6

Essence of the Case (NWS): Suppressed eruptions
Constitution: Sulphur
Miasm: Psora
Therapeutic Remedy: Sulphur LM1, 4 oz. bottle, 8 succ.

Explanation of choice of rubrics:

The NWS contains many remedies. Normally I would include all the remedies of the NWS in my repertorizing. Here I make an exception because of the size of the rubric. I scored only the remedies at this point that are in the two delusions, keeping in mind that if another remedy scores high in the next rubrics, I always can go back to this rubric and check if that remedy is in the NWS rubric.

But no matter what rubrics you choose, Sulphur obviously would have come out on top, no other remedy is even close. Notice that Sulphur is the constitution as well as the therapeutic remedy. This sometimes happens, but not necessarily. It is a point that frequently confuses my students. A patient of a Sulphur constitution might need Sulphur to cure his rash, but a Phosphorus or Calcarea patient could also need Sulphur for a rash. The connection is that a Sulphur is more susceptible to getting rashes and needing Sulphur to cure them than patients of other constitutions.

Sample Case 3: Ms. Ellie, CC1 headaches

Comments: Obviously this case is different from the two previous ones: we have two CCs dating from two different dates. One should always consider the timeline and see what CC is the last to appear as it should be addressed first. Her first complaint, a physical one, dates back from her childhood. The second one, more recent, is mental/emotional in nature and dates back to her vaccinations. To treat the last chronic layer, the practitioner therefore needs to make a "10 rubric" choice corresponding to this layer. In other words, her first complaint, headaches should not be reflected in the choice of rubrics, but has to be repertorized by the practitioner when the first complaint (related to the vaccination) disappears.

Rubrics

1. Mind, delusion, body is brittle, K22
2. Mind, delusion, body is delicate, K22
3. Mind, delusion, body is thin, K22
4. NWS, Vaccinations; Generalities, Vaccinations, after, K1410
5. Mind, confusion, identity, as to his, K15
    loses his way in well-known streets, K15
6. Mind, weeping, music, from, K94
7. Mind, Abdomen, alive, sensation of something, K541
8. Generalities, night, 3 a.m., K1343
9. Sleeplessness, from anxiety, K 1253, after midnight, 4 a.m.
10. Body is fragile (in delusions listed above)

Rem.	1	2	3	4	5	6	7	8	9	10	Score
Arsenicum					2				3		2/5
Malan.					3						1/3
Silica					3						1/3
Sulphur					3	1		1		1	4/6
Thuja	1	1	1	3	2	2	3	2	2		9/17
Phos.						1				1	1/1
Alum.					3						
Glonoin					2						
Graphite							3				
Nat-c.						2			1		
Croc.								3			

Essence of the Case (NWS): Vaccinations

Constitution: Phosphorus

Therapeutic Remedy: Thuja LM1, 8 oz. bottle, 2 succ.

Remarks: By taking the layers in account it is not difficult to find the simillimum, Thuja. Normally I would not use three such similar rubrics as my first three choices; they are essentially different ways of saying the same thing and should be combined. But in this short case there are no other rubrics referring to the current condition rather than the underlying constitution.

If we made the mistake of including rubrics referring to her constitution, Phosphorus would receive an artificially inflated score because so many aspects of this case really reflect her constitution. Her smiling even when she has great problems, love for travel, for seances, her fears especially of thunderstorms, loquacity, and the modalities of her headaches are all Phosphorus. But it will be the second remedy to be used after she battles the current serious mental/emotional problems triggered by the vaccination. Knowing her Phosphorus constitution is important for assessing her sensitivity, however. So we give her an 8 oz. bottle with only 2 succussions. After she completes her Thuja layer, we will give her Phosphorus in an LM potency, as a therapeutic remedy for her headaches. We will finish with Phosphorus 10M, 1 pellet dry, to strengthen her constitution.

Sample Case 4: David M., CC: impotence and inadequacy

Assessment: The first time I met this patient, what struck me was how sexual issues came up all the time. He felt inadequate in many things in his life, but the most devastating things for him had to do with sex (first wife gay, jealous about other men when he sees them with attractive women, no sexual demands in his marriage, the agonizing result of his operation in the form of his partial impotence, his obsessive thoughts of sex, etc.). At the same time, one can feel his helplessness and also his tendency to avoid confrontation. He does not want to stand up for himself and take the bull by the horns. He also has a total lack of self-confidence with great performance anxiety in everything he undertakes, especially new things. And how he was humiliated by his ulcerative colitis, how it isolated him even more and broke down his self-esteem. His second wife pushed him further down with her degrading remarks. We want to tell him, "Fight" but there is too much fear to take an initiative, it really expresses cowardice. We can see we don't need a stubborn or self-confident remedy. I think, the rubric, "unable to reach his destination" perfectly describes this patient's life. Here is my choice of rubrics:

1. Delusion, music, evening, hears the music heard in the day, K29
2. Mortification, ailments after, K68
3. Mind, confidence, want of self, K13 (also the CC)
4. Mind, fear, destination, of being unable to reach his, K44
5. Mind, fear, happen, something will, K44
6. Mind, fear, failure of business, NWS list and K45
7. Mind, cowardice, K17
8. Sleep, unrefreshing, 4 a.m., K1255
9. Genitalia, male, erections, incomplete K695
10. Stomach, desires, sweets, K486

Other possible rubrics:
Mind, timidity, K88
Mind, fears, forsaken, K49
Mind, fear, high places, K45
Mind, feels unfortunate, K91
Mind, anxiety, chagrin, after, K5
Mind, company, desire for, K12
Mind, lamenting, K61
Sleep, unrefreshed, K1254
Stomach, desires, cold drinks, K484
Gen., heat, sensation of, K1366

Remedies	1	2	3	4	5	6	7	8	9	10	Score
Lycopodium	1	3	2	1	1	3	3	2	3	3	10/22
Aurum	2	2				1					3/5
Aur-m	2										
Colocynth	3					1					
Ignatia	3	1				1		1			
Nat. mur.	3	1			2	1	1	2	1		7/10
Palladium	3	1									
Ph-ac	3				2	1		2			4/8
Pulsatilla	2	2				2					
Staphysagria	3							1			
Silica		2				2					
Psorinum					2						
Ambr-gr						3					

Essence of the Case (NWS): Mortification
Therapeutic Remedy: Lyc. LM1, 4 oz. bottle, 12 succussions.

The patient is really a Calcarea: physically large/overweight (described as "robust" in high school), had separation anxiety from mother when entering school, teased and bullied by peers, was a nice easy-going person according to others. Calcareas have a high sex drive and can't tolerate high pressure like that in business. Since he is a "slow reactor," I gave him a 4 oz. bottle with a high number of succussions. Students familiar with Lycopodium will see so many indications for Lycopodium that you might suspect it is a made-up case, but it is not, and it has not been altered in any way to increase the Lycopodium rubrics. It is quite possible that the patient might need one of the grief remedies later. However, the patient responded magnificently to an LM of Lycopodium: he became more confident, taking control at work as well as in his relationship with his wife (who was also a patient of mine and complained about his "refound ability" to stand up for himself). Lycopodium makes sense when you consider all the sexual remarks he keeps making and his total feeling of impotence on all levels, as well his fear of failure (Lycopodium is the top remedy for performance anxiety, especially sexually).

We know that according to the traditional Sulphur-Calcarea-Lycopodium sequence, we should start with Calcarea. But we do not in this case because all the symptoms point to

Lycopodium. If there had been any doubt between Calcarea and Lycopodium, we would have started with Calcarea and followed it up with Lycopodium.

Sample Case 5: Management Principles

1. Phosphoric acid: she is Never Well Since grief (she had lost her parents and her husband, then the clincher was losing her only child when he moved away), and it matches the painless diarrhea, plus it is close to her Phosphorus constitution. The essence of the case is the total loss of communication with her dearest and nearest people in life. Her parents and husband had died, and when her son moved away to another state, it took all the strength out of her. Phosphorus stands for communication, sympathy, friends, neighbors, restlessness and fears. Phosphoric acid is one of the two top remedies for homesickness (the other being Capsicum), and it is the Phosphorus element which contributes the sense of unbearable longing for communication with loved ones. The Phosphoric acid patient can feel the lack of communication with a loved one so deeply that another patient of mine was hospitalized for hyperventilation after his girlfriend's father forbade him to talk to her. Phosphoric acid solved these attacks immediately. Of course the Acidums stand for exhaustion. Phosphoric acid stands for emotional exhaustion, which is understandable in this patient who reacts on the physical level with painless diarrhea (a keynote for this remedy). (Picric acid stands for mental exhaustion and Muriatic acid for physical exhaustion). According to Jan Scholten, the Acidums stand for a desire for unity.[1] Unity was definitely broken in this patient (her whole family had left), so the hurriedness of an Acidum was expressed with diarrhea (intestinal hypermotility), even when she was asleep.

Potency/dosage: 1. Ideally, LM1, 8 oz. bottle, 2 succussions, 1/2 tsp. for first dose, then adjust based on the reaction to this dose. We are treating this case as a chronic, not acute case, because the acute attacks are only exacerbations of a chronic miasmatic state.

2. Take only one pellet dry.

3. He should have asked, "Have you ever experienced this symptom (grief) before?" The answer would have been yes, she had. He would then have known that it could be considered a similar aggravation (if she was still experiencing the grief) or a return of old symptoms (if she was not aware of her grief). In either case it indicated a favorable reaction to the remedy. He should not have changed the remedy. He suggested Nat. sulph., but fortunately the patient did not follow his advice.

What happened? She had a strong reaction to Phosphoric acid 200c (which lasted for 2 weeks, one of the reasons we prefer an LM potency). But three months later, she still had no return of diarrhea, and this time when she felt that her grief came back, she took 1 pellet of 6c which was enough to keep her on course for at least four months.

This example shows how important it is to know basic principles of case management. By failing to ask a very basic question, the other homeopath could have sent this patient on the wrong road.

Sample Case 6: Joe, CC rage

The dominant syphilitic miasm can be seen in his complaints about and hatred of almost everyone, especially the police, and his violent, destructive anger (throwing things, vulgar and intentionally hurtful words, tipping over desks in school, altercations with his co-workers). Even his physical expressions, although minimal (because the center of gravity in the case is on the emotional plane), are mostly syphilitic: temporal headaches (< night, > cold), cracking in the jaw bone, and bleeding hemorrhoids with a feeling of a "torn rectum." Other syphilitic emotional expressions include his depression and lack of ambition (which means he has given up, seeing no use in struggling any more). This syphilitic despair is also expressed in his refusal to take medications and remedies ("nothing is going to help me anyway") which can also be seen as a form of syphilitic self-destructive behavior. His isolation and hiding are syphilitic (he had only one friend at school, avoided others, wanted to work by himself). It is interesting to note that he reacted in a syphilitic way when locked up in his father's van, going berserk and destroying the interior. Most young people would react to finding their brother dead with shock, fright or tears. Even as an adult, he could not understand that the police had been trying to protect him at the accident scene, and instead reacted with violence and anger towards them. Also striking is his reaction to frightening or vexing situations: even as a seventh-grader, he would not flee but would stay and fight, reflecting the syphilitic miasm. His all-consuming hate is definitely syphilitic.

The patient had a dormant syphilitic miasm, revealed in his family background, which was triggered by the shock of finding his brother dead. His mother has alcoholism, a stroke in one eye (one of the main targets of the syphilitic miasm), and a destructive tear in her colon The brain aneurysm represents a structural deformity of the vessels as well as a syphilitic weakness in the walls. The father's three major heart attacks are clearly syphilitic because the first one happened at age 49. Apparently the motorcycle accident triggered the father's syphilitic miasm as well, leading to violent, abusive behavior. The surviving brother has not escaped the syphilitic poison: atrophy or rather dystrophy of the shoulder muscles. The older brother would have had the syphilitic miasm too, and his accident could possibly have resulted from self-destructive recklessness in riding his motorcycle.

There is no doubt that this patient needs an anti-syphilitic remedy. What will happen if he does not receive this treatment? He is on a collision course with catastrophe: either he will kill or he will be killed. He has come dangerously close in his many altercations, especially with the police. Which one of the anti-syphilitics? Let's find out with our ten rubrics.

Possible rubrics:

NWS	Ailments from anger, *or*
	Ailments from vexation; *or, to be more precise,*
	Ailments from anger with indignation, K2
Mental/emotional	Mind, censorious, critical (especially regarding authority) K10
	Mind, anger over his mistakes, K2
	anger, violent, K3
	anger, morning, K2
	Mind, intolerant of contradiction, K16
	Mind, quarrelsome, K70
	Mind, rage, K70
	Mind, mania, K63
	Mind, hatred, unmoved by apologies, K51
	Mind, hatred of persons, who had offended, K51
	Mind, irritability, when questioned, K59
	Mind, cursing [verbally abusive], K17
	Mind, anger, violent, K3
	Mind, delirium, raging, K60
	Mind, aversion to company, K12
	Mind, contrary, K16
	Mind, anxiety, health, about, K7
Generalities	Ear, noises, cracking, K295 [during breakfast, when chewing]
	Rectum, constipation, alternating with diarrhea, K607
	Rectum, pain, tearing, K629

Analysis: The Never Well Since is the most important. Until the incident with the police after his brother's death, he just was a normal kid, although showing some of his contrary, stubborn behavior. The Never Well Since is definitely the vexation, the cruelty he felt when he was locked up. I am not using "ailments from grief" since even after all these years, when you ask him about the incident, he singles out "being locked up in the van" as the most horrible thing done to him. He does not express the loss of his brother as the most devastating event. We have to ask how we would expect most seventh-graders to react when finding their brother's dead body. Instead of staying there for 20 minutes, most would run and get help from their father (who was nearby). This would have been a psoric reaction (looking for support).

What else is peculiar, outstanding and striking? His hatred of the police: he has not forgiven them for how they treated him 30 years before. One would expect that looking back at the event as an adult, he would understand that the police were trying to shield him from the unbearable sight of his brother's dead body. But he is unforgiving. His foul language also stands out; it seems to be the biggest outlet for his anger. Interesting, too, that he complains about relatively minor physical symptoms: hemorrhoids, headaches, some itchy rashes, reflecting his "anxiety about his health." He certainly became a loner, preferring to work by himself. He also shows stubborn, contrary behavior. His anger is certainly expressed with great violence, and we need to use rubrics reflecting his anger since it is his Chief Complaint.

As for physical symptoms, the rubric for constipation alternating with diarrhea is too big, containing too many remedies, so we will save it in case we need it for differential diagnosis. The cracking noises in the ear can be used as a rubric because it is more peculiar and more consistent for him, since it has been present as long as he can remember.

Here is a possible choice of 10 rubrics:
1. NWS vexation, Ailments from anger (NWS list and K2)
2. Mind, anger, violent, K3 (the Chief Complaint)
3. Mind, intolerant of contradiction, K16
4. Mind, hatred, persons, of, who had offended; unmoved by apologies, K51
5. Mind, cursing, K17
6. Mind, irritability, when spoken to, K59
7. Mind, anxiety, about health, K7
8. Mind, aversion to company, K12
9. Mind, contrary, K16
10. Ear, noises, cracking, when chewing, K295

Remedies	1	2	3	4	5	6	7	8	9	10	Score
Aurum	2	3	3	2		1		2	1		7/14
Ignatia	3	1					1	3	1		
Lycopodium	2	2	3		2			2	1		6/12
Nux vomica	3	3	2		2	1	1	3	2		8/17
Nitric acid	3	3		3	3	2	3		2	3	8/22
Platina	3							2			
Staphysagria		3	3				1	1			
Sepia	1	1	3			2	2	2	1		7/12
Sulphur	1	1		1		2	1	2	2	1	8/11
Anacardium	3	1		3			3				
Nat. mur.	2	1		2	1	1		3		2	7/12

Essence of the Case (NWS): vexation, anger

Miasm: syphilitic

Explanation of choices of some rubrics: The first NWS (Ailments after anger) is too large. I limited myself to bigger polychrests, omitting acute remedies like Aconite and Colocynth and using mainly my NWS list in Appendix 2. I always keep in mind that I can come back to this rubric if on further analysis some other remedies come up which I had not included at first.

For rubric #4, I used both "Hatred, persons, of, who had offended" together with the subrubric "unmoved by apologies." (The police did not actually apologize for locking him up in the van following his brother's death, but as an adult, he should have been able to understand that they were trying to act in his own best interests.)

For rubric #8 I chose a fairly large rubric ("Company, aversion to") but I only matched the remedies I already had in the previous rubrics. It would have made no difference if I had chosen a smaller rubric such as "Aversion to company, amel., when alone," or "avoids the sight of people."

Differential Diagnosis: Obviously, Nux vomica and Nitric acid are the two top contenders. Before we do the differential diagnosis, I want to comment on some of the other remedies.

Nat. mur.: The Nat. mur. etiology is there (heartbreak upon the death of brother), but a Nat. mur. would be more likely to react by becoming a crusader for a cause, whether by publicizing the case or working to pass laws so that others will not be hurt in similar circumstances. This man reacts with violence and outrage, not in the style of a Nat. mur., who is more sophisticated. More importantly, Nat. mur. is only a 1+ antisyphilitic. (He does have some of Nat. mur.'s syphilitic traits like isolation and vindictiveness.)

Sulphur: Sulphur often comes up in a differential diagnosis simply because it appears in Kent more than any other remedy. It covers all the miasms, which is an argument in its favor. But Sulphur would work hard and get on with his life. A Sulphur usually does not hold on to so much hatred as this unforgiving man does.

Anacardium: of course there is the typical cursing and anger of an Anacardium, but an Anacardium state usually stems from rape, abuse, or (especially) dictatorial parents. And Anacardium is not anti-syphilitic.

Aurum scores rather high and is a great anti-syphilitic remedy. In my opinion, if we did not give this patient a remedy, he could easily progress to an Aurum state with a possible tendency to suicide. So we hope never to need this remedy, but we will keep it on the back burner.

That leaves us a choice between Nux vomica and Nitric acid. We do not automatically choose Nitric acid because it has the highest score; we have to make a differential diagnosis between these two remedies and see which one matches the patient the best. These two remedies do have a lot in common, as can be seen by the following chart.

Nitric acid	**Nux vomica**
Syphilitic 3+	Syphilitic 0 (or at the most, 1+)
Pest because of internal dissatisfaction	Pest because of imbalanced life
Unfit for company	Can work with others if in charge
Chilly 2+	Chilly 3+
Fissures, cracks, ulcerations, stitches	Convulsions, twitches, neuralgic symptoms
Discharges offensive	Breath foul
Craving fat (3), spicy food (2)	Craving fat (2), spicy food (2)
Cracking in jaw when chewing	No cracking in jaw when chewing
Anxiety about health; sense of defeat, nothing can be done	Life is struggle but uses drugs, food, alcohol, power to survive
Unrefreshed sleep (worry about health)	Unrefreshed sleep (theorizing)
Sx < at night and upon awaking	Sx < upon awaking
Sensitive to noise	Sensitive to noise
Unforgiving, hatred	Moves on, too busy
No courage to continue, apathy leading to isolation	Is a fighter, strong work ethic, workaholic, any problem resolved by sheer effort
Irritable (lost all ambition)	Irritable (out of ambition)
Worry about health	Worry about business
Hypersexuality (perverse)	Hypersexuality, impotence
Suicidal but fear of death	Suicidal with gun, in rage
Contrary, obstinate	Contrary, obstinate

Looking at these comparison, Nitric acid is clearly the top choice. We also know that this man fits the profile of a Nitric acid patient (the "pest" who is never pleased with the remedy and does not cooperate with treatment, believing it cannot possibly work). Knowledge of the miasmatic state makes it the top choice without doubt: it is strongly anti-syphilitic, which we need.

Choice of potency: As much as I love LM potencies, its choice for this patient was not correct. He is in an excitable state, is not in touch with his feelings, and he is just the type of person who might take too much. He is too unbalanced to handle the changes of a LM potency. What saved him from overdosing is that he is an unbalanced syphilitic person, not believing that anything will make him better, and thus did not continue the remedy. But if he had been in a psoric mood (as most of us would be after such trauma), he definitely would have overdosed himself and the case would have become more complicated. In a case like this, a 200c or 1M is much better, giving the patient Sac. lac. to take along for self-medication if he wanted it.

Nitric acid 1M was given. Reaction: two days later, he said, "I could run for President, I feel that good." This one dose held for 1 month.

Next move: My student gave Nitric acid 50M for fear it might be his last chance to give him a remedy he really needed, considering his track record for not taking medications. (I would have preferred to repeat 1M, then give 10M two times as needed before going to 50M; we should not be influenced by pressure from patients.) Fortunately the patient did not aggravate because he is a hypo-reactive Calcarea. He reverted to the natural state of a Calcarea: gentle and calm. Now he is even asking for his next remedy.

I feel that if we lose a patient because of non-compliance after doing everything correctly, too bad for the patient. In this case we were lucky that we were dealing with a low-reacting patient. If we had the simile instead of the simillimum, a 50M potency could have created many accessory symptoms, not exactly what we want with a patient already anxious about minor symptoms. The simillimum could have created a similar aggravation, i.e. an outburst of rage, which could have been destructive to himself or those around him.

Prognosis: The prognosis is good if the patient is followed up well. Without this Nitric acid he could have eventually slipped into a depressed, suicidal Aurum state. Syphilinum has to be considered in case of a miasmatic block. Because of the heavy syphilitic background, I expect that Syphilinum will be needed in the future, although it should not be given before it is indicated and not before the indicated antisyphilitic remedy (Nitric acid in this case) stops working. We can, if needed, go up to Nitric acid MM, two times and then start from 200c again. 200c should have been used first in this patient instead of 1M. His test dose of 30c was so successful that we would not expect an aggravation from 200c, so this is no reason to start with 1M. But everything worked out all right. And we wonder what other healing modality could offer such great success in this case in such a short time, without suppressing symptoms.

Sample Case 7 for Miasmatic Analysis: Ms. C. from Egypt

Psoric miasmatic traits: There are plenty of them. *Worry* about her immediate family, school. Sleeps with mom in bed (looking for support); tiredness, fainting when exercising. Energy better after eating. Sympathetic, never would leave a friend. Feels more secure at home with mother, does not want to be pushed, it makes her nervous. Wants someone to take care of her all the time (looking for support again). Quickly satiety when eating. Anxiety about her feelings. Her great sense of responsibility towards her family. Feels neglected by her friend.

Sycotic miasmatic traits: Less present. Fibroadenoma left breast (suppressed); poor memory (which can be syphilitic too); energy much better at night, prefers to stay up late; cold extremities; anemia. Mainly physical expressions. Jealousy is usually sycotic but can be syphilitic (if there is stalking behavior or the desire to kill) or psoric (jealousy of others' collections or possessions). In this case it is sycotic (based on her passionate love for M.).

Syphilitic miasmatic traits: More active and outspoken. First there is the strong syphilitic background of the father: HTN, early sudden death. Poor memory. Aversion to company, does not like people to know who she is (hiding). Silent crying (hiding). Obsessive tidiness. "Hates" a mess. Loathing of life (not very happy with my life, I do not care about my life). Feeling of being stuck, feels suffocated, no way out (but still cries out for help, so has not given up entirely). Symptoms worse at night (worry, anxiety). Sadness. Obviously we have an active syphilitic miasm on a strong psoric background. Our remedy will have to be an anti-syphilitic miasmatic one.

Analysis according to the ten rubrics: What are the peculiar, strange and rare symptoms? And in particular, do we see any delusions and NWS?

The first thing that got my attention was the worry she exhibited for her mother and sister (to the point of leaving her bed and checking on them). This shows a great sense of *duty*, going back as far as age 4 and increasing when her father died. In my opinion, she took over the *male* role in her family at that point, which represents a form of compensation and early responsibility. This gives me my first delusion: "Delusion, neglects her duty." Secondly, a very strong feeling, bordering on the delusion: even when her friend tries to keep the friendship as normal as possible (of course she had less time now for C. since she was engaged, and possibly she wanted to pull away from the intimate relationship they had), C. felt that she lost the affection of M. Her feelings for M. are very strong, always expressed in her dreams when her unconsciousness is no longer suppressed as she tries to do during the day. From there the second delusion, *she has lost the affection of her friend*. The NWS seems to be clear: "Ailments from disappointed love" with the subrubric, "Lovesick for her own sex." We also could use "Ailments from grief" (but we will not because it overlaps too much with the other rubrics we have chosen). Furthermore, she tries hard to suppress her feelings and her anger towards M. for not having a close relationship any more. This gives us "Ailments from suppressed anger."

What else stands out? As time goes on, there is more despair and sadness in this patient, to the point of "loathing of life" ("I do not care about my life, I am not very happy with my life"). In her despair she even thinks her feelings are wrong in the eyes of God ("my feelings upset God"), which reflects her religious convictions. And without any doubt she is tidy, even picking up after other people, certainly unusual for a teenager. Her CC (the dysmenorrhea) comes last, not very important as it is really a physical expression of her emotional struggle with her newly-discovered sexual orientation.

How did she react to the previous remedies? The first remedy really did nothing, not surprisingly because there is very little of Pulsatilla in this case (in fact she reacts in the exact opposite way of a Pulsatilla by being emotionally closed). The second remedy is debatable. If she reacted to the second prescription it was only to put her more in touch with her feelings, which is possible since Phosphorus stands for communication. It is debatable whether these remedies can even be called similes. Let us examine the ten rubrics to find a better remedy for this desperate young woman.

1. Delusion, neglects her duty, K30
2. Delusion, she has lost the affection of her friend, K20
3. Ailments from disappointed love, K63
4. Ailments from jealousy, K60
5. Ailments from suppressed anger, K2
6. Loathing of life, K62 (also look at "Loathing of life in evening")
7. Lovesick, for her own sex, K63
8. Religious, K71
9. Conscientious about trifles, K16
10. CC Menses, painful (dysmenorrhea), protracted, excessive

Remedies	1	2	3	4	5	6	7	8	9	10	Score
Aurum	3	2	2		1	3		2	1		7/14
Cyclamen	1										
Hyoscyamus	1		3		1	3	3		1		6/11
Ignatia	1		3		2	1			3		5/10
Lycopodium	2								2		
Natrum ars.	1										
Pulsatilla	1				2	2		2	1		5/8
Causticum			1								
Cocculus											
Lachesis			2		3	2	2	3			5/12
Hura		1									
Nat. mur.						3	1				
Phos. acid											
Staphysagria					3						
Sepia					1	2		2	1		4/6

Analysis: We need to do a differential diagnosis between the two top antisyphilitic remedies that come up, Aurum and Lachesis (both 3+ antisyphilitic). First we can ask, what is common to both remedies in this patient? Ailments from disappointed love, loathing of life, religious affections, and her aversion to talking (which is the opposite of Lachesis' usual loquacity but Lachesis can also be aloof). What speaks for Lachesis which is not covered by Aurum? Ailments from jealousy and the sense of constriction in the chest which expresses the sense of being trapped. (Lachesis is well known for a constricted feeling in the throat, but it can appear anywhere in the body.) Love for her own sex is outstanding in this case, and Lachesis is one of only four italic remedies in the rubric (which has no black-type remedies).

On the other hand, Aurum reflects her despair and hopelessness, which stand for dejection and grief, seeking solitude; in Aurum the memory is greatly affected; there is self-reproach, prolonged anxiety and unusual responsibility (one of the etiologies of Aurum). Aurum is peevish and indisposed to talk. The future always looks dark for Aurum. One thing I saw in this case right away was her conscientiousness, industriousness (she says she works very hard in school and takes very good care of her family), religiousness, perfectionism: all these stand for Aurum. And of course this loss of her love, the heartbreak, is a classic Aurum etiology:

the loss of the one thing which is most important in the patient's life. I think these characteristics reflect this patient.

Let us look again at the qualities which Aurum and Lachesis share in the case.

Ailments from disappointed love: Lachesis has an excess of energy seeking for an outlet, and this patient does not express this quality. She does not react to her grief in a Lachesis way, which could include stalking and active jealousy, even killing; finding an alternative outlet through meditation or religion; or becoming very haughty or very talkative. C. does not seem to have done any of these things. Aurum typically reacts to grief by seeking solitude, which she has done.

Loathing of life: Aurum has this characteristic much more intensely than Lachesis; in fact, Aurum is one of the top remedies for this condition. We must be concerned about the patient when we see this issue becoming more and more outspoken over the past year and a half.

Religious affections: Lachesis expresses this quality by overcompensating, by becoming overly religious, for example by preaching against sex or by taking a vow of celibacy. Lachesis has the delusion of being in direct communication with God, expressed by the rubric "Delusion, is under a powerful influence," K28. Aurum expresses religious affections by being very dutiful, respectful, and guilt-ridden, which is much more reflective of this patient. In a way we should not have even scored 3 points for Lachesis under this rubric, because the patient does not express her religious affections in a Lachesis way.

Aversion to talking: Aurum seeks solitude out of grief and heartbreak. Lachesis patients can be reserved but they do not necessarily avoid people. Lachesis is normally loquacious and if she cannot be, she needs to find another outlet. We do not see any other outlet for this patient, whereas the provings of Aurum have "dejected and full of grief, seeks solitude," which is very reflective of this patient.

Prescription: No doubt she needs Aurum now. If she lived close to me, I would give her LM potencies of Aurum, but I will settle on 200c.

I think this Aurum layer will go back quite far in her life. She seems to have felt an unusual sense of responsibility already at age 4; one wonders if it had to do with the depressive moods of her father. What is underneath the layer of Aurum? Lachesis (which does match the patient in many ways)? Sulphur (her possible constitution)? Time will tell, but for now, we hope that Aurum restores her love for life.

Sample Case 8: 35-year-old woman with facial twitching

My initial assessment:

What struck me in this case was the patient's childish behavior, always asking for permission to say or do something, with a cowering expression on her face and in her body language. One might consider this behavior "timidity," but in a 35-year-old woman I would see it as a consequence of the humiliation she suffers from her husband and previously from her mother. I realized this had more to do with cowardice than with timidity, accentuated by a total lack of confidence which was evident in this case. She seems to be afraid of new situations, as my student was the first homeopath she had ever consulted. I also noticed that she seemed to feel vulnerable in situations where she could be easily hurt. She says, "I get blamed by everybody." Then there is the incident at work in which she overreacted to her supervisor. When asked why she reacted this way, she said, "I thought she was going to hit me." I translated this into "Delusion, is about to receive an injury," K28.

It is obvious what her constitution is. In her love for the theatre, dancing center stage; her aspirations to become an art therapist; her great clairvoyance and sensitivity towards exterior impressions; her great need to talk to someone when upset; her description of herself learning "like a sponge"; and her appearance much younger than her years, Phosphorus shines through. We must make sure that we do not confuse these characteristics of her innate constitution with the symptoms we need to prescribe on. And we must take her extreme sensitivity into account when selecting the potency of the remedy (LM1, 8 oz., 2 succ., 1/2 tsp.) Obviously her Phosphorus "fire" has been almost extinguished by the domineering and abusive behavior of the husband.

The severity of her Chief Complaint expresses the intensity of her internal turmoil. Obviously we want to prescribe on her internal mental/emotional state, with the confidence that the matching remedy will take care of its external expression. If by any chance this Chief Complaint is covered by the simillimum, so much the better.

Choice of rubrics:

Delusions	Delusion, is about to receive an injury, K28
	Delusion, vanish, seems as if everything would, K34
	(i.e. she has vanishing thoughts while speaking)
NWS	Ailments from mortification, K68
Mental/emotional	Mind, mistakes in reading, K66
	Mind, confusion from mental exertion, K15
	Mind, cowardice, K17

Mind, confidence, want of, K13

Mind, irresolution, K57

Face, expression, anxious-looking, K374

Chief Complaint   Face, twitching, K395

Remedies	1	2	3	4	5	6	7	8	9	10	Score
Arsenicum	1							2	3	2	4/8
Aurum			2		2	1	2	1			5/8
Ignatia			3					3	2		
Lachesis	1						1	3			
Lycopodium	1	1	3	2	2	3	2	2	2	3	10/21
Mercury	1		1	1		1	1	2	1		
Nat. mur.			3		2	1	1	2		2	6/11
Nux vomica	1		1		2		1		2	1	6/8
Pulsatilla			2		2	1	2	2		1	6/10
Silica	1			1	2	1	2	2		3	7/12
Staphysagria			3		2						
Sulphur	1		2		2	1	1	2	2	1	8/12

The remedy is clearly Lycopodium, which we could see already in the etiology (humiliation), which beats her into cowardice; in her lack of confidence, especially when confronting new tasks; her reading problems, mental confusion, and vanishing of thoughts; and her 4-8 pm aggravation time. She has some Pulsatilla and Silica in her behavior, but they do not match the etiology. Her Phosphorus constitution explains all of her symptoms and traits which are not covered by Lycopodium. Lycopodium is even a 3 for her Chief Complaint.

Miasmatically, her case is clearly psoric: the mental/emotional state is one of weakness, looking for support (reassurance) and lack of self-confidence to the extreme of cowardice; she has a worried and anxious expression on her face; and her Chief Complaint is neuralgic. Lycopodium is a 3+ antipsoric.

Solutions to Cancer Cases

Cancer Case 1: Mrs. K, tumor of the uterus

Choice of rubrics: We look first for delusions, any strange-rare-peculiar symptoms, and a Never Well Since, but we do not see any of these rubrics in the case. (The palpitations which are worse from lying but not from exercise are unusual, the opposite of what we would expect. But we do not have a single rubric which covers this characteristic. We will use this symptom as an elimination point at the end, as explained later on.) We go next to the mental/emotional symptoms, then to the physical generals, with their page numbers in Kent: Rubrics for her weakness ("Prostration," "Lassitude") are too large to be useful.

    Weeping from music, K94

    Weeping < when alone K93

    Sadness from music, K77

    Sensitive to noise, K79

    Offended easily, K69

    Drawing sensation in lumbar region, K926, < excitement, < menses

    Headache (heaviness) on vertex, K171, during menstruation, K172 > lying, > open air K135, < standing, K148, < after eating K172.

    Palpitations, < sitting, lying on side, K875, < especially after slightest emotional excitement (*translated as:* attention is directed to anything, when, K874) but not < walking K877

    Bread gives headache: Generalities, food, farinaceous food aggr, K1363

    Sweets give headache: Generalities, sweets, aggr., K1364.

    Before warm and > open air, K 1344, now chilly in bed: Generalities, heat, vital, want of, K1366

    Flatus odor of rotten eggs, < after milk, K548

    Rectum, flatus offensive, K618,

    Distension, abdomen, flatus amel., K545

    Rectum, constipation, insufficient, incomplete stools, K608

    Stomach, desires, salt things, K486

Miasmatic assessment: Almost all the symptoms are psoric: weakness, fears, hypersensitivity to noise, digestive disturbances, headaches, unrefreshed sleep. This is why it was a slow growing tumor.

Selection of rubrics:
1. Weeping from music, K94
2. Sadness, music, from, K77
3. Sensitive to noise, K79
4. Offended, easily, K69

Note: I would like to have had more emotional symptoms, but there are no more except the tendency to depression, which is too general to be helpful. Therefore, I will have to look for peculiar physical symptoms, by preference generals. What do we have?

I am not using the drawing sensation in lumbar region because the rubric is too big, as are the rubrics for her menstrual disturbances. But what is peculiar is that there are palpitations when the patient is lying which are not present while walking, in other words on exertion (K875). So the rubric, "Palpitations, exertion," K875 can be used as a differential if we have two or three top remedies at the end. Usually I would not do negative prescribing, but in this case the combination of < lying and not < exercise is so unusual that we would prefer our top remedy not to appear in the latter rubric. Continuing with the choice of rubrics:

5. Chest, palpitations, lying on side, K875
6. Chest, palpitations, attention is directed to anything when, K874
7. Generalities, food, farinaceous food aggr, K1363
8. Abdomen, flatulence, milk, after, K548
9. CC: Cancer of uterus, K715

"Flatus, offensive" has too many remedies to be useful; instead, it can also be used to help make a differential diagnosis among the top remedies at the end. The same with the patient's chilliness ("Generalities, heat, vital, lack of"). Also notice that the tumor is placed at the bottom of the hierarchy as the Chief Complaint. In other words, even if the remedy does not appear in this rubric, but it is the simillimum according to the other rubrics, I would use it and expect good results.

When we look at this patient, we know we will need a remedy for a person sensitive to noise and music, who weeps when alone (silent grief), is easily offended, has a tendency to depression (sadness) and constipation or ineffective stool, who reacts to sweets and breads, who likes salt and who has palpitations more in rest than in movement. There is no doubt that this group of symptoms draws you to the Natrum group of remedies. Which one? Nat. mur., Nat. carb., and Nat. sulph. all have many of these characteristics. The 10 rubrics (actually 9 are enough to solve this case) will help us make the choice; we will still need to read about the two top remedies in the Materia Medica.

Remedies	1	2	3	4	5	6	7	8	9	Score
Graphites	3	2	0	2					3	4/10
Kreosotum	2	2	0	0					3	
Nat. carb.	2	2	2	1*	2	1	2	2	2	9/16
Nat. sulph.	1	2	2	0			3	2		5/10
Thuja	2	1	0	0					3	
Nat. phos.		1	1	0						
Sabina		2	0	0						
Nux vomica	1	1	3	3		1				
Nat. mur.			2	2	1		3		2	5/10

*According to Schroyens' *Synthesis Repertorium*

Conclusion: Nat. carb. is a clear winner, but I would advise the practitioner to read about Nat. sulph. and Nat. mur., which were in the top group as predicted. The other remedy in the running is Graphites. Upon reading about all these remedies, Nat. carb. would come out first. It even covers the tumor (although I was not concerned about that). It is chilly, it has the offensive flatus, and certainly a tendency to depression like all the Natrums. It is a 3+ antipsoric remedy which fits this tumor. The runner-up was Nat. mur., but this does not show up in the rubrics "weeping and sadness from music" which are so outspoken here. Nat. mur. loves classical music but does not weep with it because it expresses her moods. The author of this case gave Nat. carb. 200c. My choice of course would have been Nat. carb. LM1.

Cancer Case 2, businessman with cancer of the stomach:

Remedy A: Chelidonium. It has the well-known keynote of pain under the right shoulder blade (upon which you almost can prescribe immediately); it also has " Abdomen, constriction, string, as if by a," K542 (black type remedy, the only other one is Caust.), and "Stomach, pain, heat amel." K513. The author claims that in the clinic he has also verified on numerous occasions the improvement of pain in the stomach from bending backwards. Indeed we should add it to Kent, p. 512; we see Belladonna there, which of course has the aggravation from a jar. But Chelidonium fits better. The aggravation time of Chelidonium is from 4-10 p.m., well within the range of the patient's complaint.

Remedy B: Arsenicum, of course. All the keynotes are there, especially "Restlessness, wants to go from one bed to another," K73, and "Restlessness, driving out of bed," K73.

Remedy C: Belladonna, without any doubt.

Remedy D: Lycopodium, no doubt.

Remedy E: a little trickier, but the new symptom showed by the Vital Force is a peculiar one: "Stomach, eructations, salty," K496 has only a few remedies of which only two are italics. We prefer *Carbo animalis,* a well-known cancer remedy and a burning remedy.

Remedy F: Phosphorus, of course.

Remedy G: Carbo veg. ("Abdomen, flatulence," K548, and "Rectum, flatus, hot, during diarrhea," K618).

Remedy H: Sulphur, of course!

Remedy I: Zincum. You can't miss this great remedy for nervous prostration, and the fidgety feet are a give-away.

Remedy J: Sulphur again. We must finish with an antipsoric, and Sulphur is the king of the antipsorics.

Remarks: It is interesting to see that CM potencies were often used in spite of the advanced pathology. However, the zigzag method of prescribing used was more like acute prescribing, and in this sense an argument could be made for the high potencies. In spite of the different similes used, the Vital Force, relieved somehow from its suppressive forces, was always able to keep throwing new symptoms up, indicating the next remedy each time. Would LM potencies have worked better and faster? Based on my own experience, I am sure they would; and they would probably have worked longer in each case, especially considering how much suppression the patient had experienced. Nevertheless, this is a wonderful example of a cure according to Hering's Laws.

Cancer Case 3, middle-aged woman with cancer of the breast:

Remarks: Would Nitric acid have helped if it was given first? We will never know, but Dr. Carleton prescribed on the symptoms provided by the patient. If anything, this case shows how a diligent and careful examination is necessary. It is marvelous to see, however, how each remedy given was followed by improvement and showed the way to the next prescription. In fact, the Vital Force seemed to throw symptoms out which are well known even to the beginning homeopath.

Remedy A: Sulphur, of course!

Remedy B: Lachesis greatly indicated.

Remedy C: Bryonia with its great keynote < from motion.

Remedy D: Nitric acid for its great keynote, "sensation of needles or wire."

Cancer Case 4: Maria with metastatic breast cancer

Analysis: We can determine the family miasmatic background by looking at the family history, then look at the timeline to determine what events created or triggered the different miasms.

Looking at the father and mother: The mother reached old age with CHF (so she must be very psoric) in spite of having had bouts with strong syphilitic miasmatic expressions (psychotic depression, cataracts) as well as sycotic ones (varicose veins, shingles). Somehow her strong psoric background must have kept the other miasms in check, even when she had cancer of the uterus (which must have been psoric, as it was not fatal). But all three miasms were present in her. The father had mainly a syphilitic background: he died suddenly from CVA, had three heart attacks at young age, and finally had cancer, too.

So we have a strong syphilitic and cancer background in both parents. Because of this we can almost expect to find the syphilitic background in all the children. In fact we find that none of the siblings escaped the powerful poison of the syphilitic miasm: the oldest sister has had depression and three miscarriages, the next has had IDDM and depression, the only brother has depression, and the youngest sister has breast cancer with mets to the brain (mixed miasm including syphilitic).

As for our patient, she was born with the syphilitic miasm, but the sycotic miasm was dominant from age 7 to age 34, activated by the smallpox vaccination. The sycotic miasm expressed itself (as sequelae of the vaccination, although this would not be acknowledged by allopathy) in many sycotic manifestations: encephalitis, rheumatic fever, prolapsed valve. Some other unfortunate events brought this miasm even more to life: gonorrhea from her husband, repeated vaccinations (DPT, BCG), leading to initial infertility, warts (burned off, another suppression), fibrocystic breasts and a cyst on the left ovary. How much would this patient have benefited from Thuja/Medorrhinum from a young age on!

Perhaps even more traumatic to the Vital Force than the physical miasmatic triggers were the emotional traumas she suffered: the separation of her family when she was young, her years in the orphanage, and the years of emotional, physical, and/or sexual abuse, beginning at age 3 and continuing in her schooling and in her marriage. The resulting humiliation, indignation, and suppressed anger undoubtedly helped fuel these miasms, ultimately leading to cancer. In her cancer we see a combination of the syphilitic miasm from her family background with a strong sycotic miasm stamped on her by her life experiences. The cancer is both sycotic (worse from dampness) and syphilitic (metastasized to the bones of cranium and spine, causing deep bone pains).

Prescription: It would be a mistake to prescribe according to the miasmatic diagnosis: the remedy would be too hard on the Vital Force. This situation requires lesional prescribing. It is not difficult to see what remedy she needs now: she has great anxiety and great fear of being alone, to the point that she even seeks company which has a negative effect on her. She needs people around her, probably to relieve her anxiety. She still is in a psoric state (has not given up hope, asks for help, looks for support from people) which is a positive sign. I wonder if she has that strong psoric background of her mother. She takes Ativan for her anxiety, is best lying down with many pillows, is very chilly. No doubt a dose of Arsenicum album (LM or 200c) is required to reinforce her Vital Force and give her some well-needed rest. Arsenicum is truly a great remedy for any stage for almost any cancer, when indicated. Aurum may be the next remedy coming up, because it covers depression and intractable pain. The cancer has taken on life of its own (one-sided disease), and lesional prescribing with Arsenicum is necessary. Especially with an LM potency, which can bring suppressed cases into remission or cure, we just have to wait and see what this remedy will do. But this case reflects very well the result of consecutive suppressions fueling the miasms present. It certainly helps to make the case for anti-miasmatic prescribing *before* one has children.

APPENDIX FIVE

Homeopathy and Traditional Chinese Medicine

Similarities Between Two Great Healing Modalities

Hahnemann's concept of the Vital Force; the natural laws of healing he observed and which Hering codified in his Laws; and even the examination of the patient in homeopathy are so similar to those in Traditional Chinese Medicine (TCM) that it is hard to believe that Hahnemann was not influenced by TCM. We do know that in his search for an alternative to the noxious medicine of his day, Hahnemann was eager to learn systems of medicine from around the world, including the ancient Greek and Arabic. We also know that Hahnemann "had a liking for the Chinese, and his favorite topics for conversation were the natural sciences aned conditions in other countries."[1] And we know that reference books on TCM would have been available to Hahnemann; for example, Willem ten Rhyne's *Secrets of Chinese Medicine* was published in 1671. I find it surprising that Hahnemann does not quote from the Chinese texts, although he quotes extensively from Arabic and Greek texts.

Why did Hahnemann condemn acupuncture and moxabustion (burning a special combination of herbs) in the foreword of the *Organon*? He included both modalities in a list of "obnoxious counter irritants" (which also included setons and cautery, i.e. allopathic suppresssive treatments).[2] His mistake was understandable because little was known at that time about dermal-spinal reflexes, or acupuncture in general for that matter. Acupuncture works on an entirely different principle than suppressive allopathic treatments, but apparently Hahnemann did not know that. Several textbooks of acupuncture were published in Germany in the nineteenth century, but most appeared after Hahnemann's death. And acupuncture was not *practiced* in Europe until the early twentieth century (or at least, not practiced correctly). In 1907 Soulié de Morant, the French consul at the Chinese imperial court, became the first Westerner to be granted the title of "Physician in Traditional Chinese Medicine." He brought acupuncture to France, publishing *Précis de la vraie acupuncture Chinoise (Treatise on True Chinese Acupuncture)* in 1934.

Acupuncture, in continuous use for approximately five thousand years,[3] is effective because it redirects and normalizes the flow of the body's healing energy, what TCM calls "chi" and homeopathy calls the Vital Force. Roger Schmidt believes that acupuncture "determines physio-pathological changes in the patient similar to the effects following the administration of a homeopathic drug."[4] Hahnemann definitely supported the use of complementary modalities like galvanism, mesmerism, and the use of magnets (discussed in Aphorisms 286-290), which are energetic healing modalities like acupuncture. Hahnemann also recommends adjunctive modalities which stimulate the Vital Force like hydrotherapy, enemas, and gentle electric shocks (not strong shocks as in modern electroconvulsive therapy). Hahnemann says that this type of stimulation can remove obstructions and suppressions of the Vital Force. Acupuncture aims at the same effect, removing blockages to the flow of "chi" (what we call "stagnation of Qi" in TCM).

Many homeopaths tell their patients not to have acupuncture while under homeopathic treatment, on the basis that Hahnemann forbade it. As we have seen, Hahnemann probably was misinformed or misunderstood acupuncture. I believe that if Hahnemann knew enough about acupuncture he would definitely have recommended it. I have treated thousands of patients with both modalities and have found the action of each one enhanced the other.

However, I have found homeopathy to be so much more effective that for many years I have only used homeopathy and have not felt the need to use acupuncture on my patients. I can help many more patients and help them more effectively with homeopathy, because with acupuncture we need to treat patients weekly or even several times a week, whereas with homeopathy we can see patients once a month or every few months. With homeopathy we can go deeper to the mental and emotional planes. More importantly, we can eradicate the miasmatic basis of disease.

At this point, if a patient came to me who was seeing an acupuncturist and feeling some benefit, I would not prevent him from continuing. (This does not usually happen, because if patients are seeing results with one modality they do not usually seek out another.) If the patient did continue acupuncture, I would want to be sure that the acupuncturist did not give palliative treatment for a healing reaction or for symptoms exteriorized by the Law of Hering, which could risk suppressing the symptoms. If we want to allow our patients to have acupuncture treatments in addition, we should work with acupuncturists who we know and trust, because palliative acupuncture treatments can be suppressive just as superficial homeopathy can be. (For example if a patient picks up a "cold-flu" combination in the health food store to stop the nasal discharge caused by a healing reaction, it can block the beneficial action of a chronic remedy.)

If a patient were beginning homeopathic treatment with me and considering starting acupuncture too, I would recommend waiting until we had seen the reaction to the remedy. At that point I would expect that in most cases the patient would no longer feel the need for acupuncture. In any case, I always ask patients not to start any other modality at the same time as the remedy, because we need a clear assessment of the reaction to the remedy.

We may never know whether Hahnemann was inspired by TCM. The important issue to me is whether we homeopaths can learn anything from TCM which can help us with our patients. I have had the opportunity to study a number of different healing modalities and I have found that each one has something to offer in treating our patients. I have found TCM to be especially helpful to my homeopathy practice and in this chapter I hope to distill the essence of what is useful so that my fellow homeopaths can benefit without having to spend years studying TCM. Following are certain concepts which homeopathy and TCM have in common.

Vital Force: The concept of *Qi* or energy corresponds to the Vital Force in homeopathy and is essential in TCM. Qi is considered a universal substance, inflowing and outflowing, balancing "negative" yin and "positive" yang aspects. In TCM, illness is at once the result and the cause of a derangement of this circulation of energy. When energy fails to circulate as it should, vital organs may suffer from a deficiency or a disturbing excess of this "life force."

TCM recognizes three different forms of Qi (also spelled *chi* and pronounced "chee"). The *Wei Qi* or defense energy provides the first line of defense on the energetic level as the immune system does on the physical level; the *Ancestral Qi* or Hereditary Qi is the energetic equivalent of the genetic makeup; and the *Yong Qi* or Food Qi is the energy generated by digestion and also by respiration. Hahnemann's concept of the Vital Force is very similar to the concept of Qi, and the three specific types are addressed in his "Perfect Prescription: he warned us about the injurious effects of food, alcohol, and environment (Yong Qi), he gave us his great discovery of the miasms (Ancestral Qi), and he explains the primary and secondary effect of any trauma or trigger on the Vital Force (Wei Qi). Hahnemann even showed a deep understanding of another form of energy recognized by TCM: the *interpersonal energy,* representing the positive or negative effect which other people have on our life energy. Homeopathy even more than TCM recognizes the impact of different emotional factors (such as grief, humiliation, indignation, fears and worries) on our exposed Vital Force. As stated in the *Nei King,* an ancient acupuncture text: "Before puncturing, the practitioner should know the role of the psyche."

Examining the patient: The Chinese classic text *Zhang Zhong Jing* states: "A skillful doctor knows by observation, a mediocre doctor knows by interrogation, an ordinary doctor knows by palpation." The homeopath certainly needs to be skillful in both observations and questions, as discussed in the chapter on case-taking. The guidelines for patient examination are set forth in two ancient books, the *Sou Ouenn* and the *Nei King* (the "Organons" of TCM). We homeopaths could learn much from the *Sou Ouenn*'s Chapter 77, "Five Mistakes of Doctors":

"Doctors must know the social status of their patients: when the patient is rich, he most likely will suffer from organic disease; when he is poor, most illnesses will stem from lack of proper nourishment." We have already mentioned how city-dwellers have more problems related to diet and overuse of drugs, and how much more sensitive they become to different stimuli, including remedies, because of a continued suppression of the Vital Force. The resulting diseases are maintained by bad habits and a bad environment. These diseases, which Hahnemann says in Aphorism 77 are not true chronic diseases, require a change in lifestyle and diet rather than a remedy. Poor people, on the other hand, are likely to be in a Psorinum state (typified by poor hygiene, lack of nourishment, and malassimilation). This condition can be found in street people, concentration camp survivors, and even in abused children of alcoholic parents. Aphorisms 5 (in which Hahnemann discusses the necessity of knowing the patient's occupation, moral and intellectual character, social and domestic relations, mode of living and habits) and 77 of the *Organon* perfectly correspond to this first point from the *Sou Ouenn*.

"Ask the patient about his life-style: is he moderate or excessive in his habits; ask about emotional traumas and events: has there been severe anxiety, fear or anger?" The first part we just discussed. As you can see in the second part of this statement, the TCM practitioner looks first for *emotional, not physical* traumas. Five thousand years ago the Chinese even knew how each organ was affected by a particular emotion, as discussed later in this chapter.

"The great doctor must know first the normal pulse very well; only then can he know the correlation between the symptoms and the pathological pulse." Chinese medicine has for each of the "twelve organs" (described below) a radial pulse position, with diagnosis based in part on these pulses. Some homeopaths use pulse changes in what we call *Autonomic Reflex Testing (ART)*, based on the principle that when the correct remedy is brought into the patient's energy fields, there are measurable changes in signs such as pulse rate, rhythm and depth, respiratory rate, percussion tones of the chest and abdomen, and dilation of the pupils. The pulse in particular is tested for a sudden hesitation, then a single strong heartbeat, then a noticeable change in rhythm and volume, all of which indicate that the correct remedy has been held near the patient (behind the patient's back to avoid any interference from the patient's conscious awareness). While the acupuncturist looks for an organ imbalance through his pulse testing, the homeopath can use it to find the simillimum.

"A good physician must be able to differentiate whether a disease is caused by an Exterior Excess or by an emotional disorder. He must know that if the reason of the psychic imbalance persists (for instance an emotional shock), he can do nothing for this patient, because a calm mind is necessary for the normal

circulation of the Yong and Wei Qi." Both TCM and homeopathy require distinguishing between exterior triggers of illness (climate, diet, drugs, physical traumas, etc.) and the more common interior ones (emotions). This passage also states the importance of removing any exciting cause (*tolle causam*).

"When a doctor examines the patient, he must go back to the origin of the disease and follow the evolution [to] determine the indicated therapeutic technique." This passage from TCM warns against a common mistake of practitioners in general: focusing on the end results (diagnosing and treating the sick leaves) and forgetting the onset (the sick root). In homeopathy we give the Never Well Since the greatest value in the selection of the remedy and we follow the time line ("follow the evolution") to track down the different layers formed in the patient.

Hering's Laws: In the Eight Conditions, TCM differentiates between "Exterior" and "Interior"; and just as in Hering's Laws, the Chinese predicted a favorable prognosis when the condition goes from the interior to the exterior. In fact, we have six levels, the Six Great Meridians in TCM, with the more superficial (Yang) levels first, followed by the Yin levels. The most precious organs (Heart and Kidney, the protector of the Ancestral Chi) are in the deepest, most protected position (see Figure A5-1, The Six Great Meridians in Acupuncture). This relates to the three levels in homeopathy (see Figure 13-1, Levels of Suppression), in which the Mind is at the deepest level. Just as in homeopathy, we expect that an accurate acupuncture treatment will first bring about mental-emotional improvement and also favor the expulsion of mucus or phlegm and other discharges.

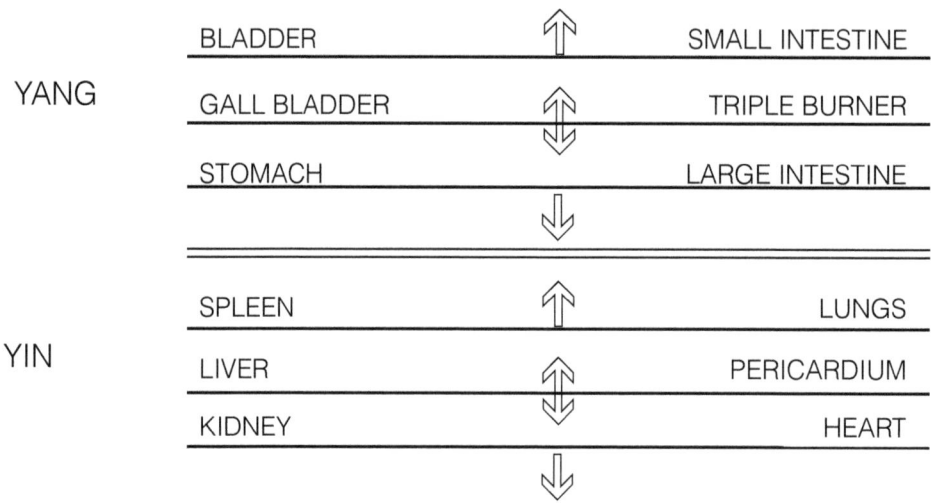

Fig. A5-1: The Six Great Meridians in Acupuncture

Organs in TCM and the Five Element Cycle

In this section, I explain the concept of organs in TCM and how to discover the organ in imbalance through the patient's symptoms. This is a wonderful tool which often allows you to choose between two or more remedies when you are close to the simillimum.

An organ in TCM is much more than the physical organ of gross anatomy (and the name of the organ is capitalized when the Chinese concept is referred to). It is a sphere of action in the body, each one associated with particular meridians of energy, a season of the year, an emotion, in fact an entire mental-emotional portrait similar to those of the polychrests. There are five "solid" or "precious" organs paired with five "hollow" organs, each pair occupying a point on the Star of the Five Elements. The Chinese observed that each organ had an activating effect on the one following it clockwise (Figure A5-2), while it has a destructive effect on the one following the arrows of the Ko cycle in Figure A5-3. If one organ is in imbalance, they found, it immediately affects the one next to it in each cycle, the Generation Cycle, as well as the one in the diagonal position, the Ko Cycle.

How does this concept help us in homeopathy? It demonstrates how all the tissues and systems of the body are intricately interrelated. It gives us another reason why we would not give one remedy for an ailment in one organ and a different remedy simultaneously for an ailment in another. They are interconnected, the expression of the same imbalance in the Vital Force, and the Star of the Five Elements can help us determine in which organ the imbalance originates.

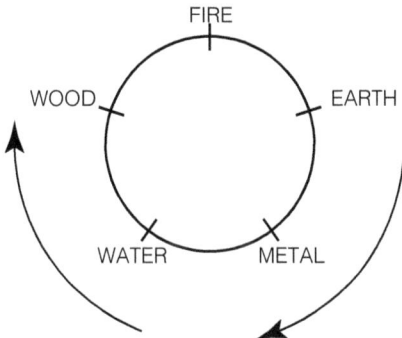

Fig. A5-2: The Generation Cycle

These five elements are by no means inert or immovable. They activate and destroy each other continuously, creating a certain equilibrium. In the Generation cycle, a certain element activates another one, which in turn, activates the next one. This always occurs clockwise.

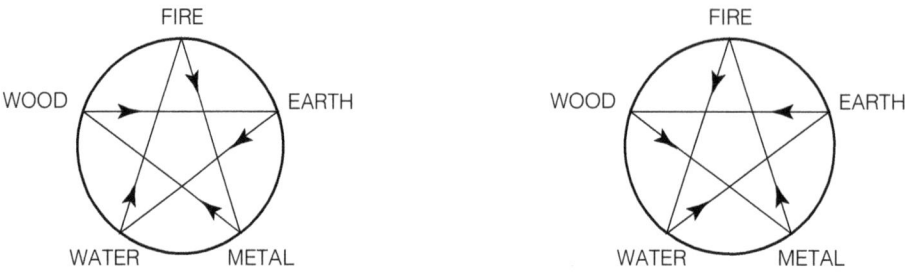

Fig. A5-3: The Ko Cycle *(left)*

To keep an equilibrium in this world, there is no production without destruction. The arrows in the diagram indicate the following cycle of how one element destroys the next: Water puts out Fire, Fire destroys (melts) Metal, Metal cuts Wood, Wood covers or hides the Earth, and Earth makes Water disappear by absorbing it.

Fig. A5-3: The Anti-Ko Cycle *(right)*

This is the opposite of the Ko cycle: a certain element becomes so strong and excessive that it reverses the Ko cycle. For example, in an excess of Earth, two elements are threatened: Water, according to the Ko cycle, but also Wood, according to the Anti-Ko cycle. Hence symptoms of both elements will appear in the patient.

The 5 Element Cycle

Here is a simple chart of the main features of the Five Element Cycle, as a reference for the portraits of the organs that follow.

Element	**Solid organ**	**Hollow organ**	**Season**	**Emotion**
Fire	Heart (H)	Small intestine (SI)	Summer	Joy, hysteria
Earth	Spleen (Sp)	Stomach (St)	Post-summer	Worry about past, present
Metal	Lung (L)	Large Intestine (LI)	Fall	Worry (future), depression
Water	Kidney (K)	Bladder (B)	Winter	Fear, anxiety, indecision
Wood	Liver (Li)	Gallbladder (GB)	Spring	Courage, irritability, anger

The Lung Element

Symptoms: The Lung is considered the *Master of Qi*: the first symptom of weakness is often found in the voice. As the patient loses energy in an illness, his weak voice will reflect the deficiency of Lung energy. Of course hoarseness and aphony (loss of voice) are directly linked to an attack on this precious organ. As the Lung energy is further attacked, physical and emotional fatigue sets in. The face becomes pale and perspiration abundant. The tongue looks pale and the patient is reluctant to speak.

Wind and especially dryness weaken the Lung energy. A "wind invasion" (as the Chinese call it) will cause chills, a painful throat, headaches, sensitivity to cold, watery nasal discharge, fever, thirst, and yellow thick secretion. We recognize an Aconite picture in this situation. The tongue initially is moderately red with a thin yellow coating and as the temperature goes up, the tongue becomes drier and redder. Dryness is the biggest enemy of this organ as it will exhaust the fluids of the body. A classic example of a Lung deficiency is tuberculosis, with its low grade afternoon fevers, night sweats, insomnia, dry cough with bloody sputum, shortness of breath, lassitude, and a dark red, dry tongue with cleavages or yellow coating.

The Lung governs the *external skin and the body hair* (all but the scalp hair), while the "internal" skin or mucosae is ruled by the Spleen. All skin conditions (no matter whether the diagnosis is eczema, psoriasis, etc.) relate to a disturbance in the Lung organ. Loss of body hair (including pubic hairs, eyelashes, eyebrows), which homeopathy usually relates to the syphilitic miasm, can also be an expression of exhausted Lung Qi. If there are no other indications for the syphilitic miasm, look for a deep, long lasting emotional factor such as grief.

Mental/emotional: In Chapter 8 of the *Nei King* we read: "Too much grief and melancholy will injure the lung and obstruct the flow of the Qi." This refers to sustained or recurrent or extremely intense grief. Recurrent grief is a typical causality for a patient in a Causticum state (Causticum being a remedy on the Lung-Liver axis): the Qi on all planes is exhausted and the patient becomes paralyzed on all levels: mentally he forgets everything; emotionally he has a flat affect; he is in a daze, not weeping, not wanting to talk to anyone; and physically he feels paralyzed and totally drained of energy. This state represents the total exhaustion of the Lung Qi, in which the patient is exhausted on every level. The Lung controls the Liver in the Ko cycle of the Five Elements, so that when the Lung is weak the Liver will be involved next, expressed in this example by the muscular paralysis (because the Liver controls the muscles). Dryness is the biggest enemy of the Lung, weakening and exhausting the Lung energy; it makes sense that Causticum is worse from dryness (an unusual modality in a remedy so often used when the allopathic diagnosis is arthritis).

Once the patient has total exhaustion of the Lung Qi, they can become very difficult to live with (as the spouse of any asthma patient can attest!) Dogmatic and rigid, they want to keep tight control over every situation and not show their emotions, no matter how great a shock they may experience. Even if his wife has an affair, the Lung or Metal man will suppress his feelings for the sake of appearances so much that a physical breakdown is inevitable. The first area of weakness is the lungs, expressed as dyspnea, asthma, and other lung problems. Next is the physical support system: the spine and skeleton (because bones belong to the Kidney element, and according to the Generation Cycle, the Kidney will be weak when the Lung is weak). Debilitating rheumatoid arthritis often can be traced to a grief, and I have cured many cases of "rheumatoid arthritis" with Nat. mur. because grief was the trauma that triggered it).

A perfect example of a Metal type is the Kali carb. person—dogmatic, rigid and emotionally suppressed. He worries about the future and about his health and suffers from what he describes as "anxiety in the pit of the stomach." People who need Kali carb. are hypersensitive to everything: noise, touch, and the slightest draft (because the skin is part of the Lung element).

Time: The worst time for a Lung person is between 3 and 5 a.m., a time when asthma patients are likely to have an attack and also covering the aggravation times of the Kali family of remedies which are so useful in asthma (Kali arsenicum, Kali carb., Kali sulph.).

Causality: Sadness or grief (mourning for loss of health, quality of life, their daily routine, not grief related to affairs of the heart which are on the Kidney-Heart axis), melancholy, and depression with fear of the future; and the climatic effects of wind and dryness.

The Kidney Element

Symptoms: The Kidney and Liver are the most important organs for a normal sexual life. The Kidney Yin Qi stores *the essence,* responsible for the growth and the reproductive functions. The libido or desire relates to the Kidney Yang Qi, whose energy can be dissipated through excessive coitus or masturbation. (In homeopathy we would call this condition "Never Well Since loss of seminal fluids," with Phosphoric acid the main remedy, or "Weariness after coition," K1416, with Selenium the top remedy.) Of course an excess of Kidney Yang is what we call nymphomania in homeopathy. A weakness of Kidney Qi is also expressed in seminal discharge at night (for which Nat. mur. and Nat. phos. are major remedies). Impotence, premature ejaculation, priapism, sterility, and oligospermia all belong to a disturbance in this organ.

Kidney Yin Qi is also responsible for the production of the bone marrow, which plays an important role in the formation of blood and the bone structure and thus in the Kidney's involvement with the teeth, bones, menstrual cycle, etc. (Interestingly, in allopathic medicine the kidney is known to stimulate the bone marrow to produce red blood cells by secreting erythropoietin.) Any symptom of a calcium defect (delayed teeth formation, porous bones, osteoporosis, or maladies like osteogenesis imperfecta) belong to a disturbance in this organ as do most menstrual irregularities (amenorrhea, dysmenorrhea, metrorrhagia, etc.).

The essence, mentioned before, also reflects the hereditary/genetic Qi (what we would call the miasmatic background). This organ can be considered the most precious of all Yin organs, and Nature protects it by selecting it to be the deepest layer of Yin. (While every organ has both a Yin and a Yang aspect, the Kidney is the most Yin organ.)

Another function of the Yang aspect of the Kidney is to help the bladder to *hold the urine*. So symptoms like enuresis nocturna and to some extent incontinence belong to the Kidney. The Kidney also is related to the ears. In TCM, a chronic ear problem (such as deafness, tinnitus, or vertigo) is addressed by treating the Kidney.

Other physical symptoms include obvious kidney and bladder symptoms like edema, renal colic and cystitis; reproductive symptoms like prostatitis; bone/joint related symptoms like osteoarthritis and rheumatoid arthritis, lower back pains, and pain anywhere along the spine; and sensitivity to cold, with the patient feeling cold in general.

Mental/emotional: The predominant emotions in the Kidney person are *fear, fright and anxiety* including all kinds of phobias (agoraphobia, claustrophobia, etc.). These are very indecisive people who can't make up their minds because they strive for perfection, which is of course unobtainable. They tend to be very detail-oriented. They can be hypochondriac and overwhelm you with a list of symptoms.

The Kidney is also associated with grief, like the Lung and the Heart, but each organ expresses it in a different way. The Kidney is associated with silent grief, the Heart with hysterical grief. The Kidney person suffering from grief will not cry in public and will retain all their emotions, until their Vital Qi has to express their grief through physical symptoms like lupus, edema, herpetic eruptions, and hives. These people are *hypo*-emotional in grief, presenting a Yin picture (withdrawn into themselves, also retaining water). Heart people are *hyper*-emotional, presenting a Yang picture with hysterical outbursts and tending to be loquacious (Ignatia, Lachesis). Grief about relationships is thus on the Kidney-Heart axis. For a young sensitive girl, it can include moving away from the neighborhood where she has always lived with all her friends. (Grief about loss of health or quality of life is in the Lung element as just described.)

Kidney people are very sentimental, especially just before menses. They are sensitive to the sun and crave cold drinks. The homeopath will recognize characteristics of Arsenicum and Nat. mur. (and Apis, the acute of Nat. mur. for hives and edema) in this picture.

Causality: Fright, fear, adrenal exhaustion, masturbation or excessive sexual activity, cold temperature, winter.

> *Clinical Case:* In the onset of rheumatoid arthritis, I have almost always found either a grief or a frightful or anxious event. One 12-year-old girl with a very sensitive Phosphorus constitution was brought to me by her parents for rheumatoid arthritis which had begun in June of the previous year. All her symptoms pointed to Nat. mur., but there was no mention of a grief in her timeline. Upon inquiring I found that the family's house was sold in September, which at first did not seem to explain a RA attack three months before. But I found out that the "For Sale" sign had been on the front lawn for three months. Moving out of the house meant the loss of everything important in that young girl's life: her friends, her school, her familiar neighborhood, and the home where she had spent her entire life. I wondered aloud whether this grief might have brought on the RA, and the girl turned to her parents and said, "See? I told you so!"

The Liver Element

Symptoms: One of the Liver's most important functions is the *storage of blood*. When an increased amount of blood is required (such as in muscular activity or during menstruation), the Liver must be able to provide this required blood supply to the body. It is the organ that contains the greatest amount of blood, and thus it influences aspects of the body which need extra blood supply, such as movement, standing up, and eyesight (due to the heavy vascularization of the retina).

The Yang part of the Liver is responsible for the flow of the Qi (Vital Force) throughout the body. Anger, frustration, and irritability will block the flow of Qi and lead to its stagnation in the liver. This will lead in turn to stagnation of the Stomach Qi, creating symptoms such as nausea, dyspepsia, vomiting, and dyspepsia. (And in homeopathy one of our top remedies for these symptoms is Nux vomica, a Liver remedy). Craving for hot drinks and relief from eating hot foods are typical Liver symptoms.

The Yin part of the Liver, in addition to storing the blood, nourishes the tendons and muscles. Disturbances in these areas, such as dyskinesia, akinesia, spasms, and cramps are treated by Liver points in acupuncture (and often by Nux vomica and Mag. phos. in homeopathy, both Liver remedies).

The functioning of the eyes is affected by different organs, especially the Liver. Bleedings in the eye (Phosphorus, a Liver remedy, is a good example), dim vision, and night blindness are all related to a Liver disturbance. In the West we call the eyes the window of the soul, but according to the Chinese, the eyes are the openings of the liver.

Symptoms such as hypoglycemia, seizures, and waking in the morning feeling unrefreshed are all expressions of a disordered Liver function. Why? Seizures represent an excess of muscular activity, and muscles are controlled by the Liver; unrefreshed sleep occurs when the toxins build up at night because the liver is not processing them adequately; and we know in allopathic physiology that the liver controls the blood sugar level even more than the pancreas does.

Mental/emotional: The Liver person is a leader in his field, in command because of his knowledge and phenomenal memory, his competitive drive, and his single-minded focus on his goal. Thus he tends to be an expert, armed with the facts, just the facts. It is hard to beat him in any given subject; he has no time for small-talk and diplomacy. He has a strange mix of confidence, competence, arrogance and chutzpah, but it is backed up by knowledge and hard work. In fact, a Liver person needs to work with other Liver people, because he is likely to call the others "nothing but lazy freeloaders." He has an entrepreneurial quickness, a driven quality, and a tremendous capacity for sheer hard work. He is always multitasking, making many plans at once and pursuing them even at 3 a.m. when he tends to wake up. No wonder remedies such as Sulphur, Nat. sulph., and Nux vomica come to mind. This Liver person always takes good care of his family (if he is in balance, of course), because being a good provider is his top priority (except maybe becoming famous or accumulating ever-more money and possessions).

Causality: Anger, suppressed anger, indignation, disappointment, humiliation; alcohol, wind, spring.

The Heart Element

Symptoms: This is the most important and precious organ, together with the brain (and in fact, TCM considers the heart the seat of mental activities). In TCM it is considered the Emperor, commanding and controlling the other organs. The heart plays an important role in the *circulation of the blood,* together with the liver and spleen. In TCM, *mental disorders* and even daily neuroses are attributed to disturbed Heart Qi. *The tongue* is the opening of the heart, therefore the heart commands the speech.

A *decrease* of Qi in the Heart leads to shortness of breath, palpitations, nocturnal perspiration, lassitude, arrhythmia, and chilliness. An *obstruction* of the Qi in the Heart (when it builds up because it is blocked) leads to stuttering, hysteria, a bitter taste in mouth, insomnia, and rapid pulse.

Mental-emotional: The Heart person is all emotional: charming and entertaining from a young age, silly, smiling easily, enthusiastic but running out of gas too fast, easily impressed and therefore changing subjects at school, wanting different things, traveling to different places. This dissatisfaction, which is driven by emotion rather than reason, is found in Tuberculinum and Phosphorus. The Heart person loves beauty and is at his all-time best when creating, whether a song, a poem, a screen-play, a book, or a painting. Even if he never finds a publisher, this will not stop him from expressing all his fantasies and imaginative ideas through his artistic expression.

Of course with his great sensitivity, he is the first one to suffer from a heartbreak, claiming that he will never get over the loss of his soul-mate. Fortunately for him, his next soul-mate is always only one step away. His job (if he works) definitely has to be something he can pour his heart into. He doesn't care how much money he will earn, just how much fun he can have. Of course he is loquacious and he confides in you, the practitioner, on his first visit as if you are an old friend, not holding back, often overdramatizing, but always with a charming smile on his face. He makes you feel good, and that certainly was one of his purposes in coming. His feelings of sympathy are always focused on the person he is with, not something as serious and all-encompassing as world affairs.

Causality: Ailments from grief, heat (sunstroke), excessive joy, summer.

The Spleen Element

Symptoms: The main function of the Spleen in TCM is the transportation and transformation of blood and energy: thus it is involved with anemia and hemorrhages (because the Spleen is too weak to control the blood in the vessels). The Spleen is the main organ in the *digestion* and a balanced function provides good appetite, normal stools and adequate digestion, with imbalances leading to gastritis and anorexia.

The Spleen is also responsible for maintaining muscle strength. Disturbances of the Spleen will lead to muscle wasting and prolapse of the organs (hence Sepia with its typical prolapses and overworry, related to this element, is one of the major Spleen remedies).

Another important function is its role in *water retention,* along with the Lung and Kidney. This can be manifested at different levels: at the intestines, causing diarrhea (especially chronic morning diarrhea); at the bladder, causing anuria; and at the subcutaneous level, producing edema. Disorders of the lips and palate also belong to the Spleen, including herpes simplex I.

Other symptoms and disorders belonging to the Spleen are abdominal distention due to gas, canker sores, short menstrual cycle, and leucorrhea.

Mental/emotional: The Earth person is always good-natured, sensitive and family-oriented. He loves to take it easy, to mull things over, and to have friends over for a game of cards with plenty of food. Protected in his house, he tries to shield himself from outside "horrible" things—which, as Kent says, "affect him greatly" (Calcarea.) But he gets easily overwhelmed out of a sense of duty like Sepia. Family means everything to him, and he loves a placid, circumscribed, uneventful life. Unfortunately, his worries about present and past events make him prone to stomach disorders. His sole ambition is to succeed socially and with his usually gentle nature he is able to lend great comfort to others without probing too deeply into their souls. He does not like to argue (the opposite of the Liver person), but rather retreats into his protective shell, his house (Calcarea). He is not indifferent, he just does not like outside pressure.

Causality: Ailments from worry, sweets, dampness.

The Organ Clock in TCM

All homeopaths know the importance of the time of symptoms (mainly aggravation, sometimes amelioration), found in Generalities and also throughout the *Repertory* as a subrubric to many rubrics. It is interesting therefore to note how TCM has a similar system which can be useful to us. Where the time modality in homeopathy relates to the remedy, in TCM it relates to the organ affected. The energy (Vital Force) circulating in the organs and meridians partially stagnates in each organ for two hours, during which time it is most subject to disturbances (see Figure A5-5).

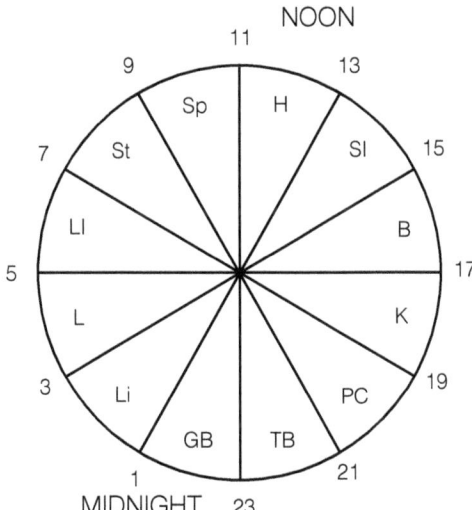

Fig. A5-5: The Organ Clock in Traditional Chinese Medicine

If a patient wakes up in the middle of the night, the acupuncturist as well as the homeopath asks the patient to look at his clock to see when the aggravation takes place. A 2 a.m. waking might signify to the homeopath the need for remedies such as Arsenicum and the Kalis, while for the acupuncturist it indicates an imbalance in Qi in the Liver organ. Gallbladder attacks usually take usually place late at night, not surprisingly for the acupuncturist (Gallbladder hours are from 9-11 p.m.). Heart attacks often occur during the opposite hours (midday-midnight connection): 11 a.m.-1 p.m. Kidney stone attacks often occur during Kidney time in the late afternoon (5-7 p.m.). It is an indication to the acupuncturist which organ to balance, but it is also a great tool to the homeopath, who, if confronted with the choice between two remedies, might consult this organ clock, and decide whether one of those two remedies has a predilective action on that organ. So the homeopath might use this at the end of his work, not the beginning.

Practical Applications

Practically speaking, the situation in which I most often use my understanding of TCM is in diagnosing a Liver condition in a patient. Many patients in modern Western society show the symptoms of needing a Liver remedy, such as indigestion, gas, the desire for hot drinks, hypoglycemia, etc. Of course, the mental/emotional issues of a Liver type are likely to be prominent, such as irritability, anger, and frustration, as well as positive characterisics such as courage, leadership and decisiveness. The patient is likely to be in a Liver situation (overworked business person, someone who depends too heavily on coffee or other stimulants or takes too many medications). When I see these symptoms, I think of the most effective Liver remedies: Sulphur, Nux vomica, Phosphorus (which although it is listed with Heart-Fire because of its mental/emotional makeup, has a strong beneficial effect on the Liver from a physiological point of view.)

Another practical application is the use of the organ clock. While the time of aggravation or appearance of symptoms points to a possible remedy in homeopathy, the organ clock in TCM can be used to see what organ is affected. If more than one remedy is indicated, and if they both have the same aggravation time, we could choose the remedy that has an organotropic action in the case. An exacerbation between 3-5 a.m. can indicate a "weakness" of the Lung organ, even in absence of overt Lung symptoms.

We can also the TCM connection between the organs and the emotions to track an unknown etiology. For example, if we see the symptoms in a case all belong to a Kidney deficiency (bone pains, lower back pains, osteoarthritis, RA, ear ringing, incontinence of urine, etc.) and the patient has forgotten or suppressed the causality of his event, this will make us think about the "Ailments from" belonging to this organ, in this case the Kidney. So we can suspect or even gently probe for an incident of fear or fright in the patient's history. Don't forget, the patient may never spontaneously express such an event preceding an attack of RA, for instance, since she thinks it has nothing to do with her condition. An understanding of the emotions and etiology connected to each organ can help us find the all-important Never Well Since.

And in cases where a patient has nothing but vague, common physical symptoms, such as hypoglycemia, headaches, insomnia, weak nails and vision, menstrual irregularities, and muscle cramping, we will use our knowledge of TCM to show us where the leakage of energy is (the Liver in this instance). In choosing a reactive remedy, we could narrow our selection to the one which is the strongest Liver remedy, i.e. Sulphur.

Last but not least, the "tongue picture" is easy to read and a very reliable source of information on the state of the patient's internal organs. It will point out the organ(s) most out of balance and under siege. Reading the tongue picture is described in Chapter 7, Case-Taking.

Notes

Most works cited are easily available from the homeopathic book suppliers; full bibliographical information is provided for the others.

Introduction

[1] Hahnemann's casebooks: *Krankenjournal* DF5 1837-1842. Transcription and translation by Arnold Michalowski (Heidelberg: Karl F. Haug Verlag). Made available by Robert Jutte, Institute of Medical History, Robert Bosch Institute, Stuttgart, Germany.

A Brief Overview of Hahnemann's Life

[1] Haehl, *Life and Works of Hahnemann,* Vol. 2, p. 23.

[2] Dudgeon, ed. *Lesser Writings of Samuel Hahnemann,* p. 243.

Chapter One: The Rapid, Gentle, and Permanent Cure

[1] Borchelt M. Potential side-effects and interactions in multiple medication in elderly patients: methodology and results of the Berlin Study of Aging. *Z Gerontol Geriatr,* 28(6):420-8 1995 Nov-Dec.

[2] *Boston Globe,* October, 19, 1998.

[3] Heikkinen T, Thint M, Chonmaitree T. Prevalence of various respiratory viruses in the middle ear during acute otitis media. *N Engl J Med,* 340(4):260-4 1999 Jan 28.

[4] Uhari M, Hietala J, Tuokko H. Risk of acute otitis media in relation to the viral etiology of infections in children. *Clin Infect Dis,* 20(3):521-4 1995 Mar.

[5] Buchman CA, Doyle WJ, Skoner DP, Post JC, Alper CM, Seroky JT, Anderson K, Preston RA, Hayden FG, Fireman P, et al . Influenza A virus-induced acute otitis media. *J Infect Dis,* 172(5):1348-51 1995 Nov.

[6] Guillemot D; Carbon C, Vauzelle-Kervröedan F, Balkau B, Maison P, Bouvenot G, Eschwege E. Inappropriateness and variability of antibiotic prescription among French office-based physicians. *J Clin Epidemiol,* 51(1):61-8 1998 Jan.

[7] Friese KH, Kruse S, Moeller H . Acute otitis media in children. Comparison between conventional and homeopathic therapy. *HNO,* 44(8):462-6 1996 Aug.

Chapter Two: The Vital Force in Health and Healing

[1] Ikematsu H, Nabeshima A, Yamaga S, Yamaji K, Kakuda K, Ueno K, Hayashi J, Shirai T, Hara H, Kashiwagi S. Clinical significance of peak body temperature, white blood cell count, and C-reactive protein level in febrile episodes among geriatric inpatients. *Kansenshogaku Zasshi,* 71(6):527-33 1997 Jun.

[2] Povoa P, Almeida E, Moreira P, Fernandes A, Mealha R, Aragao A, Sabino H. C-reactive protein as an indicator of sepsis. *Intensive Care Med,* 24(10):1052-6 1998 Oct.

[3] Barriere SL. Selection of antimicrobial regimens, in DiPiro JT, Talbert RL, Yee GC, Matzke GR, Wells BG, Posey LM (eds): *Pharmacotherapy: A Pathophysiologic Approach,* 3rd ed. Connecticut: Appleton and Lange, 1997, pp. 1953-4.

[4] Tang GJ. Similarity and synergy of trauma and sepsis: role of tumor necrosis factor-alpha and interleukin-6. *Acta Anaesthesiol Sin,* 34(3):141-9 1996 Sep.

[5] Fischler MP, Reinhart WH. Fever: friend or enemy?. *Schweiz Med Wochenschr,* 127(20):864-70 1997 May 17.

[6] Mackowiak PA, Plaisance KI. Benefits and risks of antipyretic therapy. *Ann N Y Acad Sci,* 856:214-23 1998 Sep 29.

[7] Kluger MJ, Kozak W, Conn CA, Leon LR, Soszynski D. The adaptive value of fever. *Infect Dis Clin North Am,* 10(1):1-20 1996 Mar.

[8] Larry Dossey, M.D., interview on *Body and Soul,* WGBH-TV, Boston, MA, Feb. 14, 1999. The evidence for the power of prayer is reviewed in Dr. Dossey's books, *Healing Words: The Power of Prayer in Medicine* (New York: HarperCollins, 1993) and *Be Careful What You Pray For ... You Just Might Get It* (New York: HarperCollins, 1997).

[9] Pharmaceutical Research and Manufacturers of America Annual Survey, 1997.

[10] original letter in possession of Dr. August Korndoffer in Philadelphia.

[11] Moore TJ, Psaty BM, Furberg CD. Time to act on drug safety. *JAMA,* 279(19):1571-3 1998 May 20.

[12] Packer M. End of the oldest controversy in medicine—are we ready to conclude the debate on digitalis? *N Eng J Med,* 336(8): 1997 Feb 20.

[13] Institute for Health Care Improvement. Preventing medication errors. *Medical Practice Communicator* 1998; 5(2):6)

[14] Quoted in *USA Today* editorial, Deadly Rx: why are drugs killing so many patients? April 24, 1998.

[15] Moore, Thomas J. The weakness in dispensing drugs. *Boston Globe,* June 28, 1998.

Chapter Three: Laws and Principles

[1] Kent, *Lesser Writings*, p. 326

[2] Kent, *Lesser Writings*, p. 432-434.

[3] Medical issue, Soviet Union, No. 4 (265), 1972.

[4] *Chronic Diseases*, Vol. 1, pp. xv and xvi, footnote.

[5] *Chronic Diseases*, Vol. I, p. 135.

[6] Kent, *Lesser Writings*, p. 202.

[7] Moskowitz, Richard, *The Case Against Immunizations*; Coulter, Harris, and B.L. Fisher: *A Shot in the Dark*; Murphy, Jamie, *What Every Parent Should Know about Childhood Immunizations*.

Chapter Four: Pathology

[1] *Homeopathy, the Science of Therapeutics*, p. 28.

Chapter Five: Potencies

[1] *Transactions of the American Journal of Homeopathy*, 1876.

[2] *Lesser Writings of von Boenninghausen*, p. 100.

[3] *Samuel Hahnemann, His Life and Work*, Richard Haehl, ed. p. 322.

[4] *In Search of the Later Hahnemann*, p. 138.

[5] *Lesser Writings*, p. 350-351.

[6] *Lesser Writings of von Boenninghausen*, p. 131-133.

[7] *ibid*.

[8] *Chronic Diseases*, Vol. 1, pp. 155-156.

[9] *Life and Letters of Hahnemann*, p. 368.

[10] Schmidt, Pierre. *Hidden Treasures of the Last Organon*.

[11] *Chronic Diseases*, vol. I, p. 120.

[4] International Hahnemaniann Association, 1883, *Bureau of Homeopathics*, p. 77-78.

Chapter Six: LM Potencies

[1] *Lesser Writings*, p. 350.

²*Lesser Writings of von Boenninghausen,* p. 169.

³*Life and Letters of Hahnemann,* Bradford, ed., p. 493.

⁴*Lesser Writings of von Boenninghausen,* p. 190.

⁴*Hidden Treasures of the Last Organon,* p. 3.

⁵*Chronic Diseases,* Vol. I, p. 156.

⁶Kent, *Materia Medica,* p. 543.

Chapter Seven: Homeopathic Case-Taking

¹Allen, H.C. *Keynotes of the Materia Medica with Nosodes,* p. 40.

²*Lesser Writings of von Boenninghausen,* p. 105-121.

³*Dateline,* January 1999.

⁴*The Homeopathic Recorder,* 1951, "The Use of Nosodes," pp. 295-296.

⁵Felitti VJ, Anda RF, Nordenberg D, Williamson DF, Spitz AM, Edwards V, Koss MP, Marks JS. Relationship of childhood abuse and household dysfunction to many of the leading causes of death in adults. The Adverse Childhood Experiences (ACE) Study. *Am J Prev Med* 1998 May; 14(4): 245-58.

Chapter Nine: Prescribing

¹*Kent, Lesser Writings,* p. 396.

²Footnote to Aphorism 7.

³*New England Medical Gazette,* 1877, p. 120.

Chapter Ten: Golden Rules and Special Forms of Prescribing

¹*Lesser Writings of von Boenninghausen,* pp. 304-307.

²*Lesser Writings of von Boenninghausen,* p. 213.

Chapter Eleven: Delusions

¹Kent, *Lectures on Materia Medica,* p. 408.

Notes

Chapter Twelve: Aggravations, Healing Crises, and Accessory Symptoms

[1] *Lesser Writings of von Boenninghausen,* p. 187.

[2] *The Lesser Writings of Samuel Hahnemann,* p. 388.

Chapter Thirteen: Suppression

[1] *Best of Burnett,* page 279.

[2] See A.H. Grimmer's description of many cured cancer cases in his *The Collected Works,* ed. by A.Currim.

[3] Dunham, C. *Th e Science of Therapeutics.*

[4] *Journal of International Homeopathic Association,* 1939.

Chapter Fourteen: Obstacles to the Cure

[1] *Life and Letters of Hahnemann,* Bradford ed., p. 195.

[2] *Boston Globe,* March 18, 1998.

[3] *Chronic Diseases,* vol. 1, p. 121.

[4] Clarke, J.H. *Dictionary of Practical Materia Medica* by p. 559.

[5] *Lesser Writings of Samuel Hahnemann,* p. *391.*

[6] "A Fix for Caffeine Headaches," *USA Today,* October 25, 1996.

[7] Dunham, C. *The Science of Therapeutics,* p. 462

Chapter Fifteen: Management of the Patient

[1] Kent. *Lesser Writings.*

[2] Kent. *Lectures on Homeopathic Philosophy,* p. 224.

[3] Kent. *Lectures on Materia Media,* pp. 568-569.

[4] Hahnemann, Samuel. *Chronic Diseases,*Vol. 1, p.160.

[5] *Lesser Writings of von Boenninghausen,* p. 129.

Chapter Sixteen: Palliation and Incurable Diseases

[1] *The Magic of the Minimum Dose,* pp. 96-97.

Chapter Seventeen: The Nosodes

[1] Nash, *Leaders in Homeopathic Therapeutics*, p. 288.

[2] Massimo Mangialavori. "Remedies for Grief and Loss," case conference, Still River, MA, March 1999.

[3] *Best of Burnett,* p. 70.

[4] Shepard, *Magic of the Minimum Dose*, p. 179.

[5] Kent, *Lesser Writings,* p. 227.

[6] H.C. Allen, *The Homeopathic Recorder,* Vol. LI, No. 5, May 1936.

[7] *Best of Burnett,* p. 176.

[8] Kent, *Lectures on Homeopathic Materia Medica,* p.932.

[9] Kent, *Lectures on Homeopathic Materia Medica,* p. 952.

Chapter Nineteen: The Roots of Chronic Disease

[1] *Chronic Diseases,* Vol. 1, p. 3.

[2] *Chronic Diseases,* Vol. 1, p. 6.

[3] *Chronic Diseases,* Vol. 1, p. 138.

Chapter Twenty: Psora, the Sensitizing Miasm

[1] *Chronic Diseases,* Vol. 1, p. 14.

[2] *Chronic Diseases,* Vol. 1, pp. 18-31.

[3] *Chronic Diseases,* Vol. 1, p. 8.

[4] *Life and Letters of Hahnemann,* Bradford, ed., page 184.

[5] *Chronic Diseases,* Vol. 1, p. 33, footnote.

[6] Phatak, *Materia Medica of Homeopathic Medicines,* p. 127

[7] *Chronic Diseases,* Vol. I, p. 137.

[8] *Chronic Diseases,* Vol 1, p. 136.

Chapter Twenty-one: Sycosis, the Miasm of Excess and Overgrowth

[1] Hunter, John. *Treatise on the Venereal Diseases,* 1787, p. 531, quoted in *Chronic Diseases.*

²Kent, *Lesser Writings,* p. 363.

³*Alg. hom. Zet.,* Vol.37, p. 21, 1849.

⁴*Lesser Writings of von Boenninghausen,* p. 3.

⁵*Journal of the International Hahnemannian Association,* 1890, p. 281.

⁶*Lesser Writings of von Boenninghausen,* pp. 3-4.

⁷*The Best of Burnett,* pp. 147, 148.

⁸McKane, L. and J. Kandel. *Microbiology: Essentials and Applications,* p. 606 (New York: McGraw-Hill, 1996).

⁹Luke 6:43.

¹⁰Reported in *Time,* Jan. 15, 1996.

¹¹*Nature Genetics Journal,* December 1997.

Chapter Twenty-two: Syphilis, the Destructive Miasm

¹Kent, *Lesser Writings,* p. 368.

²*Chronic Diseases,* pp. 87 and 89.

³Henny Heudens-Mast, live case conference, Winter Park, FL, January 1999.

⁴Chang, Iris. *The Rape of Nanking* (Penguin Books, 1998).

⁵Du Plessix Gray, Francine. *At Home with the Marquis de Sade.* (New York: Simon & Schuster, 1999).

⁶Study conducted by the Parkinson's Institute, Sunnyvale, California, January 1999.

⁷*Chronic Diseases,* Vol. 1, pp. 87-88.

Chapter Twenty-three: The Tubercular and Cancer Miasms

¹Grimmer, Arthur H. *The Collected Works.* A. Currim, ed.

Chapter Twenty-four: Homeopathy and Cancer

¹*Time Magazine,* cover story, April 25, 1994.

²Quoted in *USA Today,* March 8, 1999.

³Cancer undefeated, *NEJM,* May 29; 336(22) 1569-74.

⁴*JNCI* 1996, Dec. 4; 88(23) 1706-7.

⁵Research at the Mayo Clinic reported in the *New England Journal of Medicine,* quoted in the *New York Times,* Jan. 14, 1999.

⁶*British Homeopathic Journal,* April 1972.

⁷Henny Heudens-Mast, live case conference, Winter Park, FL, January 1999.

⁷Clarke, J.H. *Dictionary of Practical Materia Medica,* p. 482.

⁸*Boston Globe,* March 8, 1999: "New drugs fight sores from cancer treatment."

⁹Grimmer, Arthur H. *The Collected Works.* A. Currim, ed., p. 833.

¹⁰Clarke, J.H. "The place of homeopathic remedies in the treatment of malignant disease," *Homeopathic World,* Vol. 59, 1924, p. 210.

¹¹*Homeotherapy,* Vol. 1, 1875, p. 19.

¹²Gilchrist, J.G., M.D., "The homeopathic treatment of tumors," *T.A.I.H.,* Vol. 29, 1878, pp. 350-351.

¹³Powers, W.J. Sweasy, M.D., "Case that might have been surgical," *Homeopathic Recorder,* Vol. 46; 1931, pp. 712-714.

¹⁴Carlton, Edmund, M.D. "How to Cure Cancer," *Homeopathic World,* Vol. 68-69; 1933; pp. 446-450.

¹⁵Carlton, Edmund, M.D. "How to Cure Cancer," *Homeopathic World,* Vol. 68-69; 1933; pp. 557-559.

Appendix Three: Sample Cases

¹Scholten, Jan. *Homeopathy and the Elements.*

Appendix Five: Homeopathy and Traditional Chinese Medicine

¹Ernst Von Brunnow, a young law student who befriended Hahnemann, quoted in Cook, Trevor. *Samuel Hahnemann, His Life and Times,* p. 111.

²Hahnemann, Samuel. *Organon of the Medical Art.* O'Reilly, ed. p. 26.

³Veith, Ilza. *The Yellow Emperor's Classic of Internal Medicine* (Baltimore, Ohio: Williams & Wilkings, 1949).

⁴"A Reply to 'By Analogy'," *J.A.I.H.,* Vol. 66, No. 4, Dec. 1973.

Bibliography

Recommended Books

For first-year students in my school, I recommend the following books as a basic library.

Reading Books

Hahnemann, Samuel. *The Organon of the Medical Art* (the Decker translation/ O'Reilly edition).

Coulter, Catherine. *Portraits of Homeopathic Medicines,* vols. 1-3.

Handley, Rima. *A Homeopathic Love Story.*

—— *In Search of the Later Hahnemann.*

Tyler, Margaret. *Homeopathic Drug Pictures.*

Reference Books

Kent's *Repertory of the Homeopathic Materia Medica.*

A good basic inexpensive Materia Medica like Phatak's *Materia Medica of Homeopathic Medicines* or Boericke's *Pocket Manual of Homeopathic Materia Medica with Repertory.*

Banerjea, S.J. *Miasmatic Diagnosis.*

Yasgur, Jay. *Yasgur's Homeopathic Dictionary and Holistic Health Reference.*

A guide to acute prescribing like my *The People's Repertory.*

Additional Recommendations

Reading Books

For my advanced students, I recommend the following books, my favorites among the many which I read to assemble this book:

Hahnemann, Samuel. *Chronic Diseases*

—— *Lesser Writings* (Dudgeon, ed.).

Bradford, Thomas L., ed. *The Life and Letters of Hahnemann.*

Haehl, Richard. *Life and Works of Hahnemann.*

Allen, J.H. *The Chronic Miasms.*

Boenninghausen, C.M.F. von. *Lesser Writings.*

Burnett, J. Compton. *Best of Burnett.*

Choudhury, H. *Fifty Millesimal Potency.*

Dunham, Carroll. *The Science of Therapeutics.*

Foubister, Donald. *Tutorials on Homeopathy.*

Kent, James T. *Lectures on Homeopathic Materia Medica.*

—— *Lectures on Homeopathic Philosophy.*

—— *New Remedies, Clinical Cases, Lesser Writings.*

Roberts, H.A. *Principles and Art of Cure.*

Sankaran, Rajan. *The Spirit of Homeopathy*

—— *The Substance of Homeopathy.*

Schmidt, Pierre. *Hidden Treasures of the Last Organon.*

Reference Books

Schroyens, Frederik. S*ynthesis—Repertorium Homeopathicum Syntheticum.*

Allen, H.C. *Keynotes of the Materia Medica with Nosodes.*

Boger, C.M. *A Synoptic Key to Materia Medica.*

Clarke, J.H. *Dictionary of Practical Materia Medica.*

Farrington, E.A. *Clinical Materia Medica.*

Hahnemann, Samuel. *Materia Medica Pura.*

Hering, Constantine. *Guiding Symptoms.*

Nash, E.B. *Leaders in Homeopathic Therapeutics.*

About Dr. Luc De Schepper

Dr. Luc De Schepper, founder of the Renaissance Institute of Classical Homeopathy in Boston, Mass., is the author of twelve books on homeopathy, acupuncture, and holistic health care. He recently took a year's sabbatical from private practice as a homeopathic family physician in order to research and write this book. He has treated thousands of patients, following the principles in this book, at his family practice in classical homeopathy, located first in Red Bank, NJ and subsequently in San Diego, CA. Earlier Dr. Luc was in private practice in preventive medicine, homeopathy, and acupuncture in Santa Monica, CA, where he was the founder and director of the Mega Medical Group, Inc. For eight years he supervised a staff of 16 health care practitioners including MDs, nurses, chiropractors, nutritionists, and massage therapists. Prior to coming to the United States in 1981 he practiced acupuncture and holistic medicine in Belgium for 13 years.

Dr. Luc's books include The People's Repertory; Candida: the Cause, the Symptoms, the Cure; Acupuncture in Practice; and Full of Life. Human Condition: Critical, his introduction to homeopathy, won second prize among 3800 papers at the First Congress of World Traditional Medicine. His Musculoskeletal Diseases and Homeopathy won the Gold Cup (first prize) at the Second Congress of World Traditional Medicine. He has also written articles on homeopathy for journals including the British Journal of Homeopathy, Simillimum, and Townsend Letter for Doctors. He has appeared on numerous television shows in the United States and abroad as well as being interviewed on dozens of radio shows and giving over 100 public lectures. He gave two addresses at the 1998 convention of the National Association of Pediatric Nurse Associates and Practitioners and two addresses at the 1998 convention of the National Center for Homeopathy. Now retired from private practice, he lectures on homeopathy internationally at the invitation of homeopathic physicians around the globe. For updated information on studying with Dr. Luc, please consult his website, www.drluc.com.

Dr. Luc has medical licenses in Belgium and the United States; acupuncture licenses in the EEC countries and California. He has also studied with Robin Murphy and with the British Institute of Homeopathy under the personal tutelage of Dr. Trevor Cook. He graduated with honors from the University of Ghent School of Medicine in his native Belgium in 1971, one of only 35 students to complete the course among 770 entering students. He passed the first state acupuncture examination given in California in 1982 and was a professor at the California Acupuncture College. Dr. Luc is fluent in four languages and a competitive tennis player.

Other Books by Dr. Luc

The People's Repertory. A guide to acute prescribing for laypeople, including a mini-repertory and Materia Medica of over 100 remedies commonly used for acute complaints. It also includes an explanation of how to put acute remedies in water for better results, and a description of the half-dozen most common constitutional types.

Human Condition Critical. An explanation of chronic prescribing in homeopathy from the patient's perspective. Includes an explanation of LM potencies and how they work and basic guidance for patients on improving the Vital Force with good nutrition and a healthy lifestyle.

What About Men. A comparison of the basic personality types in the Five Elements theory of Traditional Chinese Medicine with the corresponding temperaments in homeopathy. One of the few books demonstrating the connection between homeopathy and TCM. Meant for laypeople to understand themselves and/or the men in their life.

Candida: the Symptoms, the Causes, the Cure. A best-selling book on treating candida with a sugar-free diet and nutritional supplements.

Full of Life. How to boost the immune system with a whole foods diet and supplements.

Acupuncture in Practice. A textbook for the student and an introduction to acupuncture for the interested medical professional, including a step-by-step guide to diagnosis and treatment and a discussion of frequently-encountered clinical conditions with their acupuncture interpretation and treatment plan.

TO ORDER BOOKS BY DR. LUC:

Please visit Dr. Luc's bookstore at his website at drluc.com

www.ingramcontent.com/pod-product-compliance
Ingram Content Group UK Ltd.
Pitfield, Milton Keynes, MK11 3LW, UK
UKHW062306230426
12049UKWH00005B/125